NUCLEAR MEDICINE TECHNOLOGY AND TECHNIQUES

NUCLEAR MEDICINE TECHNOLOGY AND TECHNIQUES

Edited by

DONALD R. BERNIER, C.N.M.T.

Director of Technical Education, Division of Nuclear Medicine,
The Edward Mallinckrodt Institute of Radiology,
Washington University School of Medicine,
St. Louis, Missouri

JAMES K. LANGAN, C.N.M.T.

Chief Technologist, Division of Nuclear Medicine,
Johns Hopkins Medical Institutions, Baltimore;
Assistant Professor of Nuclear Medicine Technology,
Essex Community College,
Baltimore, Maryland

L. DAVID WELLS, C.N.M.T.

Chief Technologist, Division of Nuclear Medicine,
University Community Hospital,
Tampa, Florida

with 555 illustrations

The C. V. Mosby Company

ST. LOUIS • TORONTO • LONDON 1981

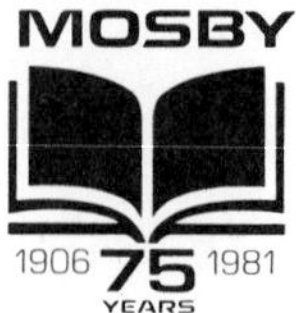

A TRADITION OF PUBLISHING EXCELLENCE

Printed in the United States of America

The C. V. Mosby Company
11830 Westline Industrial Drive, St. Louis, Missouri 63141

Library of Congress Cataloging in Publication Data

Main entry under title:

Nuclear medicine technology and techniques.

Bibliography: p.
Includes index.
1. Nuclear medicine. I. Bernier, Donald R. II. Langan, James K., 1934- III. Wells, L. David. [DNLM: 1. Nuclear medicine. 2. Nuclear medicine—Laboratory manuals. WN440 N9685]
R895.N84 616.07′575 80-17455
ISBN 0-8016-0662-4

GW/CB/CB 9 8 7 6 5 4 3 2 05/A/599

CONTRIBUTORS

PHILIP O. ALDERSON, M.D.

Director, Division of Nuclear Medicine, Professor of Radiology, College of Physicians and Surgeons, Columbia University, New York, New York

DONALD R. BERNIER, C.N.M.T.

Director of Technical Education, Division of Nuclear Medicine, The Edward Mallinckrodt Institute of Radiology, Washington University School of Medicine, St. Louis, Missouri

RICHARD J. BESCHI, B.S., C.N.M.T.

Educational Director and Instructor, Nuclear Medicine Technology Program, School of Community and Allied Health, University of Alabama/Birmingham Veterans Administration Medical Center, Birmingham, Alabama

KAREN L. BLONDEAU, C.N.M.T.

Nuclear Medicine Service, Harry S Truman Memorial Veterans Hospital, Columbia, Missouri

PAUL E. CHRISTIAN, B.S., C.N.M.T.

Technical Director, Division of Nuclear Medicine, Department of Radiology, University of Utah Medical Center, Salt Lake City, Utah

PAUL COLE, C.N.M.T.

Assistant Chief Technologist, Division of Nuclear Medicine, Johns Hopkins Medical Institutions, Baltimore, Maryland

R. EDWARD COLEMAN, M.D.

Professor of Radiology, Department of Radiology, Duke University Medical Center, Durham, North Carolina

TREVOR D. CRADDUCK, Ph.D., F.C.C.P.M.

Senior Physicist, Department of Nuclear Medicine, Victoria Hospital, London, Ontario; Assistant Professor, Division of Radiology and Nuclear Medicine and Division of Radiation Oncology, University of Western Ontario, London, Ontario, Canada

SARA JANE DAVIS, C.N.M.T.

Supervisor and Teaching Associate, Division of Nuclear Medicine, Department of Diagnostic Radiology, University of Kansas Medical Center, Kansas City, Kansas

ROBERT L. DRESSLER, Ph.D.

Professor of Chemistry, Department of Chemistry, Fort Hays State University, Hays, Kansas

EVA DUBOVSKY, M.D., Ph.D.

Professor of Diagnostic Radiology, Division of Nuclear Medicine, University of Alabama Medical Center, Birmingham, Alabama

LISA B. GOLDWORM, B.S.

Health Physicist, Washington University School of Medicine, St. Louis, Missouri

RICHARD A. GOLDWORM, M.S.

Assistant Professor of Chemistry, Cardinal Newman College, Normandy, Missouri

RICHARD A. HOLMES, M.D.

Professor of Medicine and Radiology, University of Missouri—Columbia; Chief, Nuclear Medicine Service, Harry S Truman Memorial Veterans Hospital, Columbia, Missouri

GLENN A. ISSERSTEDT, M.S., C.N.M.T.

Formerly Administrator, Department of Radiology, University of Iowa Hospitals and Clinics, Iowa City, Iowa; Presently Administrator, Department of Radiology, St. Joseph Mercy Hospital, Ann Arbor, Michigan

R. EUGENE JOHNSTON, Ph.D.

Associate Professor of Radiology, Division of Imaging, Department of Radiology, University of North Carolina, Chapel Hill, North Carolina

FRANCES N. KONTZEN, C.N.M.T.

Chief Technologist, Nuclear Medicine Service, Birmingham Veterans Administration Center; Clinical Instructor, Nuclear Medicine Technology Program, School of Community and Allied Health, University of Alabama/Birmingham Veterans Administration Medical Center, Birmingham, Alabama

EDOUARD V. KOTLYAROV, M.D., Ph.D., Sc.D.

Assistant Professor of Radiology, George Washington University; Associate Chairman, Department of Nuclear Medicine, Washington Hospital Center, Washington, D.C.

JAMES K. LANGAN, C.N.M.T.

Chief Technologist, Division of Nuclear Medicine, Johns Hopkins Medical Institutions, Baltimore; Assistant Professor of Nuclear Medicine Technology, Essex Community College, Baltimore, Maryland

ADEL G. MATTAR, M.B., Ch.B.

Professor of Medicine (Nuclear Medicine) Memorial University of Newfoundland, St. John's; Director, Department of Nuclear Medicine, Health Sciences Center, St. John's, Newfoundland, Canada

KAREN D. McELVANY, Ph.D.

Research Instructor, Division of Nuclear Medicine, The Edward Mallinckrodt Institute of Radiology, Washington University School of Medicine, St. Louis, Missouri

GAELLAN McILMOYLE, M.D.

Division of Nuclear Medicine, The Edward Mallinckrodt Institute of Radiology, Washington University School of Medicine, St. Louis, Missouri

PATRICIA A. McINTYRE, M.D.

Associate Director, Divisions of Nuclear Medicine and Radiation Health Science; Associate Professor of Medicine, Radiology and Environmental Health Science, Johns Hopkins Medical Institutions, Baltimore, Maryland

MICHAEL M. MELLO, C.N.M.T.

Director of Nuclear Cardiology, West Florida Hospital, Pensacola, Florida

MARILYN R. MUILENBURG, B.A., C.N.M.T.

Senior Staff Technologist, Division of Nuclear Medicine, The Edward Mallinckrodt Institute of Radiology, Washington University School of Medicine, St. Louis, Missouri

MARK I. MUILENBURG, B.S., C.N.M.T.

Director, Nuclear Medicine and Ultrasound, Creighton University School of Medicine and St. Joseph's Hospital, Omaha, Nebraska

MARIA V. NAGEL, B.A., C.N.M.T.

Educational Coordinator, Nuclear Medicine Technology, University of Nebraska Medical Center, Omaha, Nebraska

THOMAS J. PERSOON, M.S.

Chief Technologist, Special Chemistry Laboratory, Department of Pathology, University of Iowa Hospitals and Clinics, Iowa City, Iowa

DAVID J. PHEGLEY, B.S., C.N.M.T.

Chief Technologist, Department of Nuclear Medicine, St. Louis University Hospitals, St. Louis, Missouri

DAVID F. PRESTON, M.D.

Associate Professor of Diagnostic Radiology, Division of Nuclear Medicine, Department of Diagnostic Radiology, University of Kansas Medical Center, Kansas City, Kansas

MERTON A. QUAIFE, M.D., F.A.C.P.

Associate Professor of Radiology (Nuclear Medicine and Radiation Biology) and Medicine; Director, Division of Nuclear Medicine, University of Nebraska Medical Center, Omaha, Nebraska

FRANCINE K. SCHAFFNER, C.N.M.T.

Division of Nuclear Medicine, The Edward Mallinckrodt Institute of Radiology, Washington University School of Medicine, St. Louis, Missouri

ROGER H. SECKER-WALKER, M.B., M.R.C.P.

Professor of Medicine and Physiology, Medical Director, Pulmonary Division, Department of Internal Medicine, St. Louis University School of Medicine, St. Louis, Missouri

JAY A. SPICER, M.S.

Assistant Professor of Diagnostic Radiology (Nuclear Medicine), Division of Nuclear Medicine, Department of Diagnostic Radiology, University of Kansas Medical Center, Kansas City, Kansas

HENRY N. WAGNER, Jr., M.D.

Director, Divisions of Nuclear Medicine and Radiation Health Science, Professor of Medicine, Radiology, and Environmental Health Science, Johns Hopkins Medical Institutions, Baltimore, Maryland

SALLY J. WAGNER, M.S., R.Ph.

Research Associate, Division of Nuclear Medicine, The Edward Mallinckrodt Institute of Radiology, Washington University School of Medicine, St. Louis, Missouri

CAROLYN WEISBERG, R.N.

Clinical Nurse, Division of Nuclear Medicine, Johns Hopkins Medical Institutions, Baltimore, Maryland

MICHAEL J. WELCH, Ph.D.

Professor of Radiation Chemistry in Radiology, Division of Radiation Sciences, The Edward Mallinckrodt Institute of Radiology, Washington University School of Medicine, St. Louis, Missouri

L. DAVID WELLS, C.N.M.T.

Chief Technologist, Division of Nuclear Medicine, University Community Hospital, Tampa, Florida

To our wives

Lorraine, Mary Jane, and **Lynne**

without whose love and support

this task would never have been accomplished

and to our children

Ashley, Carol, Catherine, Chipper, John,

Kathleen, Michael, Patricia, Steven, and **Timothy**

FOREWORD

We have been waiting for this book for a long time. There are over 140 programs in nuclear medicine technology in the United States alone, turning out over 850 technologists per year. Some of these are in university medical centers; some are in community hospitals; some are affiliated with community colleges; some are at the baccalaureate level.

In most cases, students have had to search for information in textbooks designed primarily for physicians, in government documents, or in journal articles. This book, edited by three distinguished technologists with over a half-century of experience, represents the efforts of technologists, teamed up with nuclear medicine physicians to produce a single volume that covers the entire field. It covers basic and clinical science and has special features, such as chapters on patient care and the use of computers.

All the authors are involved in educational programs for technologists. Although the book is designed as the basic textbook for student technologists, others such as resident physicians will find it to be very helpful. It will also be a useful reference book to be kept at close hand after the technologist graduates and begins clinical work. Although not a detailed procedure manual, it can provide answers to many questions that arise every day.

I have long believed that a nuclear medicine technologist needs to have more different types of skills than any other person involved in the delivery of health care. Consider the various steps in carrying out a procedure: preparation of the radiopharmaceutical requires expertise in chemistry; expertise in pharmacy to ensure sterility and apyrogenicity, in radiation safety, and in accounting to keep adequate records; expertise in physics to understand the instruments and their proper use; expertise in mathematics and computers; and expertise in all the humanistic skills so necessary in caring for patients. It has been said that the best way to care *for* patients is to care *about* patients. Finally, when the day comes for the technologist to become the chief, he or she must have managerial and leadership skills.

I have never understood how so many technologists have been able to do the job so well. This book will help them to do it even better.

Henry N. Wagner, Jr.

PREFACE

The conceptual development for this textbook in nuclear medicine technology began just prior to the annual meeting of the Society of Nuclear Medicine in 1977. At the time, no textbook existed that encompassed all aspects of the curriculum in nuclear medicine technology training programs. Thus we sought to develop a book that could serve as the primary textbook employed by a student technologist during the course of training. We sincerely hope that this book meets this need.

In selecting contributors, we chose to have both a physician and a technologist collaborate on chapters devoted to clinical nuclear medicine and have selected individuals who are expert in their given subject area. We believe that the technologists contribute greatly to the scope of the technical component of these chapters because these individuals produce the images or data that the physician must interpret.

Our thanks go out to many people involved in the production of this book. To our contributors, for their time, effort, and hard work; to Drs. Barry Siegel, Larry Muroff, Daniel Biello, Philip Alderson, Henry Wagner, and Ralph Robinson for tolerating our absences from work; to the technical and secretarial staffs of our institutions; and, most of all, to our wives and children for just putting up with us.

Donald R. Bernier
James K. Langan
L. David Wells

CONTENTS

SECTION ONE

Basic sciences

Chapter 1

MATHEMATICS AND STATISTICS

Glenn A. Isserstedt

Excitement and enthusiasm are awaiting you, the student, who has elected to specialize in nuclear medicine technology until you are confronted by and reminded that you should have both a firm foundation in mathematics and the ability to apply its principles to this health-related technology. Even though most students have had prior exposure to the fundamentals of mathematics, your present level of understanding and expertise in applying these basic mathematical principles may need either revivification or fortification, or both. In this, you should not allow your enthusiasm or excitement to wane or deteriorate; however, the potentially "well-rounded" student is challenged to totally understand these basic concepts and other science relationships because they collectively form the lintel upon which the suprastructure of clinical nuclear medicine technology is based.

Not an aspect of science or its pragmatic application through technology escapes quantification. The importance of this introductory philosophy may not necessarily be initially or readily apparent. Therefore to be a further challenge, it is suggested that after reading this entire text, you at least review immediately the chapters dealing primarily with basic science. In this way, you will be able to be conversant with the fundamental parameters, which you will use constantly.

Computers and calculators have been introduced into the contemporary instrumentation available to and used in nuclear medicine facilities, and perhaps even more aspects of space-age technology will be incorporated. If nuclear medicine technologists are not cognizant of these "tools," we may very easily become the passive and physical slaves of automation without any active involvement or cerebration.

Numbers, related mathematical operations, and mathematical answers do not naturally exist but were and are generated by man to be useful to and assist him in describing quantifiable aspects of "things" with which he is in contact.

We have spent significant time during our previous educational experiences being repetitiously taught to add, subtract, multiply, and divide. In fact, in most cases, we have conditioned our minds so well to subconsciously know the relationship between numbers that we fall very easily into "number traps" when we are confronted by a confusing quantifiable problem with apparently very little practicality. One applicable way, which may be initially difficult if you are used to memorization for short-term use until after an examination, is to *think*. Mathematics is difficult for the average person because of two reasons: (1) Most texts and teachers do not illustrate mathematical operations step by step but say, "It follows that . . . ." and therefore the student must memorize to have any fluency with mathematical operations, and (2) since the student has been so busy memorizing but not knowing why or the reasoning behind it, he has not developed any skill or expertise with thinking mathematically. You do not need to be a mathematical purist or wizard to think mathematically. Before proceeding, decide that you will be self-confident and that you can and will *think*.

BASIC MATHEMATICAL MANIPULATIONS

There are four basic mathematical (that is, arithmetic or algebraic) operations or manipulations that man can perform, but even more basic to them are the two operations of addition and subtraction, with multiplication being a series of repetitive additions and division being a series of repetitive subtractions.

Addition is a mathematical manipulation that is the inverse of (undoes) subtraction and that joins individual and similar units or groups of addends, for example, $4 + 3 = 7$; microcuries + microcuries = microcuries. This operation uses a plus (+) symbol as an index of the required procedure. The result is the *sum* and is independent of the order in which the addition is performed. In other words, since the order of the units or groups can be exchanged or substituted without effect, addition is therefore said to obey the *commutative* and *associative laws*. The significance of these laws is that a list of numbers may be "added up or added down'' to check addition or to rearrange the addends in a specified or preferred order.

Subtraction is a mathematical manipulation that is the inverse of (undoes) addition and that separates individual and similar units or groups, for example, $8 - 2 = 6$; minutes − minutes = minutes. This operation uses a minus (−) symbol as an index of the required action. The result is the *difference* and is dependent on the order in which the subtraction is performed. Special names are given to the number to be diminished, the number subtracted, and the difference:

$$\text{Minuend} - \text{Subtrahend} = \text{Remainder}$$
$$220 \text{ lb} - 80 \text{ lb} = 140 \text{ lb}$$

Multiplication is a mathematical manipulation that is the inverse of (undoes) division and that requires that the *multiplicand* be increased by the *multiplier;* both of which collectively can be called factors. This operation uses a times sign (×), parentheses or round brackets ( ), a centered dot or multiplication dot (·), or juxtaposed symbols with no intervening sign, as an index of the required action. The result of the operation is called the *product*. Similarly to addition, this operation obeys the *commutative law,* which allows the factors to be rearranged to simplify multiplication, to check multiplication, or to rearrange for a preferred order.

$$\text{Multiplicand} \times \text{Multiplier} = \text{Product}$$
$$\$4.87/\text{hour} \times 40 \text{ hours/week} = \$194.80/\text{week}$$

Division is a mathematical manipulation that is the inverse of (undoes) multiplication and that determines how many times the *divisor* is contained within the *dividend;* the result of the operation or the number of times is called the *quotient*. This operation uses a division sign (÷), a ratio sign or colon (:), or a fraction bar (either / or —) as an index of the required action.

$$\text{Dividend} \div \text{Divisor} = \text{Quotient}$$
$$2080 \text{ hours/year} \div 52 \text{ weeks/year} = 40 \text{ hours/week}$$

ORDER OF OPERATIONS

Situations may present in which you will be required to translate verbal statements into mathematical expressions or to solve them. To illustrate, express this statement mathematically, ''A patient's weight in pounds (lb) that is 10 lb less than 50 kilograms (kg)''; the answer is as follows:

$$50 \text{ kg} \times 2.2 \frac{\text{lb}}{\text{kg}} - 10 \text{ lb} = 100 \text{ lb}$$

To arrive at the correct answer in this or any example, you must perform the required mathematical operations in a three-step specific sequence called the *order of operations,* which is as follows:

Step 1: Perform any required mathematical operation within any parentheses, bracket, or brace, if they are present; then

Step 2: Perform multiplications and divisions in order of appearance from left to right; and then

Step 3: Perform additions and subtractions in order of appearance from left to right.

The following example will illustrate the above specified order:

Problem: Assume that the table at which you are studying has a width of 35 inches (in) and that the length is 127 cm longer than the width. Calculate and express the perimeter in inches.

SOLUTION:

1. General: 2 (Width) + 2 (Length) = Perimeter
2. Specific:

a. $2\,(35 \text{ in}) + 2\left(35 \text{ in} + \dfrac{127 \text{ cm}}{2.54 \dfrac{\text{cm}}{\text{in}}}\right) = \text{Perimeter}$

b. $2\,(35 \text{ in}) + 2\left(35 \text{ in} + \dfrac{127 \text{ cm}}{1} \times \dfrac{1 \text{ in}}{2.54 \text{ cm}}\right) = \text{Perimeter}$

c. 2 (35 in) + 2 (35 in + 50 in) = Perimeter
d. 2 (35 in) + 2 (85 in) = Perimeter
e. 70 in + 170 in = Perimeter
f. 240 inches = Perimeter

A pair of parentheses ( ) is the simple-level symbol utilized to indicate a grouping; the second level of complexity is a pair of brackets [ ], which may include a pair of parentheses; the third level of complexity is a pair of braces { }, which may include the previous two levels. The use of all three grouping symbols is illustrated in the following algebraic expression:

$$24 - \left\{4 + \left[\frac{x}{2} + (3 + x)\right]\right\}$$

By substituting the value of 6 for x in the above example, determine the expression's value; any answer other than 8 is incorrect.

FRACTIONS IN REVIEW

Fractions consist of a numerator and denominator. In other words, a fraction represents the quotient of two integers. Several brief descriptions will be helpful.

A *numerator* is the term above or to the left of the dividing line in a fraction; the denominator is divided into this term, which is actually the dividend. A *denominator* is the term below or to the right of the dividing line in a fraction; the numerator is divided by this term, which is actually the divisor.

Fraction types

Proper or simple. The quotient is less than 1 (for example, the width of a piece of imaging film compared to its length):

14 inches/17 inches = 0.8235294

Improper. The quotient is greater than 1 (for example, the comparison of overtime pay to regular pay):

$$\frac{\$6.75/\text{hour}}{\$4.50/\text{hour}} = 1.5$$

Decimal. This fraction type may be expressed as a fraction whose denominator is a power of 10. Proper or improper fractions may be converted into a decimal fractional equivalent form by dividing the numerator by the denominator as follows:

$3/4 = 0.75 \quad 3/2 = 1.5$

Care must be exercised with the number and position of decimal places when you perform additive and subtractive manipulations on decimal fractions. Further, when multiplying decimal fractions, the number of decimal places in the product is the sum of the decimal places in the numbers multiplied.

Handling fractions

Addition and subtraction. The situation will almost never arise in your nuclear medicine technology experience wherein you are required to perform either of these manipulations with any listing of proper fractions:

1. Addition: ¾ + ½ + ⅓
2. Subtraction: ¾ − ⅜ − 3/16

However, a brief review will refresh your basic understanding and familiarization. A suggested and effective alternate method to handle these identified manipulations is to convert the proper fractions to their decimal equivalents and then proceed as indicated by the mathematical indicators or signs.

To complete the comparisons, the decimal-conversion sequence would be represented as follows (note temporary use of zeros to the right of the decimal point):

1. ¾ = 0.7500; ½ = 0.5000; ⅓ = 0.3333
2. ¾ = 0.7500; ⅜ = 0.3750; 3/16 = 0.1875

Therefore:

1. 0.7500 + 0.5000 + 0.3333 = 1.5833
2. 0.7500 − 0.3750 − 0.1875 = 0.1875

For the second example, the lowest common denominator (LCD) is 16. The required treatment and subtractive manipulation are represented as follows:

Step 1: ¾ − ⅜ − 3/16

Step 2: $\frac{3 \cdot 4}{16} - \frac{3 \cdot 2}{16} - \frac{3}{16}$

Step 3: $\frac{12}{16} - \frac{6}{16} - \frac{3}{16}$

Step 4: $\frac{12 - 6 - 3}{16} = \frac{3}{16}$

Step 5: 3/16 = 0.1875

The reasons for the examples and discussion, even though you probably will not be called upon to use these steps in clinical or didactic activities, are that you can very easily *think* mathematically and that the suggested alternate method is mathematically equivalent to the first:

$$\begin{aligned} ¾ &= 0.7500 \\ ½ &= 0.5000 \\ +⅓ &= 0.3333 \\ \hline \end{aligned}$$

Therefore, the sum is equivalent to 1.5833. You would obtain the same value but in improper fractional form by determining and using the lowest common denominator (LCD). In other words, to add fractions that initially have dissimilar denominators, a common denominator of lowest value must be found and used. From the above example, the number 24 could represent a common denominator, since it is the product of 4 × 2 × 3. However, it is not the lowest; 12 is the lowest common denominator, since each number can be evenly divided into 12. Each numerator will need to be mathematically treated in such a manner to maintain the same relationship with a new denominator of 12 as with their initial and respective denominators. The required treatment and additive manipulations are represented as follows:

Step 1: ¾ + ½ + ⅓

Step 2: $\frac{3 \cdot 3}{12} + \frac{6 \cdot 1}{12} + \frac{4 \cdot 1}{12}$

Step 3: $\frac{9}{12} + \frac{6}{12} + \frac{4}{12}$

Step 4: $\frac{9 + 6 + 4}{12} = \frac{19}{12}$

Step 5: $\frac{19}{12} = 1.583333$

Multiplication and division. Again, in your nuclear medicine technology experience you will almost never need to multiply or divide proper fractions. However, it is very conceivable that these mathematical manipulations will need to be performed on decimal fractions.

The product will need to contain a number of places to the right of the decimal equal to the sum of the decimal places in the numbers multiplied. The following will illustrate this requirement:

1.5 × \$4.50/hour = \$6.750

The quotient will generally need to contain a number of places to the right of the decimal equal to the number in the dividend minus those in the divisor:

60.000 ml ÷ 4.5 ml = 13.33 ml

UNITS

Rationale

Events that we experience in everyday living and clinical nuclear medicine have both a *quantification* portion and a *qualification* portion.

Example	Quantification	Qualification
Driving in a car	55	miles/hour
Motel lodging	\$23.75	1/day
Gamma-ray energy	140,000	eV/1
Radioactive count rate	22.2×10^{10}	counts/minute

The qualification is "what type" and the quantification is "how many." By examination of the qualification portion for each of the above examples, we observe a fraction-resembling entry. These word fractions consist of a word or numerical numerator and a word or numerical denominator. It is important to remember that accompanying all numbers or quantities there must be a qualification portion. No specific information is conveyed by this exemplary statement, "The patient's temperature is 36." Your logical response should be, "36 what?" We most likely know that it means 36 degrees Celsius but we do not know for sure. Without the qualification, the quantification is meaningless and scientifically and technically sloppy. The importance of being precise about the quality or type of data you collect or manipulate cannot be stressed enough. Suppose that you are going to administer a radiopharmaceutical to a patient for an imaging procedure, and on an injection record form you enter "150." Will you remember tomorrow or 1 year later the quality of this numerical datum? Not likely! Was it millicuries or microcuries? Without insulting your intelligence, please train and educate yourself to be totally complete about numerical data. Data need both descriptions—*what* and *how many*.

All the mathematical manipulations that apply to quantity fractions apply to quality fractions. To illustrate, solve the following quality equations by providing either the missing quality fractions or the necessary mathematical operational designations, or both:

1. $\frac{\text{Examinations}}{\text{Day}} \times \frac{\text{Days}}{\text{Week}} \times \frac{\quad}{\quad} = \frac{\text{Examinations}}{\text{Year}}$

2. $\frac{1}{\text{Minute}} \times \frac{\quad}{\quad} = {}^1\!/_1$

3. $\frac{\text{Films}}{\text{Procedure}} \; ? \; \frac{\text{Films}}{\text{Box}} = \frac{\text{Box}}{\text{Procedure}}$

In the first example, the missing quality fraction is weeks/year. From the left side, days divide out (that is, cancel out), examination remains in the numerator on the right as it is on the left, and, on the left, we must be able to divide out the weeks from the denominator by placing weeks in the numerator of the missing quality fraction, and, from the right side, we need to end with year in the denominator.

The right-hand side of the second equation is a fraction whose denominator and numerator are of the same type or value, and this equality is most frequently identified by the single number 1. However, as stated above for quality fractions, quantification portions also possess both a numerator and denominator. The missing quality fraction is minutes/1 since we need to be able to divide out minutes in order that the right-hand side results in the illustrated manner.

The third example requires that the first quality fraction be divided by the second quality fraction. When fractions are divided, the law states that the divisor is inverted and multiplied. If this is accomplished, films divide out and box moves to the numerator as is required on the right side.

As a reminder, but not illustrated by an example, is the requirement that when adding or subtracting quality fractions, a common denominator needs to be determined prior to performing the stated manipulations.

Dimensions

Physical measurement involves the comparison between an observed measure (for example, the length of this page) and that of a standard of some type (for example, a centimeter ruler). Whether by custom, legislation or agreement, various fundamental units have been identified and basically agreed upon. A physical measurement is a combined expression; a product of a number *and* a unit. Different measurements may be equivalent even though they may be represented by different numbers and different units, for example:

$$1 \text{ inch} = 2.54 \text{ centimeters} = 2.54 \times 10^8 \text{ angstroms}$$

Most of the physical quantities that you will encounter in nuclear medicine technology are derived units, the practical units that are actually defined in terms of fundamental or other basic units. In the past, numerous systems have been developed to interrelate derived units, physical laws, and fundamental units. Approximately 40 years ago, a significant transition was manifested among the fundamental mechanical units of length, mass, and time; namely the change from the cgs (centimeter-gram-second) system to the mks (meter-kilogram-second) system. Yet a third system is frequently utilized; the foot-pound-second (ft-lb-s) system. What is the relevance of this background information to studies and activities in nuclear medicine technology? The answer is, since you have no control over the form in which you will be receiving or are requested to manipulate various laboratory or clinical data, you need to understand and demonstrate an ability to mathematically translate and perform the required calculations.

In anticipation of some of your needs and activities in nuclear medicine technology, Table 1-1 identifies

Table 1-1. Selected physical units with system equivalents and interrelations

Mechanical unit	Symbol	System: mks	cgs	ft-lbm-sec*
Area	A	1 m^2	10,000 cm^2	10.758 ft^2
Length	l	1 m	100 cm	39.37 in (3.28 ft)
Mass	M	1 kg	1000 g (gm)	2.205 lb (453.4 g)
Time	t	1 sec	1 sec	1 sec
Volume	V	1 m^3 (1000 liters)	1,000,000 cc (ml)	35.28 ft^3 (264.17 gal)

**lbm*, Pound-mass (force) at a distance.

several routinely used mechanical units of physical measurement. The different systems referred to above are illustrated along with their respective units and interrelationships.

In science and technology, quantities are the measurements of properties (for example, area, velocity, volume). Logically, for consistency and comparision, measured properties must be evaluated against a common, nonvariable standard unit. To illustrate, the length and width of a clinical procedure room would be measured in meters or feet, not cubits; the former two being nonvariable standard units, whereas the cubit varies from 18 to 22 inches depending on the person obtaining the measurements.

Basic units may be manipulated to result in derived units, which may be further classified as consistent or nonconsistent.

Consistent: Require no conversion factors; calculations employing this type of derived unit are easier to perform and are more reliable, for example:

$$\text{Velocity} = \text{Meters per second} = \frac{\text{Meter}}{\text{Second}}$$

Velocity (that is, speed) is the derived unit that is generated from the basic units of meter (length) and second (time).

Nonconsistent: Require a conversion factor; calculations employing this type of derived unit are more difficult to perform and are less reliable, for example:

$$1 \text{ atomic mass unit (a.m.u.)} = 1.659 \times 10^{-27} \text{ kg}$$

$$1 \text{ curie (Ci)} = 3.7 \times 10^{10} \text{ d} \cdot \text{sec}^{-1}$$

(disintegrations per second)

In these examples, note that each derived unit (a.m.u. or Ci) is dependent on and requires a conversion factor (coefficient) used in conjunction with basic units of mass (grams) and time (seconds). Specifically, these coefficients are the respective numerical values.

Most of the units with which you will come into contact will be of the nonconsistent, derived type. Therefore, be prepared to remember conversion factors and be extra careful when performing calculations with this unit category.

In 1977, the World Health Organization recommended that the medical community throughout the world adopt the *Système International d'Unités (SI)*. As part of that recommendation and unique to the scientific, medical, and technical communities are certain word prefixes and their numerical equivalents that should be thoroughly understood and extensively utilized. Table 1-2 identifies the numerical equivalents of word and symbolic prefixes that can be combined with word units. Most frequently encountered will be the word prefix followed by the symbol for the unit. In actuality, this word-symbol combination represents a numerical product. To illustrate:

$$1 \text{ cm} = 1 \cdot \text{c} \cdot \text{m} = 1 \times (0.01) \times (\text{meter})$$

$$1 \ \mu\text{Ci} = 1 \cdot \mu \cdot \text{Ci} = 1 \times (0.000001) \times (\text{curie})$$

This format and understanding will be extremely useful when scientific notation is discussed later in this chapter. Several important points to remember about symbols and prefixes are as follows:

1. Prefixes that are numerical and multiples of 3 are preferred: 10^6, 10^3, 10^{-3}, and 10^{-6} = mega, kilo, milli, and micro, respectively.
2. Only one prefix is allowed per unit symbol:
   a. *Incorrect form:* μMg (micro-mega-gram), or $(10^{-6}) \times (10^6) \times$ (gram), needs to be rewritten to the following.
   b. *Correct form:* 1 gram, since the product of the word prefixes is numerically equivalent to 1.0.
3. In general, when expressing a fraction, the numerator should have the prefixes, if possible.
4. All unit symbols are to be written without periods (for example, sec, not sec.).
5. Symbols of units named for individuals are to be capitalized; the others are in lower-cased letters (for example, Gy = gray, but m = meters).

As a result of metrication laws (P.L. 93-380 and

Table 1-2. Numerical equivalents of word prefixes and symbols used with units

Numerical equivalent		Word prefix	Symbol
10^{18} =	1,000,000,000,000,000,000	exa	E
10^{15} =	1,000,000,000,000,000	peta	P
10^{12} =	1,000,000,000,000	tera	T
10^{9} =	1,000,000,000	giga	G
10^{6} =	1,000,000	mega	M
10^{3} =	1,000	kilo	k
10^{2} =	100	hecto	h
10^{1} =	10	deka	da
10^{0} =	1	uni-	
10^{-1} =	0.1	deci	d
10^{-2} =	0.01	centi	c
10^{-3} =	0.001	milli	m
10^{-6} =	0.000001	micro	μ
10^{-9} =	0.000000001	nano	n
10^{-12} =	0.000000000001	pico	p
10^{-15} =	0.000000000000001	femto	f
10^{-18} =	0.000000000000000001	atto	a

Table 1-3. Former and replacement units represented by symbols and numerical values

	Unit		
Measured property	**Name**	**Symbol**	**Numerical value**
Exposure to ionizing radiation	roentgen	R	$= 2.58 \times 10^{-4} \frac{\text{coulomb}}{\text{kilogram}}$ $= 1.6123 \times 10^{15} \frac{\text{ionizations}}{\text{gram of air}}$ $= 2.082 \times 10^{9} \frac{\text{ionizations}}{\text{cc of air}}$
Absorbed dose			
1. Former	rad	rad	$= 100 \frac{\text{ergs}}{\text{gram}}$
2. Replacement	gray	Gy	$= 1 \frac{\text{joule}}{\text{kilogram}}$ $= 2.39 \times 10^{-1} \frac{\text{calories}}{\text{kilogram}}$ $= 10^{7} \frac{\text{ergs}}{\text{kilogram}}$
Equivalent absorbed dose	rem	rem	$= 1 \text{ rad} = 100 \frac{\text{ergs}}{\text{gram}}$
Activity of source			
1. Former	curie	Ci	$= 3.7 \times 10^{10} \frac{\text{disintegrations}}{\text{second}}$
2. Replacement	becquerel	Bq	$= 1 \frac{\text{disintegration}}{\text{second}}$
Distances (microscopic)			
1. Former	micron	μ	$= 10^{-6}$ meter
2. Replacement	micrometer	μm	$= 10^{-6}$ meter
Distances (electron microscopic)			
1. Former	angstrom (Ångström)	Å	$= 10^{-10}$ meter $= 10^{-8}$ cm
2. Replacement	a. nanometer	nm	$= 10^{-9}$ meter
	b. picometer	pm	$= 10^{-12}$ meter
Temperature			
1. Former	Fahrenheit	°F	$= (C \times 1.8) + 32°$
2. Replacement	Celsius	°C	$= (F - 32°) \times 0.55$
Pressure (blood)			
1. Former	atmosphere	mm Hg	= 133.322 Pa
2. Replacement	pascal	Pa	= 0.0075 mm Hg = newton/meter^2

P.L. 94-168), some confusion might possibly arise based upon the legislatively mandated replacement of commonly used and familiar units such as curie, rad, rem, and others in clinical nuclear medicine. Table 1-3 identifies some of the former units that have been used in nuclear medicine and their replacements along with specified qualification factors. Day-to-day utilization can and should be made of the pragmatic information provided in Tables 1-4 to 1-7. Since the replacement units are generally unfamiliar both in magnitude and methods of manipulation, relative magnitudes expressing their relationship with the respective former units are provided in each of these four tables. In addition, mathematical formulas, which, with accompanying representative examples illustrate mathematical methods for any necessary conversions.

Your ultimate concern about these changes should not be, why did they occur? but rather, do I understand them and can I mathematically work with them in order to obviate any risk to a patient? If the answer is yes, proceed; if no, review the above material until you are fluent.

The general usefulness of the information contained in the previous four tables is as follows:

Table 1-4: Radiation protection, radiation biology and radionuclide therapy
Table 1-5: Radionuclide injection and nuclear instrumentation techniques
Table 1-6: Radiopharmaceutical preparation and clinical tracer techniques
Table 1-7: Clinical nuclear medicine with patient interaction

Additional exemplary information must be added to the information in Table 1-5 to render it more clinically relevant. Radionuclides are purchased by the activity level of the radioactive source (for example, 400 mCi ^{99m}Mo generator or 5 μCi ^{57}Co-cyanocobalamin capsules).

Subsequent to acquisition, a specific amount of the radiopharmaceutical is administered to a patient for an imaging (in vivo) procedure or combined with a biologic sample for an in vitro procedure. In these two instances, the amount is described as some portion of the basic unit, curie.

After the administration or utilization, this same radioactive material is now described in terms of count rate, which is a unit or term herein not discussed to this point. Assume that a radiation-detection instru-

Table 1-4. Relative relationship and conversion parameters for absorbed dose

Relative magnitude relationship		Conversion factors
Former	**Replacement**	
rad 1 mm × 1 mm (square)	Gy 10 mm × 10 mm (square)	To convert rad → Gy 1. $\left(\frac{\text{rad}}{1}\right) \times \left(0.01\ \frac{\text{Gy}}{\text{rad}}\right) = \left(\frac{\text{Gy}}{1}\right)$ 2. EXAMPLE: As a result of oral administration of sodium ^{131}I-iodide, 1500 rads are absorbed by the thyroid tissue. Express the equivalent absorbed dose in Gy and mGy. a. $1500\ \frac{\text{rad}}{1} \times 0.01\ \frac{\text{Gy}}{\text{rad}} = 15.00\ \text{Gy}$ b. $15\ \frac{\text{Gy}}{1} \times 1000\ \frac{\text{mGy}}{\text{Gy}} = 15{,}000\ \text{mGy}$
1 rad = 0.01 Gy		To convert Gy → rad 1. $\left(\frac{\text{Gy}}{1}\right) \times \left(100\ \frac{\text{rad}}{\text{Gy}}\right) = \left(\frac{\text{rad}}{1}\right)$ 2. EXAMPLE: As a result of oral administration of sodium ^{131}I-iodide, 5.8 Gy are absorbed by the thyroid tissue. Express the equivalent absorbed dose in rad. $5.8\ \frac{\text{Gy}}{1} \times 100\ \frac{\text{rad}}{\text{Gy}} = 580\ \text{rad}$

Table 1-5. Relative relationship and conversion parameters for source activity

Relative magnitude relationship: Former	Replacement	Conversion factors
Ci 192,353.8 mm × 192,353.8 mm (vastly larger than this) 3.7×10^{10} mm²	Bq 1 mm × 1 mm 1 mm²	To convert Ci → GBq, mCi → MBq, μCi → kBq 1. a. $\left(\frac{\text{Ci}}{1}\right) \times \left(37\frac{\text{GBq}}{\text{Ci}}\right) = \left(\frac{\text{GBq}}{1}\right)$ b. $\left(\frac{\text{mCi}}{1}\right) \times \left(37\frac{\text{MBq}}{\text{mCi}}\right) = \left(\frac{\text{MBq}}{1}\right)$ c. $\left(\frac{\mu\text{Ci}}{1}\right) \times \left(37\frac{\text{kBq}}{\mu\text{Ci}}\right) = \left(\frac{\text{kBq}}{1}\right)$ 2. EXAMPLE: 30 mCi of ^{99m}Tc-pertechnate are administered to a patient for a brain-imaging procedure. Express this quantity in MBq and GBq. a. $30\,\frac{\text{mCi}}{1} \times 37\,\frac{\text{MBq}}{\text{mCi}} = 1110\,\frac{\text{MBq}}{1}$ b. $1110\,\frac{\text{MBq}}{1} \times 10^{-3}\,\frac{\text{GBq}}{\text{MBq}} = 1.11\text{ GBq}$
1 Ci = 3.7×10^{10} Bq = 37×10^{9} Bq = 37 GBq		To convert GBq → Ci, MBq → mCi, kBq → μCi 1. a. $\left(\frac{\text{GBq}}{1}\right) \times \left(0.027027\,\frac{\text{Ci}}{\text{GBq}}\right) = \left(\frac{\text{Ci}}{1}\right)$ b. $\left(\frac{\text{MBq}}{1}\right) \times \left(0.027027\,\frac{\text{mCi}}{\text{MBq}}\right) = \left(\frac{\text{mCi}}{1}\right)$ c. $\frac{\text{kBq}}{1} \times 0.027027\,\frac{\mu\text{Ci}}{\text{kBq}} = \left(\frac{\mu\text{Ci}}{1}\right)$ 2. EXAMPLE: 74 MBq of ^{99m}Tc-labeled MAA (macroaggregated albumin) are administered for a lung-imaging procedure. Express this quantity in mCi and μCi. a. $74\,\frac{\text{MBq}}{1} \times 0.027027\,\frac{\text{mCi}}{\text{MBq}} = 2\,\frac{\text{mCi}}{1}$ b. $74\,\frac{\text{MBq}}{1} \times 10^{3}\,\frac{\text{kBq}}{\text{MBq}} = 74000\text{ kBq}$ c. $74000\,\frac{\text{kBq}}{1} \times 0.027027\,\frac{\mu\text{Ci}}{\text{kBq}} = 2000\,\mu\text{Ci}$

Table 1-6. Relative relationship and conversion parameters for microscopic distances

Relative magnitude relationship		Conversion factors
Former	**Replacement**	
micron	micrometer	To convert $\mu \rightarrow \mu m$
1 μ (vastly smaller than this)	1 μm	None needed: μ and μm are identical.

Table 1-7. Relative relationship and conversion parameters for blood pressure

Relative magnitude relationship		Conversion factors
Former	**Replacement**	
mm Hg	Pa	To convert mm Hg → Pa
11.547 mm × 11.547 mm	1 mm × 1 mm	
133.322 mm²	1 mm²	

1 mm Hg = 133.322 Pa
= 0.1333 kPa

To convert mm Hg → Pa

1. $\left(\frac{\text{mm Hg}}{1}\right) \times \left(133.322 \frac{\text{Pa}}{\text{mm Hg}}\right) = \left(\frac{\text{Pa}}{1}\right)$

2. EXAMPLE: A patient's blood pressure was 130/80. Express this pressure in Pa and kPa.

   a. $130 \frac{\text{mm Hg}}{1} \times 133.322 \frac{\text{Pa}}{\text{mm Hg}} = 17331.86 \text{ Pa}$

   b. $80 \frac{\text{mm Hg}}{1} \times 133.322 \frac{\text{Pa}}{\text{mm Hg}} = 10665.76 \text{ Pa}$

   c. $17331.86 \frac{\text{Pa}}{1} \times 10^{-3} \frac{\text{kPa}}{\text{Pa}} = 17.33 \text{ kPa}$

   d. $10665.76 \frac{\text{Pa}}{1} \times 10^{-3} \frac{\text{kPa}}{\text{Pa}} = 10.67 \text{ kPa}$

To convert Pa → mm Hg

1. a. $\left(\frac{\text{Pa}}{1}\right) \times \left(0.0075 \frac{\text{mm Hg}}{\text{Pa}}\right) = \left(\frac{\text{mm Hg}}{1}\right)$

   b. $\left(\frac{\text{kPa}}{1}\right) \times \left(7.5 \frac{\text{mm Hg}}{\text{kPa}}\right) = \left(\frac{\text{mm Hg}}{1}\right)$

2. EXAMPLE: The manometer readings for a patient are 24/12 kPa. Express these readings in mm Hg.

   a. $24 \frac{\text{kPa}}{1} \times 7.5 \frac{\text{mm Hg}}{\text{kPa}} = 180 \text{ mm Hg}$

   b. $12 \frac{\text{kPa}}{1} \times 7.5 \frac{\text{mm Hg}}{\text{kPa}} = 90 \text{ mm Hg}$

ment was so efficient that "it detected each radiative disintegration and 'counted' the number of these radiations per unit of time." From the totaled tally per time, the instrument displays a count rate, which is expressed in counts per minute (cpm). As stated above, we and the instruments have forgotten about μCi and MBg because our vocabulary is now restricted to cpm.

The following examples illustrate the conversion from *source activity (disintegrations per second) to cpm,* that is, *disintegrations to counts per minute:*

$$1 \text{ curie} = 3.7 \times 10^{10} \frac{\text{disintegrations}}{\text{sec}} \times 60 \frac{\text{sec}}{\text{minute}} =$$

$$222 \times 10^{10} \frac{\text{counts}}{\text{minute}}$$

The further subdivisions of these basic values are discussed and illustrated later under scientific notation.

EQUATIONS

By definition, an equation is a mathematical statement specifying that two expressions are equal or have the same value. The total statement, consisting of both a right and a left member, uses an equal sign (=) as a symbol to represent the conditional equality. In general, the root of an equation (for example, answer) is the conditional satisfier of the equation. As a rule for equations, whatever mathematical operation is performed on the right member (side), the same operation must be performed on the left member to retain the mathematical statement in equality. All formulas that you will encounter are literal equations in that they contain two or more unknowns or variables.

The relationship between temperatures on the Fahrenheit and Celsius scales is given by the formula (equation):

$$C = {}^5\!/_9\,(F - 32) \quad \text{or} \quad C = (F - 32) \times 0.55$$

In the above, the various Fahrenheit values determine the Celsius values in a linear manner. In other words, the relationship when graphed (discussed later) would result in a straight line.

By comparison, several other equation types are nonlinear; the most frequently encountered in nuclear medicine technology is the exponential equation whose distinguishing characteristic is that the unknown variables are used as exponents of numbers rather than as coefficients or factors. The following exponential equation is one with which you should become extremely familiar and comfortable:

$$A_t = A_0 \cdot e^{-\lambda t}$$

This equation requires solution by means of logarithms, or exponential values (Appendixes B and C, pp. 48 to 56).

RATIOS

In mathematics, a ratio, usually presenting as a fraction, is defined as a quotient resulting from the division of one quantity by another. It is imperative to remember that quantities must be of the same unit type. Since the ratio consists of a numerator and denominator, both of which have the same unit types, the quotient is actually unitless. A ratio can be expressed by any of the following equivalent indices:

1. a colon 3:10
2. "to" 3 to 10
3. a common fraction $^3/_{10}$
4. a decimal fraction 0.30
5. a percent 30%

A *proportion* is an expressed equality between two ratios as:

$$\frac{3}{4} = \frac{6}{8}$$

Additional nomenclature specific to proportions can be illustrated when this proportion is rewritten with use of the colon format.

Means

3:4 = 6:8

Extremes

Mnemonically, these terms should be easily remembered in that the means (second and third terms) are in the middle and the extremes (first and fourth terms) are on the outside. Additionally, mean as used in this context is *not* equivalent to arithmetic mean (that is, average).

Ratios and proportions are extremely useful in everyday life, since they represent linear equations or directly proportional relationships. The *proportion rule* states, "The product of the means is equal to the product of the extremes." From the above illustration:

Mean product = Extreme product

$4 \cdot 6 = 3 \cdot 8$

$24 = 24$

Remember also that when the proportion is written in fractional form, the members of the mean pair are the denominator of the first ratio multiplied by the numerator of the second ratio; the members of the extreme pair are the numerator of the first ratio multiplied by the denominator of the second ratio.

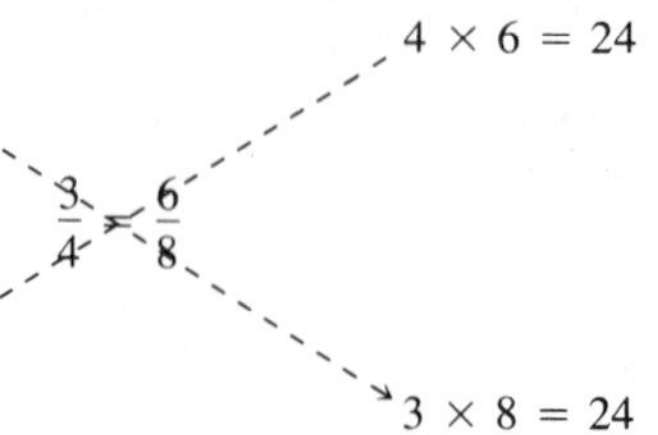

The proportion law is also extremely useful in the determination of any one of the proportional elements when the three others are known. A practical application of this relationship is illustrated in the following situation:

Problem 1: A kilogram is equivalent to 2.2 lb. What is the weight in kilograms of a 210 lb patient?
SOLUTION 1:

a. $\frac{1\text{ kg}}{2.2\text{ lb}} = \frac{x\text{ kg}}{210\text{ lb}}$

b. $1\text{ kg} \cdot 210\text{ lb} = 2.2\text{ lb} \cdot x\text{ kg}$

c. $\frac{1\text{ kg} \cdot 210\text{ lb}}{2.2\text{ lb}} = x\text{ kg}$

d. $95\text{ kg} = x\text{ kg}$
$95 = x$

Problem 2: One liter of isotonic saline solution contains 8.6 grams of solute (NaCl). How many grams of solute need to be added to 250 ml of solvent (H_2O) to produce isotonicity?
SOLUTION 2:

a. $\frac{x\text{ g}}{250\text{ ml}} = \frac{8.6\text{ g}}{1000\text{ ml}}$

b. $x\text{ g} \cdot 1000\text{ ml} = 8.6\text{ g} \cdot 250\text{ ml}$

c. $x\text{ g} = \frac{8.6\text{ g} \cdot 250\text{ ml}}{1000\text{ ml}}$

d. $x = 2.15\text{ g}$

Some background information for the next problems will be useful. One can use several methods for preparing solutions of certain concentrations or dilutions. Most of the intravenous fluids administered to patients (for example, glucose, saline) are prepared on a weight-to-volume basis—solid solute in a liquid solvent. The total volume of solution increases only negligibly from that of the original solvent since the solute dissolves. Solutions can also be prepared on a volume-to-volume basis—a liquid solute and liquid solvent. The total volume of solution is equal to the sum of the individual volumes. The solution preparation activities which you most likely will experience are not those of a pharmacist or chemist, but rather in the area of in vitro evaluation procedures. In percentage solutions, the quantity (grams) of solute present within a given volume of total solution is found when the volume (ml) and concentration (grams/ml) are calculated. For example, Lugol's solution has 5% iodine, which means that 5 g are found in a volume of 100 ml.

In dilution situations, remember that the volume and concentration vary inversely from the original to the diluted solution. In other words, as the volume increases, the concentration decreases. The amount of solute, before and after dilution, remains constant and can be related as follows:

$$\text{Amount of solute (before)} = \text{Volume}_1 \times \text{Concentration}_1$$
$$\text{Amount of solute (after)} = \text{Volume}_2 \times \text{Concentration}_2$$

Therefore:

$$\text{Volume}_1 \times \text{Concentration}_1 = \text{Volume}_2 \times \text{Concentration}_2$$

Note: In this type of problem, the SI unit system will require these changes: mole for gram, liter for milliliter, and a resulting concentration as millimole or micromole/liter. In fact, percent solutions will not be a recommended unit or description.

This same equation in proportion format is

$$\frac{\text{Volume}_2}{\text{Volume}_1} = \frac{\text{Concentration}_1}{\text{Concentration}_2}$$

In this form, both the inverse relationship and the proportion law are illustrated. This same general formula is employed in clinical nuclear medicine to calculate unknown volumes.

Problem 3: The concentration of radioactivity contained in a 2 ml syringe results in a measured count rate of 32,648 cpm. This 2 ml volume is added to a second solution of undetermined magnitude. After equilibration, the measured count rate of 1 ml of the new solution is 742 cpm. What was the magnitude of the second solution?
SOLUTION 3:

a. Substituting:
$\text{Volume}_1 = 2\text{ ml}$
$\text{Volume}_2 = x\text{ ml}$

$$\text{Concentration}_1 = \frac{32648\text{ cpm}}{2\text{ ml}} = 16324\ \frac{\text{cpm}}{\text{ml}}$$

$$\text{Concentration}_2 = 742\ \frac{\text{cpm}}{\text{ml}}$$

b. $\frac{x\text{ ml}}{2\text{ ml}} = \frac{16324\ \frac{\text{cpm}}{\text{ml}}}{724\ \frac{\text{cpm}}{\text{ml}}}$

c. $x\text{ ml} = \frac{16324\ \frac{\text{cpm}}{\text{ml}} \times 2\ \frac{\text{ml}}{1}}{742\ \frac{\text{cpm}}{\text{ml}}}$

d. $x\text{ ml} = \frac{32648\text{ cpm}}{742\ \frac{\text{cpm}}{\text{ml}}}$

e. $x = 44\text{ ml}$

Problem 4: The inverse square law states that the intensity of radiation at a distance is inversely proportional to the square of the distance from the source. The general formula is

$$\frac{I_1}{I_2} = \frac{D_2^2}{D_1^2}$$

I_1 = Intensity at distance D_1
I_2 = Intensity at distance D_2

Radiation at 680 mR/hr is measured at 8 cm. What is the intensity at 5 cm?

SOLUTION 4:

a. $$\frac{x \frac{\text{mR}}{\text{hour}}}{680 \frac{\text{mR}}{\text{hour}}} = \frac{8^2 \text{ cm}}{5^2 \text{ cm}}$$

b. $$x \frac{\text{mR}}{\text{hour}} = 680 \frac{\text{mR}}{\text{hour}} \times \frac{64 \text{ cm}}{25 \text{ cm}}$$

c. $$x \frac{\text{mR}}{\text{hour}} = 680 \frac{\text{mR}}{\text{hour}} \times 2.56$$

d. $$x \frac{\text{mR}}{\text{hour}} = 1740 \frac{\text{mR}}{\text{hour}}$$

RELATIONSHIPS

In mathematics, relationships are of one of two categories; they are either direct or inverse. The basis of the relationship is between or among variables found in physical laws or formulas.

Direct relationship

Two variables vary directly when the value of the second depends on the value of the first; in other words, if the first variable increases, the second variable will respond likewise and vice versa. A constant may be involved with the first variable in determining the value of the second variable.

EXAMPLE: Einstein's famous equation

$$E = mc^2$$

is a mathematical statement showing that the energy, E, possessed by a body of matter is directly related to the mass, m, of the body multiplied by a constant (c = velocity of light) raised to the squared power. The greater the mass, the greater the equivalent energy; the less the mass, the less the equivalent energy.

Inverse relationships

Two variables vary inversely when the product of two variables equals a constant value; in other words, as the first variable increases, the second variable must decrease in order that their product will remain equivalent to the same constant value and vice versa.

EXAMPLE: The energy of a gamma photon can be calculated by the following formula:

$$E = \frac{12.4 \text{ keV}}{\lambda}$$

when the wavelength, λ, is known. The photon's energy varies inversely with wavelength. Specifically, when the wavelength is short, the effect is that a small denominator with a constant numerator results in a larger quotient than when the wavelength is long or a large denominator.

For every formula or equation that you observe or read, ask yourself, What is the relationship of the variable present and what are the constant values, which I must remember?

NUMERICAL SIGNIFICANCE

Almost every aspect of nuclear medicine embraces quantification. In other words, numbers ranging from very small to very large will be confronted. A number can be no more accurate than the accuracy of the method or means by which it was computed or determined. Numerical computational accuracy is determined by the significance of the numbers used.

There is no question concerning the exactness or precision of discrete data. For example, the number of dynamic images taken during an in vivo procedure. Data types relating to continuous parameters of time, mass, and length present a completely different accuracy problem. Since there is a question of exactness or precision of these numbers, an estimation of the error is frequently provided. For example, you have collected from a patient 150 ml ± 0.5 ml of urine. The ± purely indicates the estimated accuracy range; in this case the magnitude is one half the basic or smallest unit measured, a milliliter.

The numerical significance or number of significant figures provides an assessment of the accuracy. Several values may assist in the determination of significance and ultimately accuracy when zeros appear with other numbers:

Rule 1: For numbers less than 1.0, zeros to the right of the decimal are significant if they follow other numbers.

EXAMPLES:

a. 0.250 has three significant figures.
b. 0.6200 has four significant figures.

Rule 2: For numbers less than 1.0, zeros to the right of the decimal are not significant if they precede the other numbers.

EXAMPLES:

a. 0.<u>00000</u>25 has two significant figures; the five underlined zeros are only place holders.
b. 0.<u>00000</u>620 has three significant figures; the five underlined zeros are only place holders.

Rule 3: For numbers greater than 1.0, the placement of the decimal and zeros determines the number of significant figures.

EXAMPLES:

a. 30.6 has three significant figures.
b. 250 has only two significant figures.
c. 506 has three significant figures.

Some confusion may arise and be based upon the difference between the number of significant figures and number of significant decimal places. To illustrate the potential confusion:

EXAMPLES:

a. 0.0028 has two significant figures but four significant decimal places.

b. 0.0000280 has three significant figures but seven significant decimal places.

c. 28.0 has two significant figures but no significant decimal places.

The solution to this potential confusion is to write the numbers in scientific notational format as discussed below.

ROUNDING OF DATA

Similar to the analogy of a chain, the accuracy of mathematical computations is predicated by the number with the least number of significant figures.

It has become practice to round numbers to an even integer when the last digit is 5.

EXAMPLES:

a. 37.35 is rounded to 37.4.

b. 72.65 is rounded to 72.6.

When the last digit is greater than 5 (that is, 6 to 9), the digit immediately to the left is increased by one digit.

EXAMPLE: 8.28 is rounded to 8.3.

When the last digit is less than 5 (that is, 0 to 4), the digit immediately to the left is left alone and remains unchanged.

EXAMPLE: 6.33 is rounded to 6.3.

As an aid to the extent of rounding, it is helpful to know the extent to which the process should be conducted.

EXAMPLES:

a. 38.8 mCi to the nearest mCi, which is 39.

b. 876,432 cpm to the nearest thousand, which is 876,000.

The net results of the process are not only the elimination of unnecessary digits, but also the resulting number is slightly less accurate.

Several rules are applicable when one performs calculations on data that are presented with differing numbers of significant figures.

Rule 1: The number of significant figures in the data and results is determined such that only one uncertain figure results.

EXAMPLE: A dose of radiopharmaceutical is to be prepared for injection. The 3 ml syringe has been predrawn for you. Your observation of the plunger and meniscus position results in a reading of 1.75 ml. How accurate is this observation? All figures are significant since the 1.0 and 0.7 are represented by actual printed scale markings; the 0.05 is determined by estimation or interpolation and is the only uncertain figure.

Rule 2: When adding or subtracting numbers with different numbers of significant decimal places, the result should have only the least number of significant decimal places.

EXAMPLE: A staff member during 1 month earned 1.25 vacation days and 0.833 sick days. Had this person utilized both, how many days would he have been gone that month?

1.25	Vacation days
0.833	Sick days
2.083	Total

Since 1.25 has two significant decimal places, there is no need to have the 0.003 in the total.

Rule 3: When multiplying or dividing numbers with different numbers of significant figures, the result should have only the least number of significant figures.

EXAMPLE: Determine the number of disintegrations per minute (dpm) for 6.4 mCi.

$$6.4 \text{ mCi} \times 3.7 \times 10^7 \frac{\text{dps}}{\text{mCi}} \times 60 \frac{\text{sec}}{\text{minute}} = 145.188 \times 10^7$$

ROOT, INDEX, POWER, EXPONENT

Occasionally, a situation will arise requiring that a number (for example, 4) be multiplied by itself repeatedly for any number of times (for example, 5 times). In other words, the mathematical expression relating to this exemplary verbal statement would be represented as follows:

$$4 \cdot 4 \cdot 4 \cdot 4 \cdot 4 = 1024$$

Mathematicians long ago developed a shorter method and an equivalent mathematical expression to the above, which is represented as follows:

$$4^5 = 1024$$

This format is based upon the identification and use of the prime factors of a number. Each of the elements in this expression has a special name:

4 = The "base number," which is the number upon which repeated multiplications will be performed.

5 = The "exponent," the number that is written in a superscript position; an exponent may possess either a + or − sign; unless stated, the sign is assumed to be positive; the exponent may be an integer or an integer with accompanying decimal component. "Exponent" and "power" may be used synonymously.

1024 = The "number," the "product" of the identified number of multiplications.

The sign of the exponent determines whether the power will be greater than one (>1.0) or less than one (<1.0). Additionally, as is illustrated later, in the

Table 1-8. Base 10 exponents, power, and inclusive number ranges for positive exponents

Exponent		Actually included numbers	
Base	**Number**	**From**	**To**
10^9	1,000,000,000	1,000,000,000.1	
10^8	100,000,000	100,000,000.1	999,999,999.999. . .
10^7	10,000,000	10,000,000.1	99,999,999.999. . .
10^6	1,000,000	1,000,000.1	9,999,999.999. . .
10^5	100,000	100,000.1	999,999.999. . .
10^4	10,000	10,000.1	999,999.999. . .
10^3	1,000	1,000.1	9,999.999. . .
10^2	100	100.1	999.999. . .
10^1	10	10.1	99.999. . .
10^0	1	1.1	9.999. . .

discussion of Table 1-8, the exponent need not always be an integer (for example, 5.0000).

In a generalized summary form

$$\text{Base}^{\text{Exponent}} = \text{Number}$$

The inverse of the process that raises a base to a specified power is the determination of a root. The root is actually the number that above was called the base. To know precisely which root is requested or how many roots are to be determined is identified by a designation called the root symbol, $\sqrt{\ }$. The only visible clue to the raising of a number to a power is the superscript position of the exponent; otherwise it may be confused with straight multiplication of another factor. The root symbol as written indicates that the square root is to be determined.

$$3^2 = 9 \qquad \sqrt{9} = 3$$

These mathematical statements are the opposite of each other. The left expression results in the squaring of the base number 3 and the right is the taking of the square root, which is the base number 3. For other than square roots, the root symbol is modified by the use of an index symbol as follows:

$$\text{Third root} = \sqrt[3]{\text{Radicand}}$$
$$\text{Fourth root} = \sqrt[4]{\text{Radicand}}$$
$$\text{Twenty-first root} = \sqrt[21]{\text{Radicand}}$$

The index numbers 3, 4, and 21, in their superscript position, determine the root of the radicand that is to be taken. If no specified index is present, the assumption is that the square root is to be determined.

Numbers with accompanying exponents may appear in the position of a numerator, denominator, or both. When in the original position of a numerator, exponents have a positive sign; when in the original position of a denominator, exponents also have a positive sign. However, toting denominators around gets tiresome and awkward not only for secretaries but also for mathematicians. To alleviate this cumbersome situation, one employs a mathematical technique that obviates the use of denominators with exponents, moves the denominator to the numerator position, and denotes that the original location was in the denominator. This technique is mathematically based upon the law of exponents relating to the division of numbers raised to powers as discussed below. Remember, we have stated that word phrases can have equivalent fractional forms.

EXAMPLES:

a. Word form
   (1) disintegrations per second
   (2) $\dfrac{\text{disintegrations}}{\text{second}}$
b. Symbolic forms
   (1) dps or d/s
   (2) $\text{d} \cdot \text{sec}^{-1}$

Note that in both word forms, even though words are used, they are treated as numbers that are raised to an undesignated, though understood, first power. In the second symbolic form, "second" is transposed from its original location in the denominator to a new location in the numerator with the designation of *both* a negative sign (−) *and* a power of 1 to indicate its new location. From Table 1-3 above and this format, three selected units could be written as follows:

$$\text{curie} = 3.7 \times 10^{10}\ \text{d} \cdot \text{sec}^{-1}$$
$$\text{becquerel} = \text{d} \cdot \text{sec}^{-1}$$
$$\text{pascal} = \text{newton} \cdot \text{meter}^{-2}$$

Yet an already frequently seen exponential equation

$$A_t = A_0 \cdot e^{-\lambda t} \quad \text{or} \quad \frac{A_t}{A_0} = e^{-\lambda t}$$

could be rewritten using the reverse of the above procedure to remove the negative sign of the exponent as follows:

$$A_t = A_0 \cdot \frac{1}{e^{\lambda t}} \quad \text{or} \quad \frac{A_t}{A_0} = \frac{1}{e^{\lambda t}}$$

Yes, the negative sign was removed, but now we have a cumbersome denominator. The value of the equation or answers obtained are not altered by this technique.

In this equation, the symbol λ is called the "decay constant." By other derivation procedures, the decay constant is equivalent to

$$\lambda = \frac{0.693}{T_{1/2}}$$

where the denominator, $T_{1/2}$, is the physical half-life time usually measured in hours and the numerator is a unitless constant. Following the above is the new formal sequence:

$$\lambda = 0.693 \cdot \text{hr}^{-1}$$

In summary, taking the reciprocal of a exponential number will result in the change of sign of the exponent.

$$\frac{1}{10^2} = 10^{-2} \qquad 2^2 = \frac{1}{2^{-2}}$$

To this point, we may have been lulled by a shallow review or simplistic generalizations. In a way, that may be correct; however, the general principles stated will always apply. The general statement, "Any number can be raised to any power," can be made. However in science and technology, the two most frequently used base numbers are *ten* (10.000) and *e* (2.7182818284). *Ten* is the base number for the briggsian (common) logarithmic system; *e* is the symbol for the irrational number 2.71828, which is the base number for the napierian (natural) logarithmic system. Logarithms are discussed below.

In Table 1-8, the base number 10 is raised by consecutive positive integers with the resulting and corresponding powers identified. Your attention is drawn to the very specific resulting relationships, for example, a single numeral increase in exponential value and very large quantum increases in the range (that is, from . . . to . . .) of the numbers included within that range. Suppose you need to determine what the exponent of 10 would be in order to achieve the number 574. By refering to Table 1-8 again, observe that the number 574 is included in the range from 100.1 to 999.999. . . . Pausing momentarily, we could locate, by percentage description, the location or position of the number (574) to the total range dimension (100.1 to 999.999). For all intents and purposes, the range dimension is 900 and the relative percentage position of 574 is 63.7% (that is, 574/900 = 0.6377). Using the same approach, we see that the relative percentage positions of 5740 and 57.4 are 63.7% and 63.7% (that is, 5740/9000 and 57.4/90, respectively). The determination of the percentage (63.7%) is not useful in determining the value of the complete exponent. The percentage serves only to indicate that, whether it is 5.74, 574, or 57,400, each of these numbers is located in the same relative position within the corresponding range 1-10, 100-1000, or 10,000-100,000, respectively. In fact, the following are the actual values of the corresponding exponents:

Number	Exponent value
5.74	0.7589
574.00	2.7589
57,400.00	4.7589

These values are obtained in Appendix B (p. 49) and will be illustrated further in the section on logarithms. As will be compared later, the percentage value denotes a linear or straight-line relationship when, in fact, exponential values are not linear.

What have we learned from this exercise and illustration in division? First, and by intuition, is that some numbers (for example, 574) are determined by exponents that have a decimal portion in addition to the integer component value of 2.00 or 3.00, for example. Second, and again by intuition, is that since the relative percentage positions are the same, the decimal portion of the corresponding exponent must be the same with only the integer number component changing 2 to 3 or 3 to 4. To illustrate that the above information is verifiable for numbers less than 1.00, Table 1-9 has been prepared. Parenthetically, there is nothing esoteric about the digits 574 nor is the mathematical validity based upon this digital sequence. These digits were chosen strictly at random and do not affect the validity of the discussion.

In Table 1-9, consecutive negative integers are placed as exponents with the resulting and corresponding numbers identified. Similarly to Table 1-8, the actual number range relating to the exponent's value is presented. Let us return to the 574 sequence and interdigitate our search in Table 1-9. Between which exponential values does the number 0.574 lie? Careful! Yes, you are correct if you said 0 and 1. Double-check yourself; find the exponential values between which the number 0.00574 lies. Correct if you said −2 and −3. Again as above, the relative location would be identical, with the only change being realized in the value of the integer.

From this background, we can now branch into a discussion of scientific notation and logarithms. You may ask, "This is all well and good, but how can I mathematically use these exponents?" The laws of expo-

Table 1-9. Base-10 exponents, powers, and inclusive number range for negative exponents

Exponent		Actually includes numbers	
Base	Number	From	To
10^{0}	1.0	1.0	0.0999. . .
10^{-1}	0.1	0.11	0.00999. . .
10^{-2}	0.01	0.011	0.000999. . .
10^{-3}	0.001	0.0011	0.0000999. . .
10^{-4}	0.0001	0.00011	0.00000999. . .
10^{-5}	0.00001	0.000011	0.000000999. . .
10^{-6}	0.000001	0.0000011	0.0000000999. . .
10^{-7}	0.0000001	0.00000011	0.00000000999. . .
10^{-8}	0.00000001	0.000000011	0.000000000999. . .
10^{-9}	0.000000001	0.0000000011	

nents need to be identified and discussed prior to their utility being demonstrated.

Laws:

1. *Multiplication.* To multiply numbers that possess exponents, simply add the exponents.
   a. General form:

$$A^{x} \cdot A^{y} = A^{x+y}$$

   b. Problem: Suppose you know the area of a square and you wish to turn it into a cube and determine its volume.

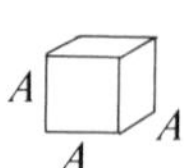

Side length $= A = 3$ cm
Area $= A^{1} \times A^{1} = A^{2}$
Volume $= A^{2} \times A^{1} = A^{3}$
Substituting: $(3 \text{ cm})^{3} = 27$ cc

2. *Division.* This rule has three possibilities.
   a. If the numerical value of the exponent of the numerator is larger than the numerical value of the exponent of the denominator, the difference is represented as the exponent of the quotient, which will be greater than 1.00.
   (1) General form:

$$x > y$$

$$\frac{A^{x}}{A^{y}} = A^{x-y}$$

   (2) Problem: If the photomultiplier tubes in an imaging device are operated at a dynode voltage of 100 volts, 2^{12} electrons are produced. However, the same photomultiplier tubes, when operated at 80 volts produce 2^{10} electrons. How many times more electrons are produced at the higher voltage?

$$\frac{100 \text{ volts} = 2^{12}}{80 \text{ volts} = 2^{10}} = 2^{12-10} = 2^{2} = 4$$

or as proof

$$\frac{2^{12} = 2\cdot2\cdot2\cdot2\cdot2\cdot2\cdot2\cdot2\cdot2\cdot2\cdot2\cdot2}{2^{10} = 2\cdot2\cdot2\cdot2\cdot2\cdot2\cdot2\cdot2\cdot2\cdot2} = \frac{4096}{1024} = \frac{4}{1}$$

   b. If the numerical value of the exponent of the numerator and denominator are the same, the difference is zero, which by definition is equivalent to the number one.
   (1) General form:

$$x = x$$

$$\frac{A^{x}}{A^{x}} = A^{0} = 1$$

   (2) Problem: Through five 2 cm layers of material A 236 mR/hour are measured and through five 2 cm layers of material B 236 mR/hour are measured. Compare the thicknesses and measured mR/hour readings for these two materials.

$$\frac{\text{Material A}}{\text{Material B}} = \frac{(2)^{5} \text{ cm}}{(2)^{5} \text{ cm}} = 2^{0} = 1$$

$$\frac{236 \text{ mR/hour}}{236 \text{ mR/hour}} = 1$$

or as proof

$$\frac{2^{5} = 2\cdot2\cdot2\cdot2\cdot2}{2^{5} = 2\cdot2\cdot2\cdot2\cdot2} = 1$$

   c. If the numerical value of the exponent of the numerator is smaller than the numerical value of the exponent of the denominator, the difference is represented as an exponent with a negative sign; the sign of the exponent can be made positive by inversion (that is, made reciprocal) with the end result of the quotient being less than 1.00.

(1) General form:

$$y > x$$

$$\frac{A^x}{A^y} = A^{-y+x} = \frac{1}{A^{y-x}}$$

(2) Problem: A radionuclide-counting instrument measures 10^5 counts per unit time from a radionuclide source calculated to radiate 10^6 counts per unit time. The instrument's efficiency may be calculated when the "observed" counts are compared to the calculated counts. What is the percent efficiency?

$$\frac{\text{Observed}}{\text{Calculated}} = \frac{10^5}{10^6} = 10^{-6+5} = 10^{-1}$$

$$10^{-1} = \frac{1}{10^1} = \frac{1}{10} = 0.10$$

$$0.10 \times 100 = 10\%$$

SCIENTIFIC NOTATION

In scientific and technologic communities, it is not unusual to use and manipulate numbers that are either very large or very small. Evidence of this is illustrated by the Tables 1-2, 1-8, and 1-9. Similar to the "shorthand" designation for powers, it should become customary for you to use a "shorthand" designation for numbers regardless of their size.

The general format utilizes a number multiplied by a base number raised to a power:

$$A \times 10^n$$

Certain specifications must be added to and clarified for the above general form:

Problem: It is estimated that the mass of a hydrogen atom is 0.0000000000000000000000016734 g.

Express this mass in scientific notational form.

1. The decimal point belonging to number A is to be relocated, if necessary, so that there is one digit remaining to the left of the decimal. Number A is 0.000000000-0000000000000016734 g; therefore:

   1.6734 grams

2. Returning to the general form, we need to add "× 10" raised to an appropriate power, which in this example is 24 since the decimal was moved 24 spaces; therefore:

   $$1.6734 \times 10^{24}$$

3. The sign, either + or −, for the exponent needs to be added. In this example, the sign will be minus because of the direction in which the decimal point was moved (for example, to the right, since the numerical value of A is less than 1.00); therefore:

   $$1.6734 \times 10^{-24}$$

Another example can illustrate a number requiring a positive exponent. By definition, a curie is

$$37{,}000{,}000{,}000 \ \frac{\text{disintegrations}}{\text{second}}$$

Even though no decimal point is written, it is assumed to be to the right of the last zero. This same numerical value written in scientific notation is

$$3.7 \times 10^{10} \ \frac{\text{disintegrations}}{\text{second}}$$

The exponent, 10, has a positive sign because of the movement of the unwritten decimal 10 places to the left. Again, this sign agrees with the fact that the number is greater than 1.00. Numbers in this format are easier to write, and calculations are easier and subsequently more reliable. Some currently available handheld calculators employ scientific notation in their display. The circuitry of the calculator is programmed to manipulate numbers in this form, but how does it know how to perform multiplications and division, either singly or in aggregate? Well, the laws of exponents as discussed and illustrated above are employed in exactly the same manner for numbers presented in this format. To illustrate, calculate the count rate per minute for a curie.

$$1 \text{ curie} = 3.7 \times 10^{10} \ \frac{\text{disintegrations}}{\text{second}}$$

$$1 \text{ minute} = \frac{60 \text{ seconds}}{\text{minute}}$$

$$3.7 \times 10^{10} \ \frac{\text{disintegrations}}{\text{second}} \ 6.0 \times 10^1 \ \frac{\text{seconds}}{\text{minute}}$$

$$22.2 \times 10^{11} \ \frac{\text{disintegrations}}{\text{minute}}$$

Building upon this example, now calculate the count rate per minute for 1 μCi. As written and verbally expressed, the prefix micro- is actually multiplied by the curie unit. Therefore

$$1 \text{ curie} = 3.7 \times 10^{10} \ \frac{\text{disintegrations}}{\text{second}} \text{ or dps}$$

$$1 \text{ minute} = \frac{60 \text{ seconds}}{\text{minute}}$$

$$1 \ \mu = 10^{-6}$$

in the combined relationship

$$\mu \quad \times \quad \text{curie} \quad \times \quad \text{Time}$$

$$(1 \times 10^{-6}) \times (3.7 \times 10^{10} \text{ dps}) \times \left(6.0 \times 10^1 \ \frac{\text{seconds}}{\text{minute}}\right)$$

multiplying the numbers

$$1 \times 3.7 \times 6.0 = 22.2$$

multiplying the exponents

$$10^{-6} + 10^{10} + 10^{1} = 10^{5}$$

be recombining, the answer can be written as

$$22.2 \times 10^{5} \frac{\text{disintegrations}}{\text{minute}}$$

To confirm your ability to work and perform calculations with scientific notation, solve the following problem:

What is the count rate represented by 0.350 millicuries? (77.7 × 10^7 dpm)

LOGARITHMS

An exponent known by yet another name is a logarithm. In fact, if the laws of exponents previously stated and illustrated were rewritten by replacement of the word exponent with the word logarithm, we would have the laws of logarithms. Unfortunately and all too frequently, most texts do not state this synonymous relationship between these laws, and most students become confused and perplexed. Logarithms can be used in the easy development of graphic axes involving large and complex numbers, in the multiplication of large and complex numbers when calculators are not available or are dysfunctional, or in the operation of a slide rule.

As stated earlier, an exponent can be stated as either positive (+) or negative (−), greater than (>), less than (<), equal to (=), or one (1), or possess a decimal portion. If we follow the above example and Table 1-9, the exponent for the base number 10, to obtain the number 574, is 2.7589. As stated, this exponent meets the criteria in that it is positive, is greater than 1, and also possesses a decimal portion. In this case, the exponent is given a special name "logarithm" and is abbreviated "log." In other words, the logarithm of 574, to the base 10, is 2.7589; or the logarithm of 574, to the base *e*, is 6.35262. Mathematically, the equivalent representations would be the following:

$$\log_{10} 574 = 2.7589$$
$$\text{or } 10^{2.7589} = 574$$

$$\ln 574 = 6.35262$$
$$\text{or } \quad e^{6.35262} = 574 \text{ or } 2.71828^{6.35262} = 574$$

The former logarithmic designation is referred to as the common or briggsian logarithms and is abbreviated "log"; the latter logarithmic designation is referred to as the natural or napierian logarithms and is abbreviated "ln." Mnemonically, these are easy to differentiate by the following simplistic relationships:

log = comm*o*n or *10*
ln = *n*atural or *n*apierian

The relationship between these two logarithmic systems for any number x is expressed as follows.

$$\ln x = 2.30 \cdot \log x$$

A corollary word to logarithm is antilogarithm, abbreviated "antilog." By definition, the antilog is the number to which 10 raised to a given logarithm is equivalent. In the natural logarithmic system antilog is never used. To illustrate by incorporating scientific notation and the law of logarithms for division:

$$10{,}000{,}000/1000 = \frac{1 \times 10^{7}}{1 \times 10^{3}} = \frac{10^{7}}{10^{3}} = 10^{4} = 1 \times 10^{4}$$

$1 \times 10^{4} = 10000 = 10{,}000$
logarithm of quotient = 4
antilog (or actual quotient) = 10,000

From the section on scientific notation, the exponent (logarithm) has an integral part that relates to the number of places the decimal point is moved and concomitantly to an equivalent range of antilogs or numbers. As further illustrated, the decimal part of the exponent (logarithm) more specifically locates a number within the antilog range. In logarithmic language, these depicted definitions prevail:

Natural-number name:	integer . decimal
Logarithm name:	characteristic . mantissa
Logarithmic value:	4 . 7193

This nomenclature is independent of whether the briggsian or napierian logarithms are being utilized.

Logarithmic tables, as frequently found in the appendices of texts, consist of lists of irrational numbers entitled as either four-place or five-place logarithms. The body of these tables consists actually of decimally arranged numbers or mantissas. Common logarithmic tables do not list characteristics; these must be supplied by the person performing the mathematical operations. Similarly, a slide rule, when used to multiply or divide, determine roots or logarithms, does not nor cannot supply the characteristic; the characteristic is supplied by *you!* Also, most tables of logarithms do not print the mantissa's decimal point, which are understood to be present. Their absence results in less clutter and improved tabular aesthetics. The left vertical border and top horizontal border form the loci of numbers from which their point of intersection is the specified mantissa value. These antilog numbers also most frequently do not have decimal points. Occasionally, these tables incorporate a proportional parts insert, which is used in interpolative determination of values not specifically determined by the intersection process. Appendix B (p. 48) is a table of four-place mantissa values. "What," you may ask, "is the difference between four- and five-place tables?" The only answer is precision and is illustrated as follows:

Number	Four-place mantissa	Five-place mantissa
4.750	.6766	.67669

The precision is in the last decimal place.

Tables of natural logarithms are used in the same manner as common logarithms except that the tabular body contains the characteristics, decimal points, and mantissas.

Assume that you have measured and calculated the data in Table 1-10 relating to the radioactive decay of a hypothetical radionuclide. By comparison, these data are plotted on linear and semilog graphic components of Fig. 1-1. By way of review, the percentage and logarithmic value of the dependent variables are plotted on the *y* axes.

The top linear graph demonstrates the negative slope and curvilinear configuration. In the bottom semilog graph, both plots demonstrate negative slopes and a straight line configuration, providing verification and demonstration of the usefulness of a semilog graph. Most of the area of the semilog graph is unused. The basis for this large void is that even though the mCi amounts of radioactivity represent a large range of numbers (antilogs), their logarithmic values are compressed to a short range since a larger range of logarithmic values correspond to numbers of many orders of magnitude greater. If in doubt, refer to Table 1-8 and reverify that small increases in the value of exponents (logs) correspond to large increases in corresponding numbers (antilogs). A different portion of the semilog graph would be used if the various amounts of activity were converted to count-rate values. To illustrate:

$600 \text{ mCi} \times 3.7 \times 10^{10} \text{ sec}^{-1} \cdot \text{Ci}^{-1} \times 60 \text{ sec} \cdot \text{min}^{-1}$

$6 \times 10^2 \cdot 10^{-3} \text{ Ci} \times 3.7 \times 10^{10} \text{ sec}^{-1} \cdot \text{Ci}^{-1} \times 6 \times 10^1 \text{ sec} \cdot \text{min}^{-1}$

$(6 \times 3.7 \times 6) \times (10^2 \cdot 10^{-3} \cdot 10^{10} \cdot 10^1) \times (\text{Ci} \cdot \text{sec}^{-1} \cdot \text{Ci}^{-1} \cdot \text{sec} \cdot \text{min}^{-1})$

$(133.2) \times (10^{10}) \times (\text{min}^{-1})$

1,332,000,000,000 counts per minute

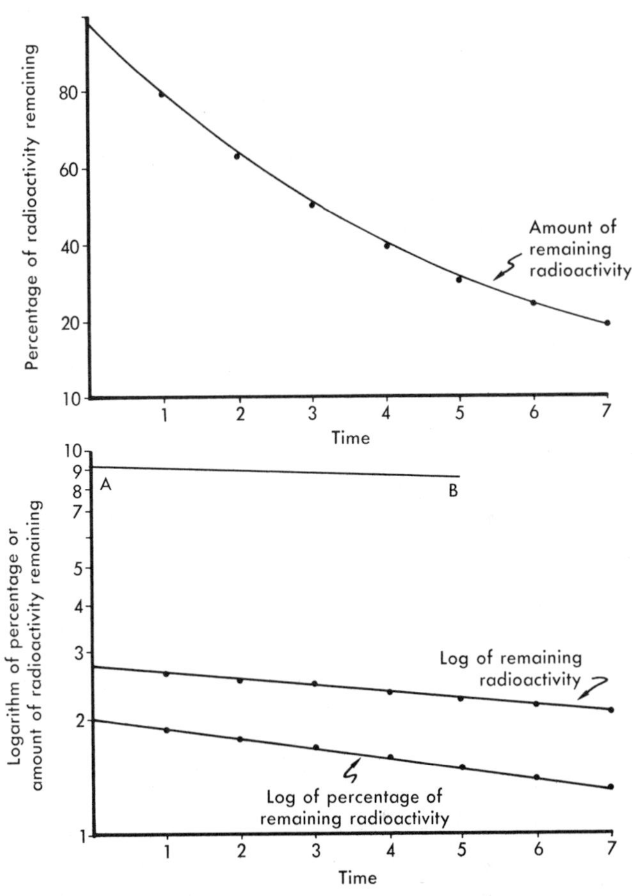

Fig. 1-1. Comparison of linear and semilog graphic plots of measured and calculated data for a hypothetical radionuclide.

Table 1-10. Measured and calculated data for hypothetical radionuclide

Elapsed time in hours	Remaining activity				
	Amount (mCi)	Percentage	Log of percentage	Log of amount
0	600	100.0	2.0000	2.7782
1	476	79.3	1.8993	2.6776
2	378	63.0	1.7993	2.5775
3	300	50.0	1.6990	2.4771
4	238	39.6	1.5977	2.3766
5	189	31.5	1.4983	2.2765
6	150	25.0	1.3979	2.1761
7	119	19.8	1.2967	2.0755

Following an identical procedure, the amount of activity at 5 hours is equivalent to a count rate per minute of 41.9×10^{10} or 41900000000.

Respective mantissas of the logarithms of these count rates are as follows:

Time: 0 hours = 133.2×10^{10} cpm = 0.1239
Time: 5 hours = 41.95×10^{10} cpm = 0.6228

In order for these values to fit on the top portion of the bottom graph in Fig. 1-1, the characteristics are adjusted accordingly:

Time: 0 hours = 9.1239
Time: 5 hours = 8.6228

with the corresponding straight line connected between points *A* and *B*. The slope and the line *AB* are identical to those at the bottom of the graph.

Logarithms and related functions can very easily be used to solve exponential equations of the general type as follows:

$$b = a^x$$
$$\log b = x \cdot \log a$$
$$\log b - \log a = x$$

A specific and related exponential equation in nuclear medicine is

$$I = I_0 \cdot e^{-\mu x}$$

which is used to calculate the emerging intensity, I, of an incident, monochromatic photon beam of incident intensity, I_0. The linear attenuation coefficient of the absorbing material is represented by μ and the thickness of the absorbing material by x.

The following discussion and procedures also hold exactly true for the exponential decay equation

$$A_t = A_0 \cdot e^{-\lambda t}$$

as well as for the formula to determine the number of radioactive atoms remaining at any specific time:

$$N_t = N_0 \cdot e^{-\lambda t}$$

Differing only in symbols, these formulas, whether by use of logarithmic tables, exponential tables, or calculators, are manipulated in exactly the same manner. The first of these three formulas will be generally and then specifically solved by use of logarithms and the following given information:

x = Absorber thickness in centimeters

$$\mu = \text{Attenuation coefficient} = \frac{0.693}{HVL} = \frac{0.693}{\text{Half-value layer in centimeters}}$$

I_0 = Incident intensity
I = Emerging intensity
$\log e$ = 0.43425

$$e^{-\mu x} = \frac{1}{e^{\mu x}}$$

$$\log e^{-\mu x} = \log 1 - \mu x \log e$$
$$I = I_0 \cdot e^{-(0.693/HVL)\,(x)}$$
$$\log I = \log I_0 + \log e^{-(0.693/HVL)\,(x)}$$
$$= \log I_0 + \log 1/e^{(0.693/HVL)\,(x)}$$
$$= \log I_0 + \log 1 - \log e^{(0.693/HVL)\,(x)}$$
$$= \log I_0 + \log 1 - \left(\frac{0.693}{HVL}\right)(x)\,(0.43425)$$
$$= \log I_0 + 0.000 - \left(\frac{0.693}{HVL}\right)(x)\,(0.43425)$$
$$I = \text{antilog}$$

Specific example

I_0 = 148 mR/hour; HVL = 15 cm;

$$\mu = \frac{0.693}{HVL} = \frac{0.693}{15}\ \text{cm}^{-1}$$

x = 25 cm

$$\log I = \log 148 + 0.0000 - \left(\frac{0.693}{15}\ \text{cm}^{-1}\right) \cdot (25\ \text{cm})\,(0.43425)$$
$$= 2.1703 + 0.0000 - (0.0462\ \text{cm}^{-1})\,(25\ \text{cm}) \cdot (0.43425)$$
$$= 2.1703 - 0.5016$$
$$\log I = 1.6687$$
$$I = \text{antilog}$$
$$I = 4.66 \times 10^1 = 46.6\ \text{mR/hour}$$

Granted the above represents, by today's instrument and accessory standards, an apparently futile and time-consuming process; nevertheless it works and is actually the basis upon which faster means and *gadgets* operate. Even though we are now satisfied with one longhand approach to these types of calculations, let us improve our efficiency somewhat and our understanding of exponential tables greatly. Appendix C (p. 50) is a table of exponential functions. Structurally, the table consists of four columns; on the left is a column, x, which can be the exponent or logarithm of any number; the second column is e^x with numbers resulting from raising 2.718 to the corresponding value of x; the third column is the listing of the determined common logarithmic values of those in the second column; and last is the e^{-x} column, which is actually the reciprocal of the second column.

Now let us determine the amount of radioactivity remaining at a specific time and use the appropriate exponential equation and Appendix C. Initially, for the radionuclide in question, there were 380 μCi with a physical half-life of 4.5 hours and the elapsed time 2 hours and 15 minutes. Mathematically, the components are equivalent to:

$$A_t = 380\ \mu\text{Ci} \cdot e^{-\left(\frac{0.693}{4.5}\right)\left(\frac{2.25}{1}\right)}$$
$$= 380\ \mu\text{Ci} \cdot e^{-0.3465}$$

As suggested above, locate the exponent value of 0.3465 in the x column. Your first observation will be that the above exponent has more significant places than listed in the table. What to do? As a suggestion, round to the next higher x value because although you are attempting to interpolate and decide what to do, the radionuclide is decaying further and the remaining amount gets smaller. Following this suggestion, locate 0.35 in the x column. Moving across to the fourth column (e^{-x}), observe the number 0.7046.

Substituting this value in the above equation, notice that the remaining activity is

$$A_t = (380\ \mu\text{Ci}) \cdot (0.70)$$
$$= 266\ \mu\text{Ci}$$

Notice the maximum and minimal values in the e^{-x} column. Maximally, this factor's value is 1.000 and minimally its value, as presented in the table, approaches 0.000 and is zero for all practical intents and purposes, though theoretically it is not true. Its significance is demonstrated as follows.

Question 1:

a. *In words:* When is the remaining activity equivalent to the original amount of activity?
b. *In symbols:* When does $A_t = A_0$?

ANSWER 1:

a. *In words:* When no time has elapsed.
b. *In symbols:* When $e^{-\lambda t} = 1.00$, so that $A_t = A_0 \cdot 1.00$.

From the answer in words, the elapsed time, t, value is zero. Therefore, again by definition, any number raised to a zero power is equal to 1.00. Numerically, this is also verified in columns two and four of the first line of the exponential tables. If $e^{-\lambda t}$ were to be greater than 1.00, the relationship would suggest that the potential to produce radioactivity were being created rather than decaying since $A_t > A_0$.

Question 2:

a. *In words:* When is all activity gone?
b. *In symbols:* When $e^{-\lambda t} = 0$, so that $0 = A_0 \cdot 0.00$.

ANSWER 2:

a. *In words:* After the passage of a significantly long time.
b. *In symbols:* When $e^{-\lambda t} = 0$, so that $0 = A_0 \cdot 0.00$.

In other words, the superficially awesome factor, $e^{-\lambda t}$, can have values no greater than 1.00 and ranges then to zero. Even in simpler terms, $e^{-\lambda t}$ is purely a percentage varying between 100% and 0%.

A very special case or situation exists when

$$A_t = \tfrac{1}{2} A_0$$

Immediately, you should know that $e^{-\lambda t}$ has a numerical value of 0.500. By using the exponential tables such that you start in column four and then go to column one, find e^{-x} value of 0.500 and what the corresponding value of x is. You are correct if you found that it is slightly more than 0.69 but less than 0.70.

Momentarily, let us shift to a brief discussion of natural logarithms, as this divergence will provide supporting information to this matter.

From the above, the following formula can be used to determine the number of radioactive atoms remaining at any specified time:

$$N_t = N_o \cdot e^{-\lambda t} \quad \text{or} \quad \frac{N_t}{N_0} = e^{-\lambda t}$$

Now, if the natural logarithm, ln, is determined for both sides of this equation, the following results:

$$\ln \frac{N_t}{N_0} = -\lambda t$$

This can be transformed by substitution:

$$N_t = (0.5)\,(N_0) \quad \text{to} \quad \ln \frac{(0.5)(N_0)}{(N_0)} = -\lambda t$$

Therefore:

$$\ln \tfrac{1}{2} = -\lambda t$$

From a table of natural logarithms:

$$\ln 0.5 = -0.69315$$
$$\ln 2 = 0.69315$$

2 is the reciprocal of ½ (= 0.5), and by such inversion, the sign of the logarithms changes when common logarithms are used:

$$\log \frac{N_t}{N_0} = 0.0000 - 0.4343\lambda t$$

Since

$$\log e = 0.4343$$

From a table of common logarithms (Appendix B):

$$\log 0.5 = -0.3010$$
$$\log 2 = 0.3010$$

From the above, then

$$\log 2 = 0.4343\ \lambda t$$

and

$$0.3010 = 0.4343\ \lambda t$$

$$\frac{0.3010}{0.4343} = \lambda t$$

$$0.693 = \lambda t$$

or by rearranging

$$\lambda = \frac{0.693}{t}$$

Since this was a special situation when t represented a passage of time whereby one half of the original activity has decayed and the other half remains, the more appropriate designation $T_{1/2}$, termed the physical half-life time, is used; therefore:

$$\lambda = 0.693/T_{1/2}$$

Mathematically, it can be demonstrated that the law of radioactive decay is a statistical law, and radioactive decay is subject to the laws of probability. The number of atoms disintegrating per second, on the average, is λN, but the actual number disintegrating per second will fluctuate around this value. The decay factor or disintegration constant, λ, is a unique characteristic of a particular radionuclide.

It is also possible to refer to the mean life or average life expectancy of the atoms of a certain radionuclide. Since the decay process is statistical, any single atom could have a lifetime from zero (0) to infinity (∞). Based upon this, the mean life is simply the reciprocal of the decay factor:

$$\text{Mean life} = \frac{1}{0.693} T_{1/2} = 1.443 \cdot T_{1/2}$$

Removing these calculations and determinations from purely the physical world and interdigitating them into the biologic world results in new aspects. Regardless of how a patient, plant or animal, receives a material, be it radioactive or not, the biologic system, with time, will "do something with the material" by either metabolizing it or excreting it from the system. The net result is that as a consequence of the operation of the biologic system alone, there will be a finite time period after which the remaining amount of material will be one half of what was originally administered, ingested or injected. This finite time period is called the biologic half-life time, T_B. Remember, this half-life period is completely independent of the physical half-life time, $T_{1/2}$. The latter may also be abbreviated as T_P. Mutual exclusiveness is operative between these two time parameters. Since these two periods, within a viable biologic system, are defined as being counted down by different "clocks," the combined, or net, period of time is called the "effective half-life time," abbreviated T_E. Each process has its own disintegration constant, λ, with the total result being

$$\lambda_E = \lambda_P + \lambda_B$$

From the earlier discussion, a substitution can be made

$$\frac{0.693}{T_E} = \frac{0.693}{T_P} + \frac{0.693}{T_B}$$

Now, dividing both members by the common factor, 0.693, one obtains the following result:

$$\frac{1}{T_E} = \frac{1}{T_P} + \frac{1}{T_B}$$

After the improper fractional forms are removed, the mathematical equivalency is

$$T_E = \frac{T_P \times T_B}{T_P + T_B}$$

The effective half-life is shorter than the physical half-life; the biologic half-life time depends on the radioactive material, the organic tissue excreting or metabolizing, and the state of health or physiologic state of the biologic organism.

PERCENTS AND PERCENTAGES

Earlier the suggestion was made that fractions could be more easily manipulated by use of their decimal equivalents, for example:

$$3/5 = 0.60 \qquad 1/7 = 0.14$$

Percents are a specific type of fraction in that their denominators have the value of 100; thus,

1. $80\% = \frac{80}{100} = \frac{8}{10} = 0.80$
2. $33\% = \frac{33}{100} = \frac{3}{10} = 0.33$

The percentage symbol, %, when attached to the numerator identifies that the denominator is 100. This follows, since percent (L. *per centum*) means per hundred. The common fractional equivalent can frequently be reduced to its simpler form and subsequently to the decimal format equivalent.

Percent values usually range from 1 to 100. This is not meant to imply that percent values of less than 1 and more than 100 cannot exist. Your primary experience with percentages will be

With words: Percentages greater than 1 and less than 100
With symbols: $1\% < 100\%$

Lesser percentage values are based upon the same rationale. To illustrate, suppose that a certain clinical datum was ¾% greater upon second measurement. To what does this percentage equate? First, reverse the above sequence and determine the decimal equivalency, which is 0.75. Secondly, we need to be concerned how 0.75 is changed, if any, by the percentage symbol. Since the 0.75 is the numerator and 100 is the denominator, if division occurs, the resulting quotient is 0.0075, which visibly assists in the verification that ¾% is less than 1% since 1% is equivalent to 0.0100 and 0.0075 is equivalent to three/fourths percent. Thirdly, the word "greater" implies that some subsequent mathematical procedure must be performed. In this context, "% greater than" suggests that the former datum could be considered as 100% and the later datum is now equal to 100% plus 0.75%. To verify that this suggestion is correct, suppose that the value of the former datum was 12.0 and that the latter's value is 12.09. If these are compared and divided as follows:

$$\frac{12.09}{12.00} = 1.0075 = \underset{(100\%)}{1.00} + \underset{(3/4\%)}{0.0075}$$

Yet another way of verifying this relationship is that the numerical difference between these values is 0.09; if this is divided by the former, then:

$$\frac{0.09}{12.00} = 0.0075$$

The resulting value is the percentage increase. Either way of comparison results in the answer and correct relationship.

Another percentage technique can be illustrated by the words "increase by." Suppose your current annual base salary is \$10,096 and that at the beginning of the next fiscal year, your salary will be "increased by" 5.2% to reflect a cost-of-living component. The numbers may be absurd; however, the technique is of primary concern. The approach can be twofold in the determination of the new salary figure. One approach is, in words, to determine five point two percent of the present salary and to add this amount to the present salary, in numbers:

$$\$10{,}096/\text{year} + \$10{,}096/\text{year} \times 5.2\% = \text{New annual salary}$$

or

$$\$10{,}096/\text{year} + \$10{,}096/\text{year} \times 0.052 = \text{New annual salary}$$

$$\$10{,}096/\text{year} + \$525\ \text{year} = \$10{,}621$$

The second approach is algebraically based upon the first. To illustrate the second, the middle equation rewritten and factored results in

$$\$10{,}096\ (1 + 0.052) = \text{New annual salary}$$

or after similar terms are combined and rewritten, it becomes

$$\$10{,}096\ (1.052) = \$10{,}621$$

Both steps are equivalent; the latter is just a shorthand method of the first. To test yourself, suppose that you work in a clinic in which the present number of in vitro procedures is 48% of in vivo procedures and that next year you expect to realize a 25% increase in the number of in vivo procedures. Calculate both the present number of in vitro procedures and the projected number of in vivo procedures if currently you perform 5820 in vivo procedures. (Answer: present in vitro = 2794; projected in vivo = 7275.) In this hypothetical situation, another mathematical clue is provided by the phrase "% of"; invariably you should know that multiplication is at hand. Note should also be directed to the fact that a percentage is a totally unitless number and purely a number. From the above several equations, no units need to be designated or manipulated for any percentage. This concept is especially meaningful when you evaluate the formula

$$A_2 = A_0 \cdot e^{-\lambda t}$$

Briefly, the factor $e^{-\lambda t}$ must be totally unitless and is actually a percentage whose value varies from 100% to 0. More attention is paid to this later.

The wording in radiation-protection situations can present several interesting problems if clarity of information is not provided or understanding rendered. Suppose that an exposure rate (measured in mR/hour) of 144 is incident upon an absorbing material (that is, matter through which photons can pass, some of which deposit energy that is absorbed). Not all photons are absorbed and on the emerging side 48 mR/hour is measured. Before tackling these numbers, let's replace the incident intensity with 100 and the emerging intensity with 40. Diagrammatically it would appear as in Fig. 1-2. These numbers are obviously chosen so that the value of the incident intensity was 100. As indicated, the reduction in intensity raises two logical questions: the first, "Is the emerging intensity *reduced by* 60%?"; the second, "Is the emerging intensity *reduced to* 40%?" The entire interpretation is predicated upon the preposition in each of these questions. It so happens that both of these questions can be answered yes.

Now, replace these intensity values with those originally stated—144 and 48, respectively. By what per-

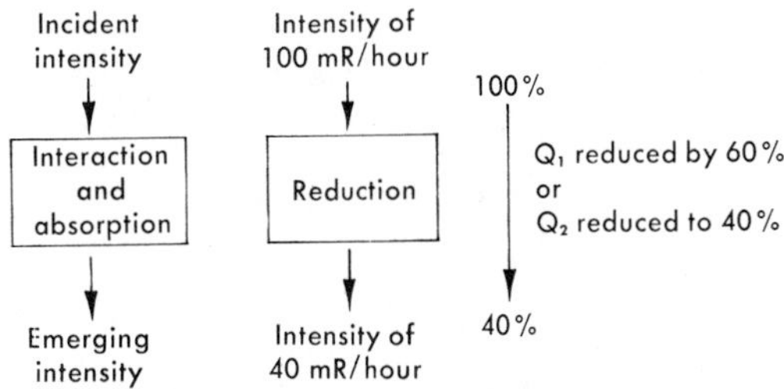

Fig. 1-2. Hypothetical radiation-reduction diagram.

CLINICAL DEPARTMENT AND PATIENT CLASSIFICATION	AVERAGE DAILY INPATIENT CENSUS					AVERAGE DAILY CLINIC CENSUS				
	July through September			Percentage of variation for 1979 census versus		July through September			Percentage of variation for 1979 census versus	
	1979	1978	1977	1977	1978	1979	1978	1977	1978	1977
NUCLEAR MEDICINE DEPARTMENT										
Private patients						12.0	13.8	8.6	A	39.5
Indigent patients						10.3	8.1	13.2	27.2	B
Total						22.3	21.9	19.8	1.8	12.6
ALL SERVICE DEPARTMENTS										
Private patients	260.8	325.6	375.1	(20.0)	(30.5)	525.6	488.3	505.2	7.6	E
Indigent patients	134.4	105.6	123.2	C	9.0	206.7	249.3	195.6	F	G
Total	395.2	431.2	498.3	D	(20.7)	732.3	737.6	700.8	H	4.5
Total bed capacity	I									
Average occupancy rate	J		94.9		K					

Fig. 1-3. Average daily inpatient census and clinical service census quarterly report—Somewhere Hospitals and Clinics.

centage is the incident intensity reduced to yield the specified emergent value? One approach might suggest that the numerical difference (144 − 48 = 96) be calculated; then what percent is this difference (96) of the entire amount (144)?

$$\frac{96}{144} = \frac{8}{12} = \frac{2}{3} = 0.66$$

Therefore the reduction is *by* 66% or *to* 33%. An alternative method would find what part the emerging intensity is of the incident intensity.

$$\frac{48}{144} = \frac{4}{12} = \frac{1}{3} = 0.33$$

Obviously, ⅓ emerges, and by deduction ⅔ was absorbed.

In the above hypothetical situation, what percent is the incident intensity of the emerging intensity; in other words, by what percentage do you need to multiply 48 to obtain 144? The answer is found by dividing

$$\frac{144}{48} = 3.00 = 300\%$$

Therefore

$$48 \times 3 = 144$$

An additional set of real-life examples further illustrates the use, incorporation, and determination of percentages. Assume that each 3 months you receive from your hospital's business office a quarterly report reflecting average daily inpatient census and clinic-service census data. Fig. 1-3 represents a hypothetical census report. The stippled area to the immediate right of "nuclear medicine department" is provided since this clinical service department has no assigned inpatient beds. Farther to the right, the average daily clinic visits by patient classification are identified for the specified quarter for the current and past 2 years. When all clinical service departments are considered, the bottom portion of the report is generated. Since some clinical services departments have inpatient beds (for example, Surgery, ICU), their average daily inpatient census data are depicted beneath the stippled area. For the entire institution, the average daily clinic visits are listed. Not all percentage values have been calculated; the intent is for you to gain practice and enhance your interpretative skills by providing these data.* As a note in this and other types of reports, decreases in percentages or amounts are generally indicated by the use of parentheses; increases are implied without the use of any accompanying symbol or desig-

*Answers:
A = (13.0); *B* = (22.0); *C* = 27.2; *D* = (8.3); *E* = 4.0; *F* = (17.0); *G* = 5.7; *H* = (0.8); *I* = 525; *J* = 75.3; and *K* = (20.6).

nation. From the identified average occupancy rate (that is, number of beds occupied) for 1977, determine the bed size of this institution; further assume that the bed size does not change. Determine the values for J and K.

Another noteworthy observation is realized when one compares the average daily clinic census values for the nuclear medicine department with those of all clinic service departments. For nuclear medicine, the variation percentages generally are larger than those for the total institution. Why? The answer is that a small value or number realizing any change (that is, increase/decrease) is very significant and with a large resulting percent value. The opposite is true for any changes in a large number. To illustrate, if there are four patients in your waiting room and one is an inpatient, you could say, "At this moment, 25% of our waiting patients are inpatients." However, if during a week, your clinic performed nuclear medicine imaging procedures on 163 patients of whom 18 were inpatients, the resulting percentage is 11.

Yet, another realistic duo situation can illustrate this relationship. In situation 1, a specimen containing a radionuclide is counted for 4 minutes and the display reads 1247; a 4-minute count without the sample reads 264. The background percentage is calculated as

$$\frac{264}{1247} = 0.211 \times 100 = 21.1\%$$

In situation 2, a different specimen is immediately counted with the same instrument and under the same conditions. The new display reading is 15,648. Now the background percentage value is calculated as

$$\frac{264}{15{,}648} = 0.016 \times 100 = 1.6\%$$

Most of these calculations have been obvious or easily done by paper and pencil; however, everyday calculations may cause you to use a calculator, many of which possess a % key. What does this key do when depressed? A simple sequence will illustrate the method when one divides 4 by 8.

GRAPHS

Mathematical equations or expressions can be pictorially represented in the form of a graph, which more clearly illustrates the relationship between variables. Commonly observed examples of graph types are linear, exponential, pie graphs, histograms, and point graphs. The type of data to be represented governs the type of graph to be used.

Linear graph—construction and rationale

The basis for the orientation and construction of a linear graph is the number scale, which is a line on which linearly and uniformly distant positions are located from a specific point called the "point of origin" (Fig. 1-4). If the number scale is positioned horizontally, it is known as a horizontal number scale; by an analogous rationale, the vertical number scale can also be designated. When these two respective scales are intersecting at right angles with their points of origins superimposed, the rudiments of the rectangular or cartesian coordinate system are formed. Numbers on either of the number scales can be positioned in opposite directions from the point of origin. The directions of right on the horizontal and up on the vertical are designated as positive (for example, +1, +2, and +3) and are respectively opposed to the directions of left on the horizontal and down on the vertical, which are designated as negative (for example, −1, −2, and −3). The plus (+) or minus (−) purely and simply note a direction from the point of origin; the number, regardless of the identifying sign designation, denotes a magnitude. More specifically and by convention, the horizontal line, in either direction from the point of origin, is called the "x axis," or "abscissa"; the vertical line, in either direction from the point of origin, is called the "y axis," or "ordinate." Together, these axes form the coordinate system of a graph and divide it into four quadrants (that is, I, II, III, IV), as illustrated in Fig. 1-5. By convention and regardless of the quadrant, one can describe a point's location on a graph by noting *both* its x and y coordinates. Given the plot in Fig. 1-6, points M and N are connected to form a straight line. The location of point M is (x_1, y_1); the magnitude of x_1 and y_1 is determined relative to the point A origin. Similarly, the location of point N is (x_2, y_2). Specifically, the respective numerical values and appropriate signs for points M and N are:

$$x_1 = +14 \qquad x_2 = +1$$
$$y_1 = +7 \qquad y_2 = -3$$

The additional and nonconnected point R, though being located on the x axis, has both coordinates (x_3, y_3), with respective values of 0 and +3. Remember that the x value is listed first and the set of coordinates is enclosed within parentheses.

Straight lines, as presented on a coordinate system, can be positioned at any angle through the origin, can be positioned at any angle and intersect both ordinates simultaneously, or can be parallel to either axis. Pre-

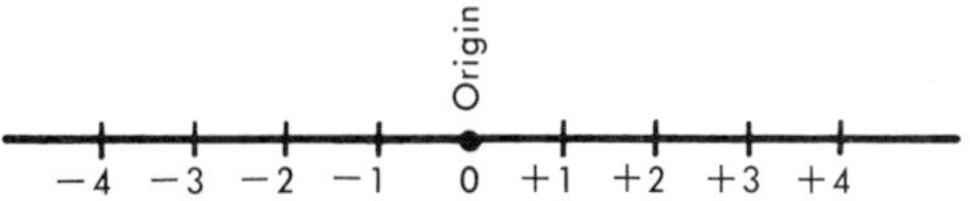

Fig. 1-4. Basic number scale.

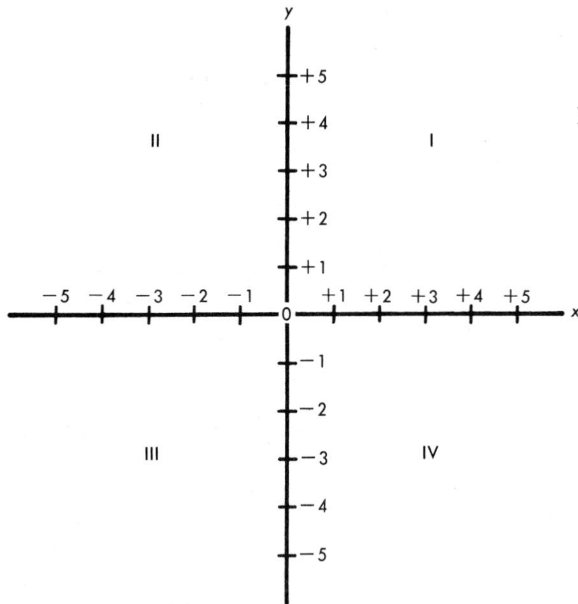

Fig. 1-5. Cartesian coordinate system.

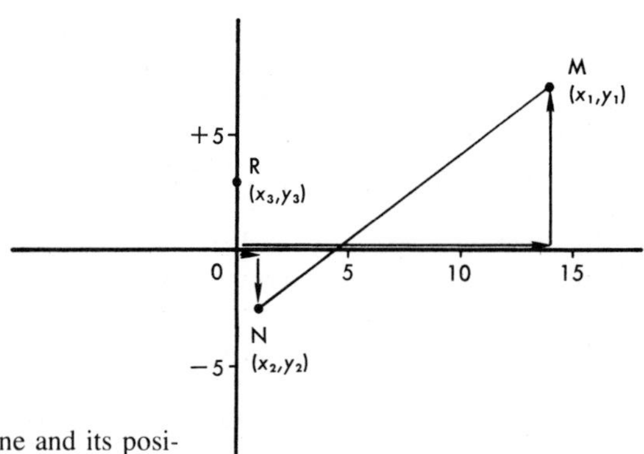

Fig. 1-6. Point coordinates to determine a line and its position.

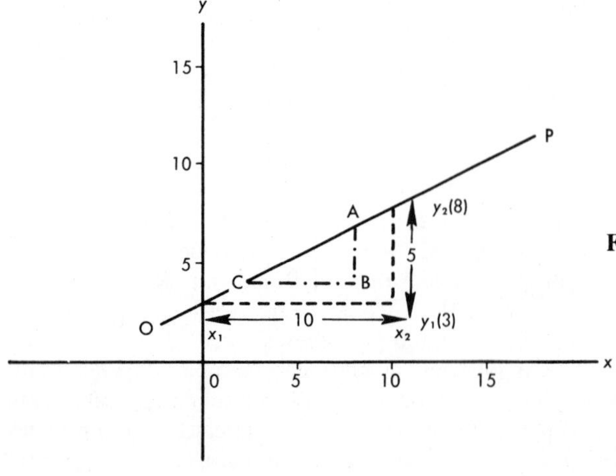

Fig. 1-7. Straight line illustrating a positive slope.

sented in such manner, the points of intersection on the x and y axes represent the numerical solutions to a linear equation in which the variables are in the first degree and whose general form is

$$y = mx + b$$

From this general form, the slope of the linear plot is m and it intercepts the y axis at b. In the rectangular coordinate system, the slope of a straight line is the constant ratio (that is, fraction) of the change of the ordinate (y axis) to the corresponding change of the abscissa (x axis) as a point moves along the line. To illustrate, Fig. 1-7 is a line, OP, whose m value (slope) is 0.5, which is calculated as follows:

$$m = \frac{(y_2 - y_1)}{(x_2 - x_1)} = \frac{8 - 3}{10 - 0} = \frac{5}{10} = 0.5$$

The vertical and horizontal legs *(dashed line)* of the apparent right triangle were drawn purely at random and have no bearing on the value of m. To support this point, similarly calculate the m value for the smaller right triangle *(ABC)*. Note that for these two cases and all others the line OP actually is the hypotenuse of a triangle.

Suppose, however, that the linear plot was represented as in Fig. 1-8. The m value (slope) for line DE is calculated as follows

$$m = \frac{y_2 - y_1}{x_2 - x_1} = \frac{5 - 10}{14 - 5} = \frac{-5}{9} = -{}^5\!/_9$$

The calculation is correct; the curiosity is that the minus (−) sign of the ratio only signifies that the line is sloped in a direction opposite to that of Fig. 1-7. The majority of graphs that you will encounter in nuclear medicine technology will have negative slopes. Generally speaking, the negative slope will relate to radioactive disintegration. The greater the ratio (for example, $-{}^5\!/_9$), the greater the disintegration rate; conversely, the lower the ratio (for example, $-{}^1\!/_4$), the slower will be the disintegration rate. This observational analysis of lines will be of significant assistance when one graphically compares different radionuclides.

When a graph represents a curvilinear line, the slope is not constant; however, an average slope, which identifies an average value between specified values of the independent variable, can be calculated.

As inferred above, linear graphs can identify not only the numerical solutions to variable unknowns in equations but also to the relationship between the variables. To illustrate the relationship aspect, we all have had some difficulty in remembering the relationship or conversion relations between temperature expressed in Celsius and Fahrenheit readings. By studying Fig. 1-9, all you must remember is that by definition the water freezes at 32° on the Fahrenheit scale, and this is equivalent to 0° C and that water boils at 212° on the Fahrenheit scale and this is equivalent to 100° C. Every other relationship after these two basic facts is by deduction and calculation.

The range of degrees between freezing and boiling is respectively 100 on Celsius and 180 on Fahrenheit. In other words, 1 degree Celsius is equivalent to 1.8 degrees Fahrenheit; conversely, 1 degree Fahrenheit is equal to 0.556 degree Celsius. The conventional two formulas are:

$$°C = {}^5\!/_9 \times (°F - 32°)$$

$$°F = (°C \times {}^9\!/_5) + 32°$$

Fig. 1-9 is a graph constructed on the above facts

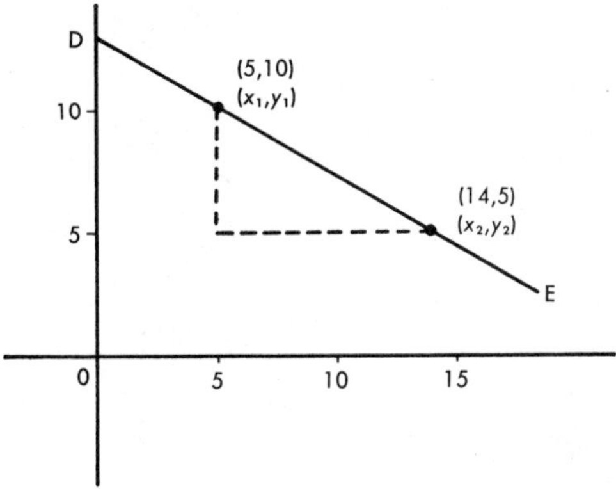

Fig. 1-8. Straight line illustrating a negative slope.

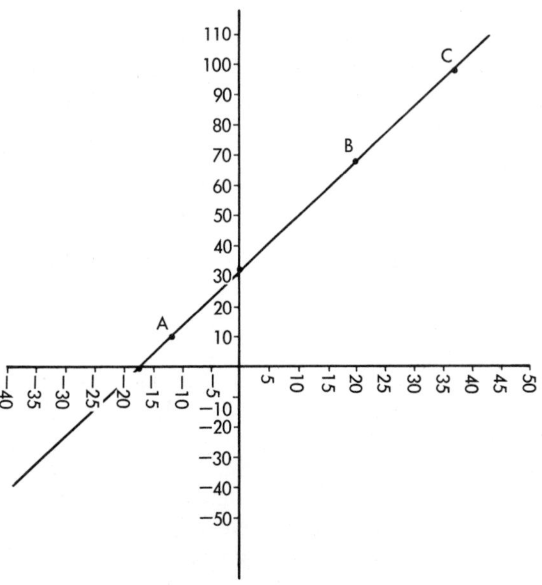

Fig. 1-9. Graphic relationship between Fahrenheit and Celsius temperature values.

and is not based upon any calculations. The entire message is that from geometry we know that two points determine a straight line. All loci along this line have coordinates that also represent other solution possibilities or relationship possibilities for the unknown. Subsequent calculations do not need to be performed. Since the line goes in two directions, any combinations of above freezing or subfreezing temperatures relationships can be extrapolated from those for a given range. When the x axis represents the Celsius scale, the y axis represents the Fahrenheit scale. Further, when the Celsius reading is zero (0), the Fahrenheit reading is +32 as noted on the y axis. When the Fahrenheit reading is zero, the Celsius reading as noted on the x axis is −17.7, that is, 0.556 − 32. Verify mathematically that points A, B, and C are in fact valid loci of relationship of this equation.

Exponential graph—construction and rationale

In comparison to a first-degree equation and to its corresponding linear graph, an exponential graph is evolved from an exponential equation that has one or more unknowns as exponents. However, in contrast, the graphically represented equivalent is not a straight line but is curvilinear, it may intersect one axis but be asymptotic to the other axis, and the graph has no constant slope since the line is curved. This phenomenon occurs when the unit dimensions on both the x and y axes are of the same type and length. The general form of an exponential equation is

$$y = a \cdot b^x$$

b is most frequently represented by a transcendental number (that is, a nonsolution number or root), called e, the base number of the natural logarithms (that is, 2.71828). The enigmatic e is derived from calculus in the differentiation of logarithmic functions and the determination of the value of the limit

$$(\lim)t \rightarrow 0\ (1 + t)^{1/t}$$

As t approaches zero, the value becomes 2.71828. By substitution, the general form now is

$$y = a \cdot e^x$$

In both general forms, a is a constant number. Unlike a linear graph, the number scales of an exponential graph do not possess either linearity or uniformity of the scale-length designations. The y-axis number scale is determined by the common or natural logarithmic values, since it is the dependent value. A graph so constructed with the y axis having a logarithmic scale and the x axis having a rectilinear scale is designated as a semilog graph. It is not absolutely dogmatic to have the axes reversed as in some special cases of dose response where the dependent variable can be plotted against a logarithmic x axis and the independent variable plotted against a linear axis. Both the rectilinear and semilog graphs are those that you will most commonly encounter and use in nuclear medicine technology; however, another type of graphic construction is possible as represented by the log-log (that is, full) graph, which is logarithmic on both axes.

The y axis of semilog graphs is defined in terms of the number of cycles; the entire length of the y axis could be one cycle, that is, from 1 to 10; it could be two cycles, that is, from 1 to 10 to 100; or it could go to five cycles. To know how many cycles to use is to know the logarithmic range of numbers represented by the dependent variable. The use of a greater number of cycles does not make the graph more accurate but to the contrary. The greatest accuracy is achieved by using only the number of cycles necessary.

Figs. 1-10 and 1-11 illustrate both the one- and two-cycle semilog graphic forms. In both of these illustrations, no specifications for the gradations of the x axis are provided, since this designation will be unique to the independent variable in each situation in which the graph would be used. The graph types illustrated in Figs. 1-10 and 1-11 would most frequently be used to represent problems in half-value layer (HVL), physical half-life ($T_{\frac{1}{2}}$), exposure rate, and red blood cell survival time.

Exponential equations, when plotted on coordinate graph paper, are represented by a curvilinear line, but on semilog graph paper the same equations are represented by a straight line. The most frequently used exponential equation again is the following:

$$A_t = A_0 \cdot e^{-(0.693/T_{\frac{1}{2}}) \cdot t}$$

The independent variables in this equation are the elapsed time, t, the physical half-life, $T_{\frac{1}{2}}$, and the original amount of radioactivity, A_0; the dependent variable is A_t, which is the amount of radioactivity remaining after the passage of the elapsed time. In other words, when this equation is plotted on a semilog graph, the elapsed time is always on the x axis and the remaining activity is always on the y axis. Rewriting the above equation and determining the natural logarithm of each side result in the following forms:

1. $\dfrac{A_t}{A_0} = e^{-(0.693/T_{\frac{1}{2}}) \cdot t}$
2. $\ln \dfrac{A_t}{A_0} = \dfrac{-0.693}{T_{\frac{1}{2}}} \cdot t \cdot \ln e$
3. $\ln e = 1$
4. $\ln \dfrac{A_t}{A_0} = \dfrac{-0.693}{T_{\frac{1}{2}}} \cdot t$

The minus sign of the right-hand member indicates that

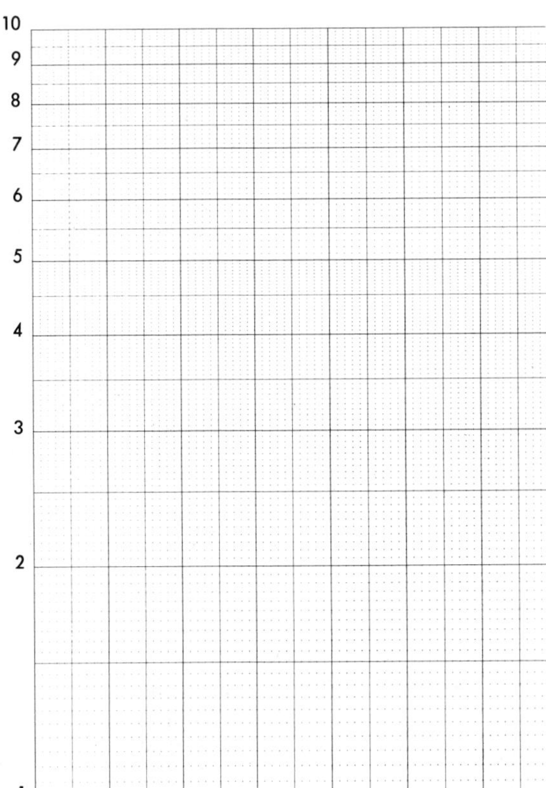

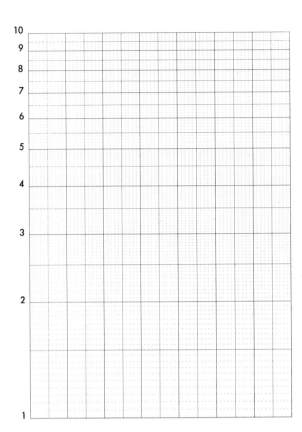

Fig. 1-10. One-cycle semilog graph paper.

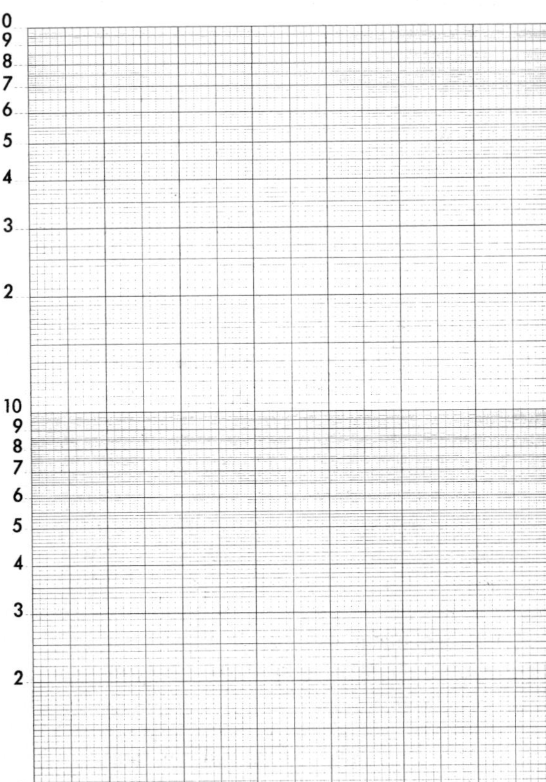

Fig. 1-11. Two-cycle semilog graph paper.

the slope of the resulting plotted line would be negative. The decay constant ($\lambda = 0.693/T_{\frac{1}{2}}$) is equivalent to the slope, as verified by the fact that the amount of radioactivity decreases as the elapsed time increases.

Graphic comparison—linear and exponential

Figs. 1-12 and 1-13 are two graphs based upon the same equation and radionuclide data. Information obtained from the interpretation of each of these graphs is the same; however, the interpreted information is easier, slightly more accurate, and more accessible from Fig. 1-13 than from Fig. 1-12. No data or relationships are lost or adversely manipulated in changing from one graphic representation format to the other. Greater ease of interpretation and graphic construction are the prime reasons for the high incidence of semilog graphs used with exponential equations.

In either the linear or exponential equations that contain two variables (x and y)

$$y = mx + b \text{ (linear)} \quad \text{or} \quad y = a \cdot b^{x} \text{ (exponential)}$$

the value of y is dependent on the values assigned to x, and conversely the value of x is not dependent on the values taken by y; in other words:

x = Independent variable
y = Dependent variable

The ability to differentiate between these variable categories is important and relates to how real-life variables are to be accurately graphed as illustrated in this situation.

Problem: During a 6-year interval, a nuclear medicine service performed the following number of clinical procedures:

Year	Total	= In vivo	+ In vitro
1973	4878	4000	878
1974	5130	3880	1250
1975	5450	3775	1675
1976	5800	3700	2100
1977	6130	3610	2520
1978	6490	3500	2990

From these data, which category represents the independent variable? Yes, it is the time period, since its value has no bearing or dependence on the number of procedures. Each of the three remaining columns illustrates dependence, since the volume of procedures depends on the year. By convention when one is graphing, the independent variable is plotted on the x axis and the dependent variable is plotted on the y axis. Following this and from the above situational data, Fig. 1-14 is prepared. Note that none of the lines actually intercepts the y axis as might be expected. A value relating to the number of procedures that could have been performed in 1972 is determined by the process of extrapolation illustrated in Fig. 1-14 by the dashed line. This estimation procedure assumes that the dependent variable varies linearly with and beyond the calculated range of the independent variable. In the above situations, a prospective estimate of the number of procedures that might be performed in 1979 could be made by extrapolation in the opposite direction. Caution must be exercised regarding the potential fault and danger of estimation beyond the calculated or known extremes of a plotted line or curve since the variables' precise relationship is not known in these remote regions.

The procedural trends as initially indicated by the tabular data above is very vividly illustrated by the respective slopes in Fig. 1-14. Another aspect illustrated is the algebraic summation effect that the individual component lines demonstrate. In other words, by knowing only two variables, one can fairly easily approximate a range value of the third solely from the graph. The precision of determining the value of the third arises from the tabular data.

Three-dimensional coordinates

To this point, the above graphic parameters have been evolved around two-dimensional, rectilinear coordinates in space in which the dimensions relate to certain quantities.

On occasion you will confront a three-dimensional problem; for example, in scintillation camera instrumentation matters. The scintillations resulting from gamma photon interactions are located in three-dimensional space and have three linear coordinates, x, y, and z, defined within a three-dimensional cartesian system. All three axes are at right angles to each other as illustrated in Fig. 1-15, which is drawn on two-dimensional paper. Any point in three-dimensional space (for example, photon interaction) can then be described in terms of its locations on the x-y plane, z-y plane, and x-z plane. Yet another practical application of this type of representation is in both B- and M-mode ultrasonographic imaging. The concept of the point of origin is the same as in the rectangular coordinate system. The linear distance (solid line) of point S from the origin can be calculated from the $x^2 + y^2 + z^2$ relationship.

One-dimensional system

Occasionally, quantifiable data and their relationships are more easily represented in a semipictorial manner. One specific type of this mode of representation is referred to as a pie graph or diagram.

Construction of this type is based upon the fact that a circle, in a one-dimensional system, has 360 degrees. Of the totally related data, each datum can be described as a percentage of the whole, which when multiplied

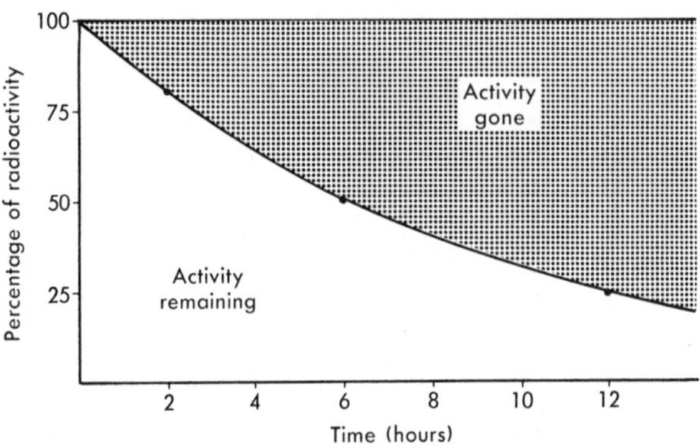

Fig. 1-12. Linear plot of radioactive exponential equation.

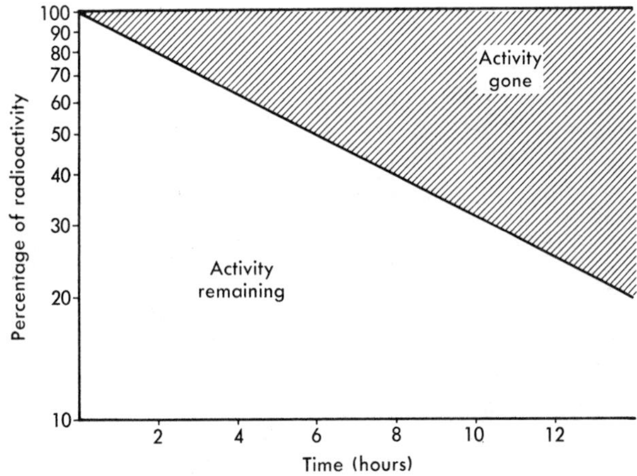

Fig. 1-13. Semilog graphic plot of radioactive exponential equation.

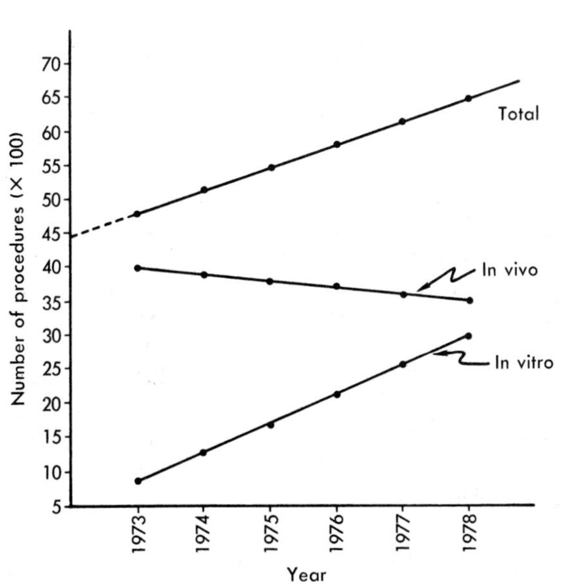

Fig. 1-14. Graphic illustration of situational data.

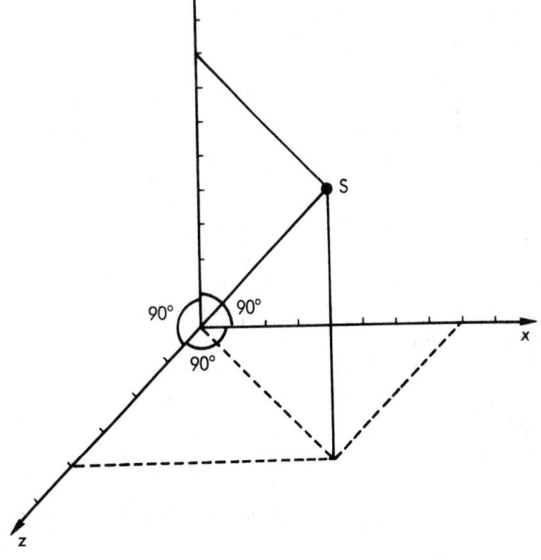

Fig. 1-15. Three-dimensional cartesian system.

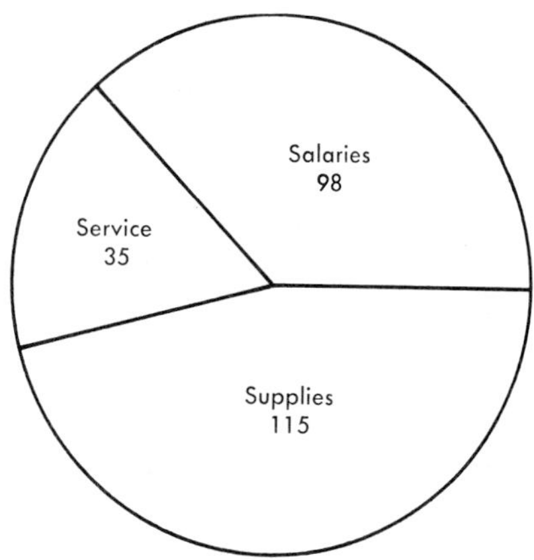

Fig. 1-16. Nuclear medicine section budget for 1978-1979 fiscal year (thousands of dollars).

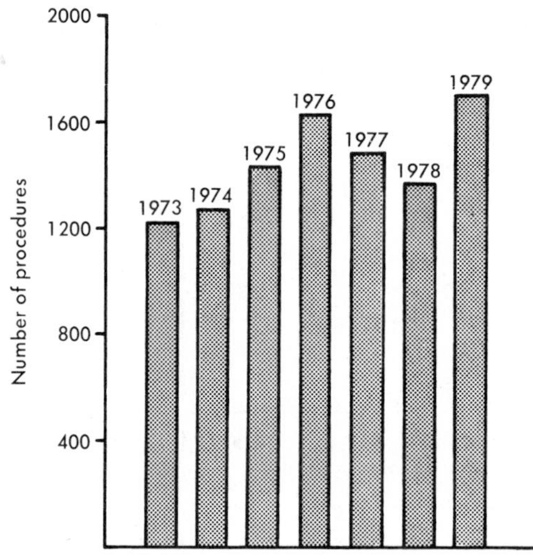

Fig. 1-17. Histogram.

by 360 degrees results in that segment of the circle equivalent to that datum's contribution to the total. A simple example will illustrate the construction of a pie graph (Fig. 1-16). Suppose you were, for the 1978-1979 fiscal year, responsible for a departmental budget. Major budget categories would be as follows:

		Percentage of total budget	Circular portion
Supplies	$115,000	46.4 × 360° =	167°
Service	35,000	14.1 × 360° =	51°
Salaries	98,000	39.5 × 360° =	142°
	$248,000	100.0	360°

By use of a protractor, Fig. 1-16 represents the pie graph resulting from the above data. Location of the necessary segmental lines is usually determined from the placement of the first line at the 3 o'clock position.

Histograms

Graphic representations based upon frequency distributions of the ranges of values of the independent variable are called "histograms," or "frequency polygons." The base width of the rectangles representing the ranges of the independent variable on the x axis is usually centered over the range midpoint. The dependent variable, incidence or frequency of the occurrence of the independent variable, determines the height of the rectangle and is equivalent to a value on the y axis.

Utilization of this graph type is found with either empirical (that is, experimental) or theoretical data. A histogram is represented in Fig. 1-17.

It can be shown easily that if the midpoint of each range is connected by a line graph (Fig. 1-18) that the total area of rectangles is equal to the area under the curve. The connecting line could be mathematically smoothed to remove the discontinuities if necessary. However, the validity of these statements is not altered by the cosmetics of the curve. Consideration of a histogram in this manner is analogous to integral calculus, which basically demonstrates the total change of the dependent variable over the range of the independent variable, which is ultimately constituted by a number of small changes.

Mechanically expanding this line of reasoning further, there are several ways in which the area can be approximated. From a plot on graph paper, a count of the number of squares below the curve could be made and the number would be multiplied by the area of each square. Another method is to physically cut from the graph the area of that portion under the graph and compare its weight with the weight of another known area.

From integral calculus, one may determine the area mathematically by dividing the portion under the graph, the boundaries of which are determined by both upper and lower limits, into small segmental rectangles. The height of these rectangles is equivalent to the dependent variable when the width (that is, differential) is equal to that small portion of the independent variable. The summation process is represented by $\int$, the integral sign. In the x-y coordinate system, the area is, in words, equal to the sum of the area of each rectangle, which is determined as the product of the height, y, and the base (that is, the value of the independent variable when the dependent variable has a precise value) between certain limits of the independent variable. In symbols, the area is determined by the following expression:

$$\int_a^b f(x) \cdot dx \quad \text{or} \quad \int_a^b y \cdot dx$$

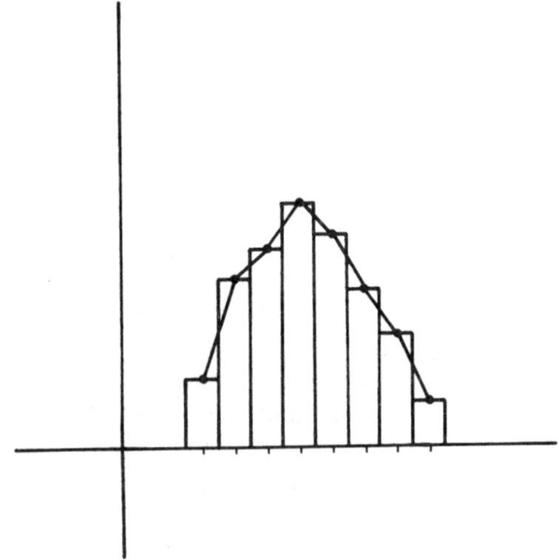

Fig. 1-18. Histogram with range midpoints connected.

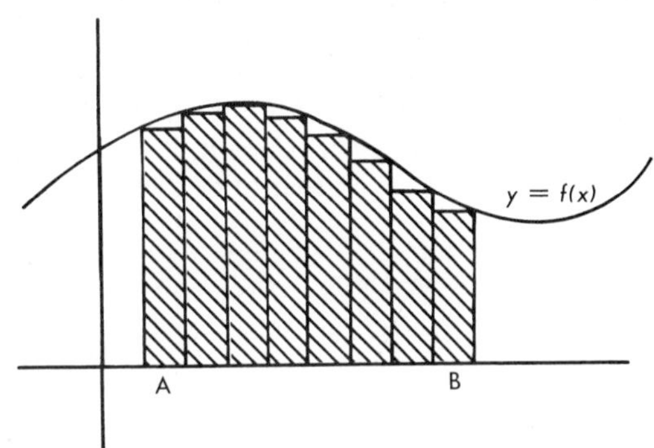

Fig. 1-19. Graphic area approximated by rectangles.

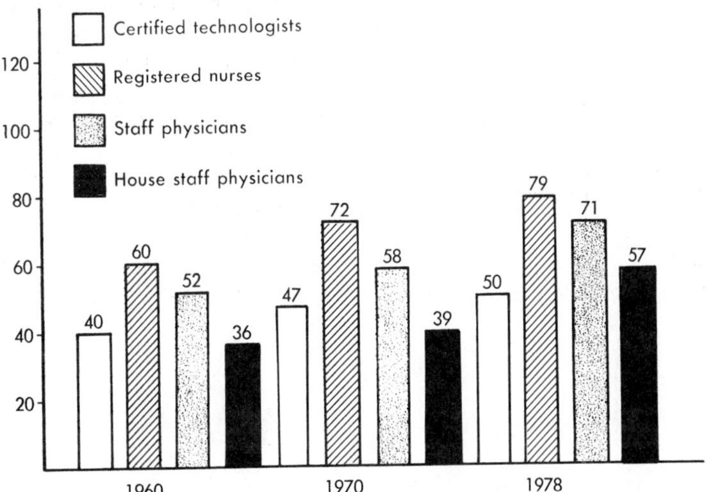

Fig. 1-20. Bar graph demonstrating professional staff growth.

Fig. 1-19 illustrates a graph that could have its area determined by the above mathematical expressions.

Bar graphs

A bar graph is a generic name for graphic representations that employ horizontal or vertical rectangles to represent the data. The spatial orientation of the rectangles does not modify the data. If the rectangles are placed in immediate juxtaposition, the previously described graphic type (histogram or frequency polygon) is generated. The width of the rectangle is generally fixed for the graph being constructed and does not represent a range; the height (if vertical) or length (if horizontal) is determined by the values of the dependent variable. Fig. 1-20 illustrates a bar graph. Both the x and y axes represent the independent and dependent variables respectively; however, note that the base width is completely independent of any factor other than personal convenience or aesthetics. A legend usually accompanies a bar graph, since the width dimension is purely arbitrary and since several types of data can be simultaneously represented.

Suppose that these rectangles were physically moved together to form a histogram. The resulting graph, after width midpoints are connected, could have the area under the curve calculated, but a meaningless number results, since the area is equivalent to the product of length and width, with the width being arbitrary. The summation of grouped or categorized data in a bar graph is simply determined arithmetically by the combination of data such as the number of professional staff for a given point in time. How many staff members were employed in 1970? Correct, if you answered 216. Differences between grouped or categorized data in a bar graph is simply determined arithmetically by subtraction of data such as the increase in the number of house staff residents between two given points in time. How many more house staff residents were there in 1978 compared to 1960? Correct, if you answered 21.

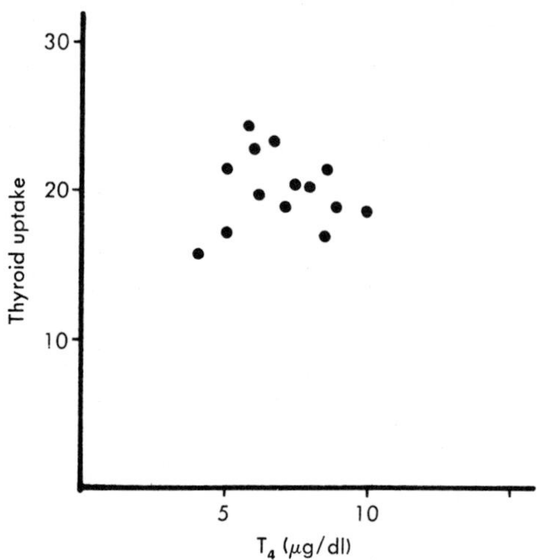

Fig. 1-21. Comparison of ^{131}I-thyroid uptake and T_4 levels in normal subjects.

Point graphs

Situations present when it is not practical to measure or calculate all values of the dependent variable when all values of the independent variable are known or calculable. In these experimental situations, a point graph (Fig. 1-21) is used and represents only preclusive values or limits. The sampled empirical information contained within this graph type can very easily be extracted and presented in tabular form. Interpolation is necessary for determination of variable relationships not specifically represented by a graph point.

Broken-line graphs

Connecting the individual data points in a point graph results in a broken-line graph when the resulting line is not linear or smoothly curvilinear. This graphic profile is represented in Fig. 1-22. As in other graphic types, the variable placement is the same. The hypothetical, though realistic, data presented illustrates yet another cumulative and algebraic aspect of graphs. As in arithmetic, the total is equal to the sum of the individual component parts. The same relationship holds true in graphing. In Fig. 1-22 the total number of patient admissions for each year is determined by the number of private-patient admissions plus the number

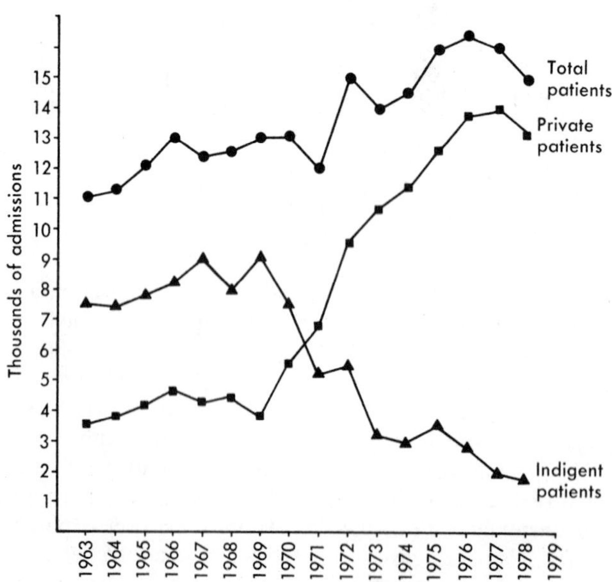

Fig. 1-22. Somewhere Hospitals and Clinics admission growth by paying classification, 1963-1978.

of indigent-patient admissions. For example in 1971, the total admission number was reported and plotted as 12,000, which consisted of 6800 private and 5200 indigent. Had the total admission line not been plotted or available, one could very easily calculate it by simply summing the individual component values and plotting their sums.

The accuracy of this graph type is frequently less than desirable. Basically, its value is to demonstrate general trends and general quantities without any finely honed precision.

Graphic accuracy

The accuracy of graphic interpretation is physically based upon the size of the graph and the number of data points selected, pragmatically upon care with which the graph was constructed, and philosophically upon the accuracy with which the data were collected and measured. The intent and purpose of this section is to suggest that the physically larger the graph type, the greater the accuracy of interpretation. Accuracy of greater than 99% is unreasonable.

Curve fitting

The real world frequently requires us to gather empirical data that are actually the collection of quantifications for both dependent and independent variables. In the analysis of this data, the construction of a graph may be required. Because of the type of dependent variable being measured, our measurement techniques and accuracy, and our understanding of the relationships between variables and related use of control, we may have data points that do not nicely lie on a straight line. The question then becomes how to determine and locate a line that most accurately reflects the relationship of the measured variables as determined by the data points.

A crude attempt at fitting a curve is the freehand method, which consists of drawing an approximating curve to fit a set of data. The major disadvantage inherent in this method is that different curves will result from different observers. From a pragmatic standpoint, the most easily determined straight-line placement is determined visibly such that there are as many points above as below the line. When data points do not appear to be on or near a straight line, a mathematical method that derives the best fit is the method of choice. Dispersed data point locations are mathematically handled such that the sum of the squares of vertical distance that each data point lies from a line is minimized. The method is referred to as "least squares."

Nomograms

Known also as alignment charts or isopleths, nomograms consist of at least two scales, oriented and constructed in such a manner that relationships between variables can be visibly and quickly determined.

Fig. 1-23 is a reproduction of a nomogram published in the *Radiological Health Handbook* (September 1960, U.S. Department of Health, Education and Welfare). This nomogram format is useful in the de-

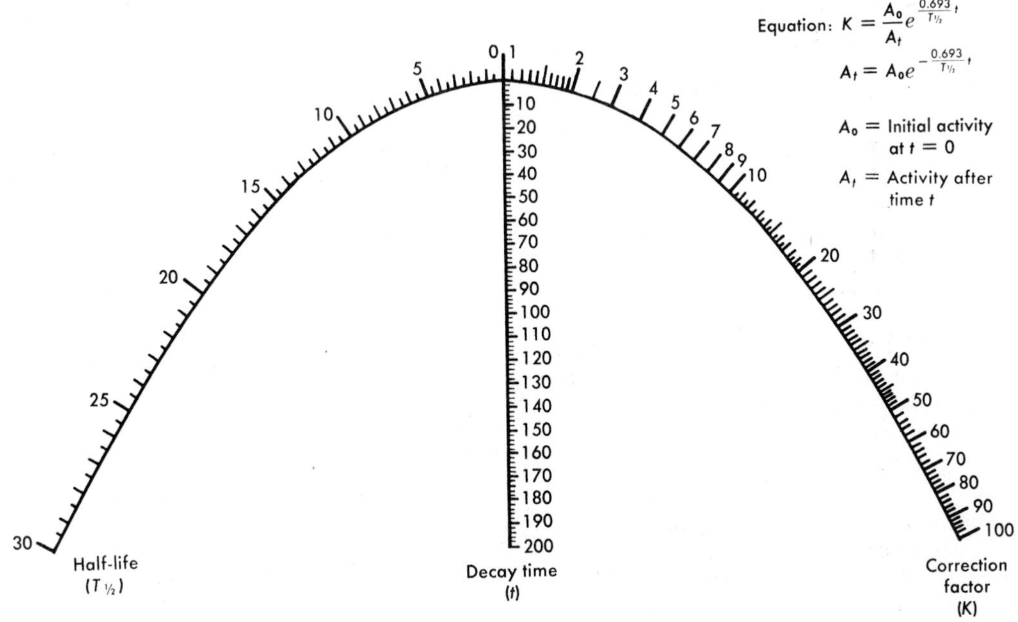

Fig. 1-23. Nomograph for radioactive-decay correction.

termination of the amount of radioactivity after a known elapsed time, the physical half-time of the radioactive source, and the original amount of activity. The two points on the half-life and decay time scales are connected by a straightedge, which must also intersect the correction factor scale, *K*. The value of the point of intersection is multiplied by the original amount to provide the calculated remaining amount.

Currently, the use of nomograms is minimal, if at all, because of the availability and speed of calculators. Basically, nomograms are only of historic note.

DIGITAL OR ANALOG DATA?

With the advent of computer technology, the sophistication of data-gathering or data-manipulating instrumentation has increased to a very high level albeit frequently requiring that the operator (you) know very little of the why and wherefore of its operation. The medical interpretations and subsequent diagnoses rendered from either in vivo or in vitro clinical procedures are no better than the instrument's ability to scientifically and accurately measure, organize, analyze, and present data and certainly are no better than the accuracy of the available data. Philosophically, there are no bad data or results; data are all good data. The quality or usefulness of the data is biased by the collector's or interpreter's expectations. The data types in nuclear medicine technology, with which you will be confronted, are either digital or analog.

Digitized data actually represents specific quantized values. For example, on Monday, your clinic performed 10 clinical procedures; on Tuesday, 8 procedures; and on Wednesday, 12 procedures. These daily quantities each represent a digital datum represented by a specific integer (whole number). However, if these digital data are collected for a longer finite time (for example, 1 week) and a daily average number of procedures is calculated for that week, the resulting numerical value, in most instances, will not be required to be represented by an integer. The instances of exception are those situations in which the daily number of procedures for each day is the same value or that the sum value is an integer multiple of the number of observations.

By comparison, the value that represents the daily average when calculated for a several-week set of observations would represent a continuum of values rather than specific integer (that is, digital) values. This continuum representation is termed "analog data."

As you proceed with your education and training, you will endlessly be confronted with the concepts of quality control (QC) and quality assurance (QA). These concepts, in real life and in the remainder of this text, form the skeleton upon which all of our efforts in the health care industry are and should be supported. Quality control almost automatically implies methods, and it is the statistical name of the game! Our active participation in the control and assurance of quality is imperative whether it be tangible (data collection) or intangible (patient care).

The material that follows is presented to you as background information, and certainly not to train you to be a statistician or quality control expert but, we hope, provide you with the basic skills and understanding to better enable you to control and evaluate the quality and accuracy of your data collections, your manipulations of the collected data, and the data you present for medical interpretation and pending patient care.

Just as in learning a new language, one usually starts by learning the names of basic things, the nouns; the accessory action words follow. Listed in Table 1-11 are the basic terms (abbreviations or symbols) we will use.

In a categorical way, the digital information or data that we collect is very limited. For example, as part of our activities as nuclear medicine technologists, we may quantify any of the following data: number of patients, amounts of radioactivity, or number of specimens. Again, the different categories are not overwhelming; however, the number of times we perform one, the categorical quantifications may seem interminable. Ergo, we need always to maintain our QC vigilance.

We desire that the count of things or events that we observe be accurate, precise, and reliable. More specifically, *accuracy* of quantification methodology or of procedural data relates to the agreement of the *observed* value with the *true* or *actual* value. In your performance of a procedure or an instrument's per-

Table 1-11. Basic statistical terms, symbols, and definitions

Symbol	Reading or pronunciation	Definition
$<$		less than
$>$		greater than
$\leq$		less than or equal to
$\geq$		greater than or equal to
$\sum$	sigma (capital)	the sum of
$\bar{x}$	*x* bar	arithmetic mean
σ	sigma (small)	standard deviation (SD)
N		number of items or events in sample size frequency
m		median, midpoint, or 50th percentile
df		degree of freedom
χ^2	chi-square	

formance, *precision* relates to your or its ability to produce results, which under comparable conditions, agree or coincide very closely. Precision adversely suffers from indeterminate errors, such as randomness of radioactive decay. You or an instrument can be precise without being accurate. No less important is the concept of *reliability*, which is a measure of both accuracy and precision in terms of variance.

From our previous and individual experiences with the physical and biologic world, we have had opportunities to replicate counts of things or events. These replicated observations were not all the same but "were close to" some average value. This problem will not end with your emergence into this field of technology utilizing radioactivity; it only gets worse because of the randomness of radioactive decay over which no person or instrument has control. Random processes can only be described by statistics. Arrangement of statistical data into ranges with specified frequencies is imperative to its analysis.

The resulting format is referred to as a frequency distribution. Suppose that you were provided with the appropriate instrumentation to "count" a sample containing a long-lived radionuclide. Your ten 1-minute observations are identified in Table 1-12. Several of the terms and symbols from Table 1-11 are used. The mean, $\bar{x}$, has been determined by division of the total number of observed counts $\sum x_i$ by the number of observations, N. Stated mathematically

$$\bar{x} = \frac{\sum x_i}{N}$$

The extent, either above (+) or below (−), to which each observed count deviates from the mean is tabulated in the third column. Note that the total deviation is equal to zero.

In this tabulation, no mode is identified. By definition, the mode is an observation occurring with the greatest frequency. Since all observations are different, with none reoccurring, there is no mode in this tabulation. A frequency distribution need not always have a mode. However, if it has only one, it is described as unimodal; having two modes is bimodal; and more than two, multimodal. A median could be calculated if necessary. Its numerical value would be found by rank, if one orders the observed counts from highest to lowest and then finds the half-way value. Had the number of observed events been odd in number, the midpoint would have been easy to determine. Since, however, the number of observed events is even in number, the midpoint would be an average value between the two adjacent observed values.

Depending on the numerical value of events and the

Table 1-12. Actual successive counting data from a long-lived radionuclide

Observation	Number of counts, x_i	Deviation $(x - \bar{x})$	Square of deviation $(x - \bar{x})^2$
1	8,038	954	910,116
2	7,530	446	198,916
3	7,347	263	69,169
4	7,044	−40	1,600
5	7,088	4	16
6	7,074	−10	100
7	6,872	−212	44,944
8	6,269	−815	664,225
9	6,951	−133	17,689
10	6,627	−457	208,849
$N = 10$	$\sum = 70,840$	$\sum = 0$	2,115,624
	$x = 7,084$		

$$\sigma = \pm\sqrt{\frac{2,115,624}{9}}$$

$$= \pm\sqrt{235,069} = \pm 485$$

or

$$\sigma = \pm\sqrt{\frac{2,115,624}{10}}$$

$$= \pm\sqrt{211,562} \pm 460$$

frequency of their occurrence, a graph depicting the overall distribution can be generated. There are generally two names associated with frequency distributions. The first, *Poisson* (or *discrete probability*) *distribution* is useful in describing the randomness of radioactive decay but is mathematically awkward to use. A graphic representation of this type of distribution is not symmetric around the mean, with the standard deviation being equal to the square or continuous probability. The second, *gaussian distribution,* though not so accurate as the first, is most widely and easily used. A graphic representation of this distribution is symmetric around the mean and is synonymously known as the normal curve, or bell-shaped curve (Fig. 1-24). In this figure, the mean is visibly

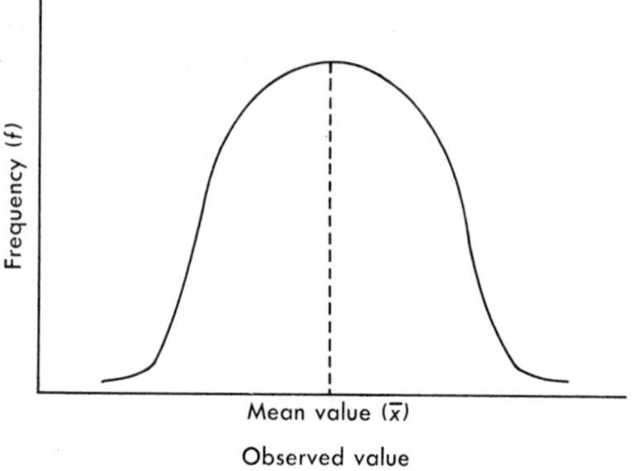

Fig. 1-24. Gaussian distribution.

a measure of the central tendency or clustering of the observed values and is equal to the square root of the variance. Variations on the theme of normal central tendency are illustrated in Fig. 1-25. By definition, skewness is that property of a distribution involving its symmetry or asymmetry. Contained within the mathematical determination of skewness is a term identified as the *standard deviation* (σ). Again by definitions, the standard deviation of a frequency distribution is a useful measure of the extent of dispersion of observed values around the mean value. Ranges and percentile ranges are yet other measures of dispersion of numerical data.

Calculation of the numerical value of the standard deviation is simply determined in words when one takes the square root of the variance, or in symbols:

$$\sigma = \pm\sqrt{\frac{\sum (x_i - \bar{x})^2}{N}} \quad \text{or} \quad \pm\sqrt{\text{Variance}}$$

The denominator of the above radicand in some texts is stated as $N - 1$ and here N. "Why?" you may ask. When $N - 1$ is used in the denominator, the resulting value represents a better estimate of the standard deviation. For large values of N, not large values of x_i, there is practically no difference between the calculated values of standard deviation. For our purposes, the single N value is adequate. Referring to Table 1-12 we find that if a gaussian distribution is assumed and the denominator is 10 (that is, N), then the standard deviation is ±485. However, if the de-

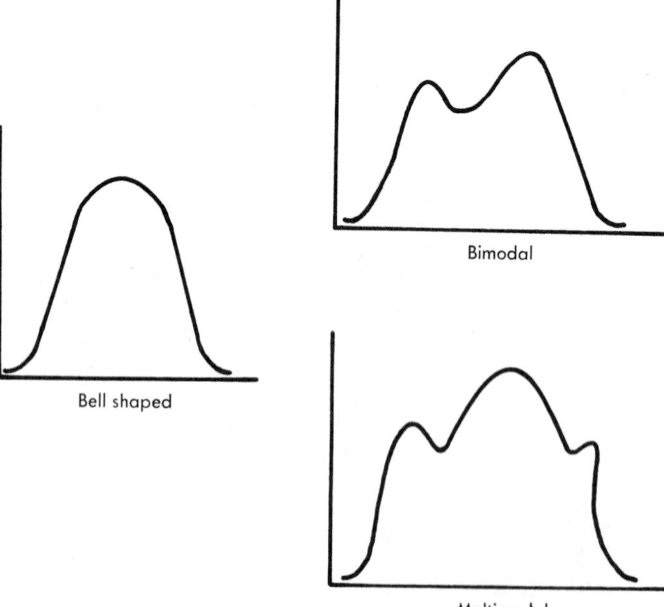

Fig. 1-25. Types of frequency distribution.

nominator is 9 (that is, $N - 1$), the standard deviation is ±460. Yes, the difference is 25, but the resulting percentage variation about the mean is ±0.3%, which is practically not significant. In comparison, the value of the standard deviation, with a Poisson distribution, is ±84.

To attempt to clarify some potentially confusing or apparently contradictory statements in other sources, we need to differentiate between the deviation of a sample and the deviation of a population.

Sample: Individual event or count, deviation (σ)

$$\sigma = \pm\sqrt{x}$$

Population: Total of all events or counts, deviation (σ)

$$\sigma = \pm\sqrt{\frac{\sum (x - \bar{x})^2}{N}}$$

Using Table 1-12 again, we find that a sample deviation could be determined for each of 10 observations. Note, however, that a deviation calculated in this manner varies; for observation 3 it is approximately 86, and for observation 9 it is approximately 83. A standard-deviation determination of this type is purely shorthand with a relatively low accuracy level. The standard deviation, however, of the entire population of observed events or counts is more accurate, more meaningful, but more time consuming to calculate than for a part of the population.

Attention should be redirected above to note that the root value can be plus or minus (±). Since the dispersion can occur or be observed in either direction around the mean, there is a need to use ±, which again purely indicates a direction on the abscissa of the graphic form of a frequency distribution. The fourth column of Table 1-12 has the variance calculated. In column three, there are deviation values with accompanying minus signs, which disappear $(-) \cdot (-) = (+)$ when squared as in column four.

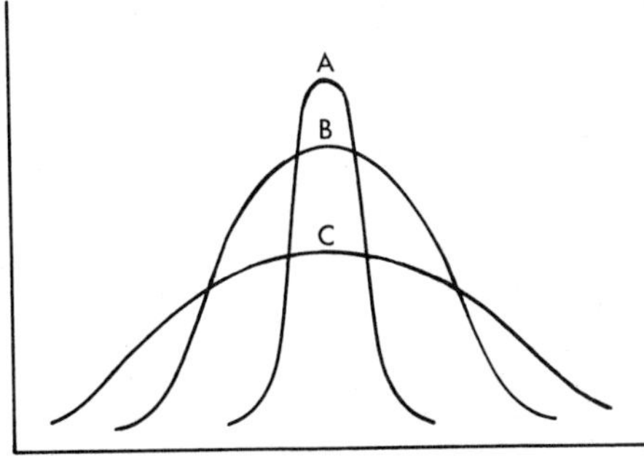

Fig. 1-26. Frequency distributions displaying identical mean values but different standard deviations.

From the above discussion, it would be an expected result to have 68% of the 10 observations have count values that when tabulated would be between 7569 (7084 + 485) and 6599 (7089 − 485). These expected 7 counts are actually 8 in number. Again to compare, we would expect to find 7 counts with values between 7544 (7084 + 460) and 6624 (7084 + 460); however, the actual count is 8.

Two distributions can have the same mean value but possess completely different dispersions or standard-deviation values as illustrated in Fig. 1-26, in which special names are associated with each of the curve types. Curve A is termed "leptokurtic"; curve B is termed "normal," or "mesokurtic"; curve C is termed "platykurtic." Adding further quantifications to the discussion and quantification of the value of the standard deviation in a normal distribution curve gives the forms in Fig. 1-27. The three percentage values differ between various sources; the variance is in the precision of the decimal places and rounding that may take place. For practical intents and purposes, little if any problem is realized from this apparent discrepancy. In gaussian or normal distributions, it turns out that in 68.3% of all the cases, events or counts will have a value equal to a minimum value of no less than the mean value minus one standard deviation ($\bar{x} - \sigma$) or greater, to a maximum value of no more than the mean value plus one standard deviation ($\bar{x} + \sigma$). In other words, approximately 34% of the observed counts or events should fall on either side of the mean value as represented by the unshaded area. Moving

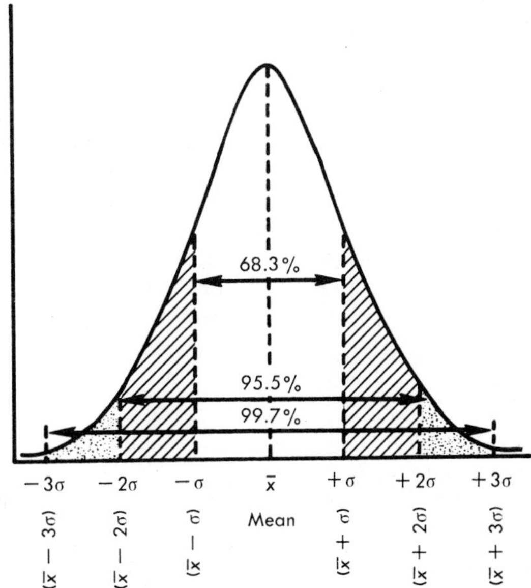

Fig. 1-27. Standard-deviation values as part of normal distribution curve.

laterally from the observed values equal to + 1σ are cross-hatched regions that represent an additional 13.6% (0.683/2 − 0.055/2) of the observed population. The percentage of the total population included to the outer limits of $+2\sigma$ is 95.5%. The remaining portion of the population, 4.2% (0.955/2 − 0.997/2), is divided equally between the two stippled areas designated as $\pm 3\sigma$. There is no formula to calculate $\pm 2\sigma$ or $\pm 3\sigma$; these values are purely additive to $\pm 1\sigma$ after it has been determined.

In the earlier part of this chapter and indirectly referred to above, dependent and independent variables exist for these types of probability distributions. In the normal or gaussian distribution, the mean $(\bar{x})$ and standard deviation (σ) are independent variables. For Poisson distributions, the mean $(\bar{x})$ is the independent variable, with the standard deviation (σ) being the dependent variable, since

$$1\sigma = \pm\sqrt{\text{Mean}}$$

to repeat and compare for normal distributions

$$1\sigma = \pm\sqrt{\text{Variance}}$$

When radioactivity is involved, the Poisson distribution is the more accurate. Suppose you had a syringe containing radioactivity and you made only one observation, which contained x counts. The determination of the standard deviation of this single value becomes

$$\pm\sqrt{x}$$

What is the usefulness of knowing the standard deviation of one observation, N, containing x counts? Assessing three different situations might assist in answering this question. Three different radioactive sources are counted under identical conditions with the observed results and calculations shown in Table 1-13.

The smaller the observed values, the higher is the relative percentage of the resulting standard deviation's value to the observed value. The usefulness of knowing the value of the standard deviation for one observation of some value is purely an assessment of this value to the true value, or for example, from Fig. 1-27, the probability that the true value of one measurement's being within one standard deviation is 68%. These odds are not too bad, approximately 2 out of 3. Quantifiable laboratory data is usually presented in the general form of

$$x \pm \sigma x$$

By example, assume that a patient's thyroid gland was being evaluated for its ability to take up radioactive iodine. This evaluation involved a 1-minute count that resulted in the number 3750. Following this generalized form, you could report this quantifiable clinical data as 3750 $\pm 1\sigma$. The standard deviation is independent of the time required to obtain the counts.

Assume that a multiple time period (for example, 5 minutes) observation was made. Now, how are the count rate (CR) and standard deviation determined? It just so happens that the following formula is what is needed:

$$\text{CR} = \frac{x \pm \sqrt{x}}{t}$$

In which the denominator is the total time and the numerator is the total number of counts observed during the total time plus or minus the square root of the total number of counts. For example, a blood sample is counted for 5 minutes, and the total number of counts was 4260. What is the count rate per minute?

$$\text{CR} = \frac{4260 \pm \sqrt{4260}}{5} = \frac{4260 \pm 65}{5} = 852 \pm 13$$

Background radiation is ubiquitous and omnipresent, and this must be remembered and considered when you evaluate statistically a sample or specimen *only*. How is the quantifiable data relating to background radiation removed from consideration? Assume that you have counted a sample for 1 minute and obtained 4900 cpm. Remember this value represents a combined value; one component (and it is to be hoped the larger) is attributable to sample radiation *only;* the remaining component is attributable to the background radiation *only*. Now under the same counting conditions only the background radiation level is determined for 1 min-

Table 1-13. Relationship between standard deviation and percentage values for varying count rates

	Counts/time (x)	Standard deviation (σ)	Percentage
Radionuclide I	40	±6.8	6.8/40 = 0.15 = 15%
Radionuclide II	100	±10	10/100 = 0.10 = 10%
Radionuclide III	100,000	±1000	$10^3/10^6$ = 0.001 = 0.1%

ute, with a resulting value of 840 cpm. Respectively, their statistical values can be calculated as follows:

$$\text{Combined} = 4900 \pm \sqrt{4900} = 4900 \pm 70$$

$$\text{Only background} = 840 \pm 29$$

To what extent then does the sample singly contribute? The counts totally attributable to the sample are 4060 (4900 − 840).
Caution! The square root of this value is ±64. The standard deviation for the sample counts alone are determined by this formula:

$$\sigma \text{ sample} = \pm \sqrt{(\sigma \text{ combined})^2 + (\sigma \text{ background})^2}$$

whereby the correct sample standard-deviation value is ±76, which is higher than the combined σ.

What confidence can be placed in statistical determinations? In other words, our observed values, calculated mean and standard-deviation values, do not exactly or precisely represent the *true value* because of some error in measurement. But just how confident do you want to be about these values in representing the *true* values? The basic level of confidence has already been discussed; this level is the standard deviation, also referred to as the standard error.

Additionally, confidence levels may also be described in terms of probable error, nine tenths error, ninety-*five* hundredths error, or ninety-*nine* hundredths error.

The level called "*probable error*" is of slightly less confidence in that it represents a 50% chance of error. Computationally, it is determined by

$$\pm 0.6745\sigma$$

By definition, a confidence level is 1.00 minus the probability of observing an error greater than a specified amount. "Why 1.00?" you may ask. The probability of an error being observed and the probability that an error will not be observed is equal to 1.00; each probability is a percentage value. A further illustration suggests that the area under the curve relating to $\pm\sigma$ represents the probability that a measurement is *not* in error (68.3% confidence level) and the remaining portion represents the probability that a measurement is in error (31.7%). Fig. 1-28 illustrates this relationship. The total area under the curve represents the above-identified probability maximum of 1.00. Similar graphs could be illustrated for 95.5% and 99.7% confidence limits; $\pm 2\sigma$ and $\pm 3\sigma$, respectively. However, it is more convenient to drop the decimal points and describe the confidence levels as 95% and 99%, respectively. The concomitant adjustments that must be made are that 2.00 ($\pm 2\sigma$) must be reduced to 1.96 and 3.00 ($\pm 3\sigma$) must be reduced to 2.58. Therefore, if one were interested in determining the population mean ($\bar{x}$) from the sample mean, the following relationship would be used for the 95% and 99%, confidence levels, respectively:

$$\bar{x} = 1.96\sigma_{\bar{x}} \quad \text{and} \quad \bar{x}\ 2.58\sigma_{\bar{x}}$$

Chi-square test

By definition, the chi-square test is a measure of the discrepancy that may exist between the *o*bserved frequency, *O*, and *e*xpected frequency, *E*. In other words, this measure is an assessment of the "goodness of fit."

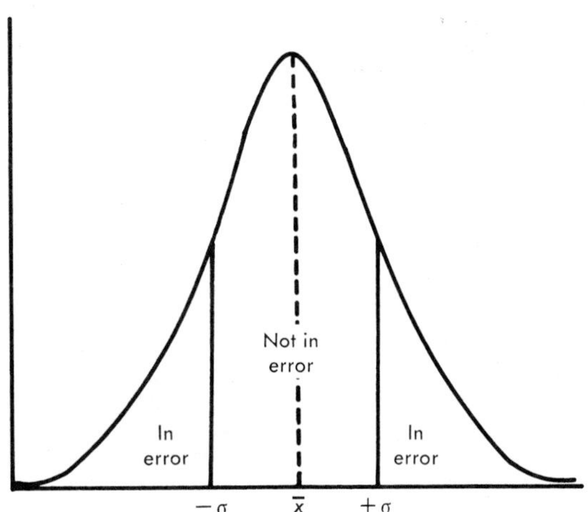

Fig. 1-28. Confidence level of 68.3% demonstrating probability in error and not in error.

In symbols:

$$\chi^2 = \frac{\sum \text{(deviations of observed from expected frequency)}^2}{\text{Expected frequency}}$$

or

$$\chi^2 = \frac{(O - E)^2}{E}$$

If $\chi^2 = O$, then there is no discrepancy with implied perfect agreement of goodness of fit. This represents its minimum value. The greater the increase in the value of χ^2, the greater the discrepancy in these frequencies.

An equivalent value to be substituted for the expected frequency is the mean, $\bar{x}$.

Therefore:

$$\chi^2 = \frac{\sum(x_i - x)^2}{\bar{x}}$$

Note that one of the basic differences between the formulas for chi-square and standard deviation is the denominator, the mean, $\bar{x}$, and number, n, respectively. The other main difference is the lack of square root extraction.

For determination of the results of counting a radioactive sample, such as that in Table 1-12, the chi-square value would be

$$\chi^2 = \frac{21156624}{7084} = 298.7$$

Oops, is that right? What does it mean? How can one use this number? Does one need to perform a square-root extraction? In reverse order: no, one does not need to take a root; remember the name is chi-square. The most common use to which these calculated chi-square values are put is in an assessment of status of operation of detection and counting instrumentation. Now, let us determine how well the counting instrument was operating. In order to learn how to do this, we must diverge momentarily to make reference to Appendix D, p. 57, which contains a chi-square distribution table. Horizontally across the top are the confidence levels. The 99% confidence level is the second from the right-hand side of the table. Vertically on the left-hand side are the number of observations. Respective chi-square values are found at the point of intersection corresponding to the appropriate column and row. Returning to the above chi-square value of 298.7 and referencing the 95% confidence level, we find that our calculated value is larger than the indicated value (298.7 > 18.3). Because of this relationship, we can feel fairly certain that our detection counting system is not operating correctly. The observed values were actually taken from a working instrument. Appropriate adjustments were made on the unit with new values as in Table 1-14. From the calculated standard deviation and the mean values, the χ^2 value is equivalent to 0.099. Returning to Appendix D, locate values at the 95% and 99% confidence levels; they are 18.3 and 23.2, respectively. Now that our newly calculated χ^2 value is *less than* the respective value in Appendix D, you can be confident that your detection/measuring instrument is operating correctly. Again, if the value is greater, you

Table 1-14. Actual successive counting data from a long-living radionuclide with correctly adjusted detection/counting instrument

Observation	Number of counts, x_i	Deviation $(x - \bar{x})$	Square of deviation $(x - x)^2$
1	4,684	25	625
2	4,586	−73	5,329
3	4,710	51	2,601
4	4,628	−31	961
5	4,727	68	4,624
6	4,643	−16	256
7	4,629	−30	900
8	4,598	−61	3,721
9	4,682	23	529
10	4,703	44	1,936
$N = 10$	$\sum = 46{,}590$	$\sum = 0$	21,482
	$\bar{x} = 4{,}659$		

$$\sigma = \pm\sqrt{\frac{21{,}482}{10}}$$

$$= \pm\sqrt{2{,}148}$$

$$= \pm\ 46.34$$

can be confident that the unit is dysfunctional. As a general statement, if the calculated χ^2 value is between the horizontal probability columns of 0.10 and 0.90, the unit is operating properly with the counts observed corresponding to a Poisson distribution.

Errors

As stated earlier, data is no more accurate than the means by which it is collected. Within the total arena of data measurement and data collection are generally two categories of types of errors. One is termed "indeterminate," which relates basically to statistical parameters; the second is "determinate," which relates basically to instrumentation, environment, or technique parameters.

Indeterminate errors are those over which you have no determining control such as the randomness of the radioactive decay process. Determinate errors are those "committed in the cockpit" and over which you have determining control, primarily in your techniques and with the instrumentation you perform the nuclear medicine procedures.

Even regulatory agencies have deemed quality control and quality assurance to be of utmost importance and have required documentation of routinely scheduled QC/QA procedures. These activities are required for institutional accreditation and licensure and specify assurance of diagnostic reliability, calibration, and preventive maintenance.

Appendix A: Table of square roots*

n	$\sqrt{n}$	n	$\sqrt{n}$	n	$\sqrt{n}$	n	$\sqrt{n}$	n	$\sqrt{n}$	n	$\sqrt{n}$	n	$\sqrt{n}$	n	$\sqrt{n}$	n	$\sqrt{n}$	n	$\sqrt{n}$
1.0	1.00	6.0	2.45	11.0	3.32	16.0	4.00	21.0	4.58	26.0	5.10	31.0	5.57	36.0	6.00	41.0	6.40	46.0	6.78
1.2	1.09	6.2	2.49	11.2	3.35	16.2	4.02	21.2	4.60	26.2	5.12	31.2	5.59	36.2	6.02	41.2	6.42	46.2	6.80
1.4	1.18	6.4	2.53	11.4	3.38	16.4	4.05	21.4	4.63	26.4	5.14	31.4	5.60	36.4	6.03	41.4	6.43	46.4	6.81
1.6	1.26	6.6	2.57	11.6	3.41	16.6	4.07	21.6	4.65	26.6	5.16	31.6	5.62	36.6	6.05	41.6	6.45	46.6	6.83
1.8	1.34	6.8	2.61	11.8	3.44	16.8	4.10	21.8	4.67	26.8	5.18	31.8	5.64	36.8	6.07	41.8	6.47	46.8	6.84
2.0	1.41	7.0	2.65	12.0	3.46	17.0	4.12	22.0	4.69	27.0	5.20	32.0	5.66	37.0	6.08	42.0	6.48	47.0	6.86
2.2	1.48	7.2	2.68	12.2	3.49	17.2	4.15	22.2	4.71	27.2	5.22	32.2	5.67	37.2	6.10	42.2	6.50	47.2	6.87
2.4	1.55	7.4	2.72	12.4	3.52	17.4	4.17	22.4	4.73	27.4	5.23	32.4	5.69	37.4	6.12	42.4	6.51	47.4	6.88
2.6	1.61	7.6	2.76	12.6	3.55	17.6	4.20	22.6	4.75	27.6	5.25	32.6	5.71	37.6	6.13	42.6	6.53	47.6	6.90
2.8	1.67	7.8	2.79	12.8	3.58	17.8	4.22	22.8	4.77	27.8	5.27	32.8	5.73	37.8	6.15	42.8	6.54	47.8	6.91
3.0	1.73	8.0	2.83	13.0	3.61	18.0	4.24	23.0	4.80	28.0	5.29	33.0	5.74	38.0	6.16	43.0	6.56	48.0	6.93
3.2	1.79	8.2	2.86	13.2	3.63	18.2	4.27	23.2	4.82	28.2	5.31	33.2	5.76	38.2	6.18	43.2	6.57	48.2	6.94
3.4	1.84	8.4	2.90	13.4	3.66	18.4	4.29	23.4	4.84	28.4	5.33	33.4	5.78	38.4	6.20	43.4	6.59	48.4	6.96
3.6	1.90	8.6	2.93	13.6	3.69	18.6	4.31	23.6	4.86	28.6	5.35	33.6	5.80	38.6	6.21	43.6	6.60	48.6	6.97
3.8	1.95	8.8	2.97	13.8	3.71	18.8	4.34	23.8	4.88	28.8	5.37	33.8	5.81	38.8	6.23	43.8	6.62	48.8	6.99
4.0	2.00	9.0	3.00	14.0	3.74	19.0	4.36	24.0	4.90	29.0	5.39	34.0	5.83	39.0	6.24	44.0	6.63	49.0	7.00
4.2	2.05	9.2	3.03	14.2	3.77	19.2	4.38	24.2	4.92	29.2	5.40	34.2	5.85	39.2	6.26	44.2	6.65	49.2	7.01
4.4	2.10	9.4	3.07	14.4	3.79	19.4	4.40	24.4	4.94	29.4	5.42	34.4	5.87	39.4	6.28	44.4	6.66	49.4	7.03
4.6	2.14	9.6	3.10	14.6	3.82	19.6	4.43	24.6	4.96	29.6	5.44	34.6	5.88	39.6	6.29	44.6	6.88	49.6	7.04
4.8	2.19	9.8	3.13	14.8	3.85	19.8	4.45	24.8	4.98	29.8	5.46	34.8	5.90	39.8	6.31	44.8	6.69	49.8	7.06
5.0	2.24	10.0	3.16	15.0	3.87	20.0	4.47	25.0	5.00	30.0	5.48	35.0	5.92	40.0	6.32	45.0	6.71	50.0	7.07
5.2	2.28	10.2	3.19	15.2	3.90	20.2	4.49	25.2	5.02	30.2	5.50	35.2	5.93	40.2	6.34	45.2	6.72	50.2	7.09
5.4	2.32	10.4	3.22	15.4	3.92	20.4	4.52	25.4	5.04	30.4	5.51	35.4	5.95	40.4	6.36	45.4	6.74	50.4	7.10
5.6	2.37	10.6	3.26	15.6	3.95	20.6	4.54	25.6	5.06	30.6	5.53	35.6	5.97	40.6	6.37	45.6	6.75	50.6	7.11
5.8	2.41	10.8	3.29	15.8	3.97	20.8	4.56	25.8	5.08	30.8	5.55	35.8	5.98	40.8	6.39	45.8	6.77	50.8	7.13

n	$\sqrt{n}$	n	$\sqrt{n}$	n	$\sqrt{n}$	n	$\sqrt{n}$	n	$\sqrt{n}$	n	$\sqrt{n}$	n	$\sqrt{n}$	n	$\sqrt{n}$	n	$\sqrt{n}$	n	$\sqrt{n}$
51.0	7.14	56.0	7.48	61.0	7.81	66.0	8.12	71.0	8.43	76.0	8.72	81.0	9.00	86.0	9.27	91.0	9.54	96.0	9.80
51.2	7.16	56.2	7.50	61.2	7.82	66.2	8.14	71.2	8.44	76.2	8.73	81.2	9.01	86.2	9.28	91.2	9.55	96.2	9.81
51.4	7.17	56.4	7.51	61.4	7.84	66.4	8.15	71.4	8.45	76.4	8.74	81.4	9.02	86.4	9.30	91.4	9.56	96.4	9.82
51.6	7.18	56.6	7.52	61.6	7.85	66.6	8.16	71.6	8.46	76.6	8.75	81.6	9.03	86.6	9.31	91.6	9.57	96.6	9.83
51.8	7.20	56.8	7.54	61.8	7.86	66.8	8.17	71.8	8.47	76.8	8.76	81.8	9.04	86.8	9.32	91.8	9.58	96.8	9.84
52.0	7.21	57.0	7.55	62.0	7.87	67.0	8.19	72.0	8.49	77.0	8.77	82.0	9.06	87.0	9.33	92.0	9.59	97.0	9.85
52.2	7.22	57.2	7.56	62.2	7.89	67.2	8.20	72.2	8.50	77.2	8.79	82.2	9.07	87.2	9.34	92.2	9.60	97.2	9.86
52.4	7.24	57.4	7.58	62.4	7.90	67.4	8.21	72.4	8.51	77.4	8.80	82.4	9.08	87.4	9.35	92.4	9.61	97.4	9.87
52.6	7.25	57.6	7.59	62.6	7.91	67.6	8.22	72.6	8.52	77.6	8.81	82.6	9.09	87.6	9.36	92.6	9.62	97.6	9.88
52.8	7.27	57.8	7.60	62.8	7.92	67.8	8.23	72.8	8.53	77.8	8.82	82.8	9.10	87.8	9.37	92.8	9.63	97.8	9.89
53.0	7.28	58.0	7.62	63.0	7.94	68.0	8.25	73.0	8.54	78.0	8.83	83.0	9.11	88.0	9.38	93.0	9.64	98.0	9.90
53.2	7.29	58.2	7.63	63.2	6.95	68.2	8.26	73.2	8.56	78.2	8.84	83.2	9.12	88,2	9.39	93.2	9.65	98.2	9.91
53.4	7.31	58.4	7.64	63.4	7.96	68.4	8.27	73.4	8.57	78.4	8.85	83.4	9.13	88.4	9.40	93.4	9.66	98.4	9.92
53.6	7.32	58.6	7.66	63.6	7.97	68.6	8.28	73.6	8.58	78.6	8.87	83.6	9.14	88.6	9.41	93.6	9.67	98.6	9.93
53.8	7.33	58.8	7.67	63.8	7.99	68.8	8.29	73.8	8.59	78.8	8.88	83.8	9.15	88.8	9.42	93.8	9.68	98.8	9.94
54.0	7.35	59.0	7.68	64.0	8.00	69.0	8.31	74.0	8.60	79.0	8.89	84.0	9.17	89.0	9.43	94.0	9.70	99.0	9.95
54.2	7.36	59.2	7.69	64.2	8.01	69.2	8.32	74.2	8.61	79.2	8.90	84.2	9.18	89.2	9.44	94.2	9.71	99.2	9.96
54.4	7.38	59.4	7.71	64.4	8.02	69.4	8.33	74.4	8.63	79.4	8.91	84.4	9.19	89.4	9.46	94.4	9.72	99.4	9.97
54.6	7.39	59.6	7.72	64.6	8.04	69.6	8.34	74.6	8.64	79.6	8.92	84.6	9.20	89.6	9.47	94.6	9.73	99.6	9.98
54.8	7.40	59.8	7.73	64.8	8.05	69.8	8.35	74.8	8.65	79.8	8.93	84.8	9.21	89.8	9.48	94.8	9.74	99.8	9.99
55.0	7.42	60.0	7.75	65.0	8.06	70.0	8.37	75.0	8.66	80.0	8.94	85.0	9.22	90.0	9.49	95.0	9.75	100.0	10.00
55.2	7.43	60.2	7.76	65.2	8.07	70.2	8.38	75.2	8.67	80.2	8.96	85.2	9.23	90.2	9.50	95.2	9.76		
55.4	7.44	60.4	7.77	65.4	8.09	70.4	8.39	75.4	8.68	80.4	8.97	85.4	9.24	90.4	9.51	95.4	9.77		
55.6	7.46	60.6	7.78	65.6	8.10	70.6	8.40	75.6	8.69	80.6	8.98	85.6	9.25	90.6	9.52	95.6	9.78		
55.8	7.47	60.8	7.80	65.8	8.11	70.8	8.41	75.8	8.71	80.8	8.99	85.8	9.26	90.8	9.53	95.8	9.79		

*From Dharan, M.: Total quality control in the clinical laboratory, St. Louis, 1977, The C. V. Mosby Co.

Appendix B: Four-place logarithms*

											Proportional parts								
N	**0**	**1**	**2**	**3**	**4**	**5**	**6**	**7**	**8**	**9**	**1**	**2**	**3**	**4**	**5**	**6**	**7**	**8**	**9**
10	0000	0043	0086	0128	0170	0212	0253	0294	0334	0374	4†	8	12	17	21	25	29	33	37
11	0414	0453	0492	0531	0569	0607	0645	0682	0719	0755	4	8	11	15	19	23	26	30	34
12	0792	0828	0864	0899	0934	0969	1004	1038	1072	1106	3	7	10	14	17	21	24	28	31
13	1139	1173	1206	1239	1271	1303	1335	1367	1399	1430	3	6	10	13	16	19	23	26	29
14	1461	1492	1523	1553	1584	1614	1644	1673	1703	1732	3	6	9	12	15	18	21	24	27
15	1761	1790	1818	1847	1875	1903	1931	1959	1987	2014	3†	6	8	11	14	17	20	22	25
16	2041	2068	2095	2122	2148	2175	2201	2227	2253	2279	3	5	8	11	13	16	18	21	24
17	2304	2330	2355	2380	2405	2430	2455	2480	2504	2529	2	5	7	10	12	15	17	20	22
18	2553	2577	2601	2625	2648	2672	2695	2718	2742	2765	2	5	7	9	12	14	16	19	21
19	2788	2810	2833	2856	2878	2900	2923	2945	2967	2989	2	4	7	9	11	13	16	18	20
20	3010	3032	3054	3075	3096	3118	3139	3160	3181	3201	2	4	6	8	11	13	15	17	19
21	3222	3243	3263	3284	3304	3324	3345	3365	3385	3404	2	4	6	8	10	12	14	16	18
22	3424	3444	3464	3483	3502	3522	3541	3560	3579	3598	2	4	6	8	10	12	14	15	17
23	3617	3636	3655	3674	3692	3711	3729	3747	3766	3784	2	4	6	7	9	11	13	15	17
24	3802	3820	3838	3856	3874	3892	3909	3927	3945	3962	2	4	5	7	9	11	12	14	16
25	3979	3997	4014	4031	4048	4065	4082	4099	4116	4133	2	3	5	7	9	10	12	14	15
26	4150	4166	4183	4200	4216	4232	4249	4265	4281	4298	2	3	5	7	8	10	11	13	15
27	4314	4330	4346	4362	4378	4393	4409	4425	4440	4456	2	3	5	6	8	9	11	13	14
28	4472	4487	4502	4518	4533	4548	4564	4579	4594	4609	2	3	5	6	8	9	11	12	14
29	4624	4639	4654	4669	4683	4698	4713	4728	4742	4757	1	3	4	6	7	9	10	12	13
30	4771	4786	4800	4814	4829	4843	4857	4871	4886	4900	1	3	4	6	7	9	10	11	13
31	4914	4928	4942	4955	4969	4983	4997	5011	5024	5038	1	3	4	6	7	8	10	11	12
32	5051	5065	5079	5092	5105	5119	5132	5145	5159	5172	1	3	4	5	7	8	9	11	12
33	5185	5198	5211	5224	5237	5250	5263	5276	5289	5302	1	3	4	5	6	8	9	10	12
34	5315	5328	5340	5353	5366	5378	5391	5403	5416	5428	1	3	4	5	6	8	9	10	11
35	5441	5453	5465	5478	5490	5502	5514	5527	5539	5551	1	2	4	5	6	7	9	10	11
36	5563	5575	5587	5599	5611	5623	5635	5647	5658	5670	1	2	4	5	6	7	8	10	11
37	5682	5694	5705	5717	5729	5740	5752	5763	5775	5786	1	2	3	5	6	7	8	9	10
38	5798	5809	5821	5832	5843	5855	5866	5877	5888	5899	1	2	3	5	6	7	8	9	10
39	5911	5922	5933	5944	5955	5966	5977	5988	5999	6010	1	2	3	4	5	7	8	9	10
40	6021	6031	6042	6053	6064	6075	6085	6096	6107	6117	1	2	3	4	5	6	8	9	10
41	6128	6138	6149	6160	6170	6180	6191	6201	6212	6222	1	2	3	4	5	6	7	8	9
42	6232	6243	6253	6263	6274	6284	6294	6304	6314	6325	1	2	3	4	5	6	7	8	9
43	6335	6345	6355	6365	6375	6385	6395	6405	6415	6425	1	2	3	4	5	6	7	8	9
44	6435	6444	6454	6464	6474	6484	6493	6503	6513	6522	1	2	3	4	5	6	7	8	9
45	6532	6542	6551	6561	6571	6580	6590	6599	6609	6618	1	2	3	4	5	6	7	8	9
46	6628	6637	6646	6656	6665	6675	6684	6693	6702	6712	1	2	3	4	5	6	7	7	8
47	6721	6730	6739	6749	6758	6767	6776	6785	6794	6803	1	2	3	4	5	5	6	7	8
48	6812	6821	6830	6839	6848	6857	6866	6875	6884	6893	1	2	3	4	4	5	6	7	8
49	6902	6911	6920	6928	6937	6946	6955	6964	6972	6981	1	2	3	4	4	5	6	7	8
50	6990	6998	7007	7016	7024	7033	7042	7050	7059	7067	1	2	3	3	4	5	6	7	8
51	7076	7084	7093	7101	7110	7118	7126	7135	7143	7152	1	2	3	3	4	5	6	7	8
52	7160	7168	7177	7185	7193	7202	7210	7218	7226	7235	1	2	2	3	4	5	6	7	7
53	7243	7251	7259	7267	7275	7284	7292	7300	7308	7316	1	2	2	3	4	5	6	6	7
54	7324	7332	7340	7348	7356	7364	7372	7380	7388	7396	1	2	2	3	4	5	6	6	7
N	**0**	**1**	**2**	**3**	**4**	**5**	**6**	**7**	**8**	**9**	**1**	**2**	**3**	**4**	**5**	**6**	**7**	**8**	**9**

*From Handbook of chemistry and physics, ed. 61, Weast, R. C., editor, 1980. Used by permission of CRC Press, Inc.
†Interpolation in this section of the table is inaccurate.

N	0	1	2	3	4	5	6	7	8	9	Proportional parts								
											1	2	3	4	5	6	7	8	9
55	7404	7412	7419	7427	7435	7443	7451	7459	7466	7474	1	2	2	3	4	5	5	6	7
56	7482	7490	7497	7505	7513	7520	7528	7536	7543	7551	1	2	2	3	4	5	5	6	7
57	7559	7566	7574	7582	7589	7597	7604	7612	7619	7627	1	2	2	3	4	5	5	6	7
58	7634	7642	7649	7657	7664	7672	7679	7686	7694	7701	1	1	2	3	4	4	5	6	7
59	7709	7716	7723	7731	7738	7745	7752	7760	7767	7774	1	1	2	3	4	4	5	6	7
60	7782	7789	7796	7803	7810	7818	7825	7832	7839	7846	1	1	2	3	4	4	5	6	6
61	7853	7860	7868	7875	7882	7889	7896	7903	7910	7917	1	1	2	3	4	4	5	6	6
62	7924	7931	7938	7945	7952	7959	7966	7973	7980	7987	1	1	2	3	3	4	5	6	6
63	7993	8000	8007	8014	8021	8028	8035	8041	8048	8055	1	1	2	3	3	4	5	5	6
64	8062	8069	8075	8082	8089	8096	8102	8109	8116	8122	1	1	2	3	3	4	5	5	6
65	8129	8136	8142	8149	8156	8162	8169	8176	8182	8189	1	1	2	3	3	4	5	5	6
66	8195	8202	8209	8215	8222	8228	8235	8241	8248	8254	1	1	2	3	3	4	5	5	6
67	8261	8267	8274	8280	8287	8293	8299	8306	8312	8319	1	1	2	3	3	4	5	5	6
68	8325	8331	8338	8344	8351	8357	8363	8370	8376	8382	1	1	2	3	3	4	4	5	6
69	8388	8395	8401	8407	8414	8420	8426	8432	8439	8445	1	1	2	2	3	4	4	5	6
70	8451	8457	8463	8470	8476	8482	8488	8494	8500	8506	1	1	2	2	3	4	4	5	6
71	8513	8519	8525	8531	8537	8543	8549	8555	8561	8567	1	1	2	2	3	4	4	5	5
72	8573	8579	8585	8591	8597	8603	8609	8615	8621	8627	1	1	2	2	3	4	4	5	5
73	8633	8639	8645	8651	8657	8663	8669	8675	8681	8686	1	1	2	2	3	4	4	5	5
74	8692	8698	8704	8710	8716	8722	8727	8733	8739	8745	1	1	2	2	3	4	4	5	5
75	8751	8756	8762	8768	8774	8779	8785	8791	8797	8802	1	1	2	2	3	3	4	5	5
76	8808	8814	8820	8825	8831	8837	8842	8848	8854	8859	1	1	2	2	3	3	4	5	5
77	8865	8871	8876	8882	8887	8893	8899	8904	8910	8915	1	1	2	2	3	3	4	4	5
78	8921	8927	8932	8938	8943	8949	8954	8960	8965	8971	1	1	2	2	3	3	4	4	5
79	8976	8982	8987	8993	8998	9004	9009	9015	9020	9025	1	1	2	2	3	3	4	4	5
80	9031	9036	9042	9047	9053	9058	9063	9069	9074	9079	1	1	2	2	3	3	4	4	5
81	9085	9090	9096	9101	9106	9112	9117	9122	9128	9133	1	1	2	2	3	3	4	4	5
82	9138	9143	9149	9154	9159	9165	9170	9175	9180	9186	1	1	2	2	3	3	4	4	5
83	9191	9196	9201	9206	9212	9217	9222	9227	9232	9238	1	1	2	2	3	3	4	4	5
84	9243	9248	9253	9258	9263	9269	9274	9279	9284	9289	1	1	2	2	3	3	4	4	5
85	9294	9299	9304	9309	9315	9320	9325	9330	9335	9340	1	1	2	2	3	3	4	4	5
86	9345	9350	9355	9360	9365	9370	9375	9380	9385	9390	1	1	2	2	3	3	4	4	5
87	9395	9400	9405	9410	9415	9420	9425	9430	9435	9440	0	1	1	2	2	3	3	4	4
88	9445	9450	9455	9460	9465	9469	9474	9479	9484	9489	0	1	1	2	2	3	3	4	4
89	9494	9499	9504	9509	9513	9518	9523	9528	9533	9538	0	1	1	2	2	3	3	4	4
90	9542	9547	9552	9557	9562	9566	9571	9576	9581	9586	0	1	1	2	2	3	3	4	4
91	9590	9595	9600	9605	9609	9614	9619	9624	9628	9633	0	1	1	2	2	3	3	4	4
92	9638	9643	9647	9652	9657	9661	9666	9671	9675	9680	0	1	1	2	2	3	3	4	4
93	9685	9689	9694	9699	9703	9708	9713	9717	9722	9727	0	1	1	2	2	3	3	4	4
94	9731	9736	9741	9745	9750	9754	9759	9763	9768	9773	0	1	1	2	2	3	3	4	4
95	9777	9782	9786	9791	9795	9800	9805	9809	9814	9818	0	1	1	2	2	3	3	4	4
96	9823	9827	9832	9836	9841	9845	9850	9854	9859	9863	0	1	1	2	2	3	3	4	4
97	9868	9872	9877	9881	9886	9890	9894	9899	9903	9908	0	1	1	2	2	3	3	4	4
98	9912	9917	9921	9926	9930	9934	9939	9943	9948	9952	0	1	1	2	2	3	3	4	4
99	9956	9961	9965	9969	9974	9978	9983	9987	9991	9996	0	1	1	2	2	3	3	3	4
N	0	1	2	3	4	5	6	7	8	9	1	2	3	4	5	6	7	8	9

Appendix C: Table of exponential functions*

Values of e^x, $\log e^x$ and e^{-x} where e is the base of the natural system of logarithms 2.71828 . . . and x has values from 0 to 10. Facilitating the solution of exponential equations, these tables also serve as a table of natural or naperian antilogarithms. For instance, if the logarithm or exponent $x = 3.26$, the corresponding number or value of e^x is 26.050. Its reciprocal e^{-x} is .038388.

x	e^x	$\log_{10}(e^x)$	e^{-x}	x	e^x	$\log_{10}(e^x)$	e^{-x}
0.00	1.0000	0.00000	1.000000	**0.50**	1.6487	0.21715	0.606531
0.01	1.0101	.00434	0.990050	0.51	1.6653	.22149	.600496
0.02	1.0202	.00869	.980199	0.52	1.6820	.22583	.594521
0.03	1.0305	.01303	.970446	0.53	1.6989	.23018	.588605
0.04	1.0408	.01737	.960789	0.54	1.7160	.23452	.582748
0.05	1.0513	0.02171	0.951229	**0.55**	1.7333	0.23886	0.576950
0.06	1.0618	.02606	.941765	0.56	1.7507	.24320	.571209
0.07	1.0725	.03040	.932394	0.57	1.7683	.24755	.565525
0.08	1.0833	.03474	.923116	0.58	1.7860	.25189	.559898
0.09	1.0942	.03909	.913931	0.59	1.8040	.25623	.554327
0.10	1.1052	0.04343	0.904837	**0.60**	1.8221	0.26058	0.548812
0.11	1.1163	.04777	.895834	0.61	1.8404	.26492	.543351
0.12	1.1275	.05212	.886920	0.62	1.8589	.26926	.537944
0.13	1.1388	.05646	.878095	0.63	1.8776	.27361	.532592
0.14	1.1503	.06080	.869358	0.64	1.8965	.27795	.527292
0.15	1.1618	0.06514	0.860708	**0.65**	1.9155	0.28229	0.522046
0.16	1.1735	.06949	.852144	0.66	1.9348	.28663	.516851
0.17	1.1853	.07383	.843665	0.67	1.9542	.29098	.511709
0.18	1.1972	.07817	.835270	0.68	1.9739	.29532	.506617
0.19	1.2092	.08252	.826959	0.69	1.9937	.29966	.501576
0.20	1.2214	0.08686	0.818731	**0.70**	2.0138	0.30401	0.496585
0.21	1.2337	09120	.810584	0.71	2.0340	.30835	.491644
0.22	1.2461	.09554	.802519	0.72	2.0544	.31269	.486752
0.23	1.2586	.09989	.794534	0.73	2.0751	.31703	.481909
0.24	1.2712	.10423	.786628	0.74	2.0959	.32138	.477114
0.25	1.2840	0.10857	0.778801	**0.75**	2.1170	0.32572	0.472367
0.26	1.2969	.11292	.771052	0.76	2.1383	.33006	.467666
0.27	1.3100	.11726	.763379	0.77	2.1598	.33441	.463013
0.28	1.3231	.12160	.755784	0.78	2.1815	.33875	.458406
0.29	1.3364	.12595	.748264	0.79	2.2034	.34309	.453845
0.30	1.3499	0.13029	0.740818	**0.80**	2.2255	0.34744	0.449329
0.31	1.3634	.13463	.733447	0.81	2.2479	.35178	.444858
0.32	1.3771	.13897	.726149	0.82	2.2705	.35612	.440432
0.33	1.3910	.14332	.718924	0.83	2.2933	.36046	.436049
0.34	1.4049	.14766	.711770	0.84	2.3164	.36481	.431711
0.35	1.4191	0.15200	0.704688	**0.85**	2.3396	0.36915	0.427415
0.36	1.4333	.15635	.697676	0.86	2.3632	.37349	.423162
0.37	1.4477	.16069	.690734	0.87	2.3869	.37784	.418952
0.38	1.4623	.16503	.683861	0.88	2.4109	.38218	.414783
0.39	1.4770	.16937	.677057	0.89	2.4351	.38652	.410656
0.40	1.4918	0.17372	0.670320	**0.90**	2.4596	0.39087	0.406570
0.41	1.5068	.17806	.663650	0.91	2.4843	.39521	.402524
0.42	1.5220	.18240	.657047	0.92	2.5093	.39955	.398519
0.43	1.5373	.18675	.650509	0.93	2.5345	.40389	.394554
0.44	1.5527	.19109	.644036	0.94	2.5600	.40824	.390628
0.45	1.5683	0.19543	0.637628	**0.95**	2.5857	0.41258	0.386741
0.46	1.5841	.19978	.631284	0.96	2.6117	.41692	.382893
0.47	1.6000	.20412	.625002	0.97	2.6379	.42127	.379083
0.48	1.6161	.20846	.618783	0.98	2.6645	.42561	.375311
0.49	1.6323	.21280	.612626	0.99	2.6912	.42995	.371577
0.50	1.6487	0.21715	0.606531	**1.00**	2.7183	0.43429	0.367879

Exponential functions—cont'd

x	e^x	$\log_{10}(e^x)$	e^{-x}	x	e^x	$\log_{10}(e^x)$	e^{-x}
1.00	2.7183	0.43429	0.367879	**1.50**	4.4817	0.65144	0.223130
1.01	2.7456	.43864	.364219	1.51	4.5267	.65578	.220910
1.02	2.7732	.44298	.360595	1.52	4.5722	.66013	.218712
1.03	2.8011	.44732	.357007	1.53	4.6182	.66447	.216536
1.04	2.8292	.45167	.353455	1.54	4.6646	.66881	.214381
1.05	2.8577	0.45601	0.349938	**1.55**	4.7115	0.67316	0.212248
1.06	2.8864	.46035	.346456	1.56	4.7588	.67750	.210136
1.07	2.9154	.46470	.343009	1.57	4.8066	.68184	.208045
1.08	2.9447	.46904	.339596	1.58	4.8550	.68619	.205975
1.09	2.9743	.47338	.336216	1.59	4.9037	.69053	.203926
1.10	3.0042	0.47772	0.332871	**1.60**	4.9530	0.69487	0.201897
1.11	3.0344	.48207	.329559	1.61	5.0028	.69921	.199888
1.12	3.0649	.48641	.326280	1.62	5.0531	.70356	.197899
1.13	3.0957	.49075	.323033	1.63	5.1039	.70790	.195930
1.14	3.1268	.49510	.319819	1.64	5.1552	.71224	.193980
1.15	3.1582	0.49944	0.316637	**1.65**	5.2070	0.71659	0.192050
1.16	3.1899	.50378	.313486	1.66	5.2593	.72093	.190139
1.17	3.2220	.50812	.310367	1.67	5.3122	.72527	.188247
1.18	3.2544	.51247	.307279	1.68	5.3656	.72961	.186374
1.19	3.2871	.51681	.304221	1.69	5.4195	.73396	.184520
1.20	3.3201	0.52115	0.301194	**1.70**	5.4739	0.73830	0.182684
1.21	3.3535	.52550	.298197	1.71	5.5290	.74264	.180866
1.22	3.3872	.52984	.295230	1.72	5.5845	.74699	.179066
1.23	3.4212	.53418	.292293	1.73	5.6407	.75133	.177284
1.24	3.4556	.53853	.289384	1.74	5.6973	.75567	.175520
1.25	3.4903	0.54287	0.286505	**1.75**	5.7546	0.76002	0.173774
1.26	3.5254	.54721	.283654	1.76	5.8124	.76436	.172045
1.27	3.5609	.55155	.280832	1.77	5.8709	.76870	.170333
1.28	3.5966	.55590	.278037	1.78	5.9299	.77304	.168638
1.29	3.6328	.56024	.275271	1.79	5.9895	.77739	.166960
1.30	3.6693	0.56458	0.272532	**1.80**	6.0496	0.78173	0.165299
1.31	3.7062	.56893	.269820	1.81	6.1104	.78607	.163654
1.32	3.7434	.57327	.267135	1.82	6.1719	.79042	.162026
1.33	3.7810	.57761	.264477	1.83	6.2339	.79476	.160414
1.34	3.8190	.58195	.261846	1.84	6.2965	.79910	.158817
1.35	3.8574	0.58630	0.259240	**1.85**	6.3598	0.80344	0.157237
1.36	3.8962	.59064	.256661	1.86	6.4237	.80779	.155673
1.37	3.9354	.59498	.254107	1.87	6.4883	.81213	.154124
1.38	3.9749	.59933	.251579	1.88	6.5535	.81647	.152590
1.39	4.0149	.60367	.249075	1.89	6.6194	.82082	.151072
1.40	4.0552	0.60801	0.246597	**1.90**	6.6859	0.82516	0.149569
1.41	4.0960	.61236	.244143	1.91	6.7531	.82950	.148080
1.42	4.1371	.61670	.241714	1.92	6.8210	.83385	.146607
1.43	4.1787	.62104	.239309	1.93	6.8895	.83819	.145148
1.44	4.2207	.62538	.236928	1.94	6.9588	.84253	.143704
1.45	4.2631	0.62973	0.234570	**1.95**	7.0287	0.84687	0.142274
1.46	4.3060	.63407	.232236	1.96	7.0993	.85122	.140858
1.47	4.3492	.63841	.229925	1.97	7.1707	.85556	.139457
1.48	4.3929	.64276	.227638	1.98	7.2427	.85990	.138069
1.49	4.4371	.64710	.225373	1.99	7.3155	.86425	.136695
1.50	4.4817	0.65144	0.223130	**2.00**	7.3891	0.86859	0.135335

Continued.

Exponential functions—cont'd

x	e^x	$\log_{10}(e^x)$	e^{-x}	x	e^x	$\log_{10}(e^x)$	e^{-x}
2.00	7.3891	0.86859	0.135335	**2.50**	12.182	1.08574	0.082085
2.01	7.4633	.87293	.133989	2.51	12.305	1.09008	.081268
2.02	7.5383	.87727	.132655	2.52	12.429	1.09442	.080460
2.03	7.6141	.88162	.131336	2.53	12.554	1.09877	.079659
2.04	7.6906	.88596	.130029	2.54	12.680	1.10311	.078866
2.05	7.7679	0.89030	0.128735	**2.55**	12.807	1.10745	0.078082
2.06	7.8460	.89465	.127454	2.56	12.936	1.11179	.077305
2.07	7.9248	.89899	.126186	2.57	13.066	1.11614	.076536
2.08	8.0045	.90333	.124930	2.58	13.197	1.12048	.075774
2.09	8.0849	.90768	.123687	2.59	13.330	1.12482	.075020
2.10	8.1662	0.91202	0.122456	**2.60**	13.464	1.12917	0.074274
2.11	8.2482	.91636	.121238	2.61	13.599	1.13351	.073535
2.12	8.3311	.92070	.120032	2.62	13.736	1.13785	.072803
2.13	8.4149	.92505	.118837	2.63	13.874	1.14219	.072078
2.14	8.4994	.92939	.117655	2.64	14.013	1.14654	.071361
2.15	8.5849	0.93373	0.116484	**2.65**	14.154	1.15088	0.070651
2.16	8.6711	.93808	.115325	2.66	14.296	1.15522	.069948
2.17	8.7583	.94242	.114178	2.67	14.440	1.15957	.069252
2.18	8.8463	.94676	.113042	2.68	14.585	1.16391	.068563
2.19	8.9352	.95110	.111917	2.69	14.732	1.16825	.067881
2.20	9.0250	0.95545	0.110803	**2.70**	14.880	1.17260	0.067206
2.21	9.1157	.95979	.109701	2.71	15.029	1.17694	.066537
2.22	9.2073	.96413	.108609	2.72	15.180	1.18128	.065875
2.23	9.2999	.96848	.107528	2.73	15.333	1.18562	.065219
2.24	9.3933	.97282	.106459	2.74	15.487	1.18997	.064570
2.25	9.4877	0.97716	0.105399	**2.75**	15.643	1.19431	0.063928
2.26	9.5831	.98151	.104350	2.76	15.800	1.19865	.063292
2.27	9.6794	.98585	.103312	2.77	15.959	1.20300	.062662
2.28	9.7767	.99019	.102284	2.78	16.119	1.20734	.062039
2.29	9.8749	.99453	.101266	2.79	16.281	1.21168	.061421
2.30	9.9742	0.99888	0.100259	**2.80**	16.445	1.21602	0.060810
2.31	10.074	1.00322	.099261	2.81	16.610	1.22037	.060205
2.32	10.176	1.00756	.098274	2.82	16.777	1.22471	.059606
2.33	10.278	1.01191	.097296	2.83	16.945	1.22905	.059013
2.34	10.381	1.01625	.096328	2.84	17.116	1.23340	.058426
2.35	10.486	1.02059	0.095369	**2.85**	17.288	1.23774	0.057844
2.36	10.591	1.02493	.094420	2.86	17.462	1.24208	.057269
2.37	10.697	1.02928	.093481	2.87	17.637	1.24643	.056699
2.38	10.805	1.03362	.092551	2.88	17.814	1.25077	.056135
2.39	10.913	1.03796	.091630	2.89	17.993	1.25511	.055576
2.40	11.023	1.04231	0.090718	**2.90**	18.174	1.25945	0.055023
2.41	11.134	1.04665	.089815	2.91	18.357	1.26380	.054476
2.42	11.246	1.05099	.088922	2.92	18.541	1.26814	.053934
2.43	11.359	1.05534	.088037	2.93	18.728	1.27248	.053397
2.44	11.473	1.05968	.087161	2.94	18.916	1.27683	.052866
2.45	11.588	1.06402	0.086294	**2.95**	19.106	1.28117	0.052340
2.46	11.705	1.06836	.085435	2.96	19.298	1.28551	.051819
2.47	11.822	1.07271	.084585	2.97	19.492	1.28985	.051303
2.48	11.941	1.07705	.083743	2.98	19.688	1.29420	.050793
2.49	12.061	1.08139	.082910	2.99	19.886	1.29854	.050287
2.50	12.182	1.08574	0.082085	**3.00**	20.086	1.30288	0.049787

Exponential functions—cont'd

x	e^x	$\log_{10}(e^x)$	e^{-x}	x	e^x	$\log_{10}(e^x)$	e^{-x}
3.00	20.086	1.30288	0.049787	**3.50**	33.115	1.52003	0.030197
3.01	20.287	1.30723	.049292	3.51	33.448	1.52437	.029897
3.02	20.491	1.31157	.048801	3.52	33.784	1.52872	.029599
3.03	20.697	1.31591	.048316	3.53	34.124	1.53306	.029305
3.04	20.905	1.32026	.047835	3.54	34.467	1.53740	.029013
3.05	21.115	1.32460	0.047359	**3.55**	34.813	1.54175	0.028725
3.06	21.328	1.32894	.046888	3.56	35.163	1.54609	.028439
3.07	21.542	1.33328	.046421	3.57	35.517	1.55043	.028156
3.08	21.758	1.33763	.045959	3.58	35.874	1.55477	.027876
3.09	21.977	1.34197	.045502	3.59	36.234	1.55912	.027598
3.10	22.198	1.34631	0.045049	**3.60**	36.598	1.56346	0.027324
3.11	22.421	1.35066	.044601	3.61	36.966	1.56780	.027052
3.12	22.646	1.35500	.044157	3.62	37.338	1.57215	.026783
3.13	22.874	1.35934	.043718	3.63	37.713	1.57649	.026516
3.14	23.104	1.36368	.043283	3.64	38.092	1.58083	.026252
3.15	23.336	1.36803	0.042852	**3.65**	38.475	1.58517	0.025991
3.16	23.571	1.37237	.042426	3.66	38.861	1.58952	.025733
3.17	23.807	1.37671	.042004	3.67	39.252	1.59386	.025476
3.18	24.047	1.38106	.041586	3.68	39.646	1.59820	.025223
3.19	24.288	1.38540	.041172	3.69	40.045	1.60255	.024972
3.20	24.533	1.38974	0.040762	**3.70**	40.447	1.60689	0.024724
3.21	24.779	1.39409	.040357	3.71	40.854	1.61123	.024478
3.22	25.028	1.39843	.039955	3.72	41.264	1.61558	.024234
3.23	25.280	1.40277	.039557	3.73	41.679	1.61992	.023993
3.24	25.534	1.40711	.039164	3.74	42.098	1.62426	.023754
3.25	25.790	1.41146	0.038774	**3.75**	42.521	1.62860	0.023518
3.26	26.050	1.41580	.038388	3.76	42.948	1.63295	.023284
3.27	26.311	1.42014	.038006	3.77	43.380	1.63729	.023052
3.28	26.576	1.42449	.037628	3.78	43.816	1.64163	.022823
3.29	26.843	1.42883	.037254	3.79	44.256	1.64598	.022596
3.30	27.113	1.43317	0.036883	**3.80**	44.701	1.65032	0.022371
3.31	27.385	1.43751	.036516	3.81	45.150	1.65466	.022148
3.32	27.660	1.44186	.036153	3.82	45.604	1.65900	.021928
3.33	27.938	1.44620	.035793	3.83	46.063	1.66335	.021710
3.34	28.219	1.45054	.035437	3.84	46.525	1.66769	.021494
3.35	28.503	1.45489	0.035084	**3.85**	46.993	1.67203	0.021280
3.36	28.789	1.45923	.034735	3.86	47.465	1.67638	.021068
3.37	29.079	1.46357	.034390	3.87	47.942	1.68072	.020858
3.38	29.371	1.46792	.034047	3.88	48.424	1.68506	.020651
3.39	29.666	1.47226	.033709	3.89	48.911	1.68941	.020445
3.40	29.964	1.47660	0.033373	**3.90**	49.402	1.69375	0.020242
3.41	30.265	1.48094	.033041	3.91	49.899	1.69809	.020041
3.42	30.569	1.48529	.032712	3.92	50.400	1.70243	.019841
3.43	30.877	1.48963	.032387	3.93	50.907	1.70678	.019644
3.44	31.187	1.49397	.032065	3.94	51.419	1.71112	.019448
3.45	31.500	1.49832	0.031746	**3.95**	51.935	1.71546	0.019255
3.46	31.817	1.50266	.031430	3.96	52.457	1.71981	.019063
3.47	32.137	1.50700	.031117	3.97	52.985	1.72415	.018873
3.48	32.460	1.51134	.030807	3.98	53.517	1.72849	.018686
3.49	32.786	1.51569	.030501	3.99	54.055	1.73283	.018500
3.50	33.115	1.52003	0.030197	**4.00**	54.598	1.73718	0.018316

Continued.

Exponential functions—cont'd

x	e^x	$\log_{10}(e^x)$	e^{-x}	x	e^x	$\log_{10}(e^x)$	e^{-x}
4.00	54.598	1.73718	0.018316	**4.50**	90.017	1.95433	0.011109
4.01	55.147	1.74152	.018133	4.51	90.922	1.95867	.010998
4.02	55.701	1.74586	.017953	4.52	91.836	1.96301	.010889
4.03	56.261	1.75021	.017774	4.53	92.759	1.96735	.010781
4.04	56.826	1.75455	.017597	4.54	93.691	1.97170	.010673
4.05	57.397	1.75889	0.017422	**4.55**	94.632	1.97604	0.010567
4.06	57.974	1.76324	.017249	4.56	95.583	1.98038	.010462
4.07	58.557	1.76758	.017077	4.57	96.544	1.98473	.010358
4.08	59.145	1.77192	.016907	4.58	97.514	1.98907	.010255
4.09	59.740	1.77626	.016739	4.59	98.494	1.99341	.010153
4.10	60.340	1.78061	0.016573	**4.60**	99.484	1.99775	0.010052
4.11	60.947	1.78495	.016408	4.61	100.48	2.00210	.009952
4.12	61.559	1.78929	.016245	4.62	101.49	2.00644	.009853
4.13	62.178	1.79364	.016083	4.63	102.51	2.01078	.009755
4.14	62.803	1.79798	.015923	4.64	103.54	2.01513	.009658
4.15	63.434	1.80232	0.015764	**4.65**	104.68	2.01947	0.009562
4.16	64.072	1.80667	.015608	4.66	105.64	2.02381	.009466
4.17	64.715	1.81101	.015452	4.67	106.70	2.02816	.009372
4.18	65.366	1.81535	.015299	4.68	107.77	2.03250	.009279
4.19	66.023	1.81969	.015146	4.69	108.85	2.03684	.009187
4.20	66.686	1.82404	0.014996	**4.70**	109.95	2.04118	0.009095
4.21	67.357	1.82838	.014846	4.71	111.05	2.04553	.009005
4.22	68.033	1.83272	.014699	4.72	112.17	2.04987	.008915
4.23	68.717	1.83707	.014552	4.73	113.30	2.05421	.008826
4.24	69.408	1.84141	.914408	4.74	114.43	2.05856	.008739
4.25	70.105	1.84575	0.014264	**4.75**	115.58	2.06290	0.008652
4.26	70.810	1.85009	.014122	4.76	116.75	2.06724	.008566
4.27	71.522	1.85444	.013982	4.77	117.92	2.07158	.008480
4.28	72.240	1.85878	.013843	4.78	119.10	2.07593	.008396
4.29	72.966	1.86312	.013705	4.79	120.30	2.08027	.008312
4.30	73.700	1.86747	0.013569	**4.80**	121.51	2.08461	0.008230
4.31	74.440	1.87181	.013434	4.81	122.73	2.08896	.008148
4.32	75.189	1.87615	.013300	4.82	123.97	2.09330	.008067
4.33	75.944	1.88050	.013168	4.83	125.21	2.09764	.007987
4.34	76.708	1.88484	.013037	4.84	126.47	2.10199	.007907
4.35	77.478	1.88918	0.012907	**4.85**	127.74	2.10633	0.007828
4.36	78.257	1.89352	.012778	4.86	129.02	2.11067	.007750
4.37	79.044	1.89787	.012651	4.87	130.32	2.11501	.007673
4.38	79.838	1.90221	.012525	4.88	131.63	2.11936	.007597
4.39	80.640	1.90655	.012401	4.89	132.95	2.12370	.007521
4.40	81.451	1.91090	0.012277	**4.90**	134.29	2.12804	0.007447
4.41	82.269	1.91524	.012155	4.91	135.64	2.13239	.007372
4.42	83.096	1.91958	.012034	4.92	137.00	2.13673	.007299
4.43	83.931	1.92392	.011914	4.93	138.38	2.14107	.007227
4.44	84.775	1.92827	.011796	4.94	139.77	2.14541	.007155
4.45	85.627	1.93261	0.011679	**4.95**	141.17	2.14976	0.007083
4.46	86.488	1.93695	.011562	4.96	142.59	2.15410	.007013
4.47	87.357	1.94130	.011447	4.97	144.03	2.15844	.006943
4.48	88.235	1.94564	.011333	4.98	145.47	2.16279	.006874
4.49	89.121	1.94998	.011221	4.99	146.94	2.16713	.006806
4.50	90.017	1.95433	0.011109	**5.00**	148.41	2.17147	0.006738

Exponential functions—cont'd

x	e^x	$\log_{10}(e^x)$	e^{-x}	x	e^x	$\log_{10}(e^x)$	e^{-x}
5.00	148.41	2.17147	0.006738	**5.50**	244.69	2.38862	0.0040868
5.01	149.90	2.17582	.006671	5.55	257.24	2.41033	.0038875
5.02	151.41	2.18016	.006605	5.60	270.43	2.43205	.0036979
5.03	152.93	2.18450	.006539	5.65	284.29	2.45376	.0035175
5.04	154.47	2.18884	.006474	5.70	298.87	2.47548	.0033460
5.05	156.02	2.19319	0.006409	**5.75**	314.19	2.49719	0.0031828
5.06	157.59	2.19753	.006346	5.80	330.30	2.51891	.0030276
5.07	159.17	2.20187	.006282	5.85	347.23	2.54062	.0028799
5.08	160.77	2.20622	.006220	5.90	365.04	2.56234	.0027394
5.09	162.39	2.21056	.006158	5.95	383.75	2.58405	.0026058
5.10	164.02	2.21490	0.006097	**6.00**	403.43	2.60577	0.0024788
5.11	165.67	2.21924	.006036	6.05	424.11	2.62748	.0023579
5.12	167.34	2.22359	.005976	6.10	445.86	2.64920	.0022429
5.13	169.02	2.22793	.005917	6.15	468.72	2.67091	.0021335
5.14	170.72	2.23227	.005858	6.20	492.75	2.69263	.0020294
5.15	172.43	2.23662	0.005799	**6.25**	518.01	2.71434	0.0019305
5.16	174.16	2.24096	.005742	6.30	544.57	2.73606	.0018363
5.17	175.91	2.24530	.005685	6.35	572.49	2.75777	.0017467
5.18	177.68	2.24965	.005628	6.40	601.85	2.77948	.0016616
5.19	179.47	2.25399	.005572	6.45	632.70	2.80120	.0015805
5.20	181.27	2.25833	0.005517	**6.50**	665.14	2.82291	0.0015034
5.21	183.09	2.26267	.005462	6.55	699.24	2.84463	.0014301
5.22	184.93	2.26702	.005407	6.60	735.10	2.86634	.0013604
5.23	186.79	2.27136	.005354	6.65	772.78	2.88806	.0012940
5.24	188.67	2.27570	.005300	6.70	812.41	2.90977	.0012309
5.25	190.57	2.28005	0.005248	**6.75**	854.06	2.93149	0.0011709
5.26	192.48	2.28439	.005195	6.80	897.85	2.95320	.0011138
5.27	194.42	2.28873	.005144	6.85	943.88	2.97492	.0010595
5.28	196.37	2.29307	.005092	6.90	992.27	2.99663	.0010078
5.29	198.34	2.29742	.005042	6.95	1043.1	3.01835	.0009586
5.30	200.34	2.30176	0.004992	**7.00**	1096.6	3.04006	0.0009119
5.31	202.35	2.30610	.004942	7.05	1152.9	3.06178	.0008674
5.32	204.38	2.31045	.004893	7.10	1212.0	3.08349	.0008251
5.33	206.44	2.31479	.004844	7.15	1274.1	3.10521	.0007849
5.34	208.51	2.31913	.004796	7.20	1339.4	3.12692	.0007466
5.35	210.61	2.32348	0.004748	**7.25**	1408.1	3.14863	0.0007102
5.36	212.72	2.32782	.004701	7.30	1480.3	3.17035	.0006755
5.37	214.86	2.33216	.004654	7.35	1556.2	3.19206	.0006426
5.38	217.02	2.33650	.004608	7.40	1636.0	3.21378	.0006113
5.39	219.20	2.34085	.004562	7.45	1719.9	3.23549	.0005814
5.40	221.41	2.34519	0.004517	**7.50**	1808.0	3.25721	0.0005531
5.41	223.63	2.34953	.004472	7.55	1900.7	3.27892	.0005261
5.42	225.88	2.35388	.004427	7.60	1998.2	3.30064	.0005005
5.43	228.15	2.35822	.004383	7.65	2100.6	3.32235	.0004760
5.44	230.44	2.36256	.004339	7.70	2208.3	3.34407	.0004528
5.45	232.76	2.36690	0.004296	**7.75**	2321.6	3.36578	0.0004307
5.46	235.10	2.37125	.004254	7.80	2440.6	3.38750	.0004097
5.47	237.46	2.37559	.004211	7.85	2565.7	3.40921	.0003898
5.48	239.85	2.37993	.004169	7.90	2697.3	3.43093	.0003707
5.49	242.26	2.38428	.004128	7.95	2835.6	3.45264	.0003527
5.50	244.69	2.38862	0.004087	**8.00**	2981.0	3.47436	0.0003355

Continued.

Exponential functions—cont'd

x	e^x	$\log_{10}(e^x)$	e^{-x}
8.00	2981.0	3.47436	0.0003355
8.05	3133.8	3.49607	.0003191
8.10	3294.5	3.51779	.0003035
8.15	3463.4	3.53950	.0002887
8.20	3641.0	3.56121	.0002747
8.25	3827.6	3.58293	0.0002613
8.30	4023.9	3.60464	.0002485
8.35	4230.2	3.62636	.0002364
8.40	4447.1	3.64807	0002249
8.45	4675.1	3.66979	.0002139
8.50	4914.8	3.69150	0.0002035
8.55	5166.8	3.71322	.0001935
8.60	5431.7	3.73493	.0001841
8.65	5710.1	3.75665	.0001751
8.70	6002.9	3.77836	.0001666
8.75	6310.7	3.80008	0.0001585
8.80	6634.2	3.82179	.0001507
8.85	6974.4	3.84351	.0001434
8.90	7332.0	3.86522	.0001364
8.95	7707.9	3.88694	.0001297
9.00	8103.1	3.90865	0.0001234
9.05	8518.5	3.93037	.0001174
9.10	8955.3	3.95208	.0001117
9.15	9414.4	3.97379	.0001062
9.20	9897.1	3.99551	.0001010
9.25	10405	4.01722	0.0000961
9.30	10938	4.03894	.0000914
9.35	11499	4.06065	.0000870
9.40	12088	4.08237	.0000827
9.45	12708	4.10408	.0000787
9.50	13360	4.12580	0.0000749
9.55	14045	4.14751	.0000712
9.60	14765	4.16923	.0000677
9.65	15522	4.19094	.0000644
9.70	16318	4.21266	.0000613
9.75	17154	4.23437	0.0000583
9.80	18034	4.25609	.0000555
9.85	18958	4.27780	.0000527
9.90	19930	4.29952	.0000502
9.95	20952	4.32123	0.0000477
10.00	22026	4.34294	0.0000454

Appendix D: Percentage points, chi-square distribution

$$F(\chi^2) = \int_0^{\chi^2} \frac{1}{2^{\frac{n}{2}}\,\Gamma\left(\frac{n}{2}\right)}\, x^{\frac{n-2}{2}}\, e^{-\frac{x}{2}}\, dx$$

n \ F	.005	.010	.025	.050	.100	.250	.500	.750	.900	.950	.975	.990	.995
1	.0000393	.000157	.000982	.00393	.0158	.102	.455	1.32	2.71	3.84	5.02	6.63	7.88
2	.0100	.0201	.0506	.103	.211	.575	1.39	2.77	4.61	5.99	7.38	9.21	10.6
3	.0717	.115	.216	.352	.584	1.21	2.37	4.11	6.25	7.81	9.35	11.3	12.8
4	.207	.297	.484	.711	1.06	1.92	3.36	5.39	7.78	9.49	11.1	13.3	14.9
5	.412	.554	.831	1.15	1.61	2.67	4.35	6.63	9.24	11.1	12.8	15.1	16.7
6	.676	.872	1.24	1.64	2.20	3.45	5.35	7.84	10.6	12.6	14.4	16.8	18.5
7	.989	1.24	1.69	2.17	2.83	4.25	6.35	9.04	12.0	14.1	16.0	18.5	20.3
8	1.34	1.65	2.18	2.73	3.49	5.07	7.34	10.2	13.4	15.5	17.5	20.1	22.0
9	1.73	2.09	2.70	3.33	4.17	5.90	8.34	11.4	14.7	16.9	19.0	21.7	23.6
10	2.16	2.56	3.25	3.94	4.87	6.74	9.34	12.5	16.0	18.3	20.5	23.2	25.2
11	2.60	3.05	3.82	4.57	5.58	7.58	10.3	13.7	17.3	19.7	21.9	24.7	26.8
12	3.07	3.57	4.40	5.23	6.30	8.44	11.3	14.8	18.5	21.0	23.3	26.2	28.3
13	3.57	4.11	5.01	5.89	7.04	9.30	12.3	16.0	19.8	22.4	24.7	27.7	29.8
14	4.07	4.66	5.63	6.57	7.79	10.2	13.3	17.1	21.1	23.7	26.1	29.1	31.3
15	4.60	5.23	6.26	7.26	8.55	11.0	14.3	18.2	22.3	25.0	27.5	30.6	32.8
16	5.14	5.81	6.91	7.96	9.31	11.9	15.3	19.4	23.5	26.3	28.8	32.0	34.3
17	5.70	6.41	7.56	8.67	10.1	12.8	16.3	20.5	24.8	27.6	30.2	33.4	35.7
18	6.26	7.01	8.23	9.39	10.9	13.7	17.3	21.6	26.0	28.9	31.5	34.8	37.2
19	6.84	7.63	8.91	10.1	11.7	14.6	18.3	22.7	27.2	30.1	32.9	36.2	38.6
20	7.43	8.26	9.59	10.9	12.4	15.5	19.3	23.8	28.4	31.4	34.2	37.6	40.0
21	8.03	8.90	10.3	11.6	13.2	16.3	20.3	24.9	29.6	32.7	35.5	38.9	41.4
22	8.64	9.54	11.0	12.3	14.0	17.2	21.3	26.0	30.8	33.9	36.8	40.3	42.8
23	9.26	10.2	11.7	13.1	14.8	18.1	22.3	27.1	32.0	35.2	38.1	41.6	44.2
24	9.89	10.9	12.4	13.8	15.7	19.0	23.3	28.2	33.2	36.4	39.4	43.0	45.6
25	10.5	11.5	13.1	14.6	16.5	19.9	24.3	29.3	34.4	37.7	40.6	44.3	46.9
26	11.2	12.2	13.8	15.4	17.3	20.8	25.3	30.4	35.6	38.9	41.9	45.6	48.3
27	11.8	12.9	14.6	16.2	18.1	21.7	26.3	31.5	36.7	40.1	43.2	47.0	49.6
28	12.5	13.6	15.3	16.9	18.9	22.7	27.3	32.6	37.9	41.3	44.5	48.3	51.0
29	13.1	14.3	16.0	17.7	19.8	23.6	28.3	33.7	39.1	42.6	45.7	49.6	52.3
30	13.8	15.0	16.8	18.5	20.6	24.5	29.3	34.8	40.3	43.8	47.0	50.9	53.7

*Reprinted with permission from Beyer, W. H., editor: CRC standard mathematical tables, ed. 25, Boca Raton, Florida, 1978. Copyright The Chemical Rubber Co., CRC Press, Inc.

Chapter 2

PHYSICS OF NUCLEAR MEDICINE

Glenn A. Isserstedt

The rudimentary substructure of contemporary nuclear physics was originally formed as a result of the attempt to learn of and understand the chemical properties of matter or the behavior of different atoms in their union and separation. Dalton's atomic theory developed around the laws of chemical combination and resulted in the concept of atomic weight. Subsequently, a combined ordering of the elements and their properties resulted in the periodic chart of the elements and the concepts of atomic number and structure. Interesting is the fact that many of the early investigators of physics and chemistry laboriously arrived at their conclusions, which many of us today take for granted, by deduction of empirical data and without the aid or assistance of sophisticated analytic instrumentation.

In 1803, John Dalton proposed an atomic theory of matter concerning atomic structure. This hypothesis was to account for scientific facts and observations relating to the laws of chemical combination: specifically, the constancy of weights in a chemical reaction as described by the law of conservation of matter, the combining weights of chemicals by the law of definite proportions, and the law of multiple proportions or the law of reciprocal proportions—both describing the quantitative relationship between combining elements. His was the first, though inaccurate, table of atomic weights.

Approximately 8 years later, Amedeo Avogadro suggested that there was a difference between atoms and molecules. Additionally, he suggested that the same number of molecules are contained in equal volumes of gases at the same temperature and pressure. The qualitative aspect of the number of molecules is the mole (gram molecular weight), and quantitatively it is equivalent of 6.025×10^{23} grams · mole^{-1}. His findings made it possible to develop a correct table of atomic weights. The interdigitated findings of other physicists resulted in the value of the electron as the unit of electric charge and thereby made it possible to quantify the number of atoms in a gram. The electrical force of the electron explained, along with the atomic number, the union and separation behavior of atoms.

The term "atom" was not original with Dalton or Avogadro but dates back to the early Greek philosophers. According to atomic theory, an atom is the smallest particle of matter that exhibits the characteristic chemical properties of an element, a collection of atoms of one type that cannot be decomposed (chemically) into simpler units but can, often spontaneously, change or be transformed into other elements by a radioactive process. Characterization of atoms is by physical properties such as nuclear charge (that is, atomic number), nuclear stability, and nuclear mass. Modern mass spectrographic analysis suggests that the nuclear charge is the fundamental chemical characteristic of the atom of an element type.

Most of the information about the atomic or nuclear theory has come about in the last four decades.

ATOMIC AND MOLECULAR WEIGHTS

Although the terms "atomic mass" and "atomic weights" are practically used interchangeably, there exists a theoretical difference between the two. A rank ordering of the natural elements from the lightest to the heaviest would list hydrogen and uranium, respectively. An additional 13 elements have been artificially produced. What is the standard unit by which all atomic weights are compared? The basic or standard atomic weight unit is the atomic mass unit (a.m.u.), which is defined as one twelfth the mass of the carbon-12 atom. In the past, oxygen was used as a standard; however, since 1960 carbon 12 has been the comparative unit. Using Avogadro's number, 12.000 grams (1 mole) of this form of carbon will contain 6.025×10^{23} atoms; therefore, 1 a.m.u. is equivalent to 1.66×10^{-24} grams ($1/6.025 \times 10^{23}$).

Molecular weight is simplistically the summation of the individual weights of the number of different atom types comprising the molecule. One can determine the weight in grams of a simple atom or molecule by dividing the gram-atomic or gram-molecular weight by Avogadro's number. The gram-atomic weight of hydrogen is 1.008 and its gram-molecular weight is 2.016 (1.008×2) since this gaseous molecule is diatomic. Hence, the atomic weight of one atom of hydrogen is 1.67×10^{-24} grams ($1.008/6.025 \times 10^{23}$); for gold 3.26×10^{-22} grams ($197.0/6.025 \times 10^{-23}$); and for lead 3.42×10^{-22} grams ($206.0/6.025 \times 10^{-23}$). This relationship holds for the three states of matter—solid, liquid, or gas. These numbers do seem extraordinarily small, in fact, so small that our minds do not even have a grasp as to their magnitude (smallness). Yet another physical aspect of an atom is its physical dimension (size). An estimate of the size of atoms or molecules is made from the molecular weight and density. Given that water has a molecular weight of 18 and a density of 1 gram $\cdot$ cc^{-1}, then one gram-molecular weight occupies 18 cc^3 and contains 6.025×10^{23} molecules. The approximate volume for each molecule then is 3×10^{-23} cm^3. Transposing this volume to a spherical volume, which is about one third smaller, or 2×10^{-23} cm^3, one can determine the radius from the relation

$$\frac{4}{3}\pi r^3 = 2 \times 10^{-23}\text{cm}^3$$

$$r = 1.7 \times 10^{-8} \text{ cm}$$

Another relationship that estimates the magnitude of nuclear radii is

$$R = k\sqrt[3]{M}$$

where M is the mass number and $k = 1.5 \times 10^{-13}$ cm.

You need not memorize this value; however, in later chapters radiopharmaceutical particle sizing and detector crystal structure in instrumentation, to mention a few, also involves the use of extremely small dimensions as well, and you should, as best as possible, develop a sensitivity and appreciation for these minute aspects.

PERIODIC SYSTEM OF ELEMENTS

Retrospectively, the most successful attempt to categorize different types of elements by physical and chemical properties was made by Mendeleev. In his tabulation and those periodic charts used today, the horizontal rows are called *periods* and the vertical columns are called *groups* or *families*. In the groups, elements listed vertically have similar chemical properties. Groups are number I to VIII; the first seven groups are subdivided into subgroups A and B. The specific A subgroup number (I-VII) provides the number of electrons in the outermost orbital location. Group D elements are those in which there is a maximum number of electrons (8) in the outermost orbital location. The underlying rationale for the periodic classification is the atomic number, to which the atomic weight is approximately proportional (Fig. 2-3).

ATOMIC MODELS

Generally, what is known about the atom is known by deduction and intuition rather than by direct observation. The early investigators, upon whose foundations modern science is built, did not have governmental grants or equipment, but they "knew" that the atom must have some structure. From differing experiments and interpretations, different ideas relating to the structure of the atom developed. Perhaps the most widely popularized concept and easily understood because of its relevance to more easily observed phenomena and the structure of systems was the idea of atomic structure as described and espoused by Niels Bohr in 1913. Simply stated, the concept develops a model of the atom and divides the total region of the atom into two portions; nuclear and extranuclear. The principle entities believed to comprise the extranuclear region are free space and orbital electrons likened to the planetary bodies around the sun. Initially, the principle entities believed to comprise the nuclear region were the protons and neutrons. Since then, the actual nuclear constituency has become more complex and contains other forms of matter. The principle entities—protons, neutrons, and electrons—are termed elementary particles, since they are the primary building blocks of an atom and they have mass and occupy space just as do other forms of matter. These nuclear entities are also known as "nucleons." Bohr's classic atomic model is illustrated in Fig. 2-1. Bear in mind that no one has seen an atom. Bohr's model is just that—only an idea of how the atom might appear—and is based upon interpretations of experimental data. However, this model does not answer all questions raised by experimentation.

Several of the other nuclear concepts are fascinating

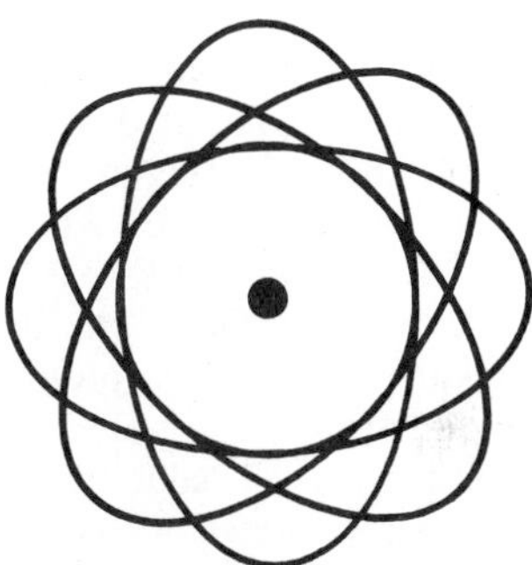

Fig. 2-1. Bohr's atomic model with central nuclear region surrounded by extranuclear region.

and interesting and do explain some experimental data. The liquid-drop or compound-nucleus model was suggested in the late 1930s by Bohr and Wheeler because they believed that the nucleons were tightly packed as opposed to the nucleus having empty space. This model somewhat accurately explains the interaction of bombarding neutrons with nuclei, nuclear fission mechanisms, and nuclear binding energies. In contradistinction, the shell model identifies that the nucleons could exist and be located in shells. Some evidence for this idea is based on the odd-even rule in which the majority of stable (nonradioactive) nuclei have an even number of nucleons. Also, when radioactive nuclei contain even numbers of neutrons and protons, their physical half-life time is greater than those of related isotopes.

ATOMIC STRUCTURE

Starting outside and working inward, the following information relates to the three elementary particles.

Electrons

From the early studies by Faraday, he inferred that there was an elementary unit of electricity. Stoney identified this unit and named it "electron" about 10 years prior to the discovery of x rays by Roentgen. Additional characteristics and properties of the electron were identified through experimentation with cathode rays. Electrons are negatively charged, travel in straight lines unless deflected, can be deflected by either electrical fields or magnetic fields, possess kinetic energy about one tenth the velocity of light, and have a rest mass equal to about 1/1850 that of a hydrogen ion, or 9.1×10^{-28} grams, or 0.00054 a.m.u. Symbolically, electrons located in or arising from the extranuclear region are represented as e or e^-. Orbital electrons may also be called "negatrons."

Protons

From scientific studies of positive rays, the lightest particle that was ever found had the same mass as a hydrogen atom. This charged particle possessed an electric charge equal in magnitude to that of an electron but of opposite polarity. The hydrogen nucleus was given the name "proton." Having a positive electrical charge, protons can be deflected by electrical and magnetic fields, though not so easily as electrons since their mass is 1850 times greater, specifically 1.67×10^{-24} grams. Note that a proton's rest mass, as identified here, is the same value as identified in the above discussion for the value of an atomic mass unit (a.m.u.). Actually, a proton has a mass equal to 1.00759 a.m.u. The number of protons in the nucleus of each atom type is the atomic number for that element, which is symbolized by the letter Z. When the number of protons within a single atom equals the number of electrons in that atom, the atom is electrically neutral, since the positive and negative electrical charges are equal, with the net effect being zero or electrically neutral.

Neutrons

In the early 1920s, Rutherford suggested that a neutron was actually a particle of matter resulting from the physical combination of an electron and a proton, with the electrical charges canceling. This idea gave rise to the designation "±" for a neutron within the nucleus of the atom. Since the particle has no net electrical charge, its path cannot be deflected by electrical fields. In 1932, Chadwick demonstrated the existence of neutrons by using bombardment of atomic nuclei with alpha particles and cloud-chamber studies. Experimental results have shown the mass of a neutron to be 1.00898, which is slightly greater than that of a proton. However, for all practical intents and purposes, the mass of a neutron, just like for protons, is considered 1. The number of neutrons in the nucleus of each atom type is the neutron number and is symbolized by the letter N. Atom types do not have a constant N number as they would have a specific Z number. The N number can vary and forms the basis for the various isotopic forms of elements, which are discussed later.

As a result of possessing slightly greater mass than a proton, a neutron demonstrates instability because of an excess mass-energy equivalency. Neutrons are categorized by the kinetic energies that they possess, for example, thermal neutrons, fast neutrons, prompt or delayed neutrons. Considering the latter two types, prompt neutrons are those released from the nucleus of an atom coincident with a fission process. Delayed neutrons are those that are released from the nucleus of an excited atom subsequent to a fission process. An example of the subsequent radioactive release or emission is beta decay. Upon release, the kinetic energy of the neutron and the type of material determine what course of actions will result. Bombardment of materials with neutrons, their capture, and the analysis of the end products form the study of activation analysis. This process is fairly common and results in the emission of gamma rays. No changes in proton number or chemical identity occurs.

Returning to Rutherford's suggestion, quantum mechanics and electron spin resonance studies provide specific reasons why electrons cannot exist or be present within the nucleus. Therefore, one must conclude that at the instant of decay a beta particle, which did not previously exist, is created. The process of neutron decay results in the formation of a beta particle, a new proton, which also did not previously exist, and a neutrino. Changes in nuclear constitution are referred to as transmutation. Beta particles are indistinguishable from electrons with which they can become involved. Symbolically, they are distinguished as β^- and e^-, respectively, only to designate their site of origin. Neutrinos are discussed later.

MASS-ENERGY RELATIONSHIP

From Einstein's theory of relativity, mass and energy are interchangeable and related by

$$E = mc^2$$

where c is the velocity of light measured in centimeters per second, mass is measured in grams, and E is expressed in ergs. The total energy possessed by a body of matter is the summation of its potential-energy and kinetic-energy components. A body at rest has no kinetic-energy component; its total energy is equal to its rest-mass equivalency.

Kinetic energy is energy that a body possesses because of its motion and is calculable by the equation $E = \frac{1}{2}mv^2$. If a beta particle or electron is ejected from an atom by a decay or interactive process and its energy is 100 keV, the respective velocity slightly exceeds one half the velocity of light.

Potential energy is attributable to a body because of its relative position. Additional energy is required to raise the body to a higher location, with energy being released in the move to a lower location. The normal location of extranuclear electrons and the possible transpositions they can undergo result in changes in their potential-energy values.

In nuclear reactions, the energy release is much greater than the amount from an ordinary chemical reaction. To illustrate, the energy equivalency of 1 gram of matter is determined from the above formula as follows:

$$\begin{aligned} E &= 1 \text{ g} \times (2.99 \times 10^{10} \text{ cm/sec})^2 \\ &= 8.94 \times 10^{20} \text{ cm}^2 \cdot \text{sec}^{-2} \cdot \text{g} \end{aligned}$$

Since 1 BTU $= 1.06 \times 10^{10}$ ergs, this energy equivalent is 8.5×10^{10} BTU, or 3.3×10^5 kilocalories.

Yet another relationship exists, since the erg is not an easily used dimension in nuclear reactions. The convenient unit is the electron volt, which is equivalent to 1.6×10^{-12} erg. Therefore, 1 keV is equal to 1.6×10^{-9} erg and 1 MeV is equal to 1.6×10^{-6}. With these values, the mass-energy relationship becomes

$$\begin{aligned} E\,(\text{MeV}) &= m\,(\text{g}) \times \frac{8.99 \times 10^{20} \text{ cm}^2 \cdot \text{sec}^{-2}}{1.6 \times 10^{-6} \text{ erg} \cdot \text{MeV}^{-1}} \\ &= 5.61 \times 10^{26} \end{aligned}$$

From the rest mass of an electron, 9.1×10^{-28} g, the equivalent energy value is as follows:

$$\begin{aligned} E &= 5.61 \times 10^{26} \frac{\text{ergs}}{\text{g}} \times 9.1 \times 10^{-28} \text{ g} \\ &= 0.511 \text{ MeV} \end{aligned}$$

Substitution of atomic mass units for grams gives the following energy relationship for a proton:

$$\begin{aligned} E\,(\text{MeV}) &= 1.66 \times 10^{-24} \text{ g} \times 5.61 \times 10^{26} \\ &= 931 \text{ MeV} \end{aligned}$$

In other words, the a.m.u. equivalent of a neutron is

$$\begin{aligned} E\,(\text{MeV}) &= \frac{931 \text{ MeV}}{\text{a.m.u.}} \times 1.0089 \\ &= 939 \text{ MeV} \end{aligned}$$

We shall return to this quantifiable discussion later in the discussion of nuclear binding energies and mass defect.

THE ISO BUSINESS

In 1816, Prout suggested that the measures of atomic weight were, in fact, whole numbers. It was later found, as we know today, that there are atom types that do have different atomic masses even though they belong to the same element type; consequently they possess the same atomic number, Z, and chemical properties. These elements with the same Z number and chemical properties but different A numbers were given a general name by Soddy in 1913, about the same time as Bohr developed his concept of atomic structure. The generic name was isotope, which when literally translated from Greek means the 'same *(iso-)* place *(topos)*' on the periodic table of elements. This term is common and frequently referred to; however, another term, "nuclide," is more accurate, is used interchangeably, and is being used more. By definition then, a radionuclide is an atom type distinguished by its nucleons' energy, which exists for a finite period of time.

In the above discussion, atomic mass numbers were defined as the number of nucleons in the nucleus. Atomic masses of nuclides are defined in terms of their relative mass as compared to that of carbon, which has an atomic mass of 12.000 and an atomic mass number, A, of 12 since it has Z and N of 6, respectively. In this case by definition and in other situations by result, the atomic mass are very close to whole numbers (that is, integers). As will be discussed below, the atomic mass for a nuclide cannot be calculated by simple summation of the nuclear constituent masses. The actual mass is less than calculated. Why? Read below.

From a chemist's standpoint, the A number of a nuclide is based upon the mass of a mixture of the various forms of this nuclide; the mixture representing the relative percentage of natural abundance of these forms. To illustrate, the element iodine (Z = 53) has 15 identified nuclidic forms, only one of which is naturally occurring and is not radioactive. In fact, all nonradioactive iodine (100%) occurring in nature is represented by the form that has an *A* of 127. By comparison, a close atomic and elemental neighbor, tin (Z = 50) has 21 identified nuclidic forms, of which 10 are nonradioactive and naturally occurring. By percentages, the top five by incidence or abundance account for only 87.4% of all naturally occurring tin. On the contrary, however, a nuclide of tremendous importance in nuclear medicine, technetium (Z = 43) does not have any naturally occurring nuclidic forms. Of its 22 different forms, all are radioactive and arise as a product of another decay process or artificially from man-induced radioactivity.

Numbers of electrons, in the un-ionized state, do not change for nuclides but are equal in number to the Z number for that form. Chemical properties are also the same and consequently nuclides of the same type cannot be separated. However, the physical property of mass changes and consequently a mass spectrograph could be used to separate the various nuclidic forms.

In nuclear medicine and other physical sciences, elements are symbolically represented by their chemical symbols, which are used on the periodic chart and which consist of one or two letters only, the first of which is capitalized and the second, if present, is lowercased. Atomic mass numbers are represented as a number in superscript position to the left of the chemical symbol. Older texts and source material used the right side. This designation was moved left so as to not interfere with the valence designation. The atomic numbers, however, are represented as a number in the subscript position, also to the left. The generalized form would appear

$$^{A}_{Z}X$$

The *N* number is usually not designated, but one may easily calculate it by subtracting *Z* from *A*.

Additional terms with the *iso-* (Gr. 'equal') prefix are known but infrequently used in clinical jargon. For reference, these terms relate to the nuclear configuration and are called "isobars, isotones, and isomers." Specific but brief definitions follow. *Isobars* ('equal weight') are nuclides that have different Z (protons) and *N* (neutrons) but have the same *A* (mass) numbers. If the *N* number remains the same with the *A* and *Z* numbers varying, they are *isotones* ('equal tension'). If all physical attributes are the same but only the level or amount of nuclear energy varies, the forms are called *isomers* ('equal parts'). Isomeric forms are easily distinguished because of the tag-along lower case *m* used with the *A* number.

Examples of these forms of nuclear configurations are listed in Table 2-1. Since their use arises infrequently, a mnemonic aid is illustrated by the boxed similarities: for isotopes, the *P* and *Z*, since the *Z* num-

Table 2-1. Nomenclature and examples of variations of nuclear configurations

Name	Examples	Nuclear configuration		
		A (mass)	**Z (protons)**	**N (neutrons)**
Isoto[p]es (same element)	$^{131}_{53}I$	131	[53]	78
	$^{127}_{53}I$	127	[53]	74
	$^{125}_{53}I$	125	[53]	72
Isob[a]rs (same mass)	$^{131}_{53}I$	[131]	53	78
	$^{131}_{54}Xe$	[131]	54	77
	$^{131}_{55}Cs$	[131]	55	76
	$^{131}_{56}Ba$	[131]	56	75
Isoto[n]es (same neutron number)	$^{53}_{24}Cr$	53	24	[29]
	$^{54}_{25}Mn$	54	25	[29]
	$^{55}_{26}Fe$	55	26	[29]
	$^{56}_{27}Co$	56	27	[29]
	$^{57}_{28}Ni$	57	28	[29]
Isom[e]rs (same attributes except energy level by gamma-ray emission) (*m* = metastable)	$^{99m}_{43}Tc$	99	43	56
	$^{99}_{43}Tc$	99	43	56
	$^{113m}_{49}In$	113	49	64
	$^{113}_{49}In$	113	49	64
	$^{133m}_{54}Xe$	133	54	79
	$^{133}_{54}Xe$	133	54	79

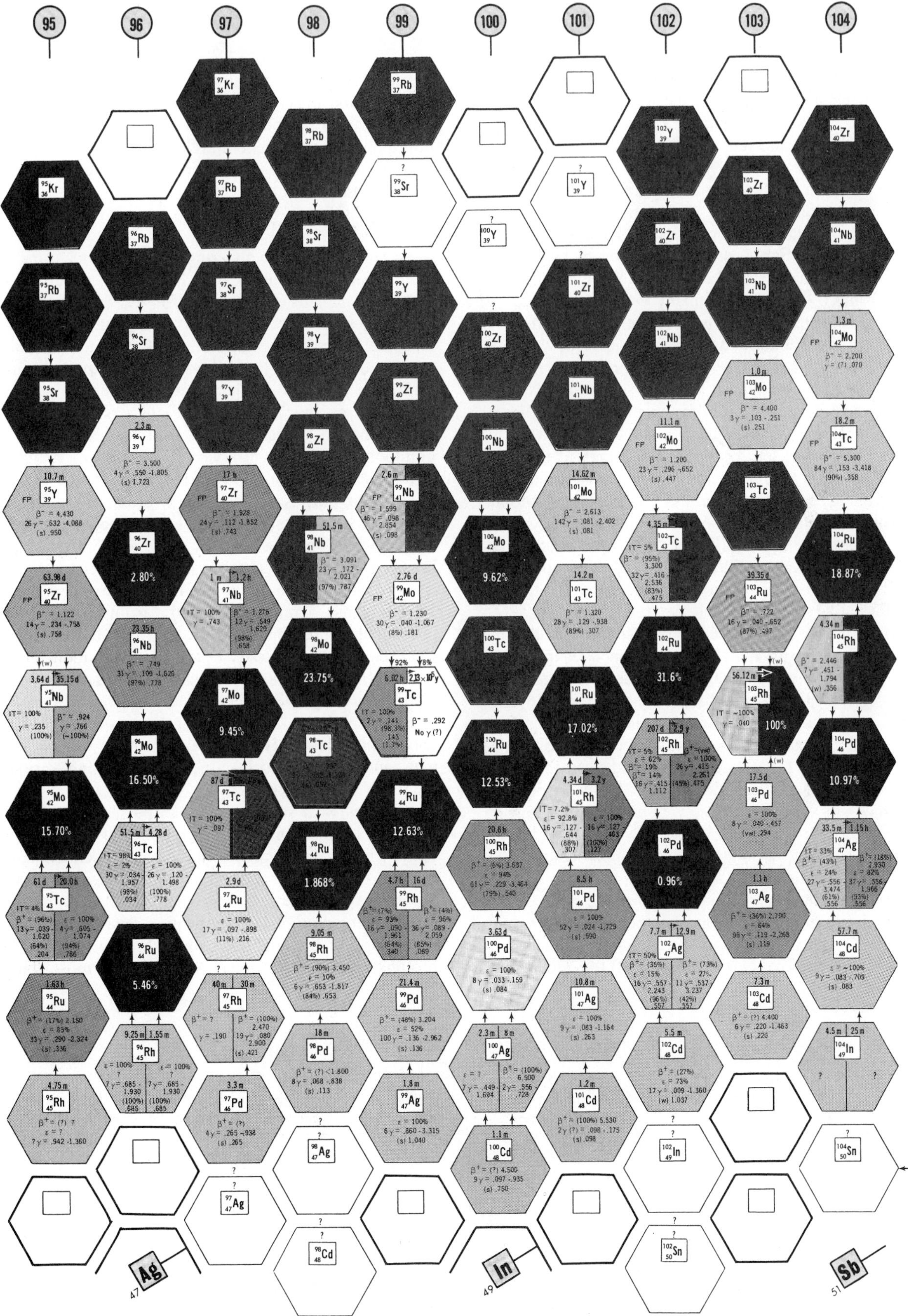

Fig. 2-2. Trilinear chart of the nuclides. *Black background* represents stable forms; *dark- to light-shaded areas* indicate instability. (Courtesy Mallinckrodt, Inc., St. Louis, 1979.)

ber is actually the number of *p*rotons; for iso*bars*, the *A* and the *A*; for iso*tones*, the *N* and the *N*; and for iso*mers*, the singly identified *E*, which suggests that all physical parameters *except* *e*nergy are the same. The *m*etastable nuclidic form designated by the lower case *m* has a higher level of nuclear energy than its genetically related form. The form with the lower nuclear potential-energy value is considered the ground state. Isomeric forms that also happen to be isotopic and isobaric exist for measurable time intervals ranging from 10^{-10} seconds to many years.

More illustrative of this information is the trilinear chart of the nuclides, a selected portion of which is found in Fig. 2-2. Each hexagon represents a nuclidic form. Vertically adjacent neighbors represent isobars; obliquely adjacent neighbors from upper left to lower right represent isotones; and obliquely adjacent neighbors from lower left to upper right represent isotopes. Atomic mass numbers are circularly identified and horizontally positioned across the top, and atomic numbers are squarely identified and obliquely positioned originating in the lower left. Within each hexagon is a square, which identifies the appropriate nomenclature with symbol and numbers. Of specific and relative importance is the relationship of ^{99}Mo and ^{99}Tc and the detailed data contained within the appropriate hexagons. These two nuclides represent the workhorses of clinical nuclear medicine. In regard to molybdenum 99, its physical half-life is 2.76 days and is itself a fission product, demonstrating both beta and gamma modes of decay. The energies (MeV) and percentage for particulate (β^-) and electromagnetic (γ) radiations are identified. The location for technetium 99 is split vertically, with the left side listing isomeric transition (IT) 100%. Precisely, this means that of the approximate 92% of molybdenum that decays into this radionuclidic form, all of it (100%) decays into the radionuclidic form on the right, which decays into a nuclidic form of ruthenium (Ru), which represents only 12.63% of the natural abundance of this element. The two segments of the technetium hexagon represent the isomeric forms as identified in Fig. 2-2 and previously discussed. Note that the isomeric form of technetium does not decay into ruthenium or any other element but releases only gamma energies from its nucleus, 90% of which have an energy value of 140 KeV.

NUCLEAR STABILITY

Perhaps you are wondering why so much time is being spent on an atom, which we have never seen, and on its nucleus. It somewhat follows that we should since the name of our study is both nuclear physics and nuclear medicine technology. Let's face it, without nuclei and their instability, we would probably be without a profession. Therefore, it is imperative that we know as much about these matters as we can. This is not to suggest that the extranuclear region is unimportant; to the contrary, it is, but not in a radioactive sense. The importance of this extranuclear region is, for our purposes, basically twofold: first, this is where chemical bonding occurs, and second, it is in this region where the majority of types of interactions between matter and energy (radiations) occur.

Now, returning again to the nucleic considerations, we could use a reference like the trilinear chart and learn that approximately 280 of all nuclides do not represent or demonstrate a propensity for radioactive decay. In other words, the nuclei of these nuclides distributed among 83 elements demonstrate a state of nuclear stability. The remaining approximately 1500 known nuclides individually exhibit their varying extents and types of nuclear instability through various modes of radioactive decay.

Nuclides with stable nuclei can be placed into two categories: those with an even number of protons and those with an odd number of protons. Subsequent subdivisions could analogously be made with even and odd numbers of neutrons, the other nucleon. Summarily, this classification and quantification data are listed in Table 2-2. Stable nuclides with both even numbers of protons and neutrons are most stable and most abun-

Table 2-2. Categorization data of nuclides demonstrating nuclear stability

Number of nucleons			Number of stable nuclei	Number of elements	Average number of nuclides per element	Abundance and stability
Z	N	A				
Even	Even	Even	168			Most
Even	Odd	Odd	59	43	53	Intermediate
			227			
Odd	Even	Odd	53			Intermediate
Odd	Odd	Even	4	40	1.4	Least
			57			

dant. In direct opposition is the situation of the nucleus having odd numbers of both protons and neutrons, which results in the least abundance and the least stability within the nucleus. "Upon what does this relationship depend?" you may ask. The most salient aspect appears to be the dependent relationship of the binding energy upon the atomic mass, A, and the atomic charge, Z. We have discussed A and Z numbers, but what is binding energy? Well, we need to digress in order to return to this point and continue properly.

From our early experiences, we have learned that when the north poles of two magnets are brought into proximity, they repel; whereas, when a north and a south pole are brought together, we have attraction. The same concept applies to electrical situations. A path of electrons (e^-) cannot be deflected by adjacent conductive metal plates that are given a negative ($-$) bias; however, the path can be deviated when these same conductive plates are given a positive ($+$) bias. Axiomatically, we have learned and can again state: "Opposite charges attract and like charges repel." What then is in a nucleus that, as a force, holds the protons and neutrons together? Logically, we could state that the nucleus should "explode" because of the repulsive forces resulting from the high density of like electrical charges. Again, logically, we can deduce that this attractive force must and does exist because stable nuclei do exist. These nuclear forces must be very intense, of great magnitude, and active over a very short range (that is, 10^{-12} average nuclear diameter). Also, it would appear that these forces experience tripartition: proton $\leftrightarrow$ proton, proton $\leftrightarrow$ neutron, and neutron $\leftrightarrow$ neutron. Measurement and quantization of these nuclear forces results in millions of electron volts (MeV); the average binding energy per nucleon is 8 MeV. By comparision, this force is much greater than the energy requirement to remove (ionize) an electron from its extranuclear location; measured in keV units. In response to Coulomb's law (electrostatics), the force, F, between two electrically charged bodies (q and q') is directly dependent on the product of their charges and inversely dependent on the square of the distance, r, separating the two bodies in a vacuum:

$$F = q \cdot q'/r^2$$

In general, these nuclear forces are called "binding energy."

From what we have learned so far, it would appear easy to determine the total atomic mass of a nuclide's nucleus simply by knowing the masses of its *free and individual* constituent parts and respective numbers of its constituents. But it does not work that way when combining to constitute an atom. In actuality, their combined atomic mass is less than the sum of its free constituent parts. This mass difference (decrease) is termed "mass defect." From Einstein's relativity theory, this deficit of mass has an energy equivalency that is termed the "binding energy." During a nuclear reaction, energy is either released or consumed. If released, the reaction is said to be exergonic; if energy is consumed, the reaction is said to be endogonic.

"Fine," you say, "but what relevance does this have?" For all practical intents and purposes there is none, but it does explain which nuclei will most probably be stable and those that will exhibit instability.

Within an isobaric series as illustrated in Fig. 2-2, two interesting aspects can be observed relating the nuclear stability to the A and Z numbers. Attention should be directed to the inserted legend. The first aspect can be demonstrated within the A series of 96. Note that there are three stable nuclides, which are naturally occurring: $^{96}_{40}Zr$, $^{96}_{42}Mo$, and $^{96}_{44}Ru$ (zirconium, molybdenum, and ruthenium, respectively). Also, observe that these nuclides are separated by two Z numbers; in almost all isobaric series, this separation aspect holds true. Nuclidic forms separating nuclearly stable forms demonstrate or possess nuclear instability. In other words, within that same series $^{96}_{41}Nb$ and $^{96}_{43}Tc$ (niobium and technetium, respectively) are radioactive. Does this relationship hold true for all nuclides in Fig. 2-2? The second aspect is best demonstrated within the range of A series 90, 91, 93, 95, 97, 99, 101, 103, or 105. We will choose the 99 series, since it has daily relevance in nuclear medicine technology. Within this isobaric series $^{99}_{44}Ru$ is the only nuclide demonstrating or possessing stability. In Fig. 2-2 note the relationship of the arrows for nuclides listed above ($^{99}_{40}Zr$ and $^{99}_{43}Tc$) and for those nuclides listed below ($^{99}_{46}Pd$ and $^{99}_{45}Rh$). For those six radionuclide forms above, the arrows point downward; for those three radionuclidic forms below, the arrows point upward. What is the significance? In this configuration of presentation, those nuclides above undergo radioactive decay to ultimately achieve nuclear stability by the ejection of a beta particle (β^-). The modes of radioactive decay for those nuclides below are emission of a positron (β^+) or else electron capture in order to ultimately achieve nuclear stability. Thus the dependent relationship between the binding energy and the A and Z numbers.

Another visual presentation that may assist in representing nuclear stability is found in Fig. 2-3 with accompanying information in Table 2-3. The tabulated neutron range values correspond to the plotted points in Fig. 2-3. The cross-hatched regions on either side of the stable nuclide range are called the "domains" of radionuclides. Radionuclides represented by the area of *D1* eventually achieve nuclear stability by under-

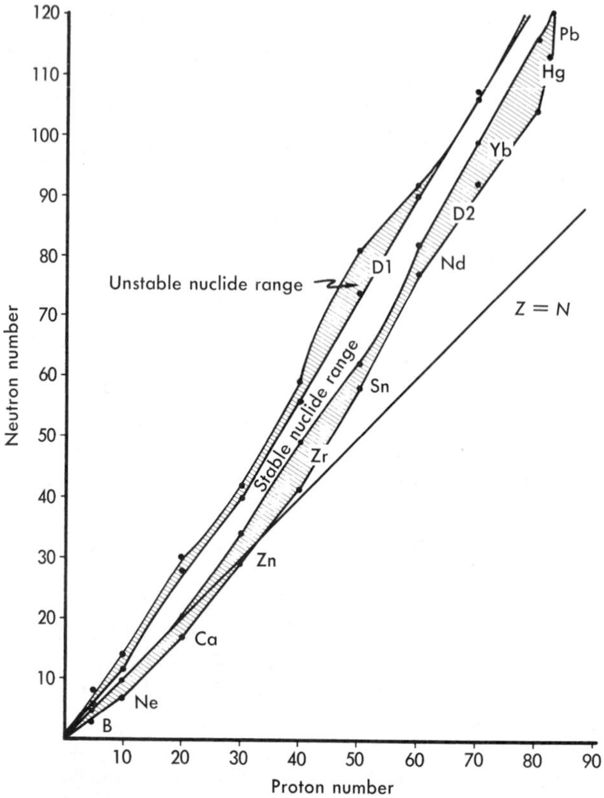

Fig. 2-3. Neutron-proton ratio with resulting indices of nuclear stability of nuclides.

Table 2-3. Selected nuclides with *N/P* ratio ranges

Element	Symbol	Z	Neutron range		N/P ratio	
			Low	High	Low	High
Boron	B	5	5	6	1	1.2
Neon	Ne	10	10	12	1	1.2
Calcium	Ca	20	20	28	1	1.4
Zinc	Zn	30	34	40	1.13	1.33
Zirconium	Zr	40	50	56	1.25	1.4
Tin	Sn	50	62	74	1.24	1.48
Neodymium	Nd	60	82	90	1.37	1.5
Ytterbium	Yb	70	100	106	1.43	1.51
Mercury	Hg	80	116	124	1.45	1.55
Lead	Pb	82	114	132	1.39	1.61

going a radioactive decay process termed "beta decay." In other words, at any point in the *D1* domain, the nuclei may be described as being "neutron rich." In comparison, radionuclides represented by the area of *D2* are "neutron poor" and eventually achieve nuclear stability by undergoing decay processes such as electron capture or positron emission. Also remember that if a nucleus demonstrates neutron richness, it concomitantly demonstrates proton poverty; the nuclide that is neutron poor is also proton rich.

If there were as many neutrons as protons, a 1:1 ratio would result and be graphed accordingly as in Fig. 2-3. When the *N/P* ratios for selected nuclides are calculated, they represent a range from 1:1 for boron to 1:1.6 for lead. Reference to a chart of the nuclides would illustrate that all elements above lead ($Z > 82$) have only radionuclide forms. The four natural radioactive series have, as the last four respective nuclidic forms into which they decay, a stable form of lead, of which only four stable forms occur naturally. These transmutational processes were not what the alchemists were desiring! In any event, for $Z > 20$, the N/P increases beyond 1:1. The usefulness of the N/P ratio is that it is basically a benchmark against which to compare nuclear stabilities and to suggest possible radioactive decay processes. By its very nature, this concept is not dogmatic.

In general then, a nucleus that is neutron rich will achieve stability by losing one of its surplus neutrons by this reaction.

$$n \rightarrow p + \beta^- + \tilde{\nu}$$

As a result, a proton, which did not previously exist, is created. The mass of the new element is the same since the practical mass of a neutron and proton are the same. The type or form of radiation from this decay process is the ejection from the nucleus of the β^- particle. Remember, it is physically the same as an electron except for its site of origin, and, prior to the decay of the neutron, it did not exist. To account for conservation laws for momentum and energy, the remaining particle is the antineutrino, which has no electrical charge and even less mass than an electron has. Remaining but nonspecific amounts of energy are shared between the beta particle and antineutrinos. Of significant clinical and biologic importance is the kinetic energy of the β^- particle.

A nucleus that is neutron poor, if personified, would desire to reduce its proton surplus. Accomplishment of this desire is through two possible processes:

$$p \rightarrow n + \beta^+ + \nu$$

or

$$p + e^- \rightarrow n + \nu$$

The first process is termed "emission of a positron," and the second is termed "electron capture." Common between these two processes is the accounting for and release of a neutrino and also that the Z number is reduced by one with the atomic mass remaining the same. Positron emission is the ejection of a particle physically comparable to a β^- particle or to an orbital electron, except it is of opposite electrical charge. An annihilative interaction is the ultimate fate of a positron with an energy release of two 0.511 MeV photons.

In the second, an orbital electron, because of the opposite electrostatic charges and the position of the electron relative to the nucleus at a specific moment in time, may be captured and combined with a proton. This process is generally referred to as electron capture. The incidence of this process is inversely related to the distance the electron is from the nucleus.

NEUTRINO

As stated, the neutrino, ν, is extraordinarily small and has no electrical charge. Therefore, when it, as a particle of matter, interacts with other particles of matter, the result is very small. The rest-mass energy equivalent of an electron is 0.511 MeV, or 511 keV, as compared to about 250 eV for a neutrino. The prefix *anti,* such as in *anti*neutrino ($\tilde{\nu}$), when used in conjunction with an elementary particle indicates another particle with certain symmetric characteristics.

EXTRANUCLEAR REGION—CONFIGURATION AND CONSTITUENTS

The lonesome electrons seem to be the sole occupants of this region. As we have learned, most of the mass of an atom resides within the region called the nucleus. Just as there is no envelope or skin surrounding the nucleus, neither is there such an entity around the circumference of the atom and placing a boundary on it.

Consistent with Bohr's concept of the atom the electrons that "belong" to an atom migrate, either circularly or elliptically, around the nucleus. Specific paths called "orbits" were originally described; however, contemporary quantum mechanics call these locations "energy levels." Closest to the nucleus is the first energy level, which has been given quantum number 1, with adjacent levels having successive numbers. These quantum-number locations are related to the previous alphabetic locations as in Fig. 2-4. Thinking of the energy levels as circles is easiest when one attempts to discuss the distance from the nucleus, an electron's velocity, and number of orbits around the nucleus per second. Magnitudes of these parameters in the closest level are the radius of 10^{-9} cm, electron velocity of 10^8 cm/sec, and revolutions of 10^{15} in contrast to these magnitudes for the fourth level out with a radius of 10^{-8} cm, an electron velocity of 10^7 cm/sec, and revolutions around the nucleus of 10^{13} times/sec. No one need memorize these values; only appreciate how small and how fast! It logically stands to reason that the fourth level has the greatest circumference and consequently the lower velocity and revolution values. If the radius of level 1, that is, the K shell, is 10^{-9} cm and the size range of an electron is 10^{-13}, 1000 electrons could be lined up in the linear space between the center and the circumference.

According to the Pauli exclusion principle, only one electron can have the same set of quantum numbers.

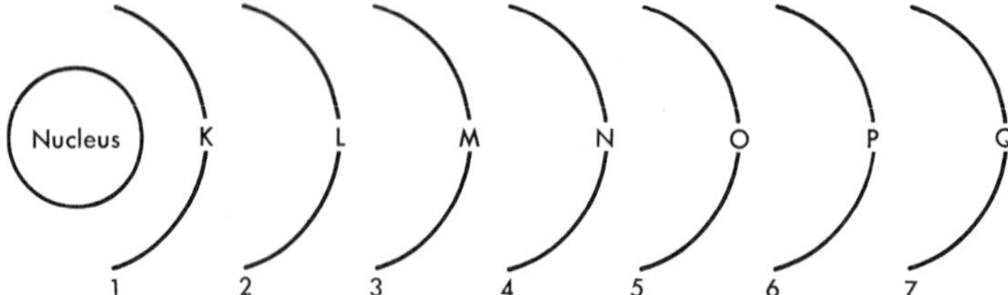

Fig. 2-4. Atomic configuration with quantum numbers.

Table 2-4. Maximum electron capacity of energy levels

Energy-level quantum number	Maximum capacity
1	2
2	8
3	18
4	32
5	50
6	72
7	98

But that statement is difficult to allow proper visualization of the structure. In simpler words, the innermost energy levels are filled with two electrons each before the outer levels are filled. Even better yet, the A-subgroup members for groups I to VII give the number of electrons in the outermost energy location; for example, group V, subgroup A elements (such as nitrogen and phosphorous) have 5 electrons in the outer locations; they could maximally have 8 in that location. Maximum numbers of electrons per energy level are listed in Table 2-4. The quantifiable relationship between the quantum number and maximum capacity is found by $2n^2$, in which n is the quantum number, or energy level. The story is not clean and easy because there are energy sublevels to each of the major ones. Specifically, these subgroups are listed for reference in Table 2-5.

As illustrated, the simplest quantum numbers from a subgroup standpoint are 1 and 7. An "s" subgroup designation regardless of quantum number indicates that 2 electrons can be located here. Electron location and designation is by the use of black dots. Designation "p" indicates 3 subgroups; designation "d" indicates five subgroups; and designation "f" indicates 7 subgroups. Subgroup designations for quantum numbers make more plausible the fact that the N shell (4) can have a maximum capacity of 32 electrons, whereas the L shell (2) can only have 8 electrons for its maximum capacity. If all energy-level locations through quantum number 5 were maximally occupied, what would be the corresponding Z number of this element as determined from the information represented in Table 2-5? In summary, an electron within an atom can be characterized by three quantum numbers; n, ℓ, and m. The n number is the principle quantum number; ℓ is the azimuthal quantum number designated by the letters s, p, d, or f, and m is the magnetic quantum number.

Electrons in the outer energy locations participate in physical activities, electron flow called electricity, and chemical activities called chemical bonding.

Physically, these outer electrons are loosely bound to the nucleus because of their long distance from the nucleus and the magnitude of the electrostatic attractive force as described by Coulomb's law. The magnitude of their adhesion to an atom is in the range of 5 to 20 electron volts. Relatively speaking, this value is insignificant compared to that for the innermost location as measured in kiloelectron volts. Therefore, the furthest removed are frequently referred to as "free electrons," and it is the movement of these electrons from atom to atom that is called electricity. In chemical considerations, these same "free" electrons are called "valence electrons." Atoms that have their outer electrons and energy locations full are extremely stable and nonreactive. Chemical properties of an element are primarily determined by the valence electrons as well as by the types of chemical bonding used in the formation of molecules and compounds. The general categories of bonding are ionic, covalent, and van der Waals. The precise type and extent of electrical interactions between ions determine the properties of the compound being formed. Are the chemical properties of nuclides and radionuclides of the same element different? If they were different, the tracer concept for use of radioactive materials would be nonexistent. Groups I and II of the periodic chart tend to give up their valence electrons to other atomic forms that are deficient in one or two electrons. When an

Table 2-5. Electron subgroup energy levels for major quantum number of locations

Quantum number	Subgroup designations	Subgroup numbers with maximum electron occupancy	Maximum capacity
1	1s	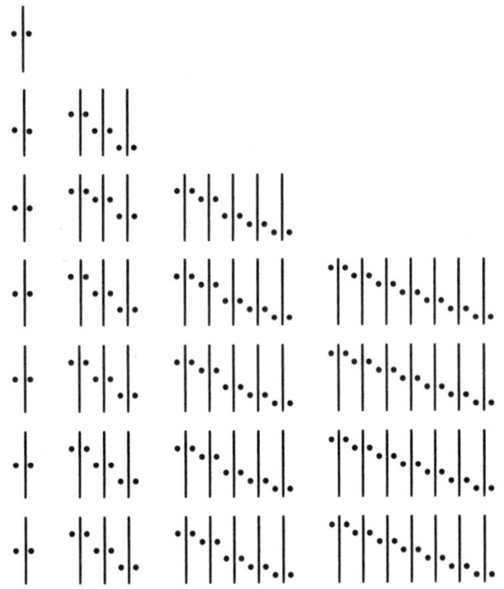	2
2	2s 2p		8
3	3s 3p 3d		18
4	4s 4p 4d 4f		32
5	5s 5p 5d 5f		32
6	6s 6p 6d 6f		32
7	7s 7p 7d 7f		32

Example:

Element:	Lawrencium	Technetium
Z:	103	43
Symbol:	Lw	Tc
Electron configuration:		
1	2s	2s
2	2s 6p	2s 6p
3	2s 6p 10d	2s 6p 10d
4	2s 6p 10d 14f	2s 6p 6d
5	2s 6p 10d 14f	1s
6	2s 6p 1d	
7	2s	

atom acquires additional electrons or donates electrons, the net result is an imbalance in the previous electrical neutrality that the atom experienced. The imbalance is negative when electrons are added (anions) and positive (cations) when electrons are donated. The entity experiencing the imbalance is termed an "ion." Cations would electrostatically be attracted to a negative electrode (cathode); anions would electrostatically be attracted to a positive electrode (anode). Ions always occur in pairs, with one ion being positive and the other negative. If an electron is removed from an atom, the electron is the negative ion and the residual atom is the positive ion. As previously described in the β^- decay process, a new proton is created, which was heretofore not present. A resulting positive imbalance exists until the new atom picks up a new electron. When is the new electron added? Routine addition of electrons takes place at the outer energy-level locations.

Somewhat the opposite situation arises from the process of positron emission with the atom having a surplus of electrons in which it must lose one to regain neutrality. In electron capture, the simultaneous loss of both a positive and negative charge maintains the electrical neutrality of the atom. This relationship is important to remember later when the interactions of ionizing radiation and matter are discussed.

Electrons experience a binding energy to their nucleus because of its intense positive attractive force for the tiny and lightweight electrons. The electrons that are the closest are most tightly held; those farthest away at the periphery of an atom are "free" electrons, which are loosely bound. The magnitude of this binding energy is dependent on the Z number and the

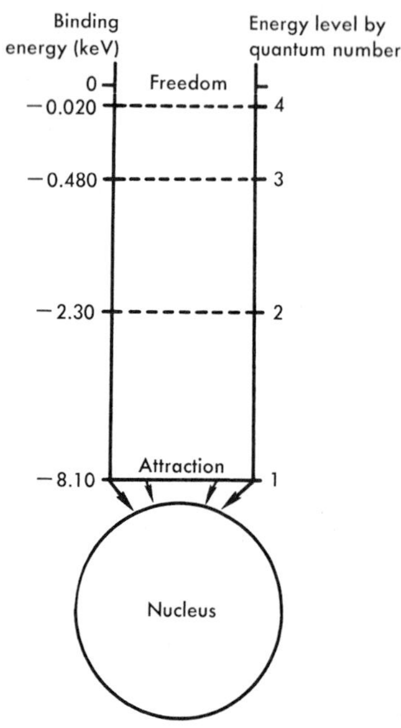

Fig. 2-5. Hypothetical binding-energy relationships.

electron's location relative to the nucleus and is equivalent to the amount of energy necessary to remove that electron from its location. Electrons can be permanently removed (ionization) or temporarily relocated (excitation) within the atom with a distinct possibility of return to their previous location. As a result of relocation, the energy difference determined by the two energy locations is released as a photon of energy called a "characteristic x ray." The binding energy is thought of as potential energy with the zero value being at the atom's outer limit and its maximum value at the K-shell location. This location is prefixed with a minus sign to designate that the energy difference between its value and the zero peripheral value would need to come from some extra-atomic source to move that electron through that distance. How can energy be released by an electron moving from the L to K levels? Well, additional energy was required to move it from the K to the L or, in other words, by going from a more negative location (K) to a less negative location (L). The move is in a positive direction (energy addition), which appears as an energy release when an electron goes from a less negative location (L) to a more negative location (K). Fig. 2-5 hypothetically illustrates this quantifiable relationship. If an electron were in energy level 1 and were relocated to energy level 2, what is the resulting energy difference?

Table 2-6. Actual electron binding energies for selected elements

Element	Z	Symbol	Electron binding energies in keV for quantum number		
			1	2	3
Iron	26	Fe	7.1	8.5	0.93
Gallium	31	Ga	10.4	1.30	0.16
Technetium	43	Tc	21.0	3.0	0.54
Iodine	53	I	33.2	5.1	1.07
Xenon	54	Xe	34.6	5.4	1.14
Thallium	81	Tl	85.5	15.3	3.7
Lead	82	Pb	88.0	15.9	3.8

Level 2	−2.3 keV
Level 1	−8.1 keV
Difference	+5.8 keV

In other words, this relocation required 5.8 keV of energy from an extranuclear source to effect this change. Conversely, if the newly arrived electron in energy level 2 is to return to energy level 1, the released photon would have what energy? (5.8 keV). These same 5.8 keV units of energy would be released as a photon. How much energy would be released if an electron from energy level 3 were relocated to energy level 2? (1.82 keV) Table 2-6 identifies actual binding energies for radionuclides used in nuclear medicine. What happens to these binding-energy values when one considers a nuclide and a radionuclide? Nothing, since the radioactive status is independent of the extranuclear electrons. For technetium, what is the actual energy difference or amount of energy released when an L-shell electron moved to the K-shell location? (18 keV) How much energy is necessary to ionize a gallium atom by removal of an M electron? (160 eV) With a separation involving 10 protons, the binding energy of the K electrons of iodine, as compared to technetium, is how many times greater? (1.58)

Behavior of electrons presents a duality, sometimes they behave as particles of matter and on other occasions, they behave as though they were waves. This topic arises as a result of the inability of Bohr's theory of the atom to account for the mechanism of photon emission subsequent to an electron changing locations. This aspect and others are accounted for in wave mechanics and from which the duality concept arises.

EXCITATION AND IONIZATION

Both of these processes can occur in physical or biologic systems. The physical system could represent the detector instruments, and the biologic system could represent the patient or any of his organs or tissues. More emphasis, however, is placed upon ionizations than excitations, though the latter plays an important role.

Ionizations may result from the collision of matter (alpha, beta, and positron particles) with matter (orbital electrons) or the collision of energy photons (gamma rays, x rays) with matter (orbital electrons). Yet another mechanism is the spontaneous disintegration of radioactive atoms (fission). Regardless of which of these interactive collisions or disintegrative actions, external energy has been given to an electron. If the energy is sufficiently larger than its binding energy value, the remaining portion is not lost but now appears as an increase in kinetic energy of that electron as it leaves the atom. Specifically, if the incident energy were 88 keV and the binding energy were 67 keV, the electron would be ejected with a kinetic energy of 21 keV.

A special adaptation and use of this term applies to *specific ionization,* which is the quantifiable number of ion pairs being created and occurring per unit length of track of the ejected electron.

Ionization processes occur in all states of matter—solids, liquids, and gases. The amount of energy to produce an ion pair is approximately 34 eV for liquids (such as a patient's soft tissue) and gases, but with slightly less for solids. A roentgen, as the former unit of exposure dose, is equivalent to the production of 1.61×10^{12} ion pairs per 715 cc of air.

Excitation is a companion (not equivalent) process to ionization and likewise embraces the absorption of external energy but not to the extent of the production of ions. The limit on absorption is the magnitude of the available and external energy rather than an intra-atomic controlling limit. In effect, the extra energy results in the temporary relocation but no removal of an electron. The excitement in the extranuclear region is temporary and short lived just as the metastability (excitement) of the nucleus. Since an electron is only moved, not removed, the total electrical neutrality of the atom is retained. Excitation events, though exceedingly short in life, can produce dissociation of chemical bonds or destroy molecular configurations, which in biologic systems can produce significant effects. In addition, chemical free radicals, which are compounds carrying a net electrical charge, can be produced. The energy that is released from the atom when the electron relocates itself and returns to a ground state is called a "low-energy photon." Excitation events usually take place with the outermost electrons, since, again, little energy is available and required. This process is extremely important in the operation of a most important "tool" to nuclear medicine, the scintillation detector. A scintillation is a tiny flash of light (photon), and it can occur in liquids or crystals. The liquid media in which scintillations can occur are called "fluors." Crystals represent a solid medium in which energy can be absorbed with subsequent released energy and relocated electrons. In a solid, electrons can be raised from a valence band to a conduction band and return to the valence state with release of a photon of energy. Depending on the wavelength of the released photon, it might be classified as visible or ultraviolet light. Specifically, these emitted photons are called "fluorescent radiation."

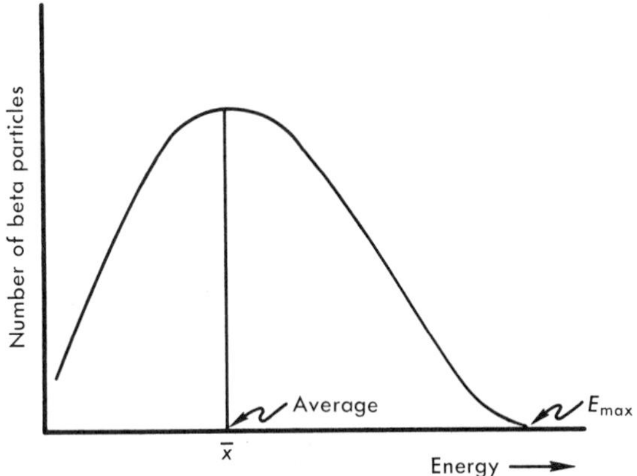

Fig. 2-6. Generalized beta-particle energy spectrum.

ADDITIONAL ASPECTS OF DECAY PROCESSES AND ENERGY RELEASE

Beta (β^- and β^+) decay

When an unstable nucleus ejects a beta particle, either β^- or β^+, kinetic energy is given to the particle. The amount of energy is dependent on the energy difference between the original nucleus *(Z)* and the resulting nucleus $(Z + 1)$ and the amount given to the antineutrino. In any event, there is some range of energy values that the beta particles may have, and this range is termed the continuous energy spectrum as compared to a simple and specific energy value. From a continuous energy spectrum, the average energy is approximately equivalent to one third the maximum energy (E_{max}). A generalized continuous energy spectrum is illustrated in Fig. 2-6. Note that this generalized graph is skewed to the right.

Why is the energy spectrum of beta particles important? Well, it just so happens that in dosimetry considerations of clinically used radionuclides of which some are beta-particle emitters, a formula to determine the dose the patient receives from the beta particles is given according to Marinelli as follows:

$$D_\beta = 73.8 \times C \times E_\beta \times T_e$$

in which C is measured in μCi/g, $\overline{E}_\beta$ is approximately one third the maximum beta-particle energy, T_e is the effective biologic half-life time, and 73.8 is a conversion constant so that the dose is given in rad units. In the NCRP Report No. 58 (A Handbook of Radioactivity Measurements and Procedures, 1978, U.S. Government Printing Office), the total average beta energy for ^{131}I is 182 keV; for ^{60}Co is 95.8 keV.

The ejection of a beta particle may not bring the resulting nucleus to a ground level. Subsequent energy release may be realized by gamma rays.

Electron capture

The actual energy level (designated by a letter) from which an electron is captured specifies the process, that is, K capture or L capture. The probability for capture from another energy level is very remote. Ionization results from the capture with subsequent relocation of an outer electron to the specific vacancy created by the capture. This process whereby proton-rich nuclei attempt to reach stability is competitive to the positron-emission process, which has the same nuclear objective. What then, in general, determines which of these two processes occurs and when? When the energy difference between the unstable nucleus and its eventual ground-state level is greater than 1022 keV (1.02 MeV), positron emission occurs; if the energy difference is less, electron capture occurs. A currently used radionuclide for clinical procedures is ^{67}Ga, which undergoes electron capture. In addition to ionization of the atom, characteristic x rays occur from energy changes resulting from electrons reshuffling to take the vacant position. As in positron emission, the capture of an electron may not completely adjust the nuclear energy problem to a ground level, a gamma ray may also be emitted.

Gamma decay

As in beta decay, the category of gamma decay has two competitive modes by which excess nuclear excitation energy is emitted from an atom.

In Table 2-1, three pairs of isomeric nuclei are identified. They differ in the aspect of their nuclear metastability, which depends only on a gamma ray, γ. In each case, the nuclei are transformed from a high energy level, by the emission of gamma ray, to a low energy level.

An alternate means of reducing nuclear energy levels or excitations is the complete transfer of energy (absorption) from the nucleus directly to an orbital electron (usually K but sometimes others), which then possesses more energy than its binding energy and is consequently ejected from the atom. This process is called "internal conversion," and the ejected electron is called a "conversion electron." It may also be referred to as "internal photoelectric effect." Symbolically and depending on the reference, these terms are represented by IC, CE, or ICE. When ionization so arises, again a reshuffling of electrons follows, with the corresponding characteristic x rays being emitted.

EXTRANUCLEAR ENERGY RELEASE

Basically, there are three energy-release processes that occur in the extranuclear region of an atom: characteristic x rays, Auger electrons, and bremsstrahlung x rays.

All x rays that are not described as bremsstrahlung x rays are in fact characteristic. Characteristic of what? Their energy properties are unique to and characteristic of the energy properties of the individual atom type in whose extranuclear regions they are conceived. What does all that mean? In each element, there are unique and specific binding-energy values for the several energy-level locations. For tungsten, they are the same if the atom came from Korea or Colorado, and any time an electron shifts or relocates between respective energy levels, the same or characteristic amount of energy will be released. The relocation of electrons is from outer locations to inner locations; not vice versa. Since characteristic x rays arise from discrete energy values, they are considered homogeneous, or monoenergetic, as compared to a heterogeneous beam emanating from a diagnostic x-ray tube, representing a range of photon energies. In general, elements have two types of characteristic x rays categorized by their absorption coefficients. The K-shell x rays are harder and experience less absorption; the L-shell x rays are softer and experience more absorption. Characteristic x rays are not described for elements with an atomic number less than 10, since the energetics (that is, $\leq$ 100 eV) is not equivalent to wavelengths within the x-ray portion of the electromagnetic spectrum. In other words, a minimum of 100 eV of energy is necessary for a classification as an x ray.

The spectrum of characteristic x rays of an element appears as the line spectrum in Fig. 2-7. A spectral configuration of this type is the result of the homogeneity factor. When a beam of x rays is heterogeneous, a continuous energy spectrum results and generally appears as Fig. 2-6.

By whichever means, be it K capture or internal conversion or Auger electrons, assume that an electron vacancy is created in the K shell. Most probably, an L-shell electron will move into this vacant position releasing energy now specifically called a K_α characteristic x ray. Had the electron come from the M shell to the K vacancy, the energy release would be greater; it would still be called a K characteristic x ray but would be designated as K_β. Possible, but not probable, is the translocation of an electron from the N shell

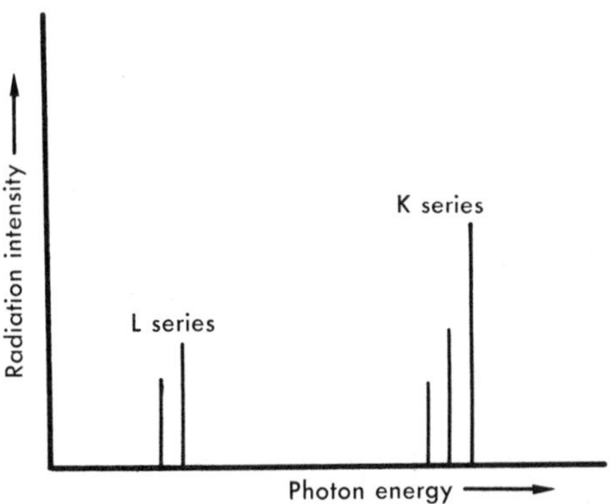

Fig. 2-7. Generalized line spectrum for characteristic x rays.

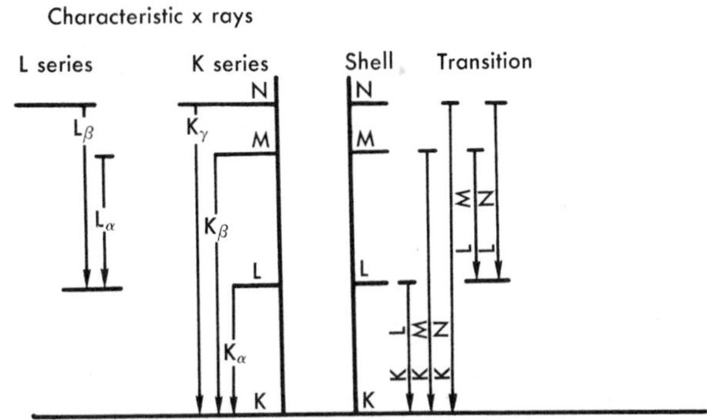

Fig. 2-8. K and L characteristic x rays of hypothetical atom.

to the K vacancy. If this condition had existed, the released energy would be the greatest in comparison to that of K_α and K_β; it would still be called a K characteristic x ray but be designated as K_γ. Why are all three called K characteristic x rays? Since the vacancy was in the K shell and all three, in this example, took turns filling it, the energy release is attributed to the difference in binding energies from its original location to the vacancy it filled. The K series then consists of K_α, K_β, and K_γ. Fig. 2-8 illustrates these relationships and designations as well as L characteristic x rays in the hypothetical atom.

Auger electrons

Assume that a photon of the characteristic x rays about which we just discussed is traversing the extranuclear region of the atom and its path is on a collision course with one of the other orbital electrons. Also, assume that the photon's energy is of a value greater than that electron's binding energy. As a result of the collision, the electron is ejected; surplus energy, if any, is given to the electron, the atom is ionized and a subsequent characteristic photon is created. In this sequence of events (Fig. 2-9) the ejected electron is called an "Auger (oh-zhay') electron." In effect, two electron vacancies occur so that the ionization effect is doubled. This process is competitive, with the emission of x rays for removing released energy in the extranuclear region of the atom. In other words, this process reduces energy levels by emitting matter as compared to the emission of a photon in x-ray production. As in the internal conversion process, Auger electrons are the result of an internal photoelectric effect.

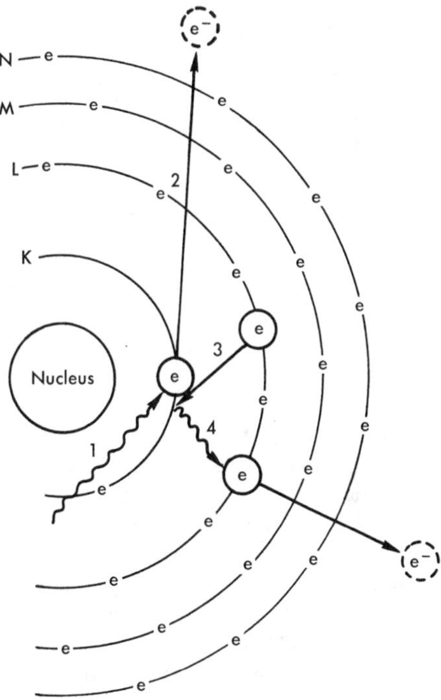

Fig. 2-9. Internal photoelectric effect producing an Auger electron. **1,** Incident photon collides with K electron. **2,** K electron is ejected from atom capable of other interactions. **3,** L electron moves to K shell. **4,** K_α characteristic of x ray is emitted and then collides with L electron. **5,** L electron, called "Auger electron," is ejected from atom.

Bremsstrahlung

Bremsstrahlung (brem'shtrah-lung; 'brake radiation') is a fancy German name that simply describes the formation of an x-ray photon as a result of a particle of matter traversing a path in such a direction that it comes under the strong and intense electrical influence of the nucleus. As a result, its path direction is changed and in effect the "brakes are applied in order to turn" onto a new path. The change in velocity (that is, deceleration) resulting from either an attraction or repulsion reduces its kinetic energy, which now appears

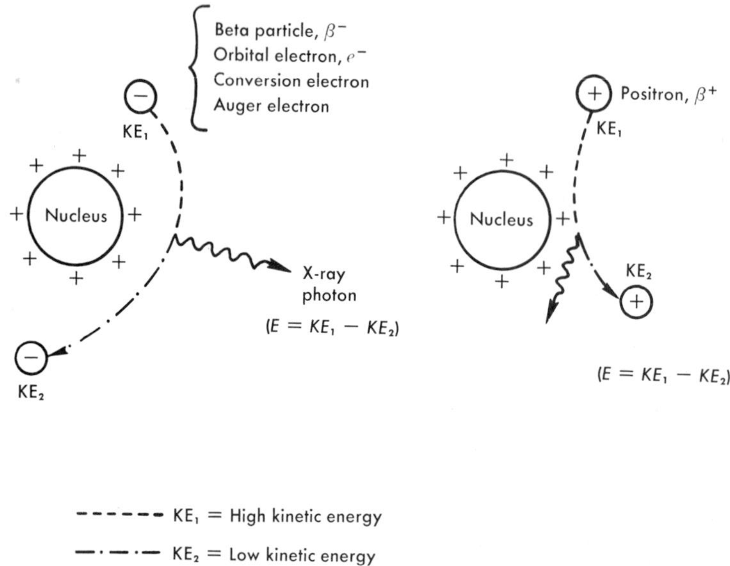

Fig. 2-10. Course changes in bremsstrahlung x-ray production.

as a photon. If the change in path is great, some of the photon's energy is manifested as x rays; if, however, the path change is very little, the photon's energy might be manifested as heat as in a diagnostic x-ray tube. The relatively large mass of the nucleus and the tiny mass of the moving particle plus the net electrostatic force (attractive) as explained by Coulomb's law in which q is great because of the high Z number multiplied by the q' of the particle, explain the extent of change in the path geometry. The limiting factor is still the distance between them (that is, its path), since this value is in the denominator and is squared.

This process of reduction of energy starts with a beta particle (β^-) or orbital electron being ejected from an atom and interacting with the positive nuclear field of an adjacent atom. The action is not just limited to the attractive force realized from a positive nucleus and negative particles. A positron (β^+) could come under the repulsive influence of the positive nuclear field of an adjacent atom. The important thing to remember is that a change in direction needs to occur so that an energy release results. In general, the energy characteristics of this type of situation is illustrated in Fig. 2-10. Observe that $KE_2 < KE_1$ and according to the law of conservation of energy the energy difference appears as an x-ray photon; the wavelength inversely depends on the radius of curvature of the path change.

ELECTROMAGNETIC ENERGY AND RADIATION

Implied in the above discussions has been the fact that those particles of matter (those having mass and occupying space) ejected from an atom represent one of the two categories of radiation. Specifically, it can be synonymously referred to as "particulate radiation" or "ionizing radiation." The adjective to "radiation" describes either the type or the results of the interaction with matter, respectively.

The other category of radiation is electromagnetic energy and both types have been generally discussed above. The respective subdivision name depends, theoretically, on the site of origin of the forms: x rays are extranuclear, and gamma rays are nuclear in origin.

Everyday common examples of electromagnetic energy with which we all have experience are heat and visible light. How many different types of electromagnetic energy are there and what is their relationship or relationships? Represented in Fig. 2-11 is a categorization of electromagnetic energies called a "spectrum," which is based upon one of the physical properties of this energy form. The property is called the "wavelength" and symbolized λ. Note the use of the Greek lambda here is not a mistake nor is it intended to have any relationship to its use as a radionuclide's decay constant.

Electromagnetic energies behave in several interesting ways. Their behavior, observed indirectly, is subsequently further categorized by the duality of wave phenomenon and corpuscularity.

X rays and gamma rays are electromagnetic waves, since they simultaneously consist of electric and magnetic fields. These electric and magnetic fields are mutually dependent, travel or propagate with the same frequency, and are in phase with each other. These interrelated wave types are illustrated in Fig. 2-12.

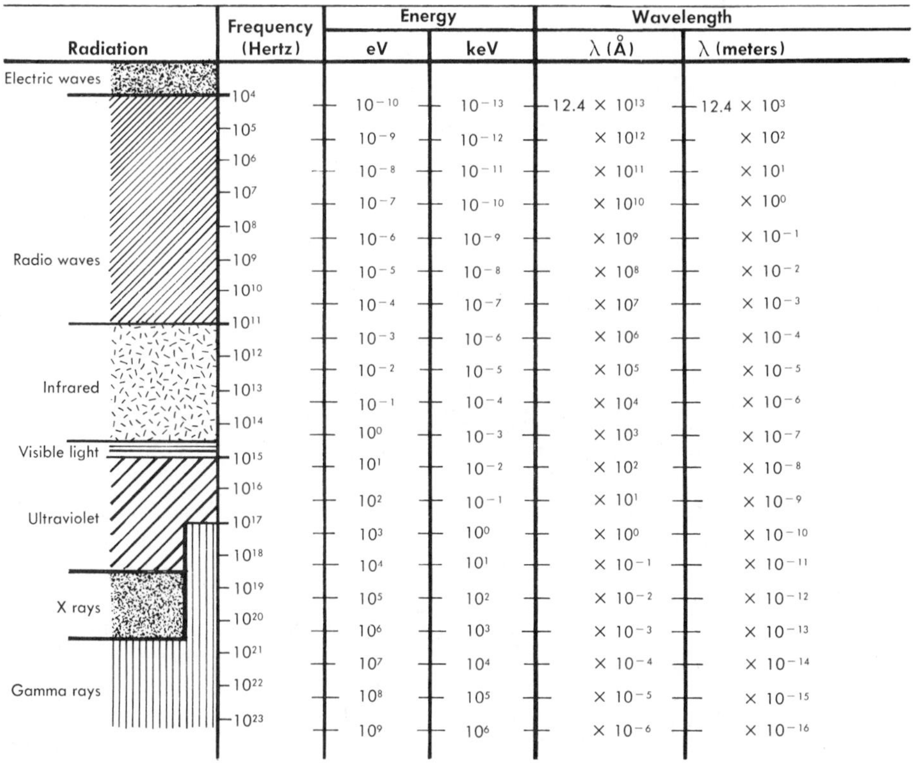

Radiation	Frequency (Hertz)	Energy eV	Energy keV	Wavelength λ (Å)	Wavelength λ (meters)
Electric waves	10^{4}	10^{-10}	10^{-13}	12.4×10^{13}	12.4×10^{3}
	10^{5}	10^{-9}	10^{-12}	$\times 10^{12}$	$\times 10^{2}$
	10^{6}	10^{-8}	10^{-11}	$\times 10^{11}$	$\times 10^{1}$
	10^{7}	10^{-7}	10^{-10}	$\times 10^{10}$	$\times 10^{0}$
	10^{8}	10^{-6}	10^{-9}	$\times 10^{9}$	$\times 10^{-1}$
Radio waves	10^{9}	10^{-5}	10^{-8}	$\times 10^{8}$	$\times 10^{-2}$
	10^{10}	10^{-4}	10^{-7}	$\times 10^{7}$	$\times 10^{-3}$
	10^{11}	10^{-3}	10^{-6}	$\times 10^{6}$	$\times 10^{-4}$
	10^{12}	10^{-2}	10^{-5}	$\times 10^{5}$	$\times 10^{-5}$
Infrared	10^{13}	10^{-1}	10^{-4}	$\times 10^{4}$	$\times 10^{-6}$
	10^{14}	10^{0}	10^{-3}	$\times 10^{3}$	$\times 10^{-7}$
Visible light	10^{15}	10^{1}	10^{-2}	$\times 10^{2}$	$\times 10^{-8}$
	10^{16}	10^{2}	10^{-1}	$\times 10^{1}$	$\times 10^{-9}$
Ultraviolet	10^{17}	10^{3}	10^{0}	$\times 10^{0}$	$\times 10^{-10}$
	10^{18}	10^{4}	10^{1}	$\times 10^{-1}$	$\times 10^{-11}$
	10^{19}	10^{5}	10^{2}	$\times 10^{-2}$	$\times 10^{-12}$
X rays	10^{20}	10^{6}	10^{3}	$\times 10^{-3}$	$\times 10^{-13}$
	10^{21}	10^{7}	10^{4}	$\times 10^{-4}$	$\times 10^{-14}$
Gamma rays	10^{22}	10^{8}	10^{5}	$\times 10^{-5}$	$\times 10^{-15}$
	10^{23}	10^{9}	10^{6}	$\times 10^{-6}$	$\times 10^{-16}$

Fig. 2-11. Electromagnetic spectrum.

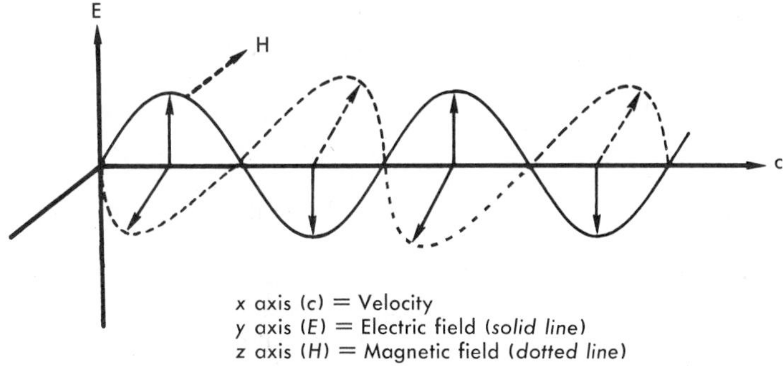

Fig. 2-12. Component energy fields of electromagnetic wave.

The field separation is 90 degrees. The height of the wave, as measured on either the E or H axes, is termed "amplitude." Referring again to Fig. 2-11, note that the aspect of comparison and designation is the wavelength. By definition, the wavelength is a linear measure of the distance between the same point in like phase. Fig. 2-13 shows that the distance, as measured in meters, centimeters, or angstroms, between these point pairs would be of equal dimensions and describe the wavelength (λ) of the propagated waves as O-O_1 or P-P_1. Additionally, the amplitude is indicated. If this figure were representing the 60-cycle alternating current (AC) used to operate nuclear medicine instrumentation, the *y* axis could represent the voltage or the current values. The wave's symbolic or graphic position above or below the *x* axis (time)

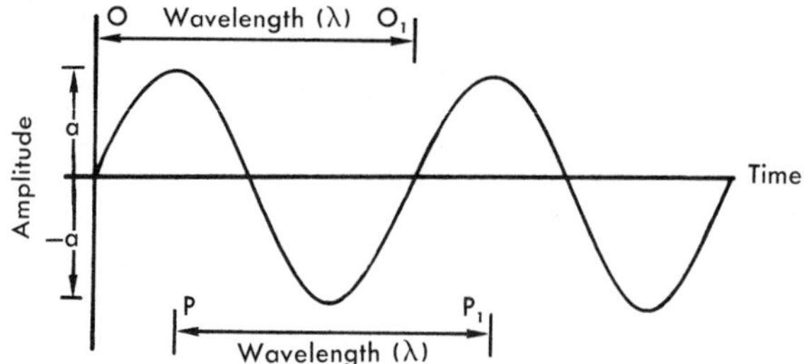

Fig. 2-13. Physical properties of propagated wave.

is important and does, in fact, indicate a direction. Again in Fig. 2-13, the wavelength distance designated by O-O_1 corresponds to a finite time on the x axis. By definition, the amount of time required to complete one cycle (that is, one λ) is called a "period" and the number of periods (that is, cycles) accomplished per second (sec^{-1}) is termed the "frequency of the propagating wave." A relatively new (and official) term, "hertz," is being used to describe the frequency. Listen to your favorite radio station's identified frequency designation. Conventional alternating current on the United States mainland is 60 hertz. Ultrasonic waves are those with a designated frequency greater than 20,000 hertz.

Since electromagnetic energy sometimes behaves as a wave, we can state its velocity and quantify its energy (in keV). All forms of electromagnetic energy commonly have the velocity, c, of light in a vacuum 3×10^{10} cm · sec^{-1} or 300,000 km · sec^{-1}, or about 186,000 miles · sec^{-1}.

Quantification of energy is based upon the wave's frequency and Plank's constant as in the following relationship:

$$E = hf$$

A more usable and workable form of this relationship is

$$E = 12.4/\lambda$$

In the latter relationship, the energy of the electromagnetic energy is expressed in kiloelectron volt units and the wavelength in angstrom units. More specific and visible then is the relationship between the energy of a wave and its wavelength or frequency. Specifically, the relationship is inverse in that when the energy is large, the wavelength must be small (that is, short), or when the energy is small, the wavelength must be large (that is, long). Verify that these relationships are validly based upon the numerical values identified in Fig. 2-11. From an appropriate reference, we could check and compare gamma-ray energies for ^{67}Ga and ^{131}I. For the former, the most abundant gamma energy is 93.3 keV, and for the latter, the most abundant gamma energy is 364 keV. Which has the longer wavelength? Wait. What does all this have to do with nuclear medicine technology? Remember that radionuclides emit gamma rays, which we now know to be waves with an energy equivalent that must be of some importance and significance when these rays, or their x-ray counterparts interact with detection instrumentation or the patient. Colors are colors to our eyes only because they represent different wavelengths. For example, the color red has a wavelength of 7000 Å, whereas the color violet has 4000 Å. Which is the more energetic?

As will be used and illustrated later, gamma rays or x rays are represented as a sinusoidal wave, of some hypothetical wavelength, and with an accompanying arrowhead to indicate that it is propagated in some direction in space (Fig. 2-14). With the four hypothetical waves illustrated, first, order them by rank from the least to the greatest energy and secondly from the shortest the longest wavelength. (respectively *J,H,K,I,* and *I,K,H,J*)

From the studies of Millikan and Einstein, who explained the photoelectric effect, there emerged a term and a definition that were necessary in the analysis of corpuscular behavior of electromagnetic energy. The term "photon" is a quantum of energy, which may be pictured as a "package" or "particle" of radiant energy. According to elementary quantum theory, a photon is regarded as a discrete quantity possessing a momentum, constantly in motion, having no electric charge, and no magnetic moment. For our purposes, photons can be created subsequent to the interaction between a particle of matter and an electrical field (for example, bremsstrahlung) or matter with matter (for example, Compton scattering). The quantum nature of radiation is evidenced in its radioactive as well as its absorptive phases. Similarly to the above wave discussion, the photon's energy is directly related to the frequency of the energy. By involving Einstein's laws of

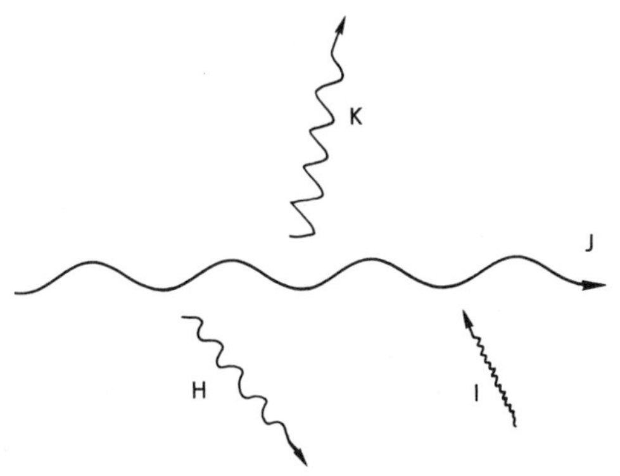

Fig. 2-14. Representation of electromagnetic energy.

mass and energy equivalency, the mass of a photon could be described as

$$m = \frac{E}{c^2} = \frac{hf}{c^2}$$

Using appropriate numerical values, we find that a radio wave whose wavelength is 2000 meters has a mass equivalence of 1.1×10^{-42} g and a 1 Å x ray has a mass equivalent of 2.2×10^{-29} g.

INTERACTIONS

On previous and numerous occasions, the concept of the interactions of radiant energy with matter or matter with matter at various levels has been mentioned. Just how meaningful and of what types are these interactive experiences? Are these interactions advantageous or deleterious? Upon what physical parameters do they depend? Have I ever experienced these interactions prior to entering this health field or are they esoteric and limited to nuclear medicine technology?

Everyday examples with which you most likely have had prior experience are numerous. One common use is a photographic camera, which is used to make a picture by the incident visible light's energy interacting with matter (that is, the emulsion on the film). When you enter a doorway with the door ''sensing'' your passage and opening for you, it is the result of the interruption of a light beam being incident upon a photoelectric cell connected to appropriate electrical circuitry. Smoke and heat detectors in buildings involve the interaction of incident energy and matter (a detection device). Information contained on this page can be transmitted either by sight or sound. The former involves interaction of electromagnetic energy (specifically, visible light) and the lens and retina of the eye; the latter involves acoustic electromagnetic energy (that is, sound waves) and the eardrum. The list that could be developed identifying these types of interactions is endless. The intent thus far is to indicate that we have all had experiences involving energy and matter, or matter and matter. The following discussion specifically presents the physical aspects involved in interactions important in nuclear medicine technology.

Interaction of charged particles with matter

Regardless of the source and the mechanism for the production of electrically charged particles of matter, when they traverse a medium (for example, air, water, soft tissue, and dense tissue), they undergo collisions (more politely interactions), which are either elastic or inelastic. The probability of charged particles being transmitted through matter without interactions is extremely low. Examples of charged particles that may undergo interactions are the alpha (α) particle and the beta (β^-, β^+) particles; an example of an electrically neutral particle that may undergo interactions is a neutron. Yet, another descriptive term to be used in this context is scattering, which denotes a change to a less orderly arrangement or a change in direction of the particles (matter) or photons (energy) because of their interaction. In general, either phrase—elastic collisions or elastic scattering—refers to a physical situation in which there is no change in the internal energy of the subsystem components or in the sum of their kinetic energies. Elastic collision, in the context of energy/matter interactions, refers to deflections, whereas inelastic collisions generally result in the production of ions or ion pairs. Attention should not be lost to the fact that the incident particle can also be completely absorbed. Further, elastic interactions release or lose no electromagnetic energy, since the total kinetic energy and total momentum of the colliding particle and atom with which it interacts remains constant. On the other hand, inelastic interactions are sometimes referred to as incoherent interactions, since there is no phase relationship between the scattered photons.

In a general sense and in a clinical setting, of what importance or usefulness is knowledge of interactions of radiation with matter? Well, for the broad categories of radiation protection, radiobiology, detection instrument operation, effective use of safe and appropriate methodologies for yourself and the patient, and accurate quantification of radionuclide concentrations resulting in images for medical interpretations, an understanding of interactions is important.

Again, thinking small to the atomic level, an incident form of radiation can interact with the nuclear region of the atom, the nuclear field, or the extranuclear region of the atom. What determines where it interacts? Simply, its ''line of sight,'' or the geometric path along which it is traveling, does the determining.

Table 2-7. Types of interactions between radiation and matter

Incident radiation	Site of interaction	Type of interaction: Elastic	Inelastic	Absorption
Alpha (α)	Nuclear			Nuclear reactions
	Nuclear field	Rutherford scattering	Bremsstrahlung	
	Extranuclear		Ionization and excitation	
Electrons (Auger, recoil, photo, β^+, β^-, conversion)	Nuclear	Rutherford scattering		Electron capture
	Nuclear field			
	Nuclear field		Bremsstrahlung	
	Extranuclear		Ionization and excitation	Annihilation radiation
Neutrons	Nuclear			Neutron activation
	Nuclear field			Nuclear reactions
	Extranuclear			
Photons (x rays, gamma rays)	Nuclear			Photodisintegration
	Nuclear field			Pair production
	Extranuclear	Bragg	Compton	Photoelectric

What determines how it will interact? The answer is much more complicated, but its mass or mass equivalency, electrical charge or lack thereof, wavelength, occurrence probability as measured in barns (10^{-24} cm^2), kinetic energy, A and Z numbers of the matter upon which the radiation is incident, and density of the material are, for our purposes, the aspects of concern in knowing the manner of its interaction or interactions.

Table 2-7 categorizes the major types of interactions between incident radiation types and the atomic regions of matter. Yes, there are blank spaces in this table. These absences are not meant to indicate that no interactions are possible. On the contrary, interaction types are possible but only those of significant academic or clinical importance are identified. The following discussion treats each type of incident radiation separately.

Alpha particles

Symbolically, the nucleus of a helium atom (^4_2He), or the Greek letter α, is used to represent this type of radiation. Since the alpha particle represents only the helium nucleus as opposed to a helium atom, it possesses a double positive ($^{++}$) electrical charge. Most alpha particles possess energy between 3 and 8 MeV and an approximate range of 3 to 8 cm in air. Since their mass is relatively large, their path in matter is approximately a straight line and because of their electrical charge, they are highly ionizing. As a charged particle moves through matter (solid, liquid, or gas), ion pairs are produced along its path. The number of pairs depends on the energy necessary to produce the pair ($\bar{x}$ 32 eV), the length of path along which the particle moves before being stopped, and the kinetic energy (MeV) of the particle. The number of ion pairs produced per track length (mm) is defined as *specific ionization*. In the case of an alpha particle, the number of ion pairs created significantly increases near the end of its path as it slows down and literally spends more time electrically influencing atoms along and in proximity to its path. Fig. 2-15 illustrates a specific ionization curve relating the number of ion pairs produced to both the distance from the radioactive source and to the range or distance from the end of the track. If the abscissa in Fig. 2-15 were differently captioned as the residual energy of the incident particle and the ordinate remained the same, the same graphic configuration would result but the graph would be called the Bragg curve. Another researcher, L. H. Gray, combined interests and efforts with Bragg and developed the Bragg-Gray formula for relating ionizations to the subsequent energy absorbed by the irradiated matter. A companion but significantly different term is *linear energy transfer* (LET), which is a quantifiable measure of the linear rate of energy loss by an incident particle such as an alpha particle or electron. The energy loss is absorbed by the atoms or molecules along or in proximity to the particle's path. An inverse relationship exists between a particle's velocity and the resulting LET. Specifically, the higher the velocity (MeV), the lower the LET value. How would the LET value of an alpha particle compare to that for a beta particle? The answer is based upon the inverse relationships between mass and velocity. By use of vertically directed arrows to indicate high(er) and

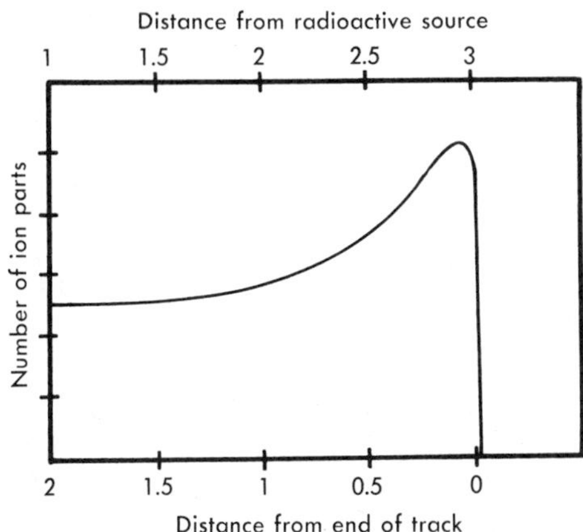

Fig. 2-15. Specific ionization curve.

low(er), the above relationships for both alpha and beta particles are as follows:

	Mass	Velocity	LET values
Alpha (α)	↑	↓	↑
Beta (β^-, β^+)	↓	↑	↓

In the scattering of alpha particles as described by Rutherford, he suggested that the angular deflections from their original path through which some alpha particles were moved was the result of electrostatic repulsive charges of the incident alpha particle and that of the nucleus of the confronted atom. This type of interaction results in no production or release of electromagnetic energy (that is, gamma rays) but only in a deflection of path geometry. However, depending on incident path geometry, the resulting deflection geometry can be of such magnitude that some of the kinetic energy of the alpha particle is released. If the energy released has appropriate wavelength dimensions, it may be classified as x rays produced by the bremsstrahlung method. For elastic interactions, the production of ionization and excitations is fairly easy to visualize by the fact that the incident alpha particle and extranuclear region of the confronted atom are oppositely charged. Consequently, the enhancement of interaction by attraction. Characteristic x-ray production can occur subsequent to the ionization of the atom. The total absorption of the incident alpha particle by the confronted atom can occur but results in nuclear transformations.

Electronic particles

As indicated in Table 2-7, several names and types of electronic particles are possible as a form of incident radiation. This listing is meant to indicate that regardless of the source of these electron type of particles, they can behave or interact similarly. Without being redundant, the site of and type of resulting interaction is determined primarily by the incident particle's path geometry relative to regions of the confronted atoms. In other words, if the negatively charged incident particle collides with a positive nucleus, Rutherford scattering is the term associated with the interaction if it is elastic and the electronic particle's path is deflected greatly. This type of interaction does have clinical importance in that the resulting great deflections of the incident particles may be up to 180 degrees (that returning in the direction from which it came). The name of the interaction type (Rutherford scattering) is most frequently replaced by the term "backscattering." This type of interaction can falsely increase the observed and measured count rate of a radioactive sample. Backscattering is primarily dependent on the *Z* number of matter upon which the radiation is incident and the energy spectrum of the incident electronic particles. As a comparative note, self-absorption of radiation by a sample results in opposite direction of falsely low observed and measured count rate. This aspect is important in sample counting and geometry.

Of practical importance is the interaction of electronic particles with the nuclear field of an atom. Again depending on geometry, the incident particle will be influenced by the attractive coulombic force of the nucleus to the extent that energy is released. You are correct in describing the released energy as x rays produced by the bremsstrahlung method. These x-ray energies represent a continuum because of the variations in the incident particles' kinetic energy and in changes of path geometry. As the *Z* number of the matter increases, the incidence and importance of bremsstrahlung interaction increases and becomes more significant. This is attributable to the increased coulombic attractive forces between a physically massive and highly positive nucleus and a physically small and singly negative particle. A beta (β^-)-particle emitting radionuclide such as ^{32}P would not be contained in or shielded from or by a material that had a high *Z* number like lead (206). On the contrary, low *Z* number materials like plastic (for example, a syringe) or pressed cardboard are both adequate and sufficient as shielding material in which this type of interaction is insignificant.

Just as for alpha-particle interaction in the extranuclear region of the atom, ionizations and excitations are possible, with resulting characteristic x-ray production from inelastic electronic-particle interaction.

The complete absorption of an electronic particle by the nucleus is possible and again depends on geometry and a particle's specific location at a given point in time. The most classic example of this type of interaction is electron capture (for example, K capture) as discussed above. If the incident electronic particle is a positron (β^+) and its path geometry causes it to interact with an orbital electron, the resulting interaction is termed "annihilation." The lifetime of a positron depends on the number of electrons in the immediate environment upon which it was incident. According to quantum physics, matter and energy can neither be destroyed but may be interconverted. The annihilative process represents the interconversion. The rest mass equivalency of the positron and negatron are identical and result in a sum of 1.022 MeV. If, at their interaction, they possess kinetic energy, the resulting energy release is the 1.022 MeV minimum plus the kinetic energy component. Also as a result of quantum mechanics, the energy released appears as two gamma photons each equally sharing the total energy of the annihilative interaction. Detection and imaging instrumentation have been designed to recognize the coincidence of these two photons as resulting from one interactive event and not two.

Neutron particles

In clinical nuclear medicine, neutrons have no role and are of no significance. However, some therapeutic treatment modalities utilize an incident beam consisting of neutrons. In Table 2-7, the significant interactions between neutrons and matter arise as a result of their complete physical absorption within the nucleus. Neutron activation has been briefly referred to previously and nuclear reactions are briefly referred to later (p. 86).

Photons

Of the major types of incident radiations and categories of interactions, clinically the most important type is photons (for example, x rays and gamma rays) and their inelastic scatterings or energy absorptions. Photons are much more penetrating, have no definite ranges, and demonstrate exponential absorption in matter.

When incident upon matter, photons may traverse it without participating in any interactions, but although this is statistically possible, it is not very probable. On the other hand, photons may totally disappear when being incident, or they may undergo interactions and change direction or undergo interaction with no change in direction.

Bragg scattering interactions are elastic and coherent in that no energy is lost and that the reradiated photon energy is in a definite phase of relationship to the incident photon energy. Use of this type of interaction is in crystallography and for determining the wavelengths of various forms of electromagnetic energies. The total absorption (μ) of photons by matter depends on the additive absorption coefficients for photoelectric (τ), Compton (σ), and pair production (K) processes as in the following equation:

$$\mu = \tau + \sigma + K$$

The total absorption value is used as the exponent in the intensity formula, as follows:

$$I = I_0 \cdot e^{-\mu x}$$

Compton effect

Known as Compton scattering, the Compton effect involves the inelastic interaction of an incident photon with orbital electrons. The interaction may also be known as modified or incoherent scattering. The process is inelastic by definition, since energy is lost by the incident photon. Diagrammatically, this type of interaction is represented in Fig. 2-16. The incident photon's wavelength is represented as λ_0; the emitted photon's wavelength is represented by λ_1. Symbolically and actually $\lambda_1 > \lambda_0$. In other words, the emitted photon is less energetic than the incident photon. The dotted line in Fig. 2-16 indicates the straight-line geometric path along which the incident photon would have traveled had not an interaction resulted. A range of energies from a maximum to a minimum are possible for the scattered photon and the recoil electron; however, their values are inversely related, since the total energy before and after the interaction must be accounted for and is the same. To illustrate, when the scattered photon's energy is high, the recoil electron's energy is low and vice versa. Actually most of this type of interaction results in values between the

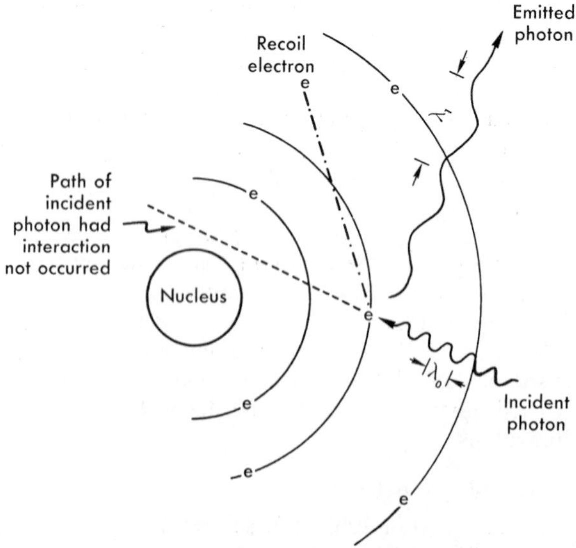

Fig. 2-16. Compton scattering.

two extremes. Since an interaction resulted, the orbital electron was ejected if one assumes that the incident photon's energy was of a value greater than the binding energy for the involved electron. Where in the extranuclear region is or does this interaction most likely occur? Generally, the photons interact with "free" electrons. What are "free" electrons? They are those whose binding energy values are low as compared to the energy of the incident photon. Further, the constituents of a patient's soft tissues such as water, proteins, and fats consist primarily of hydrogen, carbon, nitrogen, and oxygen, all of which have low Z numbers, 1, 6, 7, and 8, respectively, and as a result, the binding energies are extremely low and their electrons are considered "free," relative to the incident photon's energy. There is nothing magic about a recoil electron. It behaves the same as any electron, except it is so named to indicate its genesis. Since a recoil electron has been supplied with kinetic energy, it can now undergo the types of electronic-particle interactions described and discussed above. A recoil electron has its maximum value when the photon is scattered directly backwards as compared to the situation that would result if the recoil electron were ejected at a slight angular deflection from the dotted line in Fig. 2-16. Also, the emitted photon can undergo subsequent interactions of these categories, and since its direction is other than that for the incident photon, it is said to be scattered.

"What," you may ask, "is the significance of this type of interaction?" Resulting from this type of interaction are two subsequent phenomena—absorption and attenuation. Absorption is the deposition of energy into the matter upon which the photons were incident. Attenuation is the removal of a photon or photons by some interactive process. A special case identifying the attenuation of one half the incident photons was discussed in the previous chapter under the topic half-value layer (HVL).

Both the type of matter (not state of matter but atomic number, Z) and the incident photon's energy affect the scattering process. The extent or number of times this type of interaction occurs depends on the number of electrons present. For all materials containing hydrogen (for example, water, proteins, fats, and carbohydrates), the number of electrons is approximately twice the number for oxygen (for example, air in lungs) or calcium (bone). The doubling effect of the number happens over a relatively short range of atomic numbers. What does this mean? More Compton scattering will take place in hydrogenous materials (that is, soft tissue) than in bony material.

The other character in this scattering scenario is the recoil electron. For a given scattering angle, as the incident photon's energy increases, a significantly greater percentage of the total energy appears with the recoil electron. In other words, with low incident photon energies, most of its energy is scattered. Also, as the incident photon energy increases, the scattered photon is more likely to be traveling nearly in the same direction (that is, forward) than it would have been prior to the interaction. The frequency of scattering in a backward direction, also called back scattering, is almost as likely as scattering in a forward direction.

Photoelectric effect

In contradistinction to the Compton scattering phenomenon, the photoelectric effect involves an interaction between an incident photon and a "bound" electron. There is no scattered photon, since all the photon's energy is consumed by an orbital electron in the process of its release. In other words, the "bound" electron cannot be ejected from the atom unless the incident photon's energy is equal to or greater than the binding energy for the specific electron and to which kinetic energy is given if an energy difference exists. This relationship is given by this generalized relationship:

Incident photon's energy = Electron binding energy + Electron kinetic energy

Subsequent to the interaction, no evidence of the primary or initiating photon is evident because its energy has been completely absorbed. The result of this interaction is the formation of an ion pair; the positive ion is the electrically neutral atom from which the electron was removed and the negative ion is the removed electron. With the electron vacancy created in a bound position such as in the K or L shells, subsequent electron positional rearrangement results in the production and emission of characteristic x-ray photons. The original electrically neutral profile that the atom possessed is reachieved by the acquisition of a free and available electron.

Just as the ejected electron in Compton scattering is known by a special name, the ejected electron from this type of interaction is known as a photoelectron. Once removed from the atom, there is nothing esoteric or special about this electron or its behavior. Because of the kinetic energy that has been supplied to the photoelectron, it can now undergo the types of electronic particle interactions described and discussed above.

The complete disappearance of the incident photon's energy is clinically important for not only is the photon attenuated but also its energy is completely absorbed by the patient.

Diagrammatically, this type of interaction is represented in Fig. 2-17. As stated in words above, a bound electron (for example, K electron) is shown interacting

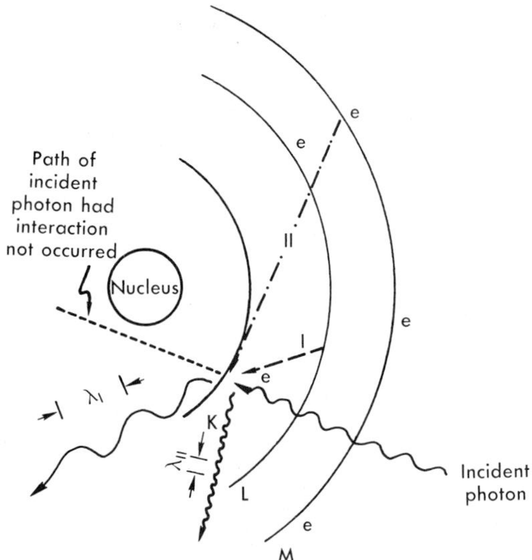

Fig. 2-17. Photoelectric effect.

with the incident photon. The geometric path of its ejection is so indicated and is in the forward position and identical to that of the photon had an interaction not occurred. With one of the two K electrons now removed, the orbital desire of the atom can be satisfied by any electron, usually one from either the L or the M shell, undergoing a physical rearrangement in its energy location. Either change I or II, as indicated in Fig. 2-17, is possible. The energy difference between orbital levels determines the unique energetic values of these characteristic x-ray photons emitted (for example, K_α or K_β). Both x-ray photons, λ_I and λ_{II}, represent the K series of the characteristic photons. Even though these two x-ray photons are each monoenergetic (that is, represent a specific energetic value), they represent two of the K x-ray spectral lines. Specifically, photon λ_I represents the K_α component and photon λ_{II} represents the K_β component. The wavelengths of these K_α and K_β photons are different because of the differences in their respective extranuclear positions and respective binding energies. To illustrate, suppose a patient previously had a diagnostic radiographic examination that used an iodine-based contrast medium. If a gamma ray was incident upon the K electron of iodine, 33 keV of its energy would be consumed in its ejection, with the balance as kinetic energy of the photoelectron. For iodine, an L electron and an M electron are bound by approximately 5 and 1 keV units of energy. The respective energy values of K_α and K_β are 28 and 32, respectively. To determine the respective wavelengths, a previously discussed formula needs to be reutilized to express the relationship between wavelength and energy as follows:

$$\lambda = \frac{12.4}{\text{keV}}$$

For K_α, the photon's wavelength is 0.443 Å (that is, 12.4/28), and for K_β, the photon's wavelength is 0.387 Å (that is, 12.4/32). Reaffirm that the diagrammatic representation of these characteristic x-ray photons in Fig. 2-17 is correct.

With the emission of characteristic x-ray photons, which is secondary to the primary photoelectric interaction, the story can become more involved when one includes the tertiary interactions resulting in the ejection of Auger electrons.

The atomic number and incident photon's energy both affect the photoelectric process. As the atomic number *(Z)* increases, so do the binding energy values for their bound electrons, and the probability of a photoelectric interaction is therefore high. A majority (that is, 80%) of the photoelectric interactions involve the K electrons. The probability of this type of interaction is proportional to Z^5. In other words, the photoelectric process is more important in materials of higher atomic number than those of lower. When one considers the energy of the incident photon, the probability is inversely proportional to the photon's energy as

$$h\nu^{7/2}$$

and greatest for energies less than 0.5 MeV. In other words, the probability of this interaction is much greater at low photon energies. In summary, the photoelectric effect is most important in the absorption of low-energy photons by heavy elements of which not too many at all are normally present in the human body (that is, the patient). However, you have had or will have an opportunity to experience this type of interaction. Photocells, either in a burglar alarm or a door sensor or in other uses employ the photoelectric process whereby light representing low incident photon energy is incident upon a heavy atomic material called a photocathode. The process releases electrons, which can be used as an electric current in other circuitry applications. This type of interaction in nuclear medicine is discussed in greater detail in other chapters.

Pair production

The remaining category of photon interaction is interaction with an electrical field. In Table 2-7, only the positive electrical field of the nucleus is suggested. However, it is theoretically possible for the photon to interact with the electrical field of the electron. For the former, the photon threshold energy is 1.02 MeV, and for the latter, the threshold energy is 2.04 MeV. From these values, it could easily be stated that this interactive process has little clinical importance in nuclear medicine because of the lower photon energies

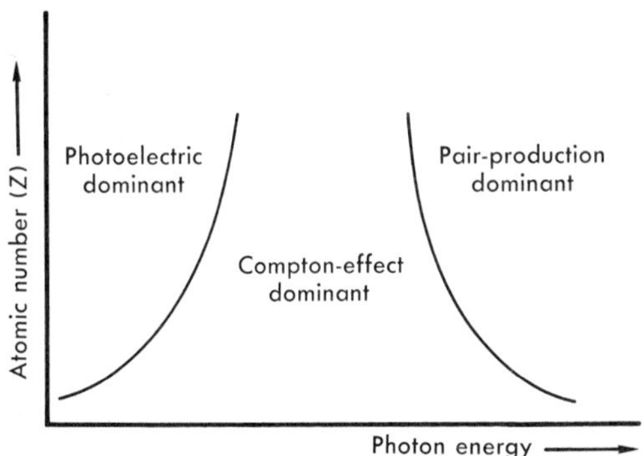

Fig. 2-18. Predominance of photon interactive types as related to photon energy and atomic number of absorber.

arising from the various and most frequently used radionuclides.

The process is interesting from the standpoint that is represents the interconversion of energy and mass. The interactive process may also be known as materialization. The greater threshold energy difference between the field of an electron and nucleus is attributable to the conservation of momentum and energy. A photon whose energy is greater than 1.02 MeV and whose geometric path brings it close to but not in contact with the nucleus can totally disappear. In the place of the photon, a pair of particles of matter are created, consequently, the name. The pair consists of a positron (β^+) and negatron (β^-) whose combined mass represents an energy equivalence of 1.02 MeV. Note the relationship between this number and the threshold energy value mentioned previously. By the creation of these two electrically charged particles of matter, their charges offset each other, but nonetheless two ions are present. From this point forward, the behavior of these two ions is as discussed above under positron emission and annihilative radiation. The probability of this type of interaction increases with atomic number, *Z*, and the corresponding increase in magnitude of the electrical field. Also, the relationship between the incident photon energy and probability of interaction is direct.

The gamma photons from the annihilative process are emitted in opposite directions (that is, separated by 180 degrees) and are of an energy value of at least 0.511 MeV, based upon the rest mass equivalencies of each of the two annihilative components. These photons are, when traversing matter, capable of undergoing any of the types of interactions discussed above.

In summary, Fig. 2-18 illustrates the predominance of these three major interaction categories as a function of incident photon energy. There is no clear diagrammatic boundary for these types of interactions but only ranges. Fig. 2-18 is a broad generalization, and the specific aspects for each type of material need to be consulted.

TYPE OF EFFECTS SECONDARY TO INTERACTIONS

The previous generalized statements state the major categories of interactions and generally what the by-products (for example, characteristic x rays, photoelectrons) of the interactions are capable of. The following statements present some specific details for these by-product interactions.

Simply stated, electrons, as a by-product, are common to the Compton scattering, photoelectric and pair-production processes. What specifically happens to these electrons as they interact with matter? As a result of electronic interaction, changes take effect. What are the categories of changes? The major categories of changes in biologic matter (for example, patient) are chemical, physical, and biologic, with the latter two being specific modifications of the chemical or electronic nature of matter. Generally speaking, ionizations, excitations, and heat are the forms of changes within these categories. Without delving into radiobiology, we find that the chemical changes are resultant from disruptions in the electrical balance and nature of matter such that free "radicals," electrically charged molecules, are produced and may cause deleterious manifestations in the finely tuned chemical mechanisms of the biologic system. Physical changes can be as simple as the direct deposition of energy into a system or indirectly from exogenic chemical reactions. Biologic changes, when viewed fundamentally, are chemically derived at the atomic or molecular level.

Transmission or attenuation

If a photon is incident upon matter and completely traverses it without interacting with the nucleus, orbital electrons or nuclear field, the photon has been transmitted, whereas if an interaction takes place and results in the photon's inability to traverse the material or produces a reduction in its energy, the photon has been attenuated.

In the previous chapter, a special case in point was raised and discussed in which the emerging intensity or radiation, *I*, was equal to one half the incident intensity, I_0, such that

$$I = \frac{1}{2} I_0$$

The thickness of material that results in these intensity relationships is the half-value layer (HVL). As a part of the intensity equation

$$I = I_0 \cdot e^{-\mu x}$$

μ is a parameter that now needs further discussion and

elaboration. Represented as an exponent, μ, the linear attenuation coefficient is the quantifiable measurement of the exponential reduction in intensity per unit dimension of material (cm^{-1}). As a corollary parameter, the mass attenuation coefficient, μ, is another quantifiable measurement that is independent of the material's density. The units of this coefficient are cm^2/g. From the following, the relationship between these two attenuation coefficients is represented:

$$\mu_{mass} = \frac{\mu_{linear}}{\text{Density}}$$

Unitizing these attenuation relationships results in the following expression:

$$\frac{cm^2}{g} = \frac{cm^{-1}}{g/cm^3}$$

Two additional attenuation coefficients, atomic and electronic, quantify the chance or probability of a photon's removal by an atom or electron per unit length of track. To compare, the quantifiable linear attenuation coefficient consists of three summated probabilities for the three major photon interactions. Literally, it is a probability or percentage value to state by how much the photon intensity will be decreased per linear distance.

Schematics of radioactive decay

Frequently referred to as decay schemes, these diagrams indicate and provide empirically derived information about the various physical parameters involved with the radioactive disintegration of a parent radionuclide into a daughter nuclide, which may or may not itself be radioactive.

Refer to Fig. 2-3 for the basic diagrammatic decay scheme. Note the shaded unstable nuclide ranges on either side of the clear stable nuclide segment. Radionuclides, if personified, would like to achieve a ground or stable nuclidic state. The achievement of stability (clear segment), from wherever the nuclide's location may be in the scheme, by emission of particulate radiation or electromagnetic radiation, or both, can occur quickly in one step or quickly in multiple steps. Note again the axis designations in Fig. 2-3. Inherent in decay schemes is the assumption that it is constructed such that its bottom is parallel to the x axis. Also the vertical placement of the parent and daughter nuclides is such that its side is parallel to the y axis. Expanding on this relationship, we can add the energy characteristics, modes, frequencies, and physical half-life periods of the decay process.

Since the disintegrating radionuclide (that is, the parent) is attempting to achieve a ground or stable state through the emission of one of both forms of radiation, it is written on top, with the daughter nuclide, which

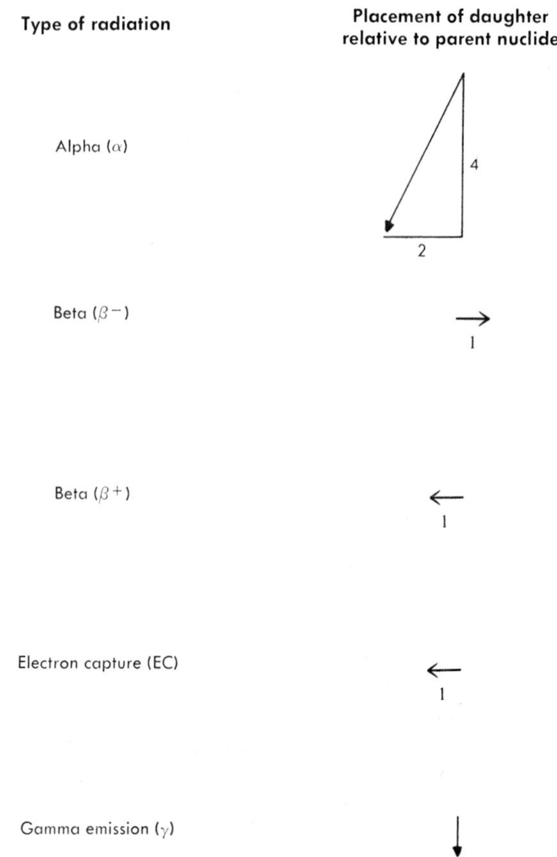

Fig. 2-19. Directional placement of daughter relative to parent in decay scheme.

is at a lower energy level, written below. Where below? Directly below, or below and to one side? The answer depends on the type of radiation that is emitted. Fig. 2-19 identifies the types of radiation and the general directional placement of the daughter relative to the parent. For the first four entries in this tabular information, triangular shapes are represented. The hypotenuse is the solid line with the arrow and indicates the relative placement of the inferiorly placed daughter. The leg of these triangles are not included in decay schemes but are represented here to denote the changes resulting from the decay process. For example, in alpha decay, the daughter nuclide's atomic number is two less than the parent's. Also, the A number for the daughter is 4 less than that of the parent's. For β^- and electron capture, these triangulate legs representing Z and A numbers are only one unit long and are not drawn to scale. The reason is that the slope of the hypotenuse is not important here but need only indicate a direction. From previous discussion, you know that the only change experienced in isomeric transi-

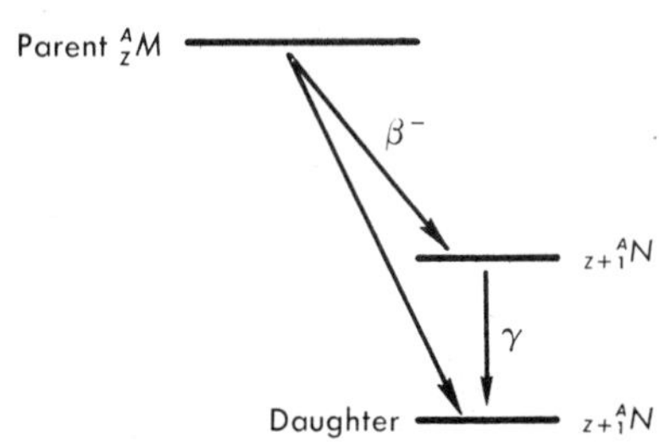

Fig. 2-20. Hypothetical decay scheme representing beta-particle emission.

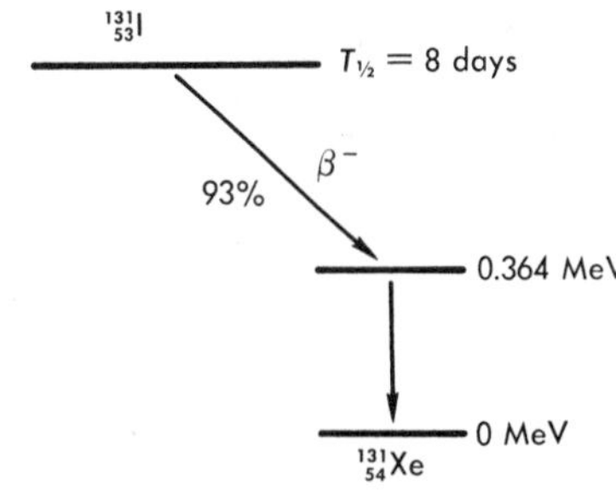

Fig. 2-21. Generalized decay scheme for iodine 131.

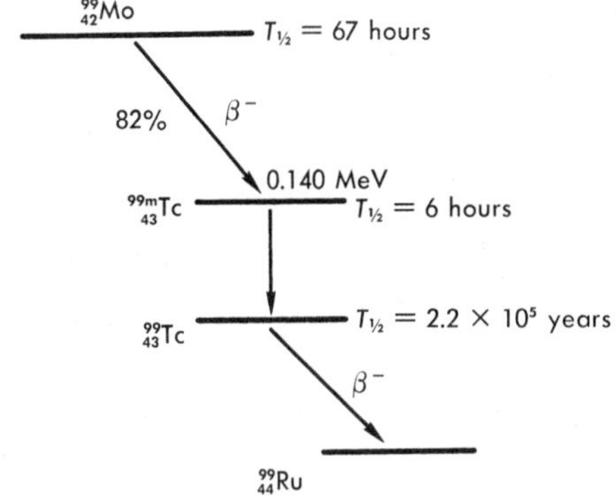

Fig. 2-22. Generalized decay scheme for molybdenum 99.

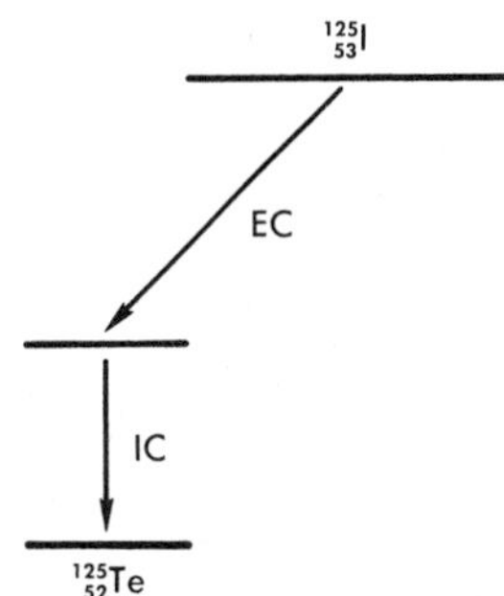

Fig. 2-23. Generalized decay scheme for iodine 125.

tions is the emission of a gamma ray to release nuclear excitation energy and is appropriately and accurately represented by a vertical arrow, which has no atomic number, Z, or atomic mass number, A, components.

Energy levels of the daughter nucleus are represented by horizontal lines directly above the ground state of the daughter with corresponding gamma-ray emission lines. These nuclear energetic lines are labeled with their monochromatic energy values as measured in keV. In Fig. 2-20, the parent radionuclide, $^{A}_{Z}M$, decays by beta-particle (β^-) emission directly to the daughter $_{Z+1}^{A}N$ as a one-step decay path, whereas another path emits a less energetic β^- particle and subsequent gamma-photon emission to deenergize the daughter nucleus. The energy release is of the daughter nucleus because the beta particle has already been released and is no longer the parental element since the Z number has changed.

The daughter may also be a radionuclide, which, in the next step of the overall decay process, becomes the parent radionuclide for that process.

Figs. 2-21 and 2-22 represent simplified but pragmatic decay schemes for ^{131}I and ^{99}Mo. Note the similarity of their respective decay schemes to that of the hypothetical decay scheme in Fig. 2-19. For ^{131}I, approximately 93% of the decay transformations are by beta-particle ejection, with the resulting xenon daughter nucleus being 364 keV units of nuclear energy above its stable state. To achieve nuclear stability, a 364 keV gamma photon is emitted, and this photon is useful and detected in clinical nuclear medicine. Approximately 82% of the nuclear transformations of ^{99}Mo occur as a result of an ejection of a beta particle to a metastable nuclear state of the daughter, technetium (Tc). Metastable nuclear energy of the daughter is released by the emission of a 140 keV gamma photon, which is of clinical significance and importance. The daughter becomes a parent by radioactively decaying to ruthenium (Ru). Note the schematic agreement of the increase in atomic numbers with earlier discussion.

By comparison, Fig. 2-23 represents the schemes for

Table 2-8. Gallium-67 photon emissions

Photons	Abundance percentage	Mean energy (keV)
Gamma 2	38	93.3
Gamma 3	21	184.6
Gamam 5	16	300.2
Gamma 6	4	393.5

the radioactive disintegration of ^{125}I, an actively used radionuclide in radioimmunoassay procedures. Initially, electron capture by the parental nucleus results in the excited state of the daughter nucleus, which then releases energy by the process of internal conversion. Subsequent to the internal conversion by the tellurium nucleus is the emission of K-characteristic x rays, which, for ^{125}I, is the means by which it is detected and quantized in addition to the characteristic x rays from the electron-capture process.

In these previously generalized radioactive decay schemes, simplicity of photon energies and percentages of abundance has been employed. Unfortunately, the real world is not that simple. The aspect of abundance and energy properties can be illustrated for a currently used clinical radionuclide ^{67}Ga as in Table 2-8. Gallium 67 decays by electron capture (EC) to ^{67}Zn.

From the excited zinc nucleus, several gamma photons can be emitted. The three most abundant average photon energies are listed as well as their percent abundance. In other words, for every 100 excited zinc nuclei, approximately 38% would have a mean energy of 93.3 keV and so forth. The most energetic photons, 393 keV, are not the most abundant as evidenced by the low percentage of approximately 4%.

Nuclear reactions

From where, besides commercial vendors, do radionuclides come? Or from where do the vendors obtain the radioactive materials to produce radiopharmaceuticals? The sources of radioactive materials are either naturally occurring or synthetically produced.

In general, the naturally occurring radionuclides have high atomic numbers ($Z \geq 80$) and belong to four series, all radionuclides of which eventually terminate their disintegration process by decaying into a stable nuclidic form of lead (Pb). These radionuclides are not of clinical significance.

The detailed energy properties and modes of synthetically produced radionuclides is beyond the scope of this book even though our clinically useful radionuclides arise by this process. Some general information and discussion will be of interest.

Artificial radioactivity involves the synthesis of nuclear instability by the interaction of a high-speed particle of matter, charged or uncharged, that is incident upon an atom's nucleus. Possessing a high kinetic energy value, the particle delivers the energy necessary to initiate the reaction.

One such exogenous reaction category is fission, in which a heavy atomic nucleus splits apart into approximately two equal portions. As identified and briefly discussed previously, the liquid-drop model of the nucleus is useful in explaining this reaction type. If the target nuclei are those of ^{235}U whose atomic number is 92, the fragmenting nuclei will have an atomic number range of 30 to 64 with the modal atomic numbers of 42 and 56, molybdenum and barium, respectively. Most of these new nuclei are radioactive, since their heavier parent had a large excess of neutrons over protons.

Fusion, by comparison, is the joining of lighter nuclei to form radionuclides. In the combination process, energy is released, which is the difference of the nuclear binding energies of the product nuclei and that of the original light nuclei.

Neutron activation is a common method for the production of radionuclides by the initiation of an incident neutron and subsequent release of a gamma photon abbreviated as (n, γ).

Chapter 3

INSTRUMENTATION

Part A: Basic instrumentation

R. Eugene Johnston

The difficulty in writing about imaging instruments is that no sooner than one has described the most recent instruments, they become outdated. The goal in this chapter is to present established basic principles of radiation detectors and at the expense of breadth, consider in some detail the "work-horse" instruments in nuclear medicine.

PRINCIPLES OF GAS-FILLED RADIATION DETECTORS

Gas-filled counter tubes were introduced as radiation detectors by Rutherford and Geiger in 1908.[20] They used an apparatus to amplify the electrical effect of ionization produced in a gas from a single alpha particle. The earliest medical applications of radioisotopes utilized gas-filled detectors for the instrumentation. With the introduction of scintillation detectors in the middle 1950s, the gas-filled detector quickly became relegated to the place of survey meters and played a secondary role in the armamentarium of nuclear medicine instrumentation.

In the modern nuclear medicine laboratory, the gas-filled detector has taken on new importance under the name of "dose calibrator." Thus the earliest detectors return as important instruments dressed in the modern clothing of digital electronics.

Ionization detectors

The simplest of the gas-filled detectors is the ionization chamber. The ion chamber is a defined volume of gas such as air at atmospheric pressure or an inert gas such as argon at one or more atmospheres of pressure in which ionization is caused by exposure of the gas to radiation. Fig. 3-1 is a cross-sectional diagram of a typical ionization chamber.

The chamber is a cylindric container that holds and defines a volume of gas. Another cylinder is located concentrically within the volume of gas and is called a "collecting electrode." A high voltage is applied between the collecting electrode and the walls of the chamber to generate an electric field throughout the gas volume.

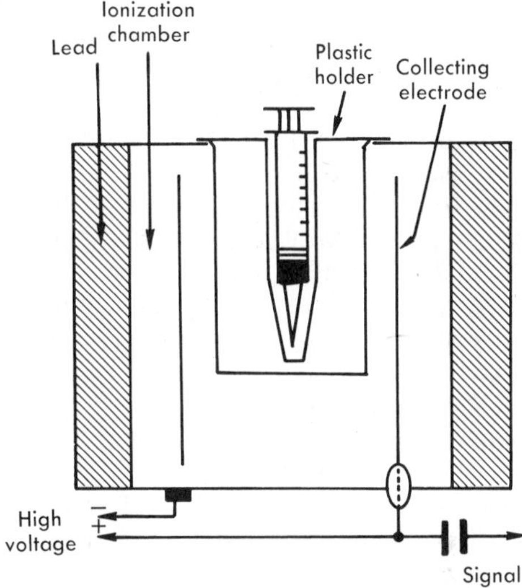

Fig. 3-1. Cross-section of typical ionization chamber used as dose calibrator.

As radiation enters the chamber, photoelectric or Compton interactions occur with a release of electrons, which cause ionization of the gas atoms. The negative ion (electron) is attracted by the electric field to the positive electrode and the positive ion is attracted to the negative electrode, which is the chamber wall. The speed at which the ions travel depends on the electric field strength (high voltage) and the mass of the ions. Since the electron is considerably less massive than the positive ion, it is collected much more rapidly than the positive ion.

If the electrical field is weak, that is, a low voltage is applied to the chamber, the ions drift apart slowly and many electrons may reattach to positive ions and therefore are not collected. This is called "recombination." As the voltage applied to the chamber is increased, the negative ions, being of smaller mass, are quickly swept away by the electric field and less opportunity exists for recombination to take place.

The collection efficiency of the ions generated in the chamber increases as the voltage is increased until all the ions that are generated in the chamber by the radiation are being collected. At this point, further increases of voltage have no effect upon ion collection, and the chamber is operating at the "saturation" voltage.

Fig. 3-2 shows how ion collection varies in a gas-filled chamber as a function of the voltage. At the "saturation" voltage the chamber is operating in the ionization region. At higher voltages secondary ionization occurs, and more ions are collected than are generated by the primary radiation. These other regions are discussed on pp. 90 and 91.

If the chamber is operated in the ionization region, the number of ions collected depends entirely on the amount of ionization taking place in the chamber, which also depends on the number of photons interacting with the detector.

If a source of radioactivity is placed in the ionization chamber, an electrical current will be generated as a result of the ionizations produced by the photons emitted from the source. If the radioactivity of the source is doubled, the number of photons emitted will double, causing twice the ionization and twice as much electrical current to flow in the circuit.

For example, a radioactive source of 1 mCi of ^{131}I will generate a current of about 10×10^{-12} amp in an ionization chamber. A source of 2 mCi of ^{131}I will generate a current of about 20×10^{-12} amp. Thus, the total current generated is directly proportional to the quantity of radioactivity in the chamber.

Radionuclides differ from one another in their mode of decay. For example, ^{51}Cr emits 10 gamma rays of 320 keV each for every 100 radioactive transitions and ^{99m}Tc emits 88 gamma rays of 140 keV for every 100 radioactive transitions.[5] Therefore, for 1 mCi of ^{99m}Tc, there are 8.8 times more photons than for 1 mCi of ^{51}Cr. Also, photons of 140 keV are more likely to interact with the gas in the ion chamber than are the more energetic 320 keV photons.

A closer examination of radiation interactions shows that most charged particles and gamma rays below about 15 keV will be stopped within the walls of the source container or the walls of the ionization chamber. Ionization of the gas in the chamber is then restricted to photons emitted from the radioactive source of greater than 15 keV. Fig. 3-3 shows the probability of gamma-ray interaction in argon gas as a function of energy. The efficiency of an ionization chamber is therefore dependent in a similar manner on photon energy.

As a result of the variation of interaction probability versus photon energy and the fact that different radionuclides emit different numbers of photons per nuclear transformation, a millicurie of one radioactive substance will not generate the same ionization current as a millicurie of a different radionuclide. Fig. 3-4 is

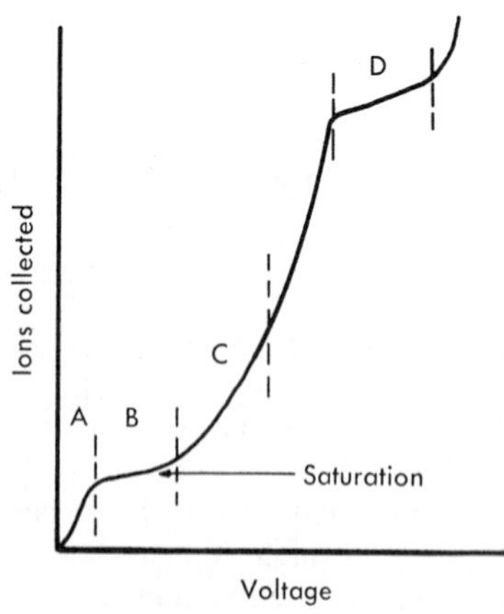

Fig. 3-2. Effect of high voltage on ion collection in gas-filled radiation detector. Region *A* is recombination region where ions formed by incident radiation may recombine before they can be collected. Ionization detectors are operated in region *B*, proportional counters are operated in region *C*, and Geiger-Müller counters are operated in region *D* of this curve.

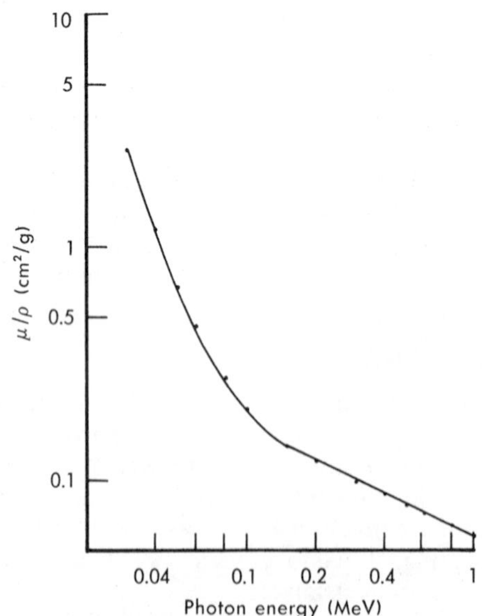

Fig. 3-3. Attenuation of photons in argon gas. As photon energy increases, a smaller ionization current will be generated in gas-filled chamber. μ/ρ, Mass absorption coefficient.

a graph showing the relative ionization current versus millicuries of radioactivity for several different radionuclides. Thus it should be emphasized that the ionization chamber must be calibrated for each and every radionuclide to be measured.

The modern dose calibrator no longer reads in units of electrical current but indicates directly in units of radioactivity as a digital readout. Fig. 3-5 shows a block diagram of a dose calibrator. The first electronic stage of an ionization chamber, when used as a dose calibrator, is a sensitive current-to-voltage amplifier. The next stage is a selector switch to allow measurement of a wide range of radioactivity levels. For example, one might assume that the voltage level required to cause the digital readout lights to record 999 is 0.5 volts. If 999 μCi of radioactivity generates 0.5 volts, then 9990 μCi of radioactivity would generate 5 volts, which cannot be recorded. The range-selector switch can be set to select a resistor value so that only 0.1 of the voltage signal goes to the read-out circuit and simultaneously switches the position of the decimal point. Now 9990 μCi will be displayed as 9.99 mCi. In this manner the instrument can be used to correctly measure and display radioactivity levels from a few microcuries up to curie amounts of radioactivity.

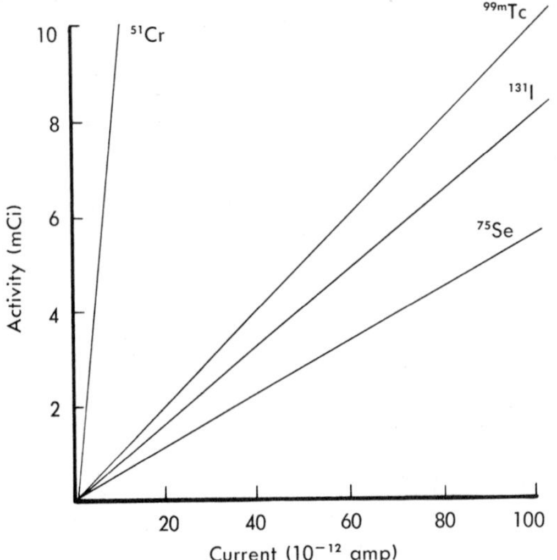

Fig. 3-4. Ionization current versus quantity of radioactivity of different radionuclides. (Data from Woods, M. J.: Int. J. Appl. Radiat. Isot. **21**:752-753, 1970.)

From the selector switch, the signal passes through another amplifier stage, which has a feedback resistor (R_n). If 1 mCi of ^{99m}Tc produces a signal of 0.5 volts and correctly displays the value, 1 mCi of ^{75}Se would generate a signal about 18 times larger because of the difference in the energy deposited in the ionization chamber. Thus, to make the display read correctly for ^{75}Se, the signal to the display must be reduced by a factor of 18. This is accomplished by choosing correctly the value for the resistor (R_n). A different resistor value for R_n must be selected for each different radionuclide. Some instruments provide a single variable resistor with a dial and corresponding calibrated dial settings for each radionuclide, whereas other instruments provide an external resistor that plugs into the instrument for each radionuclide.

Performance of a dose calibrator depends on a number of different parameters: the linearity over the activity range, sensitivity of the chamber to different source configurations, accuracy of the instrument, and precision of reproducibility. Several different studies that have been made on dose calibrators[6,7,12,22,23] demonstrate problems with some of the above parameters and emphasize the necessity for careful quality control.

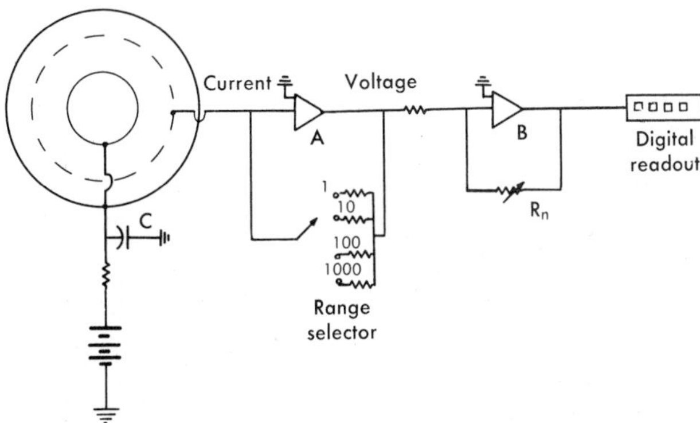

Fig. 3-5. Diagram of a typical dose calibrator. **A,** Current-to-voltage amplifier, with a range-selector switch to allow instrument to be used over wide range of amounts of radioactivity. **B,** Amplifier stage with resistor, R_n, which is used to adjust the instrument so that it will read correctly for different radionuclides. **C,** Capacitor.

Geiger-Müller detectors

The Geiger-Müller (G-M), or Geiger, counter is a gas-filled detector operated at a voltage high enough to cause multiple secondary ionization in the gas. Typically the gas is 90% argon and 10% ethanol, or 99.9% neon and 0.1% chlorine. These are known as organic- or halogen-quenched counting tubes, respectively. Fig. 3-2 describes how the ion collection varies as the high voltage of the detector is increased. The G-M region *(D)* shows a plateau and indicates a maximum level of ionization.

The mechanism that takes place within the detector chamber is briefly described. Incident radiation releases electrons when interacting with the gas molecules in the counter tube (Fig. 3-6). These released electrons are attracted toward the collecting electrodes under the influence of a very strong electric field and gain sufficient energy to cause further ionization. These secondary electrons are also accelerated to an energy level where they too cause ionization. The net result within the counting chamber is the rapid generation of an avalanche of ions swept to the collecting electrode. At this point ions completely engulf the counting chamber.

Because of the small mass of the electrons relative to the mass of the positive ions, the avalanche involves only the electrons. The positive ions are still drifting toward the cathode long after the electrons have been collected. The presence of the positive ions reduces the effectiveness of the electric field and disables the counter from further detection until the positive ions have been neutralized. The period of time during which the detector is disabled is called "dead time," or "resolving time." Fig. 3-7 illustrates the history of the electric field of a G-M counter when it detects an event. All detection systems have a limit to how fast they can detect and process radiation events. The G-M counter is a fairly slow system, with a resolving time typically around 400×10^{-6} second. A measured count can be corrected for loss of counts if the dead time of the system is known.

The basic equation that relates resolving time, τ, true count rate, m, and measured count rate, n, is as follows:

$$m = \frac{n}{1 - n\tau}$$

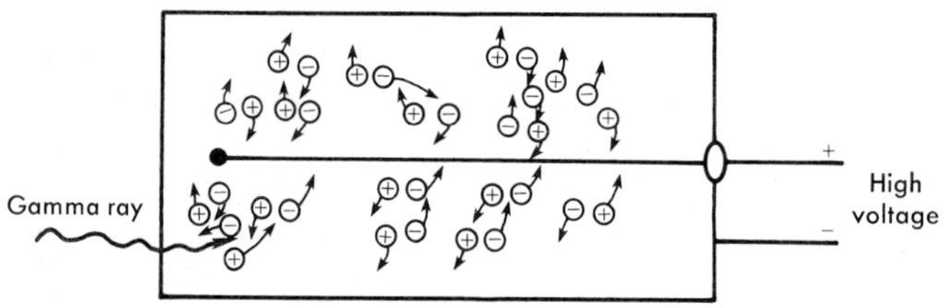

Fig. 3-6. Diagram of Geiger counter showing how single gamma ray can trigger ionization throughout entire chamber.

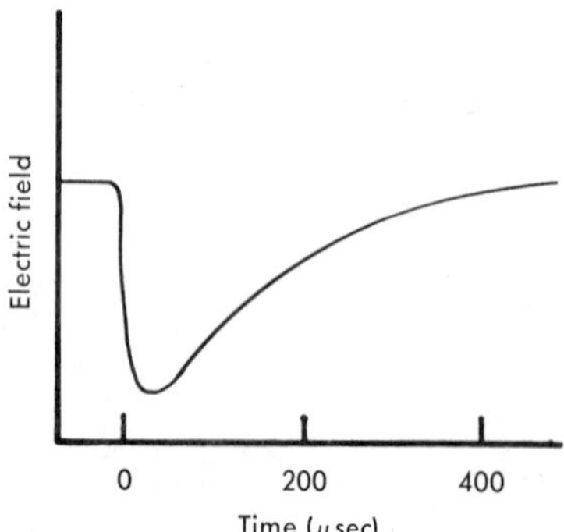

Fig. 3-7. History of electric field in Geiger counter. At time zero an event has been detected and electric field across electrodes of chamber drops significantly. Recovery of electric field is related to time it takes for ions to be collected.

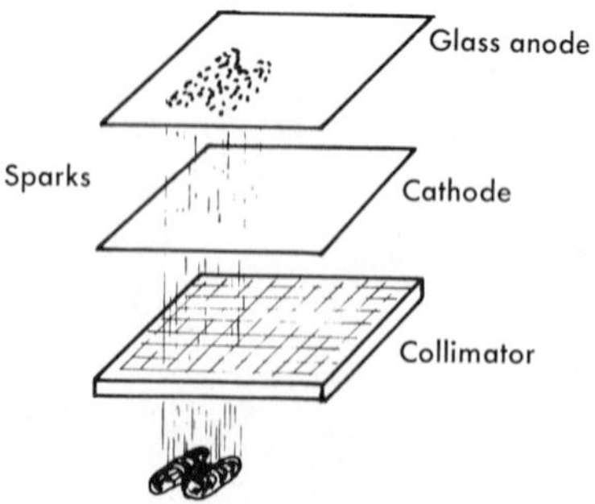

Fig. 3-8. Spark chamber. Diagram shows how gamma rays from thyroid pass through collimator, impinge on cathode, and generate sparks between cathode and anode. Sparks are viewed end-on to generate image on piece of film.

For example, if the resolving time of a G-M counter is 400×10^{-6} second, and the measured count rate of a radioactive sample is 200 counts per second, cps, then:

$$m = \frac{200}{1 - 200\,(400 \times 10^{-6})} = \frac{200}{1 - 0.08} = 217 \text{ cps}$$

In this example, the counter lost 17 counts per second.

Resolving time can be experimentally measured by the classical two-source method. For two different sources that are measured separately and together, the measurement of both sources together should give the same number as the sum of each source measured separately. Since the detector loses some of the counts, the sum will be a number smaller than the measurement of both sources separately. Using the following terms—R_1, count rate for source 1; R_2, count rate for source 2; R_{12}, count rate for both sources together; R_b count rate for the background, one can estimate the resolving time by the following equation:

$$\tau = \frac{R_1 + R_2 - R_{12} - R_b}{R_{12}^2 - R_1^2 - R_2^2}$$

Geiger counters are used in the nuclear medicine laboratory primarily to monitor for possible contamination of personnel and work areas. The disadvantages are that they cannot distinguish different energies of radiation and are relatively inefficient for gamma-ray detection, on the order of a few percent. The primary advantage of the G-M survey meter is that it is inexpensive and portable.

Spark and proportional counters

A brief discussion of two other gas-filled detector systems is included in this section because these detectors have been used in nuclear medicine and, in the case of multiwire proportional counters, could become useful in the future.

In Fig. 3-2, the ion collection as a function of detector voltage is shown. If the voltage is increased beyond the G-M plateau region, the gas within the detector breaks down and an electrical spark occurs between the electrodes. A number of investigators[9-11] took advantage of this phenomenon to construct an imaging device. Although the actual devices varied, the principle was basically the same, that is, a high voltage is applied across two electrodes such as the parallel plates shown in Fig. 3-8. A photon interacts with either the cathode or the detector gas and releases photoelectrons. Because of the high voltage across the electrodes, an avalanche of ionization is produced followed by a spark. The spark is viewed end-on as a pinpoint of light that falls on a photographic film. Spark detectors have a poor detection efficiency for photons, especially if the photon energy is much greater than around 30 keV.

Proportional counters were formerly the detector of choice when beta radiation was measured. The operating characteristics fall between the ionization region and the G-M region (Fig. 3-2). The advantage of the proportional counter is that the electric field is sufficiently strong to accelerate the primary ionization in the counter to produce an avalanche of ions, but not strong enough that the avalanche engulfs the entire chamber. The gas in the counter functions as an amplifier with a multiplication factor causing 1000 to 10,000 times more ions to be collected than those released by the initial radiation interaction.

In one type of proportional counter, beta particle–emitting sources were placed inside the chamber and counting gas continually flowed through the chamber, so that the beta particles did not have to penetrate through a window or the walls of the detector to deposit ionization in the counting gas. Modern day beta counting is mostly done with liquid scintillation systems.

Recent developments in the proportional counter as an imaging device could revive the usefulness of this detector. Kaufman et al.[10] have constructed proportional chambers by using crossed-wire grids as shown in Fig. 3-9.

Gamma rays interact with the xenon counting gas to produce photoelectrons. The electrons are accelerated to the central wires and generate ion pairs along the path. The negative ions are collected on the closest central wire, and the positive ions are collected on the closest outer wires. Thus one can determine the coordinates of the ionizing event by noting which set of wires collect the ions. These systems have reasonably good detection efficiency up to about 80 keV and a spatial resolution on the order of 1 mm.

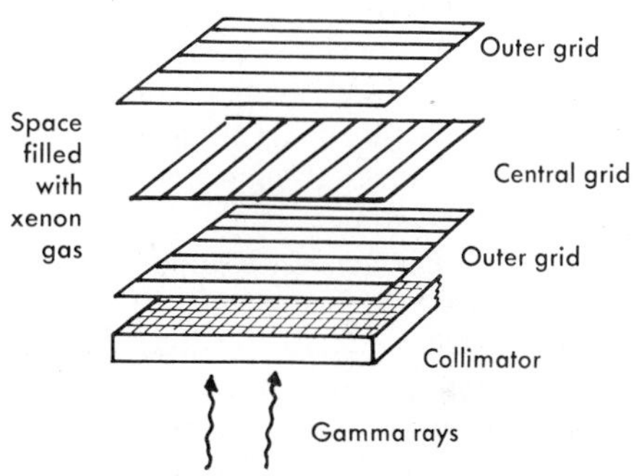

Fig. 3-9. Proportional-counter imaging system. Collimated gamma rays cause ionization in xenon gas. Location of ionization is determined from set of wires that collect ions.

PRINCIPLES OF SCINTILLATION DETECTORS

Inorganic crystal detectors and scintillation process

The scintillation detector is, and probably will remain for some time, the most important means of radiation detection in nuclear medicine. An interesting history of the development of scintillation detectors is presented by Hine.[8]

The word "scintillate" comes from the Latin *scintillare,* which means 'to sparkle.' Indeed, light flashes occur in the scintillation crystal when it is bombarded with radiation. *Luminescence* is a general term for absorption of radiation energy by matter and reemission as visible radiation. If the reemission occurs during excitation of the material or within 10^{-8} second, the process is called *fluorescence*. If the reemission occurs much later, fractions of seconds to many hours, it is called *phosphorescence*.

When a gamma ray is absorbed in a sodium iodide crystal, its energy is transferred to an electron most likely by means of a photoelectric or Compton interaction. These secondary electrons cause ionization within the crystal. The ion pairs are free to move throughout the crystal until they become "trapped" or captured by imperfections in the crystal. One can make imperfections by adding a trace of some foreign material, such as thallium atoms, to the crystal lattice. When the ion pair is captured by the imperfection, the crystal "trapping center" becomes excited (that is, gains energy) and releases this excitation energy in the form of a light photon.

For a crystal of sodium iodide, about 0.1 mole percent of thallium is added to provide imperfections. The photons are released with an energy of around 3 eV or a wavelength of about 4200 angstroms, which has a color of blue blue-violet. Somewhere between 10% to 20% of the ionization results in luminescence, and the rest of the energy is dissipated as heat within the crystal.

The total time required for this process of light emission takes on the order of 0.25 to 0.5 μsec for NaI(Tl). One should also be aware that the efficiency for light emission depends on the temperature of the crystal. A change of 8° C in crystal temperature causes a 1% change in light production.

The quantity of light generated within a crystal is directly proportional to the amount of ionization produced by the incident radiation. Thus, if two gamma rays undergo photoelectric interactions within a NaI (Tl) crystal at different times, and one gamma ray has twice the energy of the other, the higher-energy photon will produce two times the ionization and also two times the quantity of light than will the lower-energy gamma ray. If, however, a gamma ray undergoes a Compton interaction in the crystal and if the scattered photon were to escape the crystal, the quantity of ionization and thereby light output would be proportional only to the energy received by the Compton electron.

Photomultiplication

The photomultiplier (PM) tube is the device that converts light photons from a crystal into electrical pulses. The quantity of light produced in the crystal by a gamma ray is very minute, but because of the sensitivity of the phototube such tiny amounts of light can be detected and measured. The PM tube is optically coupled to the crystal and the inside face of the tube referred to as the photocathode is coated with a very thin layer of photoemissive material (Fig. 3-10). The photoemissive material releases electrons when bombarded with light. Typically it requires about 8 light photons to release 1 electron.

A series of dynodes, each at a higher electrical potential, permits the single electron to be multiplied many times over. An electric field is applied between the photocathode and the first dynode so as to attract and accelerate electrons released at the photocathode. The electrons slam into the dynode, which is also coated with a photoemissive material, with sufficient energy to release additional electrons, typically about 4. This acceleration and multiplication process takes place from dynode to dynode, with the result being a collection of approximately 1 million electrons for every electron released from the photocathode.

The average number of electrons released at the dynodes depends on the accelerating voltage applied, as well as the material coating the dynode. If the voltage is increased, the average number of electrons released per dynode increases. For example, if 4 electrons are released when voltage V_1 is applied and there

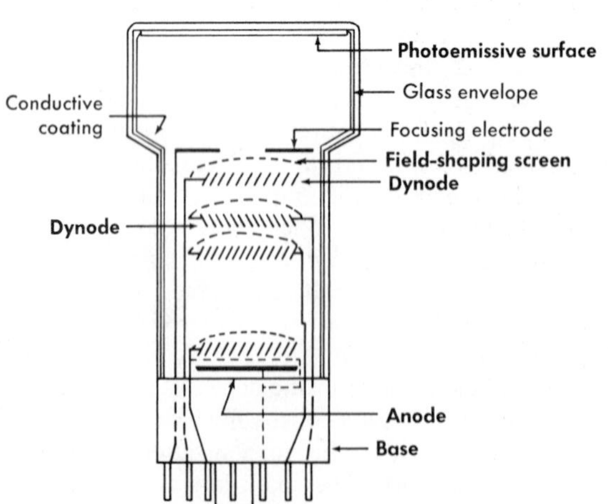

Fig. 3-10. Photomultiplier tube (PMT).

are 10 dynodes, the multiplication factor (gain) of the PM tube would be $4^{10} \cong 10^6$. If the voltage is increased by 10% to the sum $(V_1 + 0.1V_1)$, then on the average 4.4 electrons might be released per dynode and $4.4^{10} = 2.7 \times 10^6$ would be the gain of the PM tube. Thus, changing the high voltage applied to the PM tube changes the amplification of the scintillation detector.

One of the most important features of the scintillation detector is the relationship between the voltage signal coming from the detector and the energy of the incident gamma ray. If the energy of the incident gamma ray is totally absorbed within the NaI(Tl) crystal, the average quantity of light produced is proportional to the energy of the gamma ray. The average number of electrons released at the photocathode is proportional to the quantity of light in the crystal, and the size of the final voltage pulse is the gain factor of the PM tube times the number of electrons released at the photocathode. Thus, if a 100 keV gamma ray is totally absorbed in the crystal, approximately 3000 ± 50 blue-light photons will be generated; if all these photons reach the photocathode, approximately 450 ± 70 electrons will be released. If on the average 4 electrons are ejected at each dynode, then approximately $4.5 \times 10^8 \pm 0.7 \times 10^8$ electrons will be collected to generate the final voltage pulse. The variation in output voltage about the average value for 100 keV gamma rays in the example is attributable to statistical fluctuations at each stage of the process and results in a gaussian distribution of voltage-pulse height about the average value.

The literature[16,24] contains more detailed descriptions of the scintillation process and voltage conversion if you wish to pursue these topics in greater depth.

Liquid scintillation detectors

Liquid scintillation systems are used for the detection of charged-particle radiation and low-energy x-ray radiations. They are particularly suited for low-energy radiations such as the beta particles from ^3H (5.7 keV) or ^{14}C (49 keV). The advantage of the liquid scintillator is that the radioactive source is mixed directly with the scintillator material (Fig. 3-11). The mixture consists of the radioactive labeled substance, the liquid scintillator (for example, *p*-terphenyl), and a solvent. The solvent, for example, toluene, must be capable of dissolving the radioactive material, efficiently transfer the energy of the beta emission to the scintillator, and be transparent to the scintillation photons. Problems arise in liquid scintillation counting if interference occurs in the transfer of energy between the site of an event and the scintillator molecule or because of absorption of the light by materials in the solution. These interferences are called "quenching." Different techniques have been used to account for quenching effects and even more numerous approaches have been used for sample preparation. Those who find themselves involved with liquid scintillation counting should consult more detailed discussions.[17]

Besides source preparation and the source-scintillator geometry, the liquid scintillation counter also differs in regard to its instrumentation.

The light released by the scintillation material is sent in all directions within the source vial and will be seen simultaneously by both PM tubes. Thus voltage signals will be produced in both PM tubes at the same time and essentially of equal size.

Because of the very low radiation energies, the resultant voltage signals from the PM tubes are very weak and not much different from thermal noise randomly generated in the PM tubes. For reduction of the thermal noise, the PM tubes and the source-holding and -changing mechanism are all enclosed in a refrigerated compartment.

If signals are present in both PM tubes in coincidence, the logic circuit recognizes this signal as an acceptable count and a count is recorded. Noise is random and the likelihood of two pulses of the same size occurring simultaneously from both PM tubes is very small; thus a single pulse from either tube is

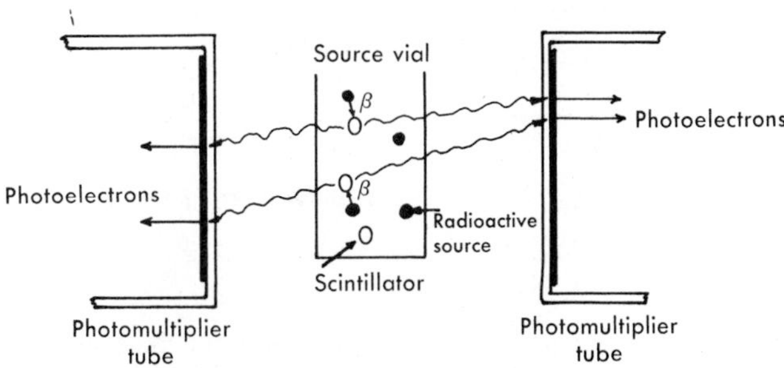

Fig. 3-11. Diagram of liquid scintillation process. Radioactive source *(solid dots)* emits beta particles, which interact with scintillator molecules and eject light in all directions.

treated as a noise signal and is not recorded as a count. The rest of the circuitry is similar to any scintillation spectrometer and is covered on p. 95.

PRINCIPLES OF OTHER DETECTORS

Lithium-drifted germanium

Among the variety of radiation detectors that may someday become important in nuclear medicine, the semiconductor is quite promising. Semiconductor radiation detectors are made of high-purity single crystals of germanium or silicon.[19]

In a semiconductor detector, ionization by the incident radiation produces electron-hole pairs. An electron is raised from its normal valence state to what is called the "conduction band," which means that the electron is free to move about through the crystal. The absence of the electron in the valence state is called a "hole," which can also in effect move about through the crystal. If a voltage is applied across the crystal, the electrons will flow toward the positive electrode and the holes will flow toward the negative electrode (Fig. 3-12, *A*). This current flow created by the incident radiation is very similar to the description of a gas-filled ionization chamber.

A piece of semiconductor material will contain a small number of electron-hole pairs that are thermally generated and with the application of a voltage will cause "noise" signals. To reduce the noise, impurities such as lithium can be drifted into the germanium to trap the thermal electron-hole pairs. To maintain the drifted state of the lithium and also to reduce thermal noise, the lithium drifted–germanium (GE[Li]) detector must be operated and maintained at liquid-nitrogen temperatures.

The major advantage of semiconductor detectors is the improvement in resolution. For germanium, it requires only 2.9 eV to produce an ion pair. Therefore, for a 100 keV gamma ray incident on this detector, approximately 34,000 electrons will be produced as compared to about 3000 blue-light photons generated in a NaI(Tl) scintillation crystal. It is this difference in numbers and the associated statistics (with one standard deviation being the square root of the number) that results in a tenfold improvement in energy resolution for the semiconductor (Fig. 3-12, *B*).

Efficiency for stopping gamma rays depends on the atomic number and the thickness of the detector material. The atomic number for germanium is 32 as compared to 53 for iodine, the effective stopping element in a NaI(Tl) detector. The ratio of absorption coefficients for 140 keV in germanium versus iodine is on the order of 1:3. Therefore the inherent detection efficiency is less for a Ge(Li) detector than for a NaI(Tl) one. To produce a Ge(Li) detector with a usable thickness of 1 cm or more that would yield a detector with an efficiency similar to the typical NaI(Tl) detector used in nuclear medicine is difficult and expensive. A detector made with extremely pure germanium, an "intrinsic germanium detector," can be made sufficiently thick to produce efficiencies comparable to that of NaI(Tl) detectors. However, the manufacture of intrinsic germanium is costly and the cooling of such detectors (intrinsic or not) with liquid nitrogen introduces engineering problems and user inconvenience. Thus, for these reasons, at this time the superior energy resolution of these detectors has not been fully utilized in nuclear medicine imaging.

Thermoluminescent detectors

Thermoluminescent detectors (TLD) are used as radiation-dose monitors. The principle of their operation in many respects is similar to scintillation systems. Instead of light being immediately released

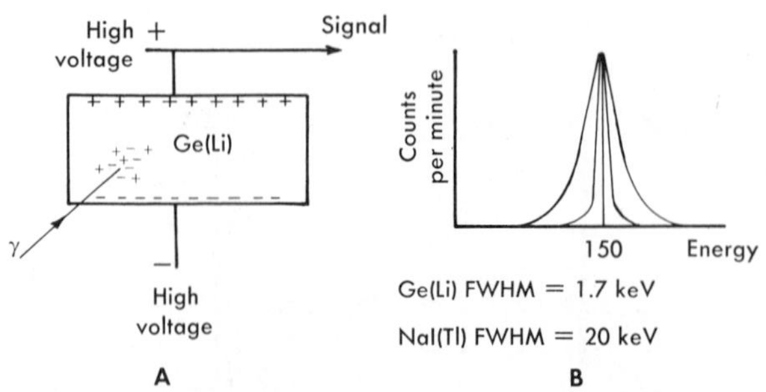

Fig. 3-12. A shows how radiation generates ionization in detector. Ions are attracted in direction of opposite polarity inducing a current flow across detector. **B** indicates difference in energy resolution between a Ge(Li) detector and a typical NaI(Tl) scintillation detector. *FWHM* is energy resolution defined by width of curve at one half maximum of count rate.

(fluorescence) or spontaneously released after a period of time (phosphorescence), the light energy is released only upon thermal stimulation (heating).

When incident radiation deposits energy in the form of ionization, electrons are released and move through the crystal (made of lithium fluoride, calcium sulfate, calcium fluoride, and so forth) until they become trapped. To release the electrons from these traps, one heats the material until the electrons gain sufficient energy to return to their original valence state, emitting light in the process. The total number of electrons originally released by the radiation, trapped, and released by heating to generate light is proportional to the radiation energy deposited in the crystal.

Lithium fluoride TLDs can measure radiation doses as low as 10 to 20 mR and are used for personnel monitoring and other dosimetry applications in the nuclear medicine laboratory. The dosimeters may be used as a lithium fluoride powder contained in a gelatin capsule, or the lithium fluoride can be pressed into small rods or chips. After exposure the lithium fluoride is heated on a small platinum pan at a controlled rate to a predefined temperature. The dosimeter is viewed by a photomultiplier tube, and the light released by the dosimeter is converted to an electrical current. The total light released and the total electric current generated are proportional to the radiation exposure received by the dosimeter.

The advantage of TLDs as compared to film for use as a radiation dosimeter is that the TLD is small, relatively energy independent, and can be used over and over.

THE NaI(Tl) SCINTILLATION SPECTROMETER

The scintillation spectrometer is an electronic device that allows the user to sort out different gamma-ray energies, that is, to analyze the spectrum of gamma-ray energies detected by the scintillation crystal. The components that make up the spectrometer system are a high-voltage supply, preamplifier, amplifier, and pulse-height analyzer. Scintillation cameras (informally gamma cameras), rectilinear scanners, and well counters all contain the facility of gamma-ray energy selection.

High-voltage supply

The photomultiplier tube achieves its electron multiplication by means of accelerating electrons from one dynode state to the next. This requires a stable source of high voltage. Distribution of the high voltage to each dynode is accomplished by division of the voltage into proportional parts with the use of resistors. Fig. 3-13 is a diagram of a high-voltage supply and the resistor network to a photomultiplier tube. If a potential difference of 100 volts is applied between two dynodes, the electrons will gain an energy of 100 electron volts and the photoelectric release of additional electrons from the dynode when it is struck depends on the accelerating voltage. For example, increasing the voltage by 10% increases the total multiplication of the phototube by approximately a factor of 2.

Because a change in high voltage causes a change in the multiplication factor or "amplification" of the PM tube, some instruments rely on the high-voltage control to adjust amplification of the complete spectrometer system.

Preamplifier and amplifier

The amplification electronics for a scintillation spectrometer has historically been discussed in two parts—the preamplifier and the main amplifier. The preamplifier is the first electronic stage and is usually attached directly to the phototube. If the detector is

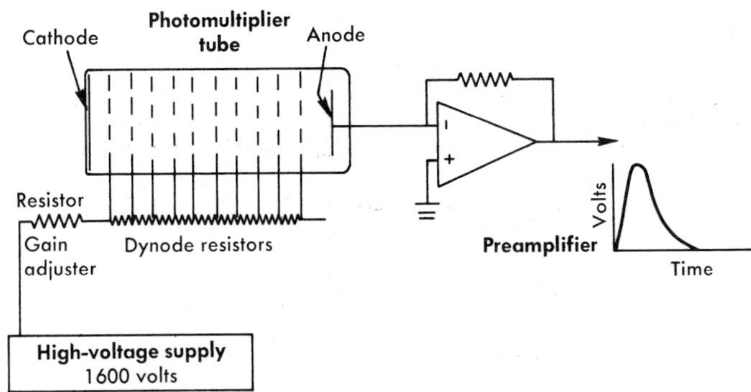

Fig. 3-13. First stage of scintillation detector. High voltage from supply is divided between dynodes by resistors. Fine adjustment of gain of photomultiplier tube can be made when value of resistor is changed.

physically remote from the majority of the electronic parts, as is the case for rectilinear scanners, well counters, and older scintillation cameras, then the preamplifier's major function is to shape the electrical pulse from the photomultiplier tube into a voltage signal and match the electrical impedance of the electronics. This impedance matching is necessary to avoid distortion and loss of the signal during its transit through the cable. In most modern camera systems the preamplifier and amplifier stages become blended together and are both located within the detector head.

The major role of the amplifier is to strengthen weak pulses coming from the preamplifier. A signal of a few volts is easier to manipulate than a signal of a few millivolts. It is also desirable somewhere within the electronics to be able to adjust the size of the voltage signals. Some instruments have two amplifier adjustments, a coarse gain, which allows the user to change the amplification by factors of 2, 10, or other multiples, and a fine gain control, which permits a continuous adjustment of amplification over a limited range.

The amplification system has some stringent requirements that it must meet. The amplifier must not change values with time or count rate once it has been set (stability). The amplifier should also amplify small signals from low-energy gamma rays exactly the same amount as it amplifies large signals from high-energy gamma rays (linearity).

Pulse-height analyzer (PHA)

One of the major features of a scintillation detector is that the output signal is proportional to the gamma-ray energy deposited in the crystal. The amplifier electronic system maintains that proportionality, and next in the system comes the pulse-height analyzer, which is designed to allow the user to select the voltage pulses that are to be recorded and that are to be rejected (Fig. 3-14).

For example, in Fig. 3-14 consider three different input signals: 1, 2, and 3 volts. If circuit *A* presents a 1.5-volt barrier, it requires a signal greater than 1.5 volts to get through; therefore the 2-volt and 3-volt pulses get through, but the 1-volt pulse is stopped. Simultaneously an alternate pathway exists by means of circuit *B*. Circuit *B* is adjusted so that it requires at least 2.5 volts to pass through, and anything less than 2.5 volts will be stopped. In circuit *B*, only the 3-volt pulse can get through. Whichever pulses get through circuit *B* go next to an inverter stage, which reverses the polarity.

The next step in the PHA is to combine signals from both circuits *A* and *B*. If a signal exists from *A* only, it continues to be recorded. If a signal exists from *B*, there will also be a signal from *A* but of opposite polarity. The signals from *A* and *B* are added together, but because of the opposite polarity, they will cancel and nothing is recorded. In this way, only voltage pulses between the level set at circuit *A* (the base-line setting or lower-level setting) and the level set at circuit *B* (upper level) will pass through and be recorded. Most often the level of circuit *B* is selected as a fixed difference in voltage greater than circuit *A* and is referred to as the "window." In the example above, the "window" spans from 1.5 to 2.5 volts (that is, it has or was set at) a width of 1 volt.

In the actual use of spectrometers, one never knows the voltage values but instead calibrates the base-line and window dials in units of gamma-ray energy (keV). The standard calibration procedure or "peaking" of a spec-

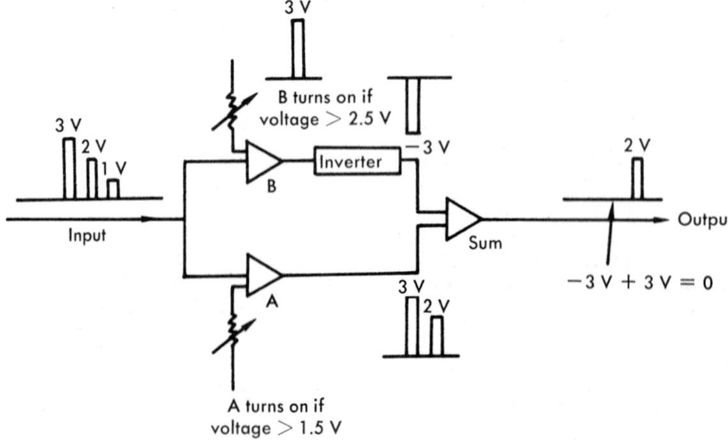

Fig. 3-14. Example of pulse-height analyzer (PHA). Input signals that pass through discriminator *A* only and not *B* will appear as output signals. Trigger levels of both *A* and *B* are adjustable on front panel of analyzer.

trometer is outlined in Fig. 3-15, which shows the distribution of counts (photopeak for a 140 keV gamma ray with the base line set at 135 and a window of 10). In Fig. 3-15, *A,* the voltage signals are not amplified enough to place the photopeak at the center of the window. In Fig. 3-15, *B,* the gain of the amplifier or high voltage has been increased so that now the photopeak is centered in the window. In Fig. 3-15, *C,* the amplifier gain or high voltage was again increased and now the photopeak has shifted away from and above the window. In Fig. 3-15, *A,* the count rate getting through the window is 800 cpm, in *B* it increases or "peaks" at a maximum of 1000 cpm, and in *C,* the count rate again drops to 800 cpm. With the base line at 135 and window at 10, adjustment of the high-voltage or amplifier gain to achieve maximum counts also calibrates the dial so that the combination of 135 on the base line and 10 on the window dials now corresponds to an acceptance "window" of 135 to 145 keV. A resetting of the base line to 120 and the window control to 40 would correspond to a "window" of 120 to 160 keV.

The spectrometer controls on scintillation cameras and some rectilinear scanners all function basically the same way but differ in labels and some technical details. For each specific instrument the user should consult the operator's manual to see how the controls for that instrument actually function.

Scalers and rate meters

The detected and analyzed gamma rays are recorded either in the form of counts or count rate. A scaler is simply an electronic counter that tabulates the accepted pulses for a selected length of time. Modern scalers are almost all based on units of 10, so that the number of counts collected for a preset time are stored and displayed directly as the number of counts, utilizing LEDs (light-emitting diodes) as the numerical display.

Rate meters are devices that continuously display an estimate of the rate at which the detector is registering radiation events. In general, there are two types of rate meters, analog and digital. The analog rate meter determines the incoming count rate by collecting the voltage pulses on a capacitor, which builds up an electrical charge. Simultaneously while the capacitor is collecting the charge, the charge is allowed to leak through a resistor such that, for a steady radiation source, the rate of charge and discharge will eventually come into equilibrium and the current flowing through the meter will then be proportional to the rate of incoming radiation pulses.

If the resistance is small, equilibrium is established quickly but is not an accurate estimate of the incoming pulse rate. The time constant associated with analog rate meters is the product of the resistance and capacitance: RC. The actual time it takes to establish equilibrium, t_e, is not the time constant value but is given by the following equation:

$$t_e = T(\tfrac{1}{2} \ln [2nT] + 0.394)$$

where T is the time constant in seconds, and n is the count rate in counts per second.

Most rate meters provide a control to select time constant values from a fraction of a second to several minutes. A short time constant enables the rate meter to respond quickly to changes in count rate but provides less accurate estimates of the true value particularly if the count rate is low. A long time constant enables the rate meter to sample the incoming count rate over a longer period of time and arrive at a much better estimate, provided that the count rate did not change during the measurement.

Digital rate meters differ from analog systems in that the continuous determination of count rate is made by storage of the actual number of counts collected in a

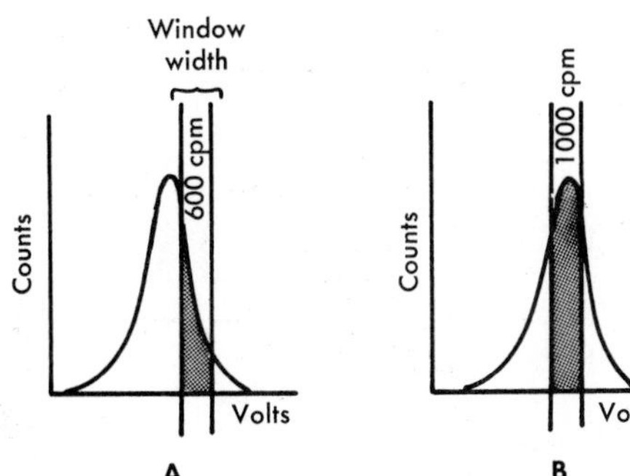

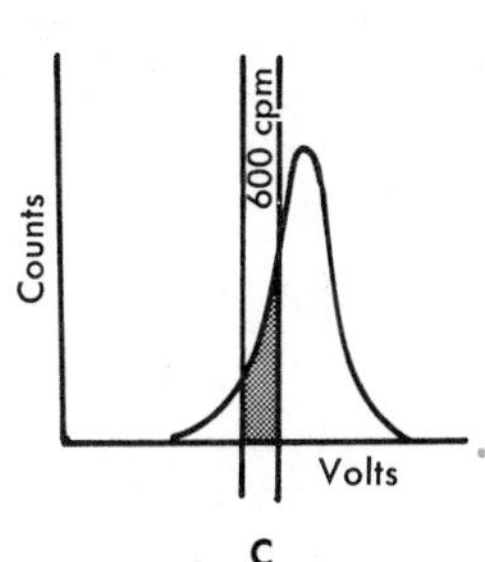

Fig. 3-15. "Peaking" a spectrometer. **A** shows distribution of voltage pulses (photopeak) too low and only pulses on the high side of distribution pass through window. **B** shows photopeak centered in window and maximum number pass through. **C** shows too much amplification and only low-voltage pulses pass through window.

defined period of time, maybe 0.1 second. While the first set of data is routed to a display or readout system, a second storage location collects the incoming signals for the next 0.1 second, by the time the second storage is ready to be read, the first storage location is available to collect counts again. The length of collecting times may or may not be set by the operator, but the major advantage of the digital rate meter is that there is no lag in response to establish an equilibrium such as for the analog rate meter.

IMAGING SYSTEMS

Rectilinear scanners

The first scanning system was built by Cassen[3] and his co-workers at UCLA in 1950. The first scans were of the thyroid gland with ^{131}I as the tracer. As the field of radionuclide scanning grew, the rectilinear scanner became more sophisticated. A selection of focused collimators became available to match the needs for high resolution and different energies. Better electronics were introduced to control scan speed, provide stability of energy window, and generate controlled photorecorded images. The rectilinear scanner probably reached its zenith as a nuclear medicine instrument about 1970 and is now being replaced by the gamma camera.

The scanner is a scintillation detector designed to view a tiny portion of the patient directly under the detector at any one time. One determines the distribution of radioactivity throughout the organ by methodically moving the detector back and forth in a "rectilinear" motion across the organ (Fig. 3-16) and recording the number of counts sensed at each location.

The scanner system can be considered as several components: (1) the scintillation detector and collimator, (2) the mechanical driving system, (3) the pulse-height analyzer, and (4) the image-recording system.

Scintillation detector and collimator. The scintillation detector has a crystal that typically ranges from 3 inches in diameter to 5 inches in diameter by 2 inches thick. Smaller diameter crystals do not provide enough sensitivity for scanning, whereas larger diameter crystals coupled to focused collimators have a very sharp, thin focal plane, which causes degeneration of resolution away from the focal plane.

One advantage of rectilinear scanners is that the crystal can be thick, and thereby gamma-ray detection efficiency is excellent over a wide range of energies. Detection efficiency (percent of incident photons completely absorbed in the crystal) for a 2-inch thick crystal of NaI(Tl) is 100% up to about 200 keV and is still 65% at 500 keV.

To achieve maximum sensitivity, multihole focusing collimators, which allowed use of as much of the crystal surface as possible, were developed. The collimator does not actually focus gamma rays but allows those gamma rays emanating from a point to reach the crystal (Fig. 3-17). Because of the construction parameters of the collimator, including the fact that each hole is of a finite size, gamma rays from radioactivity adjacent

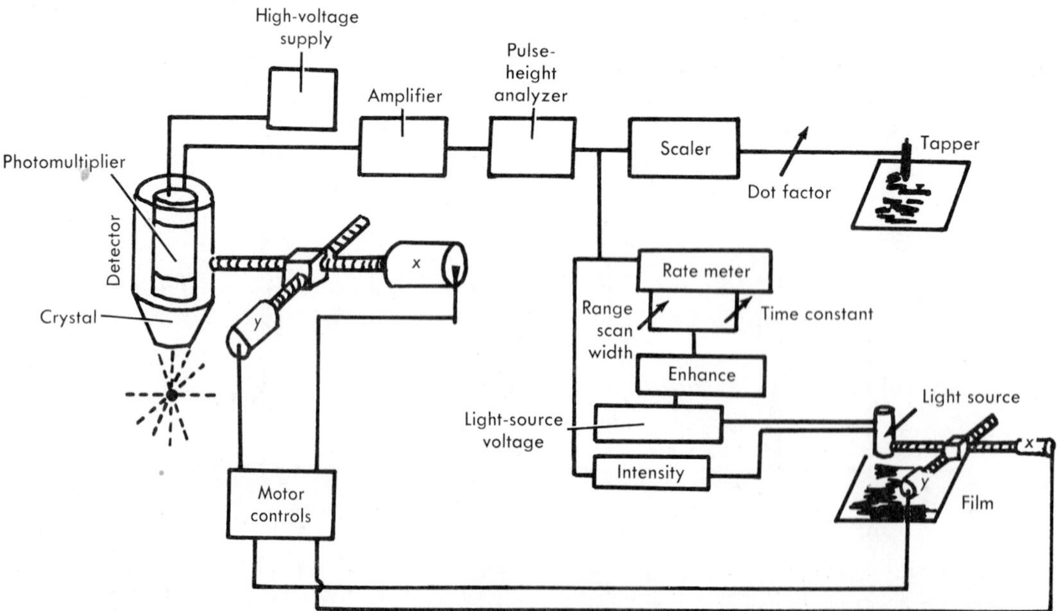

Fig. 3-16. Components of rectilinear scanner.

to that emanation point can also reach the crystal. The result is that a point will be imaged as a disk of a certain diameter. The actual resolution will be somewhat worse than the equation predicts because of scatter and possible penetration of the lead walls (septa) separating the holes. Resolution is often measured and quoted as the *f*ull *w*idth at *h*alf *m*aximum (FWHM) of a point or line source. One can measure the FWHM resolution by moving a collimated detector over a radioactive line source. The profile of counts versus location of detector relative to the line source might appear as shown in Fig. 3-18. One determines the FWHM then by locating one half the maximum counts on the curve and measuring the width of the curve (points *A* and *B* in Fig. 3-18).

Note that for the collimator in Fig. 3-18, the FWHM resolution is the same for both low- and high-energy gamma rays, but that the count profile is much lower at a distance from the central axis of the collimator. The difference in count profiles in this example is attributable to septal penetration of high-energy gamma rays with a collimator designed for low energies. Although the FWHM would indicate the same resolution, if the collimator were used to image ^{131}I gamma rays, the collimator would allow the detector to "see" gamma rays from a very wide field of view. A collimator designed for use with high-energy gamma rays can always be used to image sources of lower energy radiation but at a sacrifice of sensitivity. The higher energy collimator out of necessity must have thicker septa and therefore shield a higher percentage of the crystal from the source of gamma rays. Thus, collimators must be selected to match the specific requirements for gamma-ray energy used, resolution, and sensitivity.

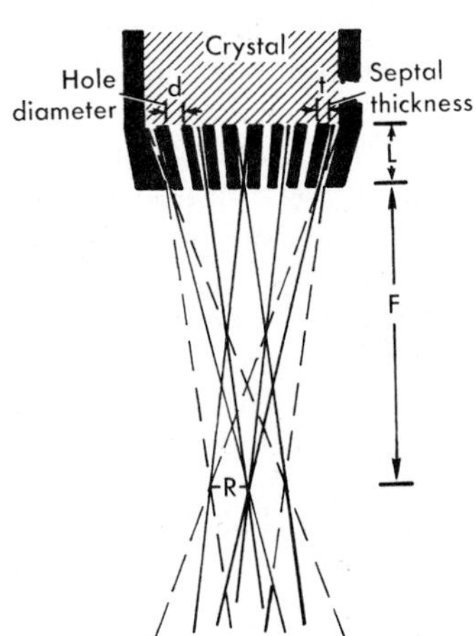

Fig. 3-17. Focused collimator. Geometric radius of resolution is given by $R = Fd/L$.

Mechanical driving system. The mechanical demands on a driving system are rather remarkable in that the system must accelerate a large mass rapidly to a set speed, maintain that speed accurately and then quickly stop, move at right angles a set distance, reverse direction, and repeat the cycle. Earlier scanners used small DC motors to power the system. It is easy to vary the speed and change the direction of a DC motor but not easy to maintain an accurate constant speed; thus not uncommon were errors in speed variation of $\pm 10\%$ or more, which were reflected in a variation of count-rate information. Later scanners used pulse-stepping motors or larger synchronous motors with more elaborate electronic control systems to accurately regulate the speed. Speed uniformity of a scanner can easily be checked by attachment of a radioactive source directly to the collimator. The number of counts recorded by the readout system per unit distance traveled should not vary along the scan line greater than the statistical variation associated with the count rate. If the number of counts per centimeter decreases, the scanner has speeded up, whereas an increase in the recorded counts per centimeter indicates a decrease in scan speed.

Pulse-height analyzer. Detected gamma rays are transformed into electronic signals through standard spectrometer electronics as described earlier in this chapter. The proper use of the spectrometer cannot be overemphasized. The signal out of the pulse-height analyzer then goes to the recording devices, which could include a scaler for recording accumulated counts and a rate meter to indicate count rate.

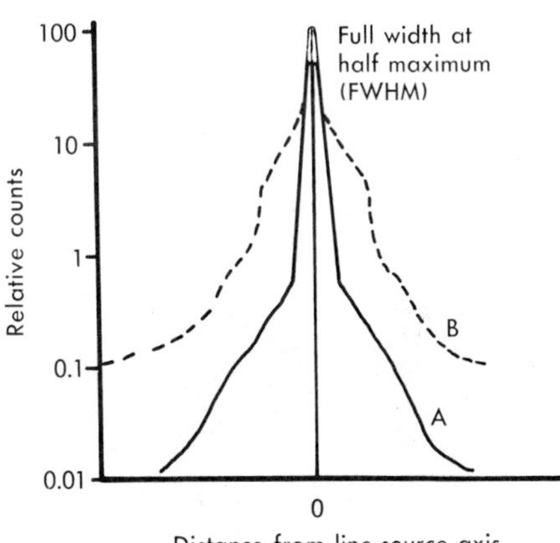

Fig. 3-18. Profile of counts from radioactive line source viewed with low-energy collimator. *A* is obtained with low-energy photon source. *B* is obtained with high-energy photon source. Full-width half-maximum (FWHM) is same, but curve *B* shows septal penetration at about 20% count rate level. In effect low-energy collimator is inadequate at limiting field of view.

The standard analog rate meter is a signal-averaging device based upon achieving an equilibrium of rate of charge and discharge of a capacitor. The time it takes to achieve equilibrium is proportional to (not equal to) the time-constant setting. To obtain reasonably accurate measurements of the count rate, one must select a long sample time (long time constant). However, when one is scanning, it is necessary to obtain count-rate information as quickly as possible to relate count rate to spatial location. Thus, inherently, the use of an analog rate meter necessitates a compromise between accurate sample information and good spatial information. A result of a lag of count-rate information behind the momentary location of the detector is demonstrated by ''scalloping'' (Fig. 3-19). The severity of scalloping depends on the time constant selected and scanner speed.

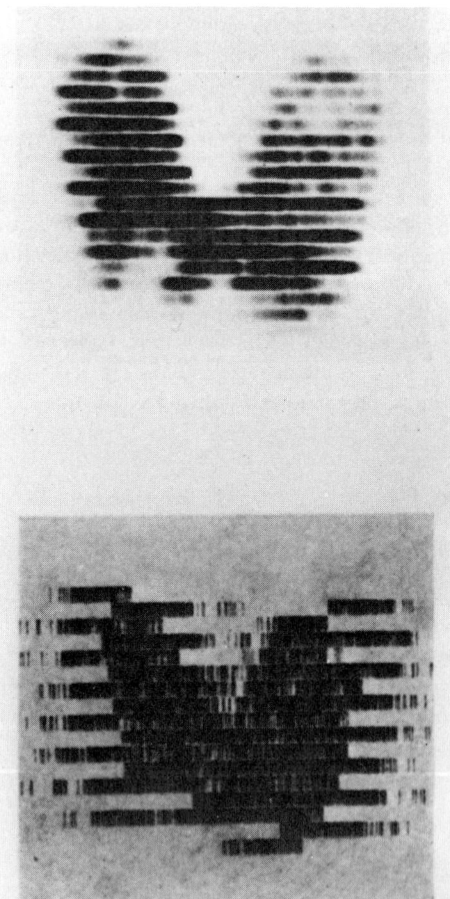

Fig. 3-19. Missetting of time constant can cause ''scalloping'' as shown. Thyroid phantom scan *at top* shows some scalloping. Scan lines are alternately displaced to right and left. *At bottom,* Thyroid scan made with time constant set at an excessively large value, which produced scalloping to extent that image is useless.

Many rectilinear scanners now incorporate digital rate meters in place of the analog rate meter. A typical digital system may involve multiple recycling scalers, which total counts for a defined time increment or scan length. The signals to the image-recording system are directly proportional to the pulses generated by the detector and reflect count-rate statistical fluctuations, but without the time lag introduced by analog rate meter circuitry.

Image-recording system. Recording devices used to form the final image are generally of two classes, those used to monitor the scan so that the operator can view the scan and make adjustments in the field during the procedure, and those used by the physician for interpretation.

The monitor display can be a simple electromechanical hammer that hits carbon paper and makes a mark on the scan paper, or it can be a storage cathode-ray scope. The photorecording display is the device that converts the electric pulses from the pulse-height analyzer into light flashes, which expose a piece of film. This is usually done by means of a small cathode-ray tube that produces a light flash within the photosensitive range of the film emulsion. The flashes are projected on the film through a light mask. The resulting exposure may be in any shape, for example, circle or rectangle, depending on the preference of the operator. However, the length of the light-mask aperture is usually chosen to match the raster step size so that the lines of the scan are contiguous.

The quality of the image is dependent on several factors. First and most important is that both the light source and the monitor-recorder source move in synchrony with the detector. This is accomplished in one of two ways. The detector and recording devices may be coupled together in a mechanical fashion; that is, they are physically attached to one another; thus if the detector moves, the recording device must also move in the same fashion. The second way is by means of an electronic coupling between the detector and the recording device such that movement of the detector and the recording device are synchronous.

Photorecorder. Photorecording systems have several controls that allow the operator to produce a film with the desired density. They control the duration of the light flash, the intensity or brightness of the flash, and the enhancement, which adjusts the linearity of film response so that blackening to the available range of count rates is facilitated. For example, the enhancement control set at 50% means that over the count rate from one-half maximum to full maximum, the entire range of film density will be seen, and the count rate from zero to half maximum will have little effect on the film. Thus the operator must be aware that he is artificially modifying data whenever he uses the enhance control and background subtraction, which allow the operator to suppress a selected range of counts from the recorded image. Some scanners use storage cathode-ray tubes as a monitor; the disadvantage of a cathode-ray tube is the lack of a life-sized hard copy upon which anatomic landmarks can be placed.

To obtain a scan that can provide meaningful information, a sufficient number of counts must be recorded per unit area of the scan in order to be statistically significant. A rule of thumb is to aim for 800 counts/cm^2. The relationship between count density and scan parameters is as follows:

$$\text{Count density (counts/cm}^2\text{)} = \text{Patient counts/min} \times \frac{1}{\begin{array}{c}\text{Scan speed}\\ \text{(cm/min)}\end{array}} \times \frac{1}{\begin{array}{c}\text{Spacing}\\ \text{(cm)}\end{array}}$$

This equation can be used to translate the count rate presented by the patient into image-count density.

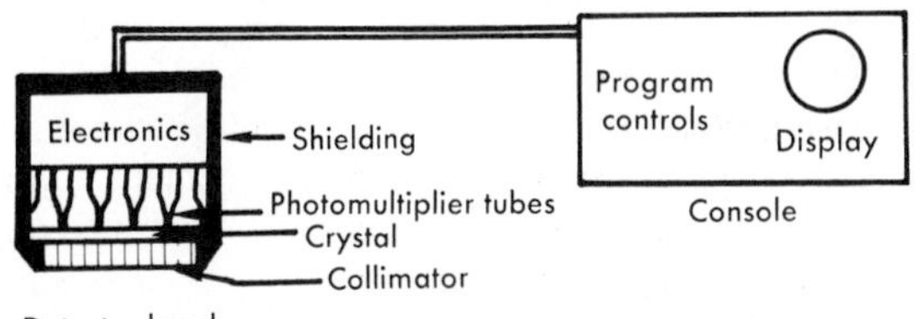

Fig. 3-20. Scintillation-camera configuration. Detector head contains collimator, crystal, photomultiplier tubes, and electronics, which determine scintillation location and photon energy. Console contains controls and display scope.

Scintillation camera

Anger camera. The scintillation camera (the term used by the National Council on Radiation Protection for the inaccurate term "gamma camera") was first designed and built in 1958 by Hal Anger at Donner Laboratory in California and has come to be known as the Anger camera. It consists of a collimator, crystal, array of photomultiplier tubes, an electronic package (analog computer) to sort out the signals to determine the location of the scintillation event that was deposited in the crystal, and a means for displaying and recording the image. Fig. 3-20 shows a general configuration of these components.

Collimators are an important part of the total camera system because they limit the gamma rays that can interact with the crystal to those that come directly from the region of interest being viewed. Thus they are a major factor in relating where the scintillation occurs in the crystal to the point of origin of the gamma ray in the patient. Collimators are discussed in greater detail later in this section.

PHOTOMULTIPLIER TUBES AND SCINTILLATION CRYSTAL. A gamma ray interacts with the sodium iodide scintillation crystal and deposits energy in the form of ionization and excitation. A portion of that energy is released in the form of fluorescence radiation as blue–blue violet light. Although the following statement is not absolutely true, we can assume that the light is released in all directions from essentially the point of gamma-ray interaction in the crystal. Fig. 3-21 shows diagrammatically how several photomultiplier (PM) tubes at different locations respond to light from the point of scintillation. As discussed earlier in this chapter, the mean value of the voltage pulse and the distribution

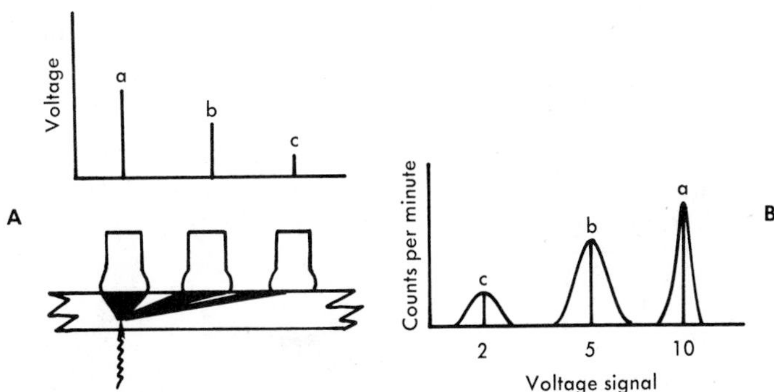

Fig. 3-21. A, Effect of distance of phototube from scintillation point. Phototube *a* is directly above scintillation point and generates voltage signal *a*. Phototubes *b* and *c* are farther from scintillation point and therefore collect less light and generate smaller signals. **B,** Smaller voltage signals are developed because phototube processed fewer photons and electrons, and so the uncertainty in mean voltage value is greater.

about the mean value is proportional to the quantity of light striking the face of the PM tube. Thus, in Fig. 3-21, PM tube *a* sees a large fraction of the light and PM tubes *b* and *c* see proportionally less. The voltage signal from *a* is larger than that from *b* or *c*. Note here that for a smaller quantity of light viewed by the PM tube, fewer electrons are generated and so a smaller voltage pulse is caused. This means poorer statistics and larger variations in the small voltage pulse. Fig. 3-21 shows this effect by the widening of the "photopeaks" generated by each tube at lower voltage levels.

The light pipe is a disk of optically transparent material that couples the PM tubes to the crystal and is empirically designed to improve the resolution and linearity of the images. The crystals used in gamma cameras are usually ½ inch thick by anwhere from 10 inches to 25 inches in diameter. The ½-inch thickness is selected so that the PM tubes are in proximity to where the gamma ray enters the crystal and the point of scintillation. Thicker crystals would provide increased counting efficiency for higher energy gamma rays by providing more opportunity for Compton interactions to take place followed by a photoelectric interaction. The advantage of increased counting efficiency is offset, however, by the larger error introduced by generation of two separated scintillation points, one for the Compton interaction, the other for the photoelectric interaction. The two separated points of light occur within the response time of the PM tubes and confuse the location of the original gamma ray so that poor spatial resolution results. Similarly, thicker crystals do not provide increased counting efficiency for low-energy gamma rays (the intrinsic photopeak efficiency for 140 keV is 90%), but because the scintillation occurs near the face of the crystal, the PM tube is farther away from the scintillation point, sees less light, generates a weaker signal, and thereby increases statistical uncertainty.

Some new cameras designed for use with low-energy gamma rays are using ¼-inch thick crystals. The intrinsic photopeak counting efficiency is decreased to about 80% for 140 keV gamma rays, with the goal of placing the PM tubes closer to the scintillation point, and thereby improving spatial resolution (Figs. 3-22 and 3-23). Some manufacturers reduce the thickness of, or completely eliminate, the light pipe between the PM tubes and crystal for the same purpose of achieving improved spatial resolution.

Another way to improve spatial resolution is to use a larger number of phototubes. The older cameras used 19 PM tubes. As the diameter of the crystal became larger, it was necessary to use more PM tubes to cover the increased size of the crystal. It was also found that when smaller diameter PM tubes and a larger number were used, spatial resolution could be improved.

An additional advantage is that a large number of small-diameter tubes placed on the crystal covers a larger portion of the crystal surface than do fewer large-diameter PM tubes (the use of hexagonal tubes can also cover a larger portion). Therefore, to increase spatial resolution and the size of the field of view, the number of PM tubes used in scintillation cameras has gone from 19 to 37 to 61 to 93 and may still increase.

PULSE-HEIGHT ANALYZER. Although the uniqueness of the scintillation camera lies in its ability to form images, part of this process requires the camera to distinguish different gamma-ray energies, just as any other scintillation detector should.

If the output signals of all photomultiplier tubes are added together, the camera will operate like any scintillation crystal viewed with a single PM tube. The size of this one signal (called the "*z* pulse") is proportional to the total energy deposited in the crystal and therefore related to the gamma-ray energy.

The *z* pulse is directed to an amplifier and pulse height–analyzer circuits, much the same as described previously in the section on scintillation spectrometers.

The camera pulse-height analyzer functions by using

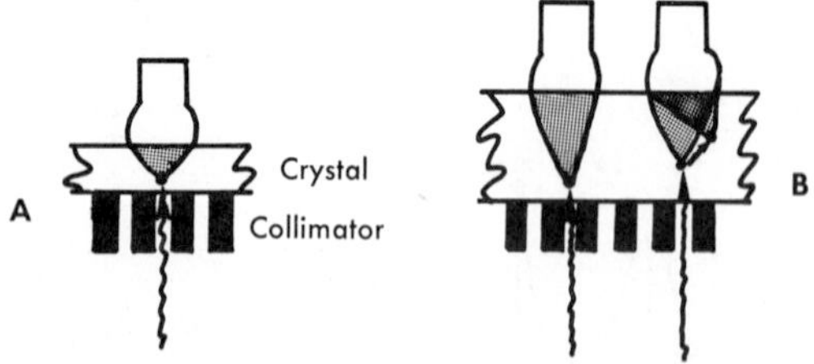

Fig. 3-22. Effect of crystal thickness. **A,** For a thin crystal, the photomultiplier tube is closer to point of scintillation and collects more light than for **B,** a thick crystal where photomultiplier tube is farther away. Thick crystal can increase probability of photon interacting by Compton effect and thereby stop more gamma rays, but Compton interactions are not desirable since there is more than one scintillation point.

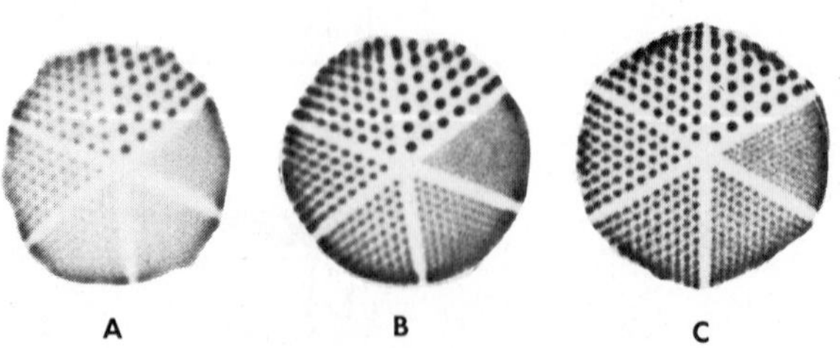

Fig. 3-23. Series of intrinsic-resolution images obtained with Anger phantom and point source of ^{201}Tl. **A,** Scintillation camera with 19 photomultiplier tubes and ½-inch crystal. **B,** 37–photomultiplier tube camera with a ½-inch crystal. **C,** 37–photomultiplier tube camera with a ¼-inch crystal.

a fixed window level and the size of the z pulse is adjusted so that it will fit through the window (Fig. 3-24).

A voltage level that corresponds to the center of the pulse-height window is set by the manufacturer; then incoming pulses are amplified by a selected factor so that the pulses of the chosen gamma-ray energy are equal to the window center–voltage level. The range of voltage levels accepted (window width) is also adjustable. The window width is calibrated in terms of percent of the "isotope" energy. This means that for a 20% window for 140 keV gamma rays, the camera will accept 140 ± 14 keV gamma rays, and a 20% window set for 365 keV gamma rays will accept 365 ± 36.5 keV gamma rays.

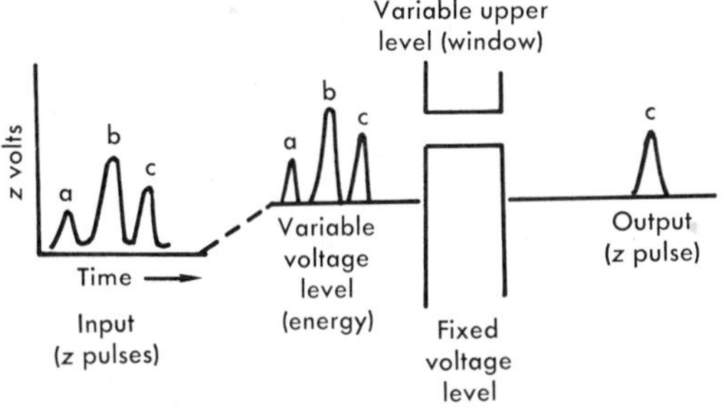

Fig. 3-24. Pulse-height analysis of the z pulse.

In Fig. 3-24 the incoming z pulses correspond to three different gamma-ray energies deposited in the crystal. The energy control has been adjusted so that only pulse c fits in the window. If the "energy" control were to be adjusted to allow the high-energy pulse, b, through the window, the voltage gain would be lowered and pulse b would get through but a and c would be too small and be stopped. Similarly, if the "energy" control were adjusted to a level so that pulse a could get through the window, pulses b and c would be too large and be stopped. The "width" of the window allows the user to adjust how critical he wishes it to be by selecting a narrow or wide band of energy pulses. The output of the pulse-height analyzer becomes labeled a "z unblank" signal and is again considered later in this section.

A very convenient feature on many of the new cameras is an *autopeaking circuit,* which when activated automatically "peaks in" the pulse-height analyzer. In simplistic terms, the auto-peak works in the manner shown in Fig. 3-25.

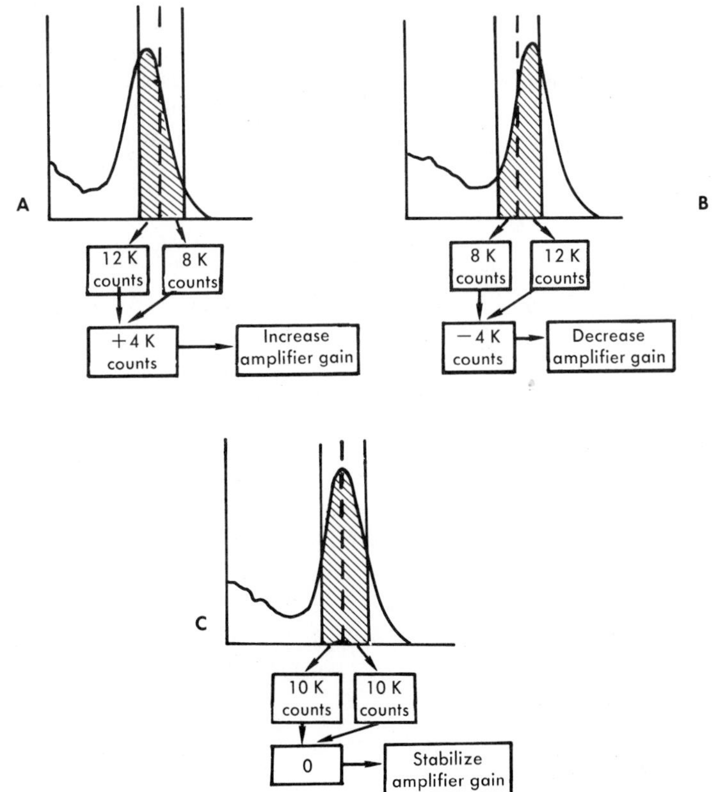

Fig. 3-25. "Autopeaking circuit." K, 1000.

The window of the pulse-height analyzer is divided into two equal parts, and the counts passing through each half are recorded and compared. If the counts are greater in the lower half than in the upper half, a difference signal or correction voltage is fed to the energy level, which in effect shifts the photopeak upward (Fig. 3-25, *A*); if the counts are greater in the upper half of the window compared to the lower half, the correction signal shifts the photopeak downward (Fig. 3-25, *B*). When the lower-count information equals the upper-count information, the photopeak is exactly centered within the window (Fig. 3-25, *C*).

Autopeaking is only a fine adjustment. The operator must first select the correct energy level so that the photopeak is located somewhere within the window. The Siemens camera, for example, has on its front panel a deviation meter, which indicates the percentage correction applied to "peak in" the signal as well as to indicate if the photopeak is located within the range of the autopeaking circuitry.

If one changes the energy selector switch or preset buttons, the camera must be repeaked. If one uses the manual energy selection controls, the autopeaking circuitry is disengaged.

LOCATING THE SCINTILLATION POINT. The clue to success of the gamma camera and to the continuing improvement in resolution is the clever electronics used for locating the position of the scintillation event in the crystal and translating that information to the display device.

Fig. 3-26 is a diagram of the electronics that trace the signals and demonstrate how a scintillation event can be located within the crystal.

The array of photomultiplier tubes that view the crystal are electronically divided into quadrants. Signals from the PM tubes in each quadrant are routed to an x and a y amplifier for that quadrant through a resistor so that the resistor can "weight" the signal according to the location of the PM tube within the quadrant. The signals from the amplifiers x_{I} and x_{IV} are added together, and the signals from the amplifiers x_{II} and x_{III} are added together. These two sums are then subtracted to generate the difference x signal:

$$\text{Diff } x = x_{I} + x_{IV} - (x_{II} + x_{III})$$

The result is an x signal that is a positive voltage if the scintillation occurred in quadrants I or IV and the size of the signal is proportional to how far away from the center of the crystal the scintillation occurred. If the result is a negative voltage, the scintillation would have occurred in quadrants II or III and again the size of the voltage is proportional to the distance from the center of the crystal along the x axis. Signals from the y amplifiers are treated the same way. The Diff y signal is a plus or minus voltage and the voltage size is related to the distance from the crystal center along the y axis.

The amplitude of the voltage pulses are not only related to x and y locations, but also depend on the gamma-ray energy deposited in the crystal. The x and y location signals for 140 keV gamma rays would be exactly one half the voltage of 280 keV gamma rays striking the crystal at exactly the same location. To

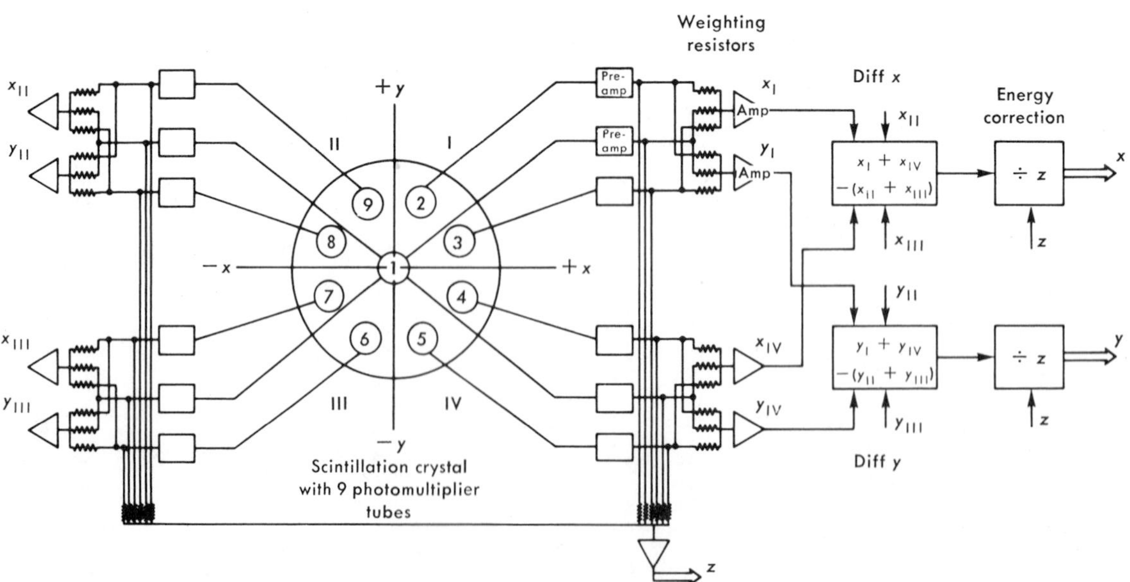

Fig. 3-26. Simplified diagram of scintillation-camera electronics.

eliminate this dependence on energy, one makes a correction by dividing the Diff x and Diff y signals by the z signal. For example, if the x and y signals were 0.1 and 0.04 volts, respectively, for 140 keV (z pulse = 0.14 volts), the x and y signals for a 240 keV (z = 0.28 volts) gamma ray would be 0.2 and 0.08 volts. Normalizing the x and y signals by dividing by z yields

$$x = \frac{0.1}{0.14} \qquad y = \frac{0.04}{0.14}$$

for the 140 keV gamma ray and

$$x = \frac{0.2}{0.28} \qquad y = \frac{0.08}{0.28}$$

for the 280 keV gamma ray. Understand that the x and y signals only reflect the position of the scintillation pulse independent of gamma-ray energy. The x and y signals are sent to the cathode-ray tube to locate the dot in the proper location on the face of the cathode-ray tube. An excellent detailed discussion of two specific camera systems is presented by Richardson.[18]

The "uniformity" of a scintillation camera refers to the response of a uniform field of radiation, and a daily check of the camera uniformity is made by inspection of the flood image. Distortions in the flood image are attributable to nonuniformity of the camera sensitivity, nonlinearity (misplacing the counts on the image), and statistical fluctuations.

Electronic techniques are available for correction of the uniformity of the flood image. There are in general two different approaches to "uniformity correction": count skipping and energy correction. Count-skipping correction involves the collection of a flood image where the counts are stored by the camera in a matrix of 64 by 64 memory cells. The memory cell with the smallest number of counts becomes the reference cell, and correction factors are calculated for all the cells and stored in the memory locations. For example, if the minimum counts were 1000 and another matrix cell had 1100 counts, the correction factor stored in that matrix cell would be $\frac{1000}{1100}$ or 0.9. As a clinical image is collected, the location of each detected count is referred to the correction matrix and the corresponding correction factor for that region is used. For example, if the matrix cell has a correction factor of 0.9 and indicates that 10% more counts were collected in the flood matrix than in the minimum cell, then in a random fashion 10% of the counts occurring in that region would be discarded or skipped.

For some camera systems, the counts are not rejected, but instead the correction factors are used to alter the intensity of the electron beam of the cathode-ray tube that is being photographed. In our example, the intensity of the beam would be reduced by 10%. The advantage is that the photographic image has been uniformity corrected but all counts remain available if a computer is attached to the camera.

A second approach to uniformity correction is to correct energy of the signals from each photomultiplier tube. The photopeak signal generated in a scintillation camera depends on the location of scintillation events within the crystal and phototubes. Fig. 3-27 shows the spectrums one might record from scintillations occurring in several locations of the crystal. To include all these legitimate signals, the window of the pulse-height analyzer must be made wider. This variation in accepted energy pulses introduces spatial distortion because the x and y signals reflect the same variations of the photopeak signals.

Energy corrections are accomplished by determination of the size of the photopeak signal at each spatial location in a 64 by 64 matrix. If the photopeak is lower or higher than the center of the selected energy window, an appropriate correction factor is stored in the matrix. As each photopeak event from a clinical study is collected, the stored correction factor for that location is used to adjust the gain so that the photopeak signal falls in the center of the energy window.

Multiple-crystal systems. Another camera system in use today, which is different from the Anger type of camera, is the Bender and Blau autofluoroscope. This system employs a mosaic of 294 NaI(Tl) crystals, ⅜ × ⅜ inches by 1½ inches long. Each crystal is independent of the other in that events that occur in one crystal are not seen by any other. The crystals are coupled to an array of photomultiplier tubes by plastic light pipes. Fig. 3-28 shows a matrix of crystals, wherein each crystal is viewed by two PM tubes—one determines the x position of the crystal and one determines the y position. If a light pulse occurs simul-

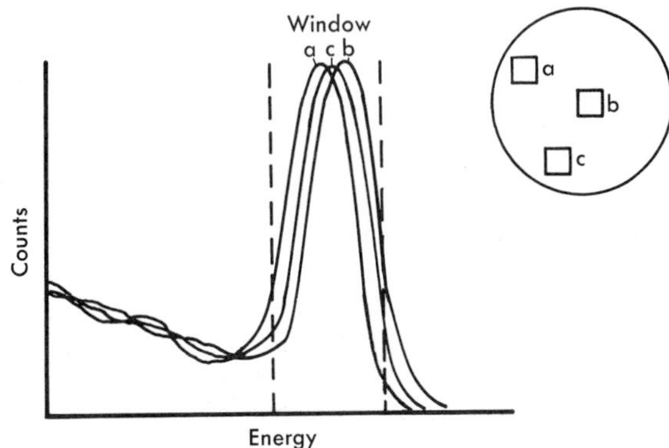

Fig. 3-27. Spectrums from three different regions of camera crystal.

taneously in row PM tube number 3 and column PM tube number 2, the gamma ray must have interacted with crystal 2,3 in the diagram.

The advantages of this system over the Anger camera is that the crystals are thicker and so the camera can be used to image high-energy gamma rays much more efficiently than the Anger camera can, and the speed at which the scintillation pulses can be processed is inherently faster than that of the Anger camera.

The inherent high speed is possible because each crystal is isolated from all the others so that when a gamma ray strikes one crystal, the processing of that event does not preempt the operation of the entire camera as it does in a single-crystal system. The processing speed becomes an important feature for doing fast dynamic studies as in nuclear cardiology.

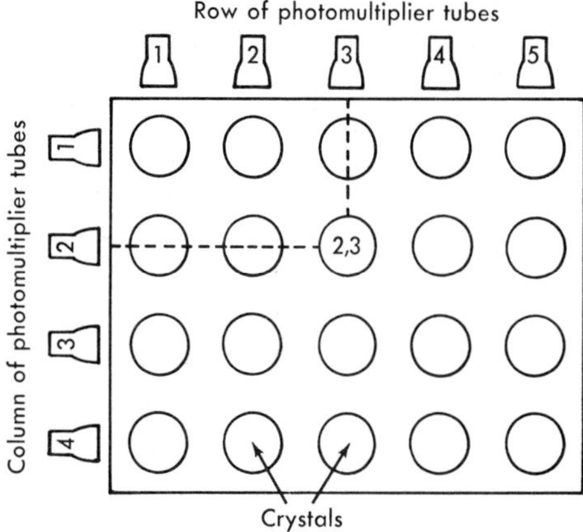

Fig. 3-28. Example of photomultiplier tube–crystal configuration for an autofluoroscope. Event that occurs in crystal 2,3 causes equal signals to be generated in column PMT 2 and row PMT 3.

The disadvantages are that the size of the field of view of these cameras is typically 8 × 11 inches and spatial resolution does not equal that achieved by the newer Anger type of cameras.

Image displays

Cathode-ray tube. The standard method for generating an image from the scintillation camera is to utilize a cathode-ray tube (CRT) to generate spots of light on the face of the tube and to photograph all the light flashes that occur over a period of time. The components of a typical cathode-ray tube are shown in Fig. 3-29.

Electrons are released from the cathode and accelerated across a high voltage, 4000 volts, between the cathode and the anode. The grid has a bias voltage that does not allow the flow of electrons from the cathode to the anode thereby blanking the cathode-ray tube. When a z-unblank signal that corresponds to an acceptable signal passing through the pulse-height analyzer appears, the grid is turned off and electrons can pass through the grid. The x- and y-position signals are sent to the horizontal and vertical deflection plates of the cathode-ray tube, which bend the beam of electrons so that the beam strikes the CRT face in a loca-

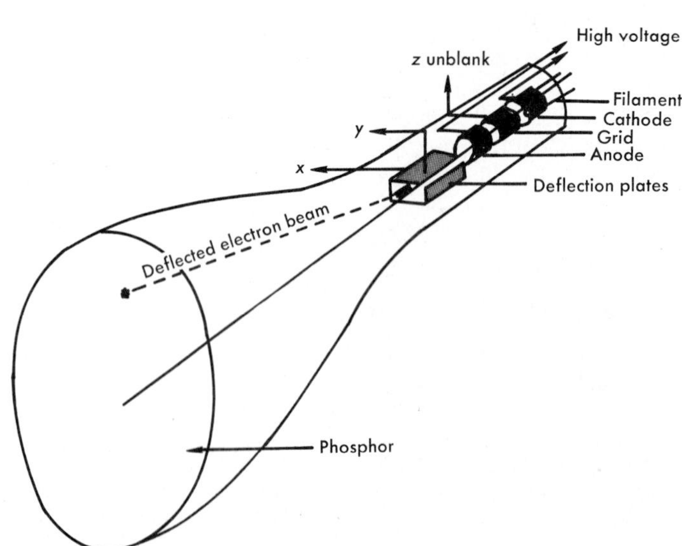

Fig. 3-29. Cathode-ray tube (CRT). Electron beam emerges from filament and strikes face of CRT in center unless beam is deflected by deflection electrodes. If a z-unblank signal is not generated, electron beam is squelched and does not strike the CRT phosphor.

tion corresponding to the location of the scintillation in the crystal.

The face of a cathode-ray tube is coated with a phosphor such that when struck by the electron beam a small dot of light is generated. The color of the dot of light is determined by the phosphor in the cathode-ray tube chosen by the camera manufacturer. P-31 is predominantly green and P-11 is blue, and the type of film should be chosen to match the color characteristics of the cathode-ray tube. Typically the size of the dot on the tube is around 0.008 inches in diameter. To generate enough light, maintain a very small dot size, and adequately expose the film, the dot must exist for about 4 μsec.

Some camera systems provide an option to magnify the image. For example, if a small organ is being studied, the majority of the camera field is wasted. Magnification allows the image of the small organ to be expanded. Two different techniques are used to accomplish magnification. One approach is to amplify the x and y signals that go to the CRT such that events occurring in the central region of the crystal are expanded to fill the face of the tube. The x and y signals from photons striking the outer edges of the crystal would be amplified beyond the outer edges of the CRT. The advantage of this system is that the magnification factor can be continuously variable from no magnification to a maximum value set by the manufacturer. The disadvantage is that in magnification mode the number of counts used to form the image is only a fraction of the counts recorded by the scintillation camera. The second approach is to choose a fixed diameter of the crystal, for example, 9 inches, and electronically reject x and y signals generated in the crystal that would correspond to events detected outside that central portion of the crystal. The x and y signals from photons striking the central 9 inches of the crystal are adjusted to generate an image utilizing the full face of the CRT. The advantage of this system is that the camera electronically functions as a small field-of-view camera and counts detected in the outer edge of the crystal are not processed. Since the outer signals are not processed, all counts registered by the camera are also recorded on the CRT and the photographed image. The disadvantage of this mode is that magnification is a fixed value with no variable stages of magnification.

Persistence cathode-ray tube. A special monitor display cathode-ray tube is used with scintillation cameras called a "persistence oscilloscope." This display has the unique feature of being able to "store" the dots from the scintillation camera long enough for an image to form on the screen. The uniformity, quality, resolution, and gray scale of these images is poor and only adequate for use as a monitor image to aid in patients positioning. The unique ability to store an image is a rather complex topic and is treated in greater depth by DeVere.[4]

Multiformat systems. With the increasing importance of dynamic studies performed with the scintillation camera, a means for rapid sequencing of images on film became necessary and this led to the development of formating systems. They also have the advantage of using sheet film.

Basically the multiformat systems employ a cathode-ray tube that forms dot images from the x, y, and z unblank camera pulses just as the standard cathode-ray tube. The major difference is that the image is minified and then electronically located systematically at different locations on the cathode-ray tube. If, for example, the format calls for four images, the original image is reduced to one fourth the size, then electronically located first in first quadrant of the tube, and then located in the second, third, and fourth quadrants (Fig. 3-30).

Because the image must be reduced in size on the cathode-ray tube to obtain multi-images, some systems use larger diameter tubes, some use specially constructed tubes with smaller dot sizes, and some add a system of lenses that open and close in sequence to achieve larger numbers of formats without reducing the images on the cathode-ray tube beyond a factor of ¼.

Because of the variation of techniques used to achieve multiformating, the comparison of CRT dot size among manufacturers is not sufficient to judge the quality of the final image on film. A factor that must also be considered in the use of a multiformat system is that some systems add a "dead-time" loss to camera-system performance. This dead-time loss can be attributable to the techniques used to deflect the electron beam.

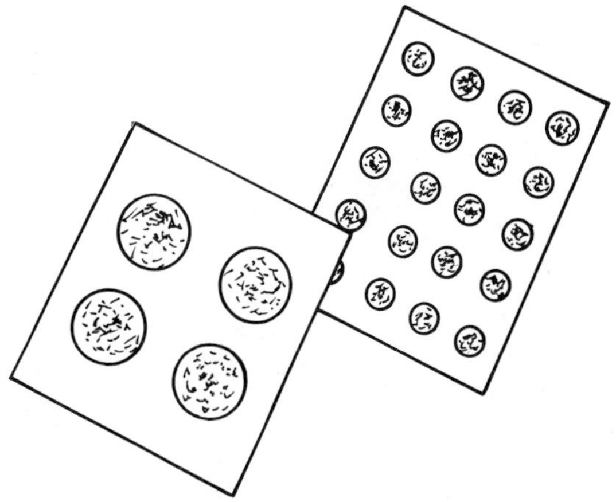

Fig. 3-30. Example of two image formats available with multiformat device.

The electronic multiformators provide the advantage of a fast, reliable means of recording dynamic images and efficient utilization of sheet film.

Collimators

Collimators are sometimes called the lenses for scintillation cameras. The comparison to optical lenses is not a good one because gamma rays are not refracted like light rays. Instead, the function of the collimator is to stop gamma rays from entering the scintillation crystal except through the holes in the collimator.

In the discussion of collimators the terms "resolution" and "sensitivity" are used to describe the physical characteristics of the collimators. Collimator sensitivity is the fraction of photons that are actually transmitted through the collimator and strike the face of the camera crystal. Spatial resolution refers to the capability of a system to produce an image in which the details are observable. We commonly measure resolution as the minimum separation that two line sources must have to be distinguished, and this is approximately the same as the full-width at half-maximum (FWHM) of a single line source. A common technique used to measure resolution is to image a bar phantom and visually determine the smallest bars that can be seen. A rule of thumb is that the FWHM of a line source is approximately twice the width of the smallest bar visualized in the bar phantom.

Multihole collimators. The standard collimator for a scintillation camera is a disk of lead with many thousands of holes penetrating the lead perpendicular to the plane of the disk. This is referred to as a parallel-multihole collimator (Fig. 3-31). For these collimators, the size of the image is independent of the distance from the subject to the collimator. As long as the source object is imaged completely within the boundaries of the collimator, the count rate remains essentially the same regardless of the distance in air between subject and camera.

Resolution is best for objects closest to the collimator face and degrades with distance away from the collimator. The frustrating story always associated with collimators is that if one wishes to attain the very best resolution one must sacrifice counts. Therefore collimators come in a variety of classes: (1) high resolution–low sensitivity, (2) medium resolution–medium sensitivity (3) low resolution–high sensitivity. In addition to these classifications, one must match the collimator to the energy of the gamma rays used. A low-energy collimator has thin lead septa and, if used with high-energy gamma rays, would allow gamma rays to enter the crystal from directions not restricted by the holes (that is, septal penetration and poor images). On the other hand, a high-energy collimator with thick septa could be used for any gamma-ray energy equal to or less than that for which it was designed. One would in the latter case unwisely sacrifice the best sensitivity and resolution because an unnecessary amount of crystal is covered with lead septa. Thus the well-equipped scintillation camera has the correct collimators for each specific use. Fig. 3-31 shows examples of both low- and high-energy collimators.

Pinhole collimators. The pinhole collimator was the first collimator used with a scintillation camera and of all collimators provides the best effective resolution. In contrast to its excellent resolution, it suffers from lack of sensitivity. For the pinhole collimator, sensitivity follows the inverse square law. Therefore the maximum sensitivity is achieved when the object is close to the collimator. Resolution and magnification also decrease as the distance between collimator and object increase. The relationship between resolution, sensitivity, and magnification is shown in Fig. 3-32.

Factors that should be noted in the use of pinhole collimators are that objects nearest the collimator are magnified more than objects farther away, sometimes referred to as "foreshortening," and sensitivity decreases for points distant from the central axis. Ob-

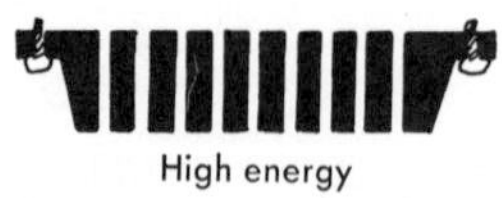

Fig. 3-31. Example of multihole parallel collimators. High-energy collimator has thicker lead septa than does low-energy collimator. Thus high-energy collimator out of necessity covers crystal with more lead than does low-energy collimator.

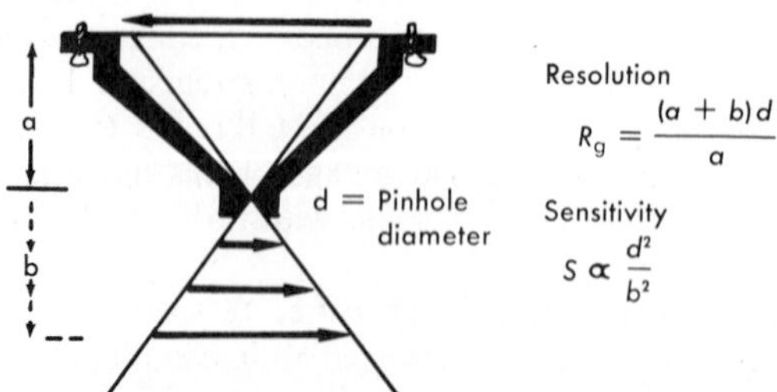

Fig. 3-32. Pinhole collimator. Object closer to collimator is imaged with greater magnification and better resolution, R_g, than is an object farther from collimator. Sensitivity, S, decreases with inverse square of distance between object and collimator.

jects located off the central axis and on different planes are imaged obliquely (Fig. 3-33) and introduce displacement distortion.

Diverging and converging collimators. The diverging collimator was designed primarily to enable 10-inch diameter cameras to view larger fields, such as lungs, kidneys, or the entire liver. The advent of large-field-of-view cameras have essentially made obsolete the diverging collimators. The diverging collimator allowed a larger geometric field of view at the cost of both resolution and sensitivity. Sensitivity and resolution get worse as the source moves away from the collimator. Fig. 3-34 shows a diagram of a diverging collimator with typical values for the relative sensitivity and resolution at different distances in air from the face of the collimator.

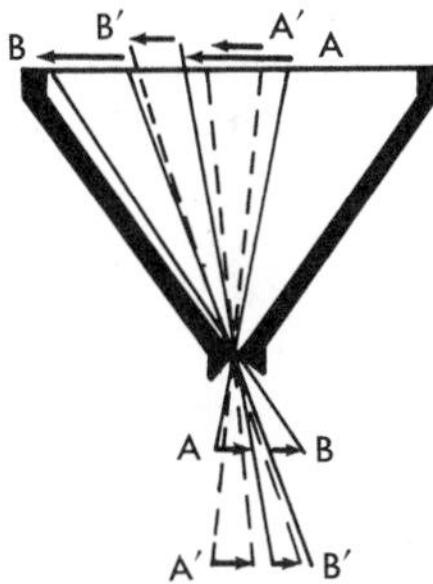

Fig. 3-33. Pinhole-collimator distortion. Apparent size of object depends on its distance from collimator. *A* and *B* appear larger than do *A′* and *B′*. *B* and *B′* appear at different locations in image and may cause confusion as to their true locations.

The converging collimator serves primarily as a compromise between the parallel-hole collimator, which can have good sensitivity, and the pinhole collimator, which provides the best resolution through magnification.

Because of the geometric magnification of objects and the fact that magnification increases as the distance between the object and collimator increases, a larger number of photons from each point within the object can pass through the collimator and thereby increase the sensitivity. Fig. 3-35 is a diagram of a converging

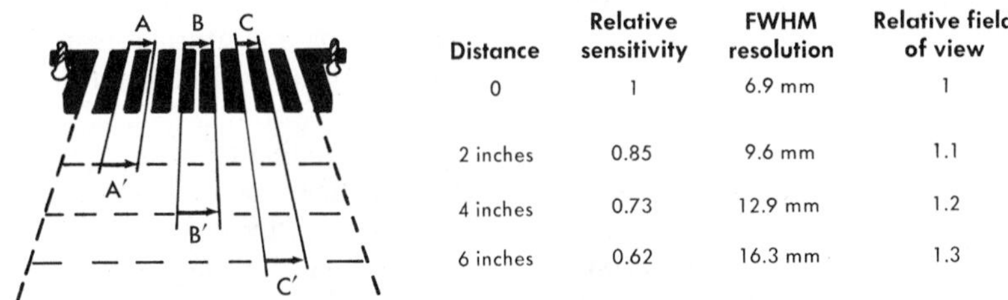

Distance	Relative sensitivity	FWHM resolution	Relative field of view
0	1	6.9 mm	1
2 inches	0.85	9.6 mm	1.1
4 inches	0.73	12.9 mm	1.2
6 inches	0.62	16.3 mm	1.3

Fig. 3-34. Diverging collimator, with typical set of parameters that show how sensitivity, resolution, and size of field of view vary with distance from face of collimator. *FWHM*, Full-width at half-maximum.

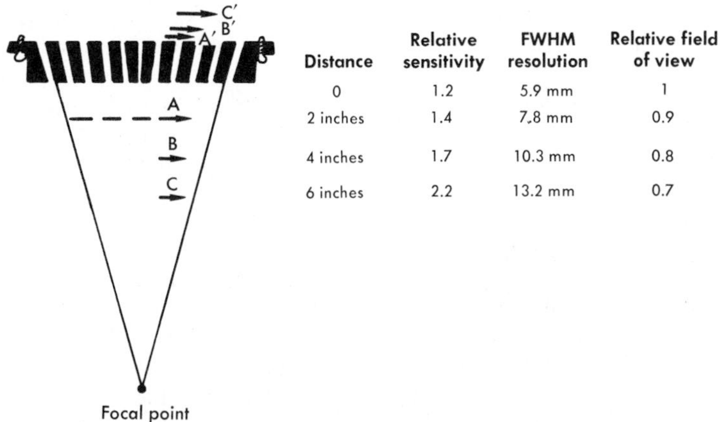

Distance	Relative sensitivity	FWHM resolution	Relative field of view
0	1.2	5.9 mm	1
2 inches	1.4	7.8 mm	0.9
4 inches	1.7	10.3 mm	0.8
6 inches	2.2	13.2 mm	0.7

Fig. 3-35. Converging collimator, with typical set of parameters that show how sensitivity, resolution, and size of field of view vary with distance from face of collimator. Objects *A, B,* and *C* are displaced and appear as different sizes in image.

collimator with a typical set of parameters. One may question why the sensitivity increases with distance from a converging collimator and in fact decreases with distance from a pinhole collimator. The difference is that the object is never viewed by more than one hole with a pinhole collimator; therefore the number of photons entering the hole from a point source decreases with the inverse of the square of the distance. But as the object moves farther away from the converging collimator, a larger number of holes are used to form the image, and the number of photons admitted to the crystal increases.

The reader should be reminded that in all discussions of collimator sensitivity no account has been taken of attenuation of gamma rays by the patient.

Special imaging systems

Total body scanners. It has always been desirable to be able to obtain images of a large portion of the body or the total body. A bone scan is an obvious case where it is desirable to view the total body; a search for metastases would be another case. Of less clinical interest, but nevertheless important, is the total body scan to obtain information about the distribution of new radionuclide labels for dosimetric purposes.

A rectilinear scanner is probably the simplest and oldest approach to total body scanning. Its major drawback is the time it takes (about 1 hour) to obtain simultaneously an anterior scan and a posterior scan. To speed up the scanning time, a number of approaches have been tried. One technique is a scanner that consists of an array of 10 NaI(Tl) crystals. Each crystal is 6.1 cm wide by 11.4 cm long by 2.5 cm thick and is coupled to its own photomultiplier tube. Each crystal is collimated by a multihole focused collimator. The scan motion consists of a lateral scan of 6.1 cm, which covers a total width for all 10 detectors of 61 cm, with a longitudinal (length-of-body) scan size up to 193 cm. Traveling at a maximum scan speed of 20 cm/min, it takes approximately 10 minutes for a total body scan.

The scanner utilizes focused collimators, which allow objects within about a centimeter on either side of the prescribed focal plane to be seen with good resolution and information closer to or farther from that depth to be blurred.

Another way to generate a total body image is to move a scintillation camera from head to toe of the patient (or move the patient in front of the camera). Most companies provide this accessory for their scintillation cameras. Total body scanning with a scintillation camera basically involves two additions to a standard system: (1) a means of mechanically moving the patient or camera from head to toe, with indexing being done once or twice and repeating the scan, and (2) electronically keeping track of the physical location of the scintillation camera to direct the cathode-ray tube's electron beam to the proper location.

The mechanical motion is easily achieved and the major difference between moving the camera versus moving the patient is the greater floor space required for the latter. With large-field cameras, adequate scan width can be achieved with two passes. Cameras of smaller field size need three passes to achieve adequately wide scans and thereby also a longer time to complete the study. Special diverging collimators have been used with smaller-sized cameras to obtain width, but the diverging collimators compromise resolution and introduce distortion. Therefore, they are not a desirable way to save scan time.

The camera field of view when operated in the body-scan mode is electronically reduced to a rectangular slit. The x-position signal from the camera is related to the location of the detected gamma ray along the length of the slit, whereas the y-position signal from the scintillation camera is modified so that it now relates to the physical location of the slit as it travels along the length of the body. A special mode of operation on multiformat-display systems can be selected so that the full length of the scan can be displayed on the film.

Most scanning camera systems allow the operator to select different total scan lengths, scan speeds, and single- or multiple-pass scans. The advantage of multiple-pass scans is that a wide scan can be achieved but at the cost of longer imaging times. Multiple-pass scans also require additional quality-control checks to avoid the "zipper" effect between the scan images.

Finally it should be noted that the second and third passes in a multiple-pass scan occur a scan period later. If there is a change in radionuclide distribution during the time of a scan pass, the two halves of a scan would represent different information. Usually total body scans do not involve such rapidly changing distributions, and this has not been a problem.

Emission tomographic systems. From the very early days of nuclear medicine, various techniques have been explored to obtain tomographic images. One of the earliest techniques was developed by Brownell[2] and colleagues and used positron-emitting radionuclides. Somewhat later Kuhl and Edwards[13] developed a tomographic scanner that could be used with a single gamma-ray emitter. The image was the distribution of activity in a transverse section. A third type of tomography was introduced by Anger,[1] where the properties of a focused collimator, rectilinear scanning, and a scintillation camera were combined to produce multiplane longitudinal sections.

For discussion, one can divide the type of tomographic systems into two general categories: (1) planar tomography, where the image corresponds to a longitudinal plane parallel to the head-to-toe axis of the patient and (2) transverse tomography where the image corresponds to a cross-section perpendicular to the head-to-toe axis of the patient. The positron camera of Brownell and Burnham[2] and the multiplane scanner of Anger are examples of planar tomography, whereas Kuhl's scanner and the newer emission computerized axial tomographic systems (ECAT, PETT, and so on) are examples of transverse tomography.

Planar tomography is based upon the principle that the instrument is designed to have a maximum sensitivity to the radioactive distribution at a selected focal plane. Radioactive objects located in this plane will result in sharp images, whereas objects located above or below that plane will be detected but the detected counts will be smeared over a larger area and result in blurred images. Perhaps the best example of planar tomography is that developed by Anger.[1] Basically the system employs a focused collimator to generate the tomographic effect and a scintillation camera to determine the location of scintillations within the crystal. Fig. 3-36 shows how point sources located at different depths from the face of the focused collimator would be imaged on the camera crystal and how the images would progress across the crystal as the scanner moves. Thus the rate of movement and distance moved by the image depends on the location of the source within the field of view of the collimator.

Reconstruction of the images is accomplished with an optical camera and independent lens systems for each plane to be imaged. Fig. 3-37 shows a simple example for two different depths. As the rectilinear scan is being generated, the film is moved in front of the cathode-ray tube in synchrony with the scanner probe. If the film moves at exactly the same velocity as the image moves across the crystal and cathode-ray tube, the image formed on the film will be sharply in focus. If the velocities are not the same, the image

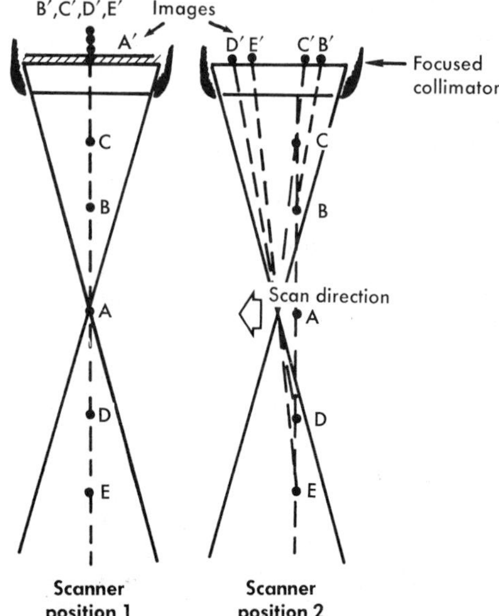

Fig. 3-36. As scanner moves to left in this figure, point-source images move across face of crystal. Sources *B* and *C*, located between collimator face and focal plane, move in direction opposite to scan direction. Sources *D* and *E*, located beyond focal plane, move in same direction as does scanner. Amount of motion of image depends on distance the source is away from focal plane.

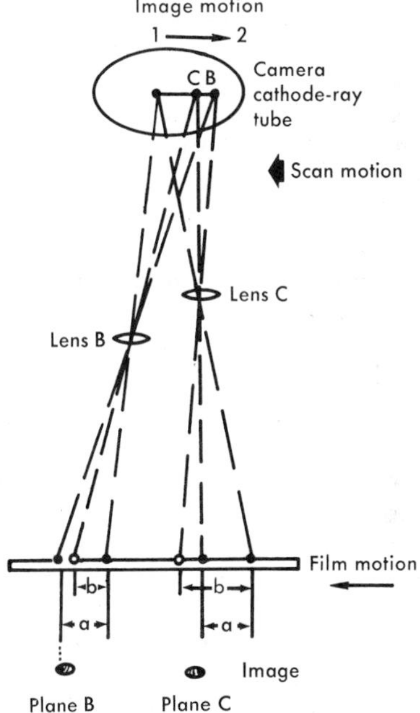

Fig. 3-37. Optical display system of Tomocamera. An example of optical read-out system for only two planes (*B* and *C*) are shown. As scanner moves, images of point sources *B* and *C* move to right on face of cathode-ray tube (CRT). Image *C* does not move so far as image *B* because of its depth from scanner (see Fig. 3-36). Lenses *B* and *C* have different focal lengths; therefore projections of image motion onto film from lenses *B* and *C* will be different. In fact, distance traveled on film by image *B* will be some value *a* seen through lens *B*, but distance traveled by image *C* will be less. Through lens *C*, image *C* will also travel a distance *a*, but image *B* will travel farther than that. If film is moved distance *a*, then image *B* will remain in focus on film viewed through lens *B*, and image *C* will remain in focus on film viewed through lens *C*. Any images not moving distance *a* on film will be blurred. In this way images of radioactive distributions at different depths can be obtained simultaneously.

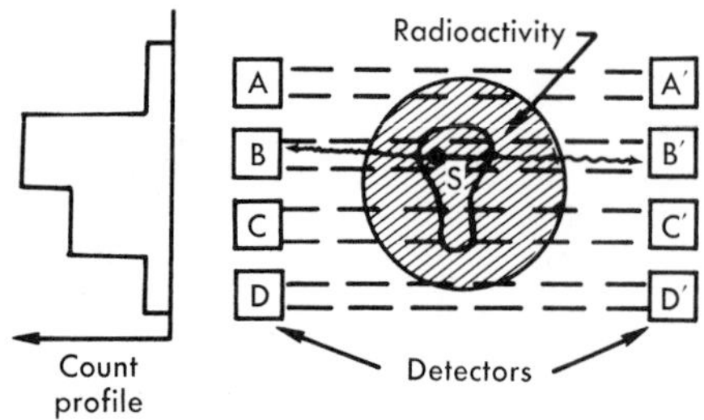

Fig. 3-38. Single profile of counts detected from radioactive distribution. Detectors *A*, *B*, *C*, and *D* are in coincidence with *A′*, *B′*, *C′*, and *D′* to detect gamma rays from positron emitters. For example, the two 0.511 MeV gamma rays emitted from point *S* travel in opposite directions and interact "in coincidence" with detectors *B* and *B′*.

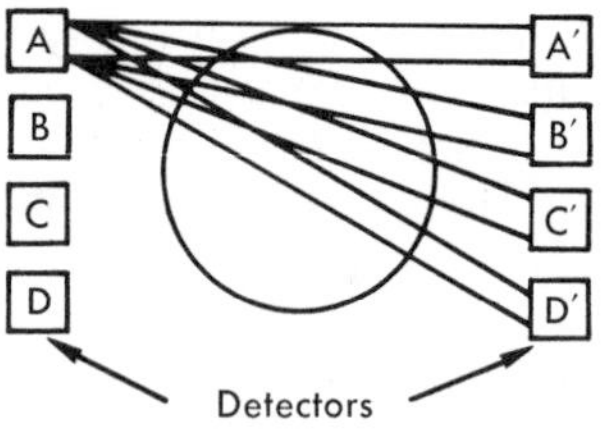

Fig. 3-39. Coincidences can be electronically established between each set of detectors to produce 16 different count profiles. In this figure only coincidence lines between detector *A* and opposite detectors are shown.

formed on the film will be blurred. Thus radioactivity on the particular plane to be imaged will result in a sharp image and radioactivity off the plane will be smeared out. The commercial version of this system provides 12 images at 12 different longitudinal planes throughout the patient's body.

Transverse tomography[15] provides a cross-sectional view of the radioactive distribution. Among the newest of these systems is the positron-emission computerized system. Not only does this approach use the principles of transverse computerized tomography but also incorporates the advantages offered by positron emitters.

To obtain a transverse tomographic image, one makes a number of measurements to obtain a profile of the emission radiation. Many profiles must be obtained at different discrete angles about the cross section of interest (Fig. 3-38). Computer algorithms essentially the same as those used for x-ray computerized tomographic scanners are used to calculate the radioactivity pattern within the cross sections. The gamma radiation from positron emission is the result of annihilation of the positron and electron essentially at the site of the radionuclide and the 0.511 MeV annihilation gamma rays are ejected at 180 degrees apart. Thus, if two detectors on opposite sides of the body each detect a 0.511 MeV gamma ray simultaneously, that is, within a few nanoseconds, it is assumed that the gamma rays were emitted from positron annihilation somewhere along the straight line connecting the two detectors (Fig. 3-38). Thus any two detectors that record two 0.511 MeV photons in "coincidence" provide information about radioactivity within a well-defined region between that pair of detectors. For example, Fig. 3-39 shows coincidences can be electronically established between any two sets of four detectors, which would result in 16 different profiles. Rotation of the detector system would generate another 16 profiles from a different set of angles. The coincidence data along with positional information is directed to a computer, which then proceeds to calculate the emission image.

Because the attenuation of gamma rays depends on the kind and quantity of material interposed between each detector pair, a correction must be made on each data point recorded. One method for correction is to experimentally measure the attenuation of 0.511 MeV radiation in the subject and correct the emission data before the computer reconstructs the image.

REFERENCES

1. Anger, H. O.: Multiplane tomographic gamma-ray scanner, Med. Radioisot. Scintigraphy. **1**:203, 1969, International Atomic Energy Agency, Vienna.
2. Brownell, G. L., and Burnham, C. A.: Recent developments in positron scintigraphy. In Hine, G. J., editor: Instrumentation in nuclear medicine, vol. 2, New York, 1974, Academic Press, Inc.
3. Cassen, B., Curtis, L., Reed, C., and Libby, R.: Instrumentation of I 131 use in medical studies, Nucleonics **9**(2):46, 1951.
4. DeVere, C.: Storage cathode ray tubes and circuits, ed. 2, Beaverton, Oreg., 1970, Tektronix, Inc.
5. Dillman, L. T., and Von der Lage, F. C.: Radionuclide decay schemes and nuclear parameters for use in radiation dose estimation, Medical Internal Radiation Dose Pamphlet No. 10, New York, 1975, The Society of Nuclear Medicine, Inc.
6. Gunther, C. W., Wilkerson, S. U., and Floriddia, D. G.: Letter to the editor, response to "Dose calibrator performance and quality control," J. Nucl. Med. Tech. **5**(3):168-169, 1977.
7. Hare, D. L., Hendee, W. R., Whitney, W. P., and Chaney, E. L.: Accuracy of well ionization chamber isotope calibrators, J. Nucl. Med. **15**(12):1138-1141, 1974.
8. Hine, G. J.: The inception of photoelectric scintillation detection commemorated after three decades, J. Nucl. Med. **18**(9): 867-871, 1977.
9. Horwitz, N. H., Lofstrom, J. E., and Forsaith, A. L.: The spintharicon: a new approach to radiation imaging, J. Nucl. Med. **6**:724-739, 1965.
10. Kaufman, L., Perez-Mendez, V., Rindi, A., Sperinde, J. M., and Wollenberg, H. A.: Wire spark chambers for clinical imaging of gamma rays, Phys. Med. Biol. **16**:417-426, 1971a.
11. Kellershohn, C., Degrez, A., and Lansiart, A. J.: Deux nouveau types de détecteurs pour camera à rayons X ou γ. Med. Radioisot. Scanning **1**:333-354, 1964, International Atomic Energy Agency, Vienna.
12. Kowalsky, R., Johnston, R. E., and Chan, F.: Dose calibrator

performance and quality control, J. Nucl. Med. Tech. **5**:35-40, March 1977.
13. Kuhl, D. E., and Edwards, R. Q.: Image separation radioisotope scanning, Radiology **80**:652-662, 1963.
14. Orvis, A. L.: Systems for data accumulation and presentation, Chapter 7. In Hine, G. J., editor: Instrumentation in nuclear medicine, vol. 1, New York, 1967, Academic Press, Inc.
15. Phelps, M. E., Hoffman, E. J., Mullani, N. A., and Ter-Pogossian, M. M.: Application of annihilation coincidence detection to transaxial reconstruction tomography, J. Nucl. Med. **16**(3):210-224, 1975.
16. Price, W. J.: Nuclear radiation detection, ed. 2, New York, 1964, McGraw-Hill Book Co.
17. Rapkin, E.: Preparation of samples for liquid scintillation counting, Chapter 9. In Hine, G. J., editor: Instrumentation in nuclear medicine, vol. 1, New York, 1967, Academic Press, Inc.
18. Richardson, R. L.: Anger scintillation camera, Chapter 6. In Rollo, F. D., editor: Nuclear medicine physics, instrumentation, and agents, St. Louis, 1977, The C. V. Mosby Co.
19. Rollo, R. D.: Detection and measurement of nuclear radiations: solid state detectors, Chapter 5. In Rollo, F. D., editor: Nuclear medicine physics, instrumentation, and agents, St. Louis, 1977, The C. V. Mosby Co.
20. Rutherford, E. R., and Geiger, H.: The charge and nature of the alpha particle, Proc. Roy. Soc. **A81**:162, 1908.
21. Stever, H. G.: Discharge mechanisms of fast G-M counters from the deadtime experiment, Phys. Rev. **61**:38, 1942.
22. Suzuki, A., Suzuki, M. N., and Weis, A. M.: Analysis of a radioisotope calibrator, J. Nucl. Med. Tech. **4**(4):193-198, Dec. 1976.
23. Timpe, G. M., Deville, T., and Shepard, J.: Letter to editor: More on dose calibrator performance, J. Nucl. Med. Tech. **5**(3):169, 1977.
24. Wagner, H. N., Jr.: Principles of nuclear medicine, Chapter 5, Philadelphia, 1968, W. B. Saunders Co.
25. Woods, M. J.: Calibration figures for Type 138-A ionization chamber, Int. J. Appl. Radiat. Isot. **21**:752-753, 1970.

Part B: Quality assurance of instruments

Marilyn R. Muilenburg and Mark I. Muilenburg

The interpretation of all diagnostic nuclear medicine procedures is based on the assumption that the performance of the system used for data acquisition is reliable and accurate. To provide evidence that data of diagnostic quality are acquired, a standardized program of routine system-performance assessment is essential. The quality control of nuclear instrumentation is the cornerstone of an effective overall nuclear medicine quality-assurance program.

The impetus to perform quality control procedures comes from a professional commitment to diagnostic excellence, the voluntary hospital accreditation process,[1] and the licensing process.[3]

The responsibility to provide reliable diagnostic data for interpretation and utilization in patient management is an important professional component of the practice of nuclear medicine technology. The responsibility for the routine performance and evaluation of quality control procedures is that of the nuclear medicine technologist.

The Joint Commission on Accreditation of Hospitals (JCAH) has recognized the need for quality control and has established policies and standards that must be met for nuclear medicine departments as part of the overall hospital accreditation process. JCAH standard III states:

> There shall be quality control policies and procedures governing nuclear medicine activities that assure diagnostic and therapeutic reliability and safety of patients and personnel.

The JCAH has interpreted this as ''instrument calibration procedures, sufficient to affirm proper performance, shall be conducted each day the instrument is used, and the results recorded'' as it relates to instrumentation.

The importance of quality control is gaining increased attention from the Nuclear Regulatory Commission (NRC) and from the agreement states during the process of radioactive material licensing. As quality control recommendations develop into regulations and join existing regulations, the performance of quality control procedures will be mandated with the force of law.

SCINTILLATION-CAMERA QUALITY CONTROL

The performance of a scintillation-camera system must be assessed daily to assure the acquisition of diagnostically reliable images. Performance can be affected by changes or failure of individual system components or subsystems and environmental conditions such as electrical power supply fluctuations, physical shock, temperature changes, humidity, dirt, background radiation, and radiofrequency interference. Testing procedures that elucidate the presence of these performance-affecting variables must be utilized.

Decision-making data to determine acceptability of camera performance can be acquired when the parameters of field uniformity, spatial resolution, linearity, and sensitivity are tested. These parameters must be tested at the time of installation to confirm specifications and provide the standard for all subsequent daily performance evaluations. It is also important to test after service has been performed on a camera.

These parameters and their importance are described as follows:

1. Field uniformity is the capability of the camera to produce an image of uniform density over the entire detector field of view when exposed to a uniform source of a gamma ray–emitting radionuclide. This checks the ability to produce accurate images of the relative radionuclide distribution in a patient. Without this assurance, the interpreting physician cannot be certain if all image abnormalities are attributable to the patient or to nonuniform performance of the camera.
2. Spatial resolution is the ability to accurately reproduce small differences in radionuclide concentrations in closely spaced areas. A transmission phantom is commonly used. The alternating patterns produce closely spaced areas of differing activity levels, which by definition allow for the analysis of resolution performance. The better the spatial resolution, the better will be the ability to detect small abnormalities manifested as different radionuclide concentrations in clinical images.
3. Linearity and spatial distortion deal with the ability to reproduce a linear activity source as a linear image and reproduce the spatial as well as geometric relations of an activity distribution. A transmission phantom with a linear arrangement of bars or holes are usually used. These phantoms are discussed on the following pages. The image produced should look exactly like the phantom. This is important in obtaining radionuclide organ images that accurately portray the true organ shape.

If these three parameters are assessed, analyzed, and compared routinely, the acceptability of camera performance can be determined.

Critical to the daily comparison of quality control images is the strict adherence to a standardized quality control program. Methods may vary slightly.

When embarking on a scintillation-camera quality control program, a department must make several decisions regarding methods and apparatus to be used. Three decisions to be made initially are as follows:

1. Is intrinsic or extrinsic testing to be employed?
2. What type of radiation source will be used?
3. Which transmission phantom will provide the desired information regarding resolution, linearity, and spatial distortion?

Intrinsic testing involves measuring the performance of the system without the collimator, whereas extrinsic determinations allow evaluation of the total system including the collimator. Is total or partial system performance to be assessed? What is the conformation of the system when patient procedures are performed? One might take the pragmatic approach and say that system performance should be tested in the same way it is used clinically.

The collimator's performance is constant, however, and requires only periodic evaluation. Extrinsic testing requires a considerably longer time to perform.

The geometric configuration of the radiation source and its quantity depend to a large extent on whether the intrinsic or extrinsic method of testing is chosen. The radionuclide used should be of a similar energy, if not the same radionuclide used most frequently for actual patient imaging. Because of the widespread use of ^{99m}Tc-labeled radiopharmaceuticals, the two most commonly used radionuclides are ^{99m}Tc and ^{57}Co.

There are advantages and disadvantages for both radionuclides. Cobalt 57 with a principle gamma-ray energy of 122 keV meets the criterion of a similar energy. The half-life of 271 days allows for longer usage before replenishment or replacement and also facilitates daily sensitivity checks. A disadvantage is the relatively high cost compared with ^{99m}Tc. Another consideration is that the energy selection or autopeaking circuitry may work well for ^{57}Co, and all parameters may appear acceptable, but the comparable circuitry for ^{99m}Tc may not be functioning properly. This could lead to a false sense of security when one sees acceptable ^{57}Co images whereas the clinical images using ^{99m}Tc might be unacceptable. This would support the case for using ^{99m}Tc as a source, since it is the radionuclide used in the majority of nuclear medicine imaging procedures. Its availability makes cost an insignificant factor. The 6-hour half-life does necessitate daily replenishment.

If camera performance is being assessed without a collimator, a small volume or point source of the chosen radionuclide is positioned at a distance of at least 1 meter from the crystal. When a collimator is used during assessment, a planar source having a uniform radionuclide distribution is placed on the collimator. Two types of planar sources are in use, a Lucite disk impregnated with ^{57}Co and a fillable flat plastic phantom.

The solid disk consists of a circular epoxy type of material with ^{57}Co dispersed uniformly throughout the disk, which ranges in diameter from 30 cm to 50 cm (Fig. 3-40). The liquid-filled planar source commonly called a "flood phantom" is usually water filled and requires replenishment. The phantom is a sealable, flat, thin-walled container usually made of Lucite. It has a circular cavity, which can be filled and then sealed (Fig. 3-41).

Thorough mixing of the radionuclide in the flood

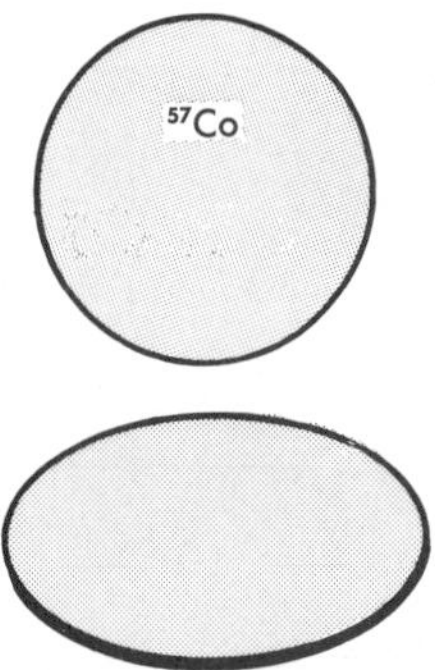

Fig. 3-40. Solid-disk flood source.

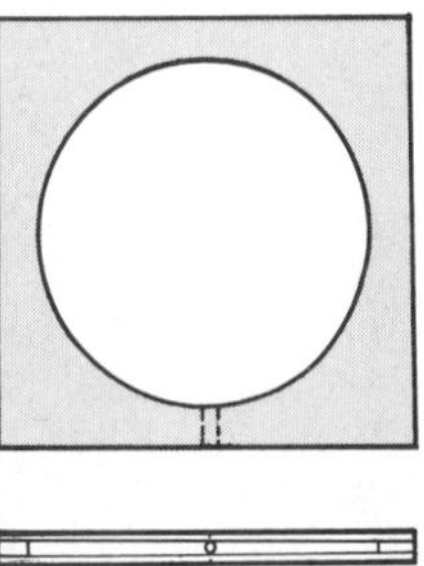

Fig. 3-41. Liquid-filled planar source (flood phantom).

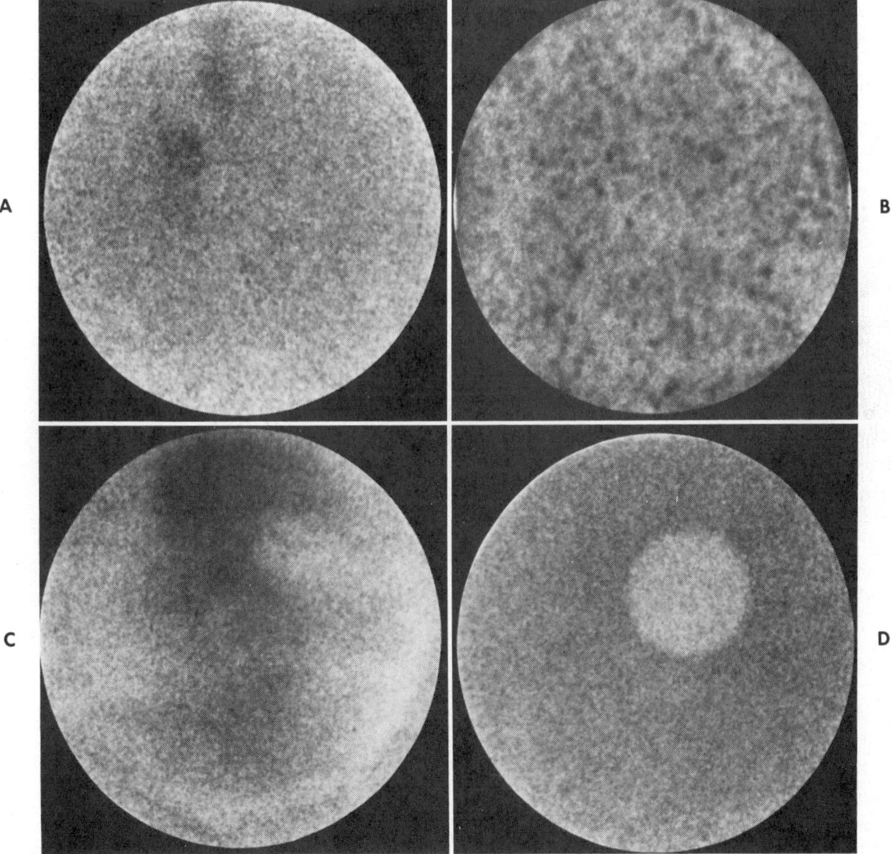

Fig. 3-42. Complications arising from improper flood phantom preparation. **A,** Adherence of macroaggregated albumin particles to inner surface. **B,** Particulate formation within liquid. **C,** Incomplete mixing of radionuclide. **D,** Air bubble simulating a photomultiplier tube malfunction.

phantom is essential, since any nonuniformity in the distribution of radioactivity in the phantom could be interpreted as a camera malfunction. When this problem is suspected on a flood-field image, the phantom is rotated 90 degrees and a second image obtained. A change in the pattern between images indicates a mixing problem in the phantom. Various examples are shown in Fig. 3-42.

Whatever source is used, the count rate should not exceed 20,000 counts per second.[4] At excessive count-

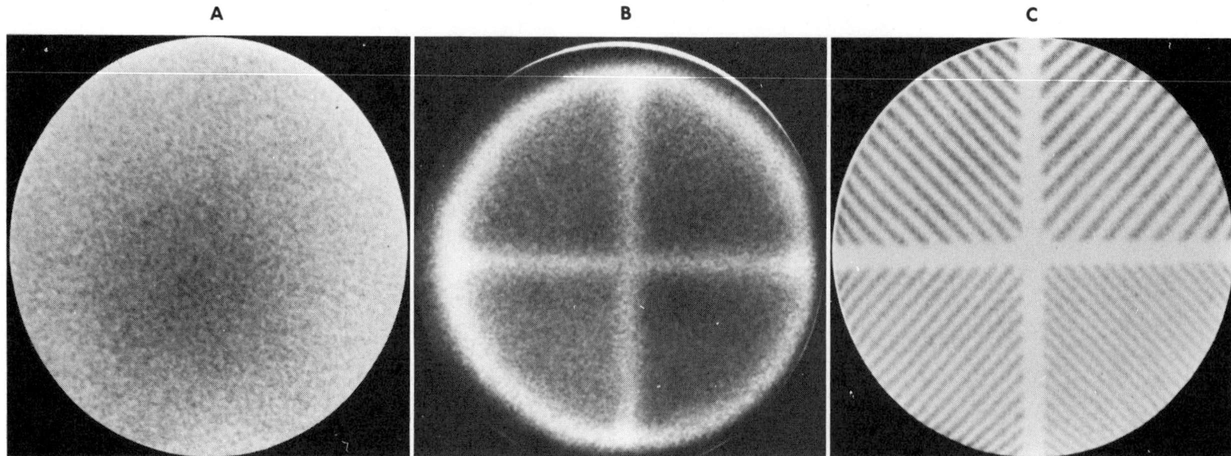

Fig. 3-43. Source quantity is important in assessing performance. **A,** Nonuniformity and, **B,** loss of resolution occur when source activity is too great. **C,** Resolution returns when activity is reduced to proper levels.

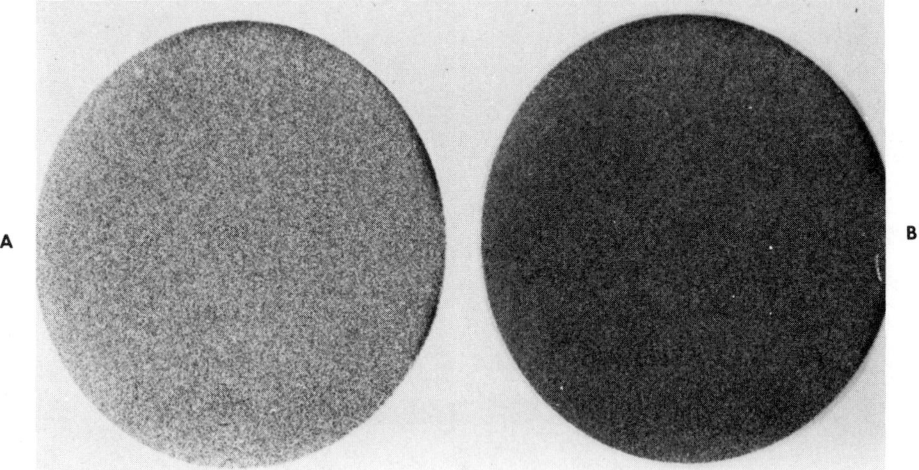

Fig. 3-44. Illustrates effect of source activity on film density. Film density increases (**A** to **B**) when source activity is doubled. All other imaging parameters are kept constant.

ing rates, poor uniformity and spatial resolution arise because of counting losses and pulse pileup (Fig. 3-43). In addition to not exceeding the correct source strength, the use of exactly the same quantity each day permits one to check the cathode ray–tube intensity. Fig. 3-44 shows that a change in source strength greatly affects film density even though all imaging parameters were kept constant. At higher counting rates, electrons from the electron gun hit the cathode ray–tube phosphor at points that have not completed phosphorescence from the last scintillation event. Therefore, the phosphor build-up effect and the increased light intensity cause increased film exposure at higher counting rates with the exposure settings kept the same. The effects of film exposure on uniformity and resolution images is illustrated in subsequent figures. In addition, maintenance of a reproducible source strength allows a quality control check on the sensitivity or counting efficiency of the system.

Phantoms for resolution and spatial distortion

Many transmission phantoms have been developed, with only a few gaining the widest acceptance.[4] An

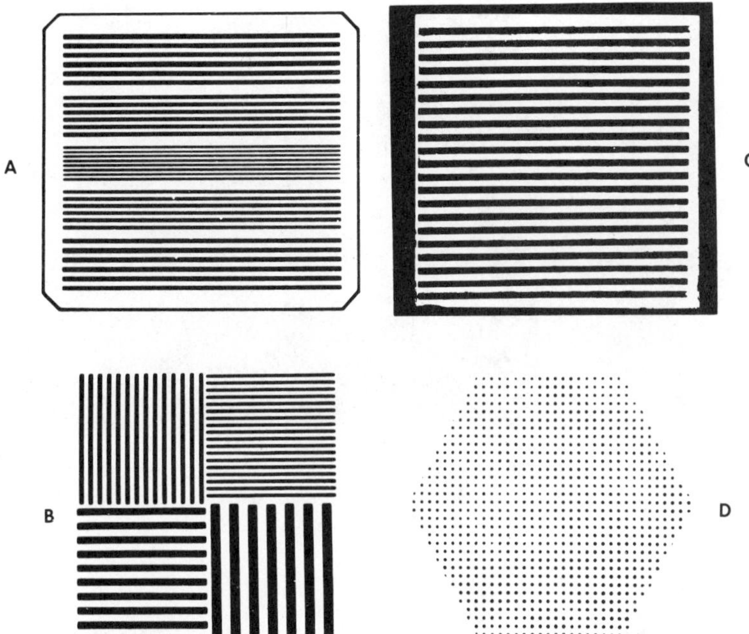

Fig. 3-45. Transmission phantoms. **A,** Hine-Duley phantom. **B,** Four-quadrant bar phantom. **C,** Parallel-line equal-space (PLES) phantom. **D,** Smith orthogonal-hole phantom. (From Rollo, F. D.: Nuclear medicine physics, instrumentation, and agents, St. Louis, 1977, The C. V. Mosby Co.)

ideal phantom would allow the accurate, simultaneous acquisition of an image that would help evaluate the parameters of uniformity, spatial resolution, linearity, and spatial distortion. To effectively assess the spatial resolution over all regions of the detector, the bars or holes must be of equal size and spacing for the entire phantom. A phantom can be used to assess spatial resolution, linearity, and spatial distortion if the bars or lines of holes extend completely across the detector, and it also must have bar or hole sizes that match the specified spatial resolution of the camera system. Four of the most widely used phantoms are pictured in Fig. 3-45 and are comparatively described.

Hine-Duley phantom

This phantom consists of five sets of 0.32 cm (⅛ inch) thick lead bars that are embedded in Lucite. The center set of bars consists of eight bars that have a width and spacing of 0.4 cm (5/32 inch). On each side of the center set there are sets of six bars with width and spacing of 0.48 cm (3/16 inch). The two outer sets have six bars at 0.64 cm (¼ inch) width and spacing. This phantom has been helpful for assessing detector uniformity, linearity, and spatial distortion of newer camera systems. Older 19-photomultiplier tube systems cannot resolve all these bars, and consequently it is impractical for older systems. Because the bars are of different widths, it does not measure spatial resolution equally over various regions of the detector.

Four-quadrant-bar phantom

In this phantom there are four quadrants with the bars arranged so that each set of bars is rotated 90 degrees from the set adjacent to it. There are four different widths of bars and spaces. The spaces and bars in each quadrant are equal. A higher resolution phantom going down to 0.32 cm (⅛ inch) bars is available for newer high-performance cameras. Measurement of the resolution of all detector regions requires imaging of the phantom in different positions, which is inconvenient. Linearity and distortion cannot be assessed, since the bars do not go completely across the face of the detector.

Parallel-line equal-space (PLES) phantom

This phantom consists of lead bars that have the same width and spacing and are embedded in Lucite. The bar width can be selected to match the lower limits of spatial resolution of the camera being evaluated. The recommended bar widths are 0.48 cm (3/16 inch) and 0.64 cm (¼ inch) for 37- and 19-photomultiplier tube cameras respectively. Two transmission images taken 90 degrees to each other provide the assessment of uniformity, spatial resolution, linearity, and spatial distortion for the entire detector area.

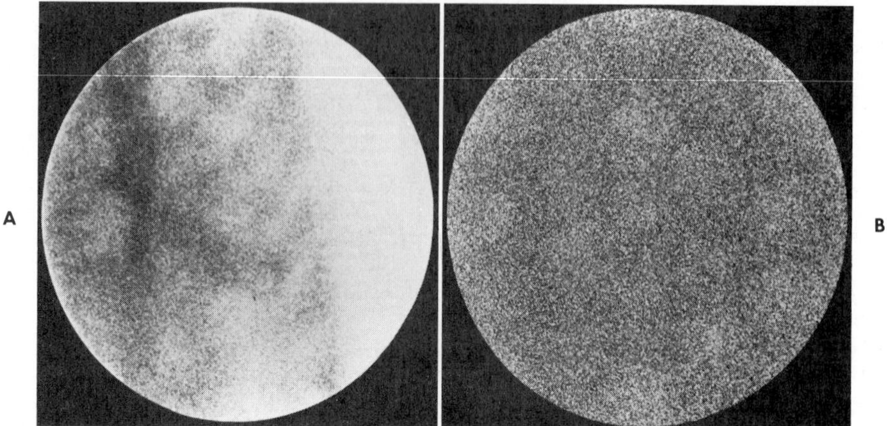

Fig. 3-46. Illustration of importance of repeaking a mobile camera after transit. **A,** ^{99m}Tc pyrophosphate cardiac image after transit. **B,** Flood-field image showing off-peak performance.

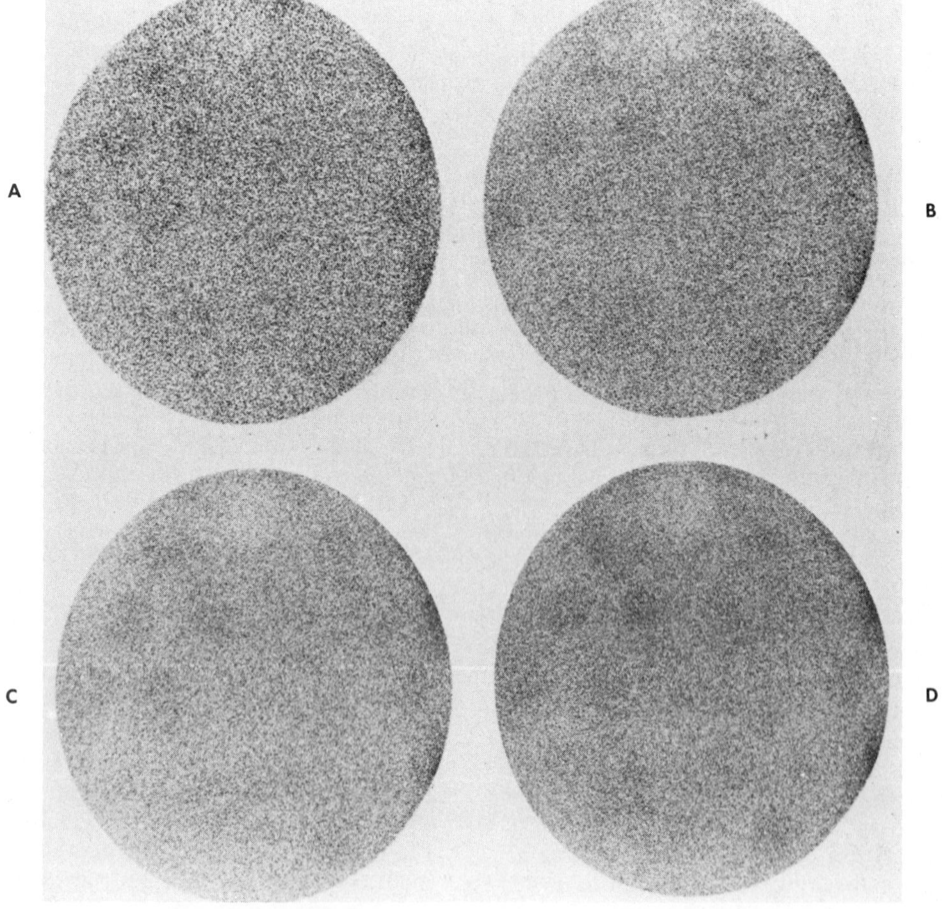

Fig. 3-47. Adequate data must be acquired to demonstrate subtle nonuniformities. **A,** 250,000 counts. **B,** 500,000 counts. **C,** 750,000 counts. **D,** 1 million counts.

Orthogonal-hole phantom

The orthogonal-hole phantom consists of a sheet of lead in which rows and columns of equal-diameter holes are arranged at right angles to one another. Phantoms are available with hole diameters 0.64 cm (¼ inch), 0.48 cm (3/16 inch), and 0.32 cm (⅛ inch) spaced at intervals of 1 cm (½ inch), 0.96 cm (⅜ inch), and 0.64 cm (¼ inch), respectively. A match of hole size to the lower limits of spatial resolution for the camera is important. A single image allows the assessment of uniformity, spatial resolution, linearity, and spatial distortion for the entire detector area. The orthogonal and PLES phantoms are considered comparable for all the parameters being assessed.

Now that intrinsic-versus-extrinsic testing, source considerations, and transmission phantoms have been discussed and decisions made, a daily quality control program for scintillation cameras can be established. One of the keys to a reliable quality control program is the standardized performance of the quality control procedures. There are a number of steps that must be taken prior to any quality control imaging. They deal with camera-system setup and are as follows:

1. *Photopeaking*. The correct energy window for the radionuclide being used must be selected and the photopeak centered in the window. If photopeaking is performed manually, the setting should be recorded. An image of the photopeak in the window is desirable. Correct photopeaking is absolutely essential for optimal camera performance. All the parameters being assessed for quality control are adversely affected if the system is off peak. The clinical ramifications of incorrect photopeaking are seen in Fig. 3-46.
2. *Orientation controls*. Image orientation must remain constant for quality control images, and so the same detector area is always recorded in the same position on the image. This is important in the evaluation of gradual performance degradation in a particular detector area.
3. *Display scope dots*. The shape and size of CRT display scope dots should be checked daily and at the time of intensity changes.
4. *Total counts*. For a standard-field-of-view camera, 1 million counts should be accumulated for a reliable image. A large-field-of-view camera requires 2 million counts for quality control images. Fig. 3-47 illustrates the importance of adequate data collection to demonstrate detector nonuniformities.
5. *Intensity*. Intensity settings must be kept constant from day to day. Differing intensities can affect the evaluation of the images by appearing to enhance or diminish the nonuniformities in detector response (Fig. 3-48). Decisions regarding spatial resolution are also made more subjective since intensity differences affect the apparent sharpness of phantom-image detail (Fig. 3-48). If intensity settings are critical for accurate quality control imaging, they are certainly no less critical for patient imaging.
6. *Photographic system*. The same image-recording devices used for patient studies are also used to record all the quality control images. A check for dust or lint on lenses and the oscilloscope face will help prevent image artifacts. These should be cleaned properly monthly. If Polaroid photography is used for image recording, the rollers should be cleaned several times daily so that debris, which can cause film artifacts and film jams, may be removed.

Upon completion of the camera-system setup, acquisition of a flood field to check detector uniformity is the next step. If extrinsic uniformity is to be evaluated, the collimator is left on and a properly prepared planar source is centered over the total detector area. Covering the collimator surface with a plastic cover or enclosing the flood phantom in a plastic bag are good practices to prevent collimator contamination.

If an intrinsic protocol has been adopted, the collimator must be removed and a point source of appropriate strength positioned at least 1 meter from the detector. The source can be positioned above or below the detector. A piece of lead under a source placed on the floor will act as an absorber for scattered radiation. *Extreme care must be taken to avoid physical shock and radionuclide contamination of the crystal*. A collimator can be removed if contaminated, but crystal contamination can shut the camera down for the day.

After source placement, the flood field is acquired and analyzed for acceptability in clinical use and any changes from previous floods. If the camera has a micropressor system for detector uniformity correction, it is critical that flood fields be acquired with and without microprocessor correction. This must be done to determine at what point detector recalibration must take place and how much the microprocessor is doing to correct nonuniformities (Fig. 3-49). If the flood field is acceptable, imaging for spatial resolution, linearity, and spatial distortion can proceed.

The selected transmission phantom is placed between the detector and source. The phantom must be against the collimator or crystal for best resolution. Resolution is decreased by the inverse square of the distance from the detector. If one is evaluating intrinsic spatial resolution, a lead mask may be used to eliminate "edge packing" from appearring on the images. The mask consists of a piece of lead with a hole in the center that corre-

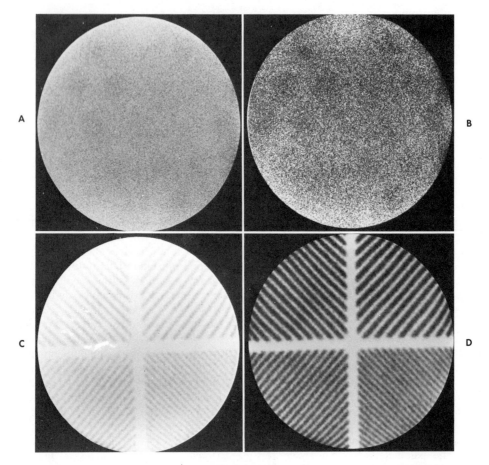

Fig. 3-48. **A** and **B** demonstrate effect of intensity differences in nonuniformity appearance. **C** and **D** show effect of intensity differences on apparent resolution with all other imaging parameters constant.

sponds to the effective field of view of the collimator.

The images must be acquired for the same counts or information density and intensity settings as those used for the flood-field images. The reasons have been illustrated previously. Only one image is required for an orthogonal phantom, whereas the PLES type of phantom requires two images to be acquired 90 degrees to each other for total detector area evaluation.

The following data should be recorded for all quality control images: date, photopeak setting, CRT intensity setting, total information density (ID), and elapsed imaging time.

Evaluation of quality control images

The flood field–uniformity images must be uniform in count density as demonstrated by uniform exposure of the total image. Any areas of increased or decreased density indicate nonuniform detector response. Edge packing, which appears as increased intensity around the edge of the field of view, is not a significant problem if it affects only the outer 10% of the field and the other 90% is uniform. An improperly set photopeak will produce nonuniform patterns whose characteristics depend on the type of scintillation camera. By rechecking the photopeak and acquiring another flood-field image, an incorrect photopeak setting can be ruled in or out as the cause of nonuniformity. If a nonuniformity still persists, one can make a determination of camera detector versus cathode-ray tube and photographic system by repeating the flood field after changing the detector orientation 90 degree. A 90-degree change in the area in question indicates a problem with the camera detector, whereas no change indicates the problem is in the cathode-ray tube or photographic system. A nonuniformity of increased intensity that persists in the same position may be from another source of radioactivity in the same or adjacent room that is not uniformly

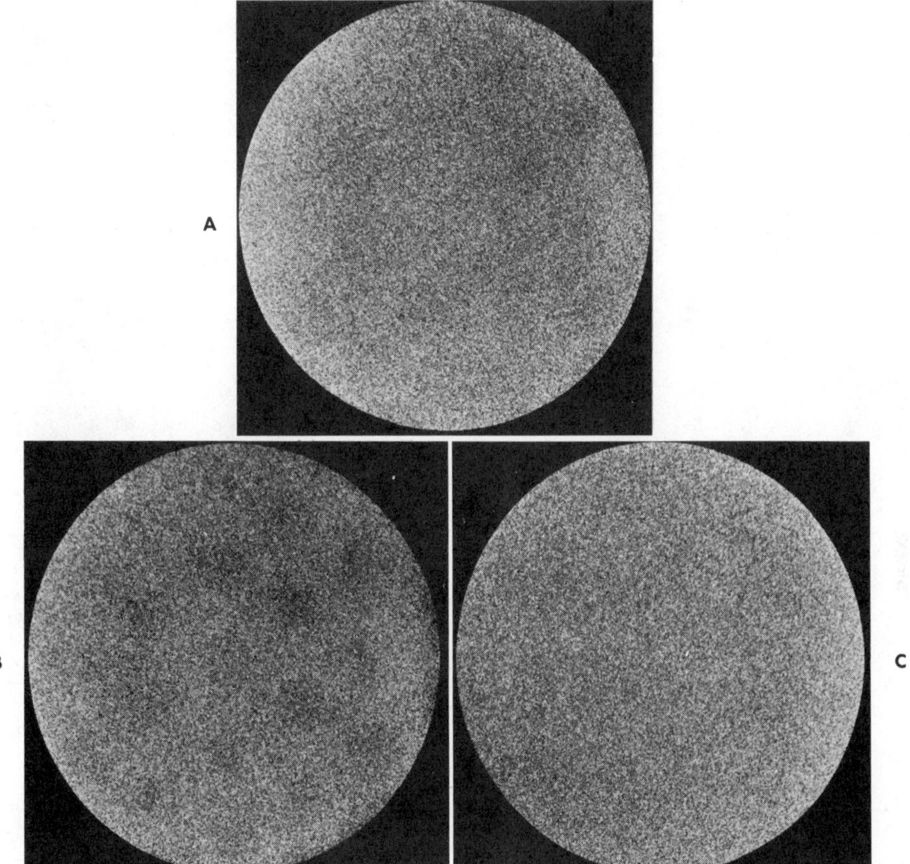

Fig. 3-49. Detector performance without uniformity correction must also be assessed. **A,** Subtle nonuniformities. **B,** Increasing nonuniformity with time. **C,** Uniformity-corrected flood of detector in **B.** Uniformity correction should not replace good detector calibration.

irradiating the detector. An improperly prepared source may also be the cause. Refer to Fig. 3-42 for examples of source-induced nonuniformities.

The cathode ray–tube face and phosphor can also be the cause of persistent problems. Debris or dust on the CRT face will produce areas of decreased intensity and can be alleviated by proper cleaning. Scratches or an area of burned-out phosphor also produce areas of decreased intensity. Dust on lenses, bad film, or debris buildup on Polaroid camera rollers also cause persistent nonuniformities. Proper cleaning and a film change usually rule out photographic system problems. If not, the persistent nonuniformity indicates oscilloscope malfunction and service personnel should be notified.

A nonuniformity that changes with an orientation-setting change indicates a detector problem and is usually caused by a mistuned photomultiplier tube. This problem usually appears as a gradual change over a few days and is best analyzed by comparisons with recent flood-field images. Complete failure of a photomultiplier tube will cause a cold area in the corresponding area of the flood-field image. A cold area can also be caused by loss of good optical coupling of the photomultiplier tube to the crystal. A diffuse cold area can be caused by a loss in the hermetic seal of the crystal. The appearance of definite lines indicates a cracked crystal and causes instant budgetary trauma because of the high cost of crystal replacement (Fig. 3-50). A cracked crystal is the common result of too rapid temperature changes or physical shock to the crystal.

If flood-field images are being acquired with the collimator on, there is the possibility that the collimator, not the detector, is responsible for nonuniformities. Radionuclide contamination of the collimator can cause hot areas (Fig. 3-51). Any collimator damage may be manifested by a variety of nonuniform-image patterns. Removing the collimator and repeating the

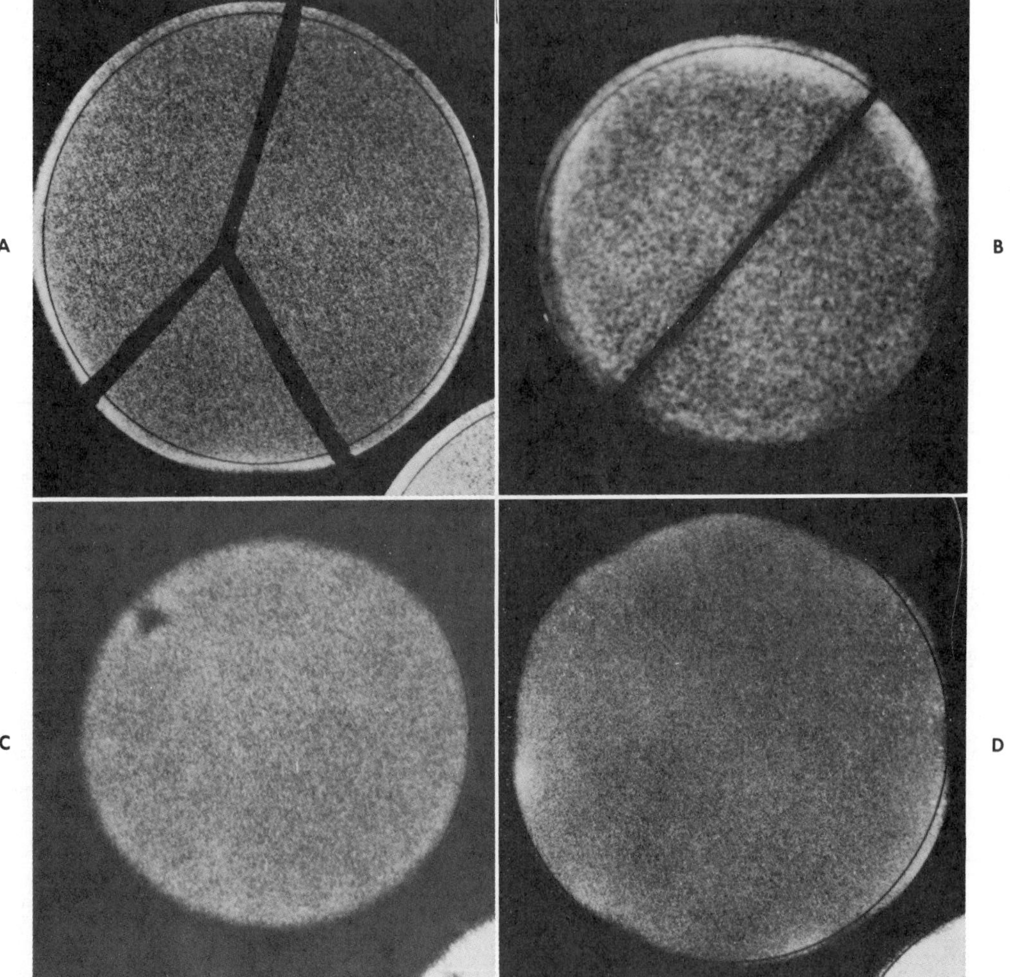

Fig. 3-50. **A,** Pattern typical for crystal cracked by impact. **B,** Typical findings associated with crack caused by severe changes in temperature. **C,** Crack caused by squeezing thumbtack between collimator and crystal. **D,** Nonuniform pattern characteristic in crystals having loss of hermetic seal. (From Rollo, F. D.: Nuclear medicine physics, instrumentation, and agents, St. Louis, 1977, The C. V. Mosby Co.)

flood-field image will help determine the cause of nonuniformity. If the nonuniformity persists, the detector is malfunctioning, and if it disappears, the collimator is the cause. Any detector malfunction requires attention by service personnel.

Loss of spatial resolution and evidence of nonlinearity or spatial distortion are best evaluated by comparison with previous quality control images acquired in an identical manner. They are manifested by loss of detail and geometric shape in the transmission phantom images. These changes are usually caused by a gradual degradation of camera system components.

A sharp decrease in spatial resolution is usually attributable to an improper photopeak setting or use of a lower resolution collimator. Photopeak readjustment or a collimator change may alleviate the resolution loss.

There are two types of spatial distortion. ''Barreling'' refers to curving of the bar image. If it occurs within the outer 10% of the detector area, it can be disregarded, since it is inherent to the detector electronics in that region. The other common distortion is ''footballing,'' occurring when the image is unequal in size in the x and y directions. This can be confirmed by the comparison of the number of bars visible in the x direction and then in the y direction after the 90-

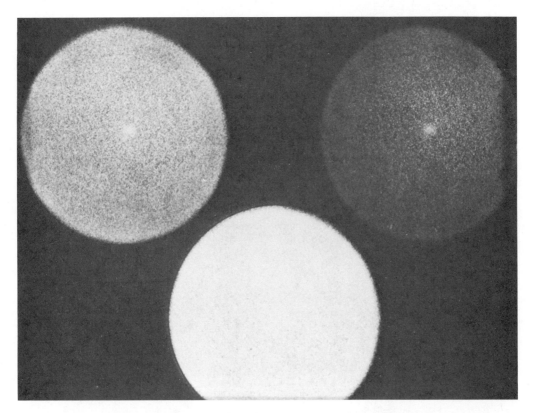

Fig. 3-51. Artifact caused by contamination of collimator with radionuclide. (From Wells, L. D., and Bernier, D. R.: Nuclear imaging artifacts, Chicago, 1980, Year Book Medical Publishers, Inc.)

degree rotation of a PLES phantom. For an orthogonal phantom the number of rows of holes in the *x* and *y* directions would be compared. In both cases the numbers of *x* and *y* bars or rows should be equal. If the numbers are unequal and the phantom was properly placed to be sure that the same numbers of bars and rows were in the detector field each time, realignment of the *x*- and *y*-positioning circuitry must be performed.

If quality control images for all parameters being assessed meet acceptance criteria, clinical imaging with the camera system can begin. If acceptable performance criteria are not met, service personnel must be contacted and repairs implemented prior to clinical use.

The fact that all parameters are acceptable in the morning, does not mean that all is well for the remainder of the working day. It is the professional responsibility of all competent nuclear medicine technologists to monitor imaging during the day, watching for changes in camera performance. Fig. 3-46 graphically demonstrates a change in photopeak adjustment during a department to patient-room move of a portable camera.

DOSE CALIBRATOR

The accuracy of the dose of radiopharmaceutical given to patients depends on the performance of the dose calibrator. An acceptable quality assurance program for radionuclide calibrators consists of a series of procedures that measure its accuracy, linearity, geometry dependence, and consistency. These quality control procedures are discussed below in detail.

Instrument accuracy[3]

This test is performed upon installation and annually thereafter.

The accuracy of the dose calibrator is measured with reference standards whose activity is traceable to the National Bureau of Standards (NBS). The instrument should be calibrated with standard sources of the radionuclide of interest whenever possible. When the use of short-lived nuclide standards is not possible, a long-lived standard of similar energy can be used, provided that the appropriate correction factors are employed. Several different radionuclides such as ^{57}Co, ^{137}Cs, and ^{133}Ba are in routine use.

By correcting the standards for decay, the exact

amount is known for comparison with the amount indicated by the dose calibrator. The average of several net-activity measurements should be compared to the activity calculated for that particular standard. If this is ±5% of the standard, the dose calibrator is functioning with acceptable accuracy.

Precision[3]

This test is performed each day that the instrument is used.

After the accuracy of the dose calibrator has been determined, the consistency of its performance is monitored by daily precision testing with long-lived standards at each of the frequently used radionuclide settings. Standards are chosen whose photon energies and activities are close to radionuclides routinely assayed. Cesium 137 (100 to 200 μCi) and cobalt 57 (2 to 5 mCi) simulating molybdenum 99 and technetium 99m, respectively, are typical examples.

A count-control chart is established for each of the radionuclide settings routinely used on the instrument. The average reading of the standard is obtained and plotted on semilogarithmic graph paper. The activity level of the standard in 10 weeks is calculated, with use of the appropriate decay schedule, and plotted. These points are connected with a straight line, which indicates the decay of the standard. Two straight lines are drawn above and below the decay line indicating the ±5% tolerance limits for precision (Fig. 3-52).

Daily readings of the standard are plotted and should fall within the ±5% lines. If a reading repeatedly falls outside of the limits, the calibrator should be taken out of service until the problem is identified and corrected.

Linearity[3]

Instrument linearity is measured at installation and quarterly thereafter.

The dose calibrator must function linearly over a wide range of activities from a few microcuries to about 2 curies. There are several methods that may be used to determine the dose-calibrator's response at different activity levels. A convenient method uses a vial of ^{99m}Tc that contains the maximum amount of activity that will be assayed in clinical practice. This is ob-

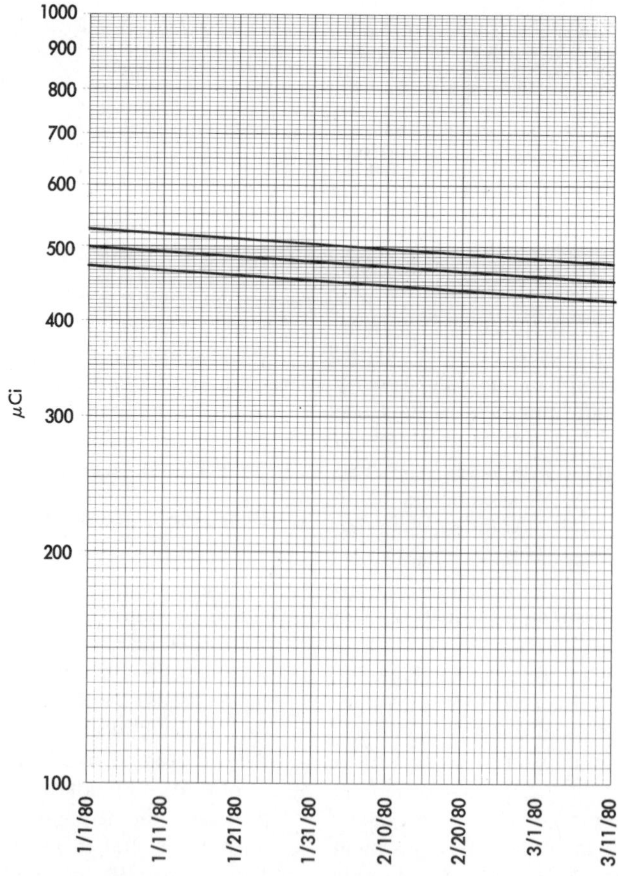

Fig. 3-52. Typical count control chart used for measurement of dose calibrator precision.

tained when the initial elution from a new generator is used and assayed at once. The vial is then assayed at frequent intervals over the next 72 hours. The observed activity versus time is plotted on semilog paper and a best-fit straight line is drawn through the points. A point is picked on the line where the accuracy of the measurement has been established by a reference standard and a straight line constructed with a slope equivalent to the half-life of ^{99m}Tc (6 hours). Compare this straight line to the line generated by the data from the observed counts. Any difference is attributable to nonlinearity of the calibrator if the ^{99m}Tc solution is not contaminated with other radionuclides.

Geometric calibration[3]

Geometric calibration is performed at installation and whenever a change is made in the type of vial or syringe used in radiopharmaceutical processing.

Changing the radionuclide sample volume or configuration can significantly affect the measurement of the sample's activity. To measure the effect of changing the volume of liquid within a vial, a 30 ml vial containing 1 mCi of ^{99m}Tc in a volume of 1 ml is used. This is assayed, and the volume is increased with water in steps of 2, 4, 8, 10, 15, 20, and 25 ml with assays being taken at each step. The net activity at each volume is determined by subtraction of the background. One of the volumes should be selected as the standard and the correction factor for each of the volumes is calculated after the ratios of the net measured activity to the standard activity are obtained.

$$\text{Correction factor} = \frac{\text{Standard-volume activity}}{\text{Volume activity}}$$

These correction factors should be plotted against the volume on linear graph paper. One can then calculate the true activity of a sample by taking the correction factor determined for that volume times the measured activity of the sample.

This procedure should be used to determine the correction factors for various types and sizes of syringes, since significant changes in the assay can occur when the radionuclide is assayed in different material or the wall thickness of the container changes.

It is important to note that the sensitivity of a dose calibrator is affected by backscattering of photons by the shielding of the unit or other adjacent objects. An erroneous activity reading may be obtained if these variables are changed after calibration of the instrument.

The dose calibrator is a tool upon which all nuclear medicine departments rely heavily. Assurance that the indicated activity on the dose calibrator is close to the true amount is important for the proper dispensing of radiopharmaceuticals to the patients in our care.

SURVEY METER

The survey meter is an essential part of a good radiation safety program. Two types of survey instruments are used in a clinical nuclear medicine unit. The ionization chamber (Cutie-Pie) is used in areas where high fluxes of radiation must be measured and the Geiger-Müller (G-M) counter, because of its sensitivity, is used for low-level surveys. They both require annual calibration and frequent precision testing with long-lived radionuclide standards. Calibration techniques are the same for both types of instruments.

Annual calibration

The standard used must be traceable within 5% accuracy to the National Bureau of Standards. The following formula expresses the relationship between activity, distance, and radiation intensity:

$$\text{mR/hour} = \frac{n \cdot I_\gamma}{S^2}$$

whereby mR/hour is radiation intensity (milliroentgens/hour), n is number of millicuries, I_γ is mR/hour at 1 foot/mCi, and S is distance in meters from the source.

This formula is used to calculate the radiation intensity at a number of distances from the standard. Readings are then made of the standard with the survey meter at those same distances. Each scale setting is calibrated over its entire range. The calculated points are plotted versus the measured readings (Fig. 3-53).

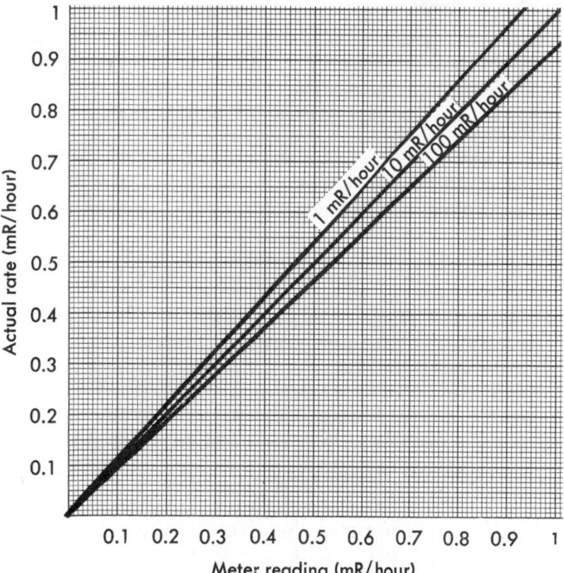

Fig. 3-53. Survey-meter calibration graph. Convert meter reading (abscissa) to actual dose rate by reading upwards to intercept point and then across to ordinate. Multiple ranges may be plotted on the same graph.

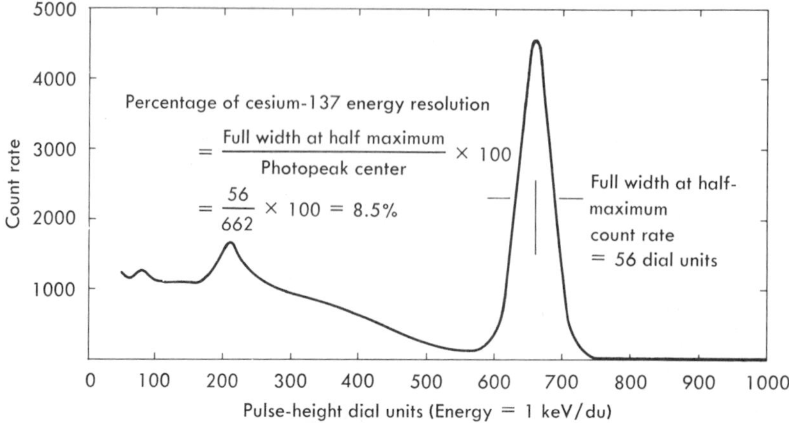

Fig. 3-54. Cesium-137 energy spectrum and energy resolution. *du,* Dial or energy units. (From Rollo, F. D.: Nuclear medicine physics, instrumentation, and agents, St. Louis, 1977, The C. V. Mosby Co.)

The line formed will allow one to determine the true dose rate from the actual reading. The graph should be minified and attached to the survey meter so that the actual dose rate can be easily ascertained while the instrument is being used.

Many departments send their instruments to qualified laboratories for calibration if they do not wish to keep a standardized source on hand.

Precision testing

A reference source with a long half-life is used at frequent intervals to check the consistency of the survey meter's performance. The initial measurement of the source is made at the time of calibration. The source is then counted with the same geometry:

1. Before each survey
2. After a battery change
3. After any maintenance

If the counts are not within 10% of the expected results, the instrument should be recalibrated.

FLAT-FIELD AND WELL TYPE OF SCINTILLATION DETECTORS

Scintillation probes employed for external organ counting and well detectors used for sample counting, like the scintillation camera, are operated on a daily basis. Both of these detection devices are almost always coupled with a gamma-ray spectrometer.

Calibration initially involves plotting an energy spectrum for a long-lived radionuclide, usually cesium 137, first by selection of a narrow window width (for example, 10 keV) and then by obtaining a series of counts at each 10 keV increment of the energy range until the principle photopeak is passed or until the count rate approaches the background level. Plotting the resultant counts on linear graph paper will yield a gamma-ray spectrum as shown in Fig. 3-54.

By measuring the full width at half maximum (FWHM) of the cesium 137 photopeak in kiloelectron volt units and dividing by the photopeak midline energy (in the same units) one may determine the percent energy resolution for that radionuclide:

$$\%\ \text{energy resolution} = \frac{\text{FWHM}}{\text{Photopeak center}} \times 100$$

Typical values for percent energy resolution should be less than 10%.[2] Ordinarily, this procedure is performed by the manufacturer, and the values obtained are furnished with the instrument. It is prudent to repeat the procedure upon installation and annually thereafter.

Daily calibration should include counting a long-lived reference source at specified window and baseline settings while either the fine gain or the voltage is adjusted. This procedure is referred to as "peaking." In other words, a series of counts at various voltage or gain settings are made until the maximum count rate is determined. The voltage or gain setting that yields the maximum or peak counts is recorded in the daily calibration log along with the maximum number of counts obtained. Background counts accumulated for a statistically sufficient time interval are recorded as well.

Any significant change in the daily calibration values should alert the technologist of a possible malfunction of the instrument. Additionally, one may perform a chi-square test of the counts from the long-lived reference source on a monthly interval to determine if the measurements fit the assumed distribution.

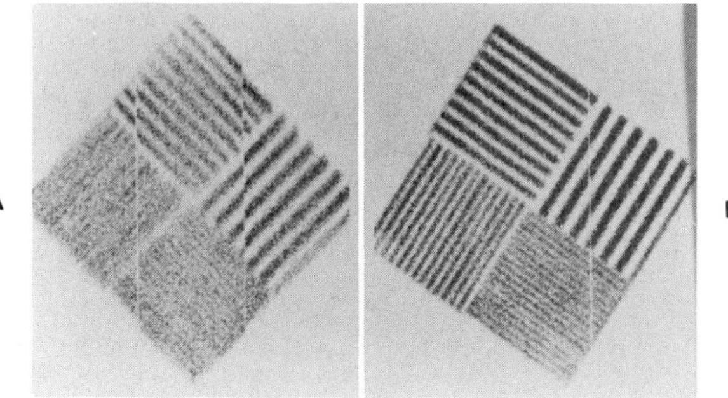

Fig. 3-55. Whole-body scan of four-quadrant bar phantoms before, **A,** and after, **B,** calibration of scintiscan electronics. (From Wells, L. D., and Bernier, D. R.: Nuclear imaging artifacts, Chicago, 1980, Year Book Medical Publishers, Inc.)

WHOLE BODY–IMAGING DEVICES

Whole body–imaging systems, whether stationary or moving detector type, can be performance tested quite easily.

A bar or hole phantom is placed on the scanning table at a 45-degree angle to the direction of scan movement. A planar flood source is placed over the phantom and a "whole body" transmission image is made (Fig. 3-55). Without disturbing either the flood source or phantom, a static image of equal count density is taken and the two images are compared. The comparison should reveal no difference in resolution or linearity. If the device is of the multiple-pass type, bar alignment at the "zipper" can be evaluated.

Quality assurance testing of whole body–imaging devices should be performed weekly.

CONCLUSION

The quality of nuclear medicine health care is directly dependent on the reliable and accurate performance of the instrumentation used for data collection and radionuclide assays. It is the professional responsibility of each certified nuclear medicine technologist (CNMT) to be able to assure the nuclear medicine physician interpreting clinical data that the data are as accurate as possible.

REFERENCES

1. Accreditation manual for hospitals, Chicago, 1970 (updated 1973), Joint Commission on Accreditation of Hospitals, pp. 113-118.
2. Johnson, R. F., Jr.: Operation and quality control of the rectilinear scanner, Chapter 9. In Rollo, F. D., editor: Nuclear medicine physics, instrumentation, and agents, St. Louis, 1977, The C. V. Mosby Co.
3. Nuclear regulatory medical guide 10.8, Guide for the preparation of applications for medical programs, Appendix D, Section 2, pp. 23-29, Washington, D.C., 1979, U.S. Nuclear Regulatory Commission.
4. Rollo, F. D., editor: Nuclear medicine physics, instrumentation, and agents, St. Louis, 1977, The C. V. Mosby Co., pp. 322-360.

Chapter 4

LABORATORY SCIENCE

Robert L. Dressler and Jay A. Spicer

In the beginning, man was created, being a fusion of two components, one spiritual and the other chemical. As has been, and is now, the well-being of each component is vital to life. Although our spiritual involvement with patients is of utmost importance, one must possess a knowledge of the chemical component of life for the successful practice of nuclear medicine.

The following discussion of the chemical principles, fundamental to an understanding of life and the diagnostic processes used in the hope of maintaining a healthy life, is not to be considered as the complete or necessary knowledge required. Because of limitations of space, the following discussion of chemistry is brief and often inadequate. Our hope and intention is that the individual instructors using this text will recognize the points that require further elucidation and will use their knowledge and talents to do so.

GLASSWARE AND INSTRUMENTATION

Glassware

The functional part of any scientific laboratory is the equipment, the most basic of which is the glassware. Fig. 4-1 shows those items most commonly used in routine laboratory manipulations.

Beakers, flasks, and graduated cylinders. The most frequently used type of glassware is the beaker. Beakers range in capacity from a few milliliters to several liters and are utilized in the preparation of solutions and as weighing vessels when a high degree of accuracy is not required.

Erlenmeyer flasks are also used in these procedures and, because of their conic shape and small mouth, offer the advantage that solutions can be prepared by swirling of the contents of the flask with little risk of spilling. This feature also makes the Erlenmeyer flask an ideal vessel for the substrate in titrations. Neither the beaker nor the flask provides the accuracy (±5% to 10%) required for precise volume measurement.

Volume measurements requiring an accuracy of ±1% to 2% can be achieved by the use of the appropriate graduated cylinder (Fig. 4-1). However, many laboratory procedures require the preparation of solutions accurate in concentration to ±0.001%. This precision can be attained by use of a volumetric flask. Flasks marked TC are calibrated to contain (that is, TC) a specific volume, depending on the size of the flask, and allow volume measurements within the accuracy limits noted above.

Pipets and burets. In the normal course of laboratory work many occasions arise where a precise volume of a solution or solvent is required and an appropriate-sized volumetric flask is not available. In such cases a small (<5 ml) or nonintegral volume is usually required, and one must resort to the use of a pipet or buret.

Pipets (Fig. 4-1) are transfer vessels that are used to measure and deliver a precise volume of solution or pure liquid. They are generally of two types: those that must be filled and drained manually, and automatic pipets, which measure and deliver a fixed volume when activated.

The ordinary pipets, which require manipulation, are of two styles: one is calibrated to deliver a fixed volume, whereas the other type is graduated and may be used to deliver any increment of volume up to the full capacity of the pipet. Both styles are available in sizes ranging from microvolumes (a fraction of a milliliter) to those having a capacity of several hundred milliliters.

Care must be exercised in the use of pipets, as some are calibrated to deliver the stated volume by normal drainage (some solution remains in the tip of the pipet), and others are calibrated to deliver the entire volume drawn into the pipet and thus require "blowing out" of the last traces of the solution. The "blow-out" pipets are identified by one or two bands placed near the top of the pipet.

Automatic pipets are especially important to the radioimmunoassay laboratory where accurately known volumes of radioactive solutions are required.

Procedures, such as titrations (p. 150), in which an accurately measured but unknown volume of solution

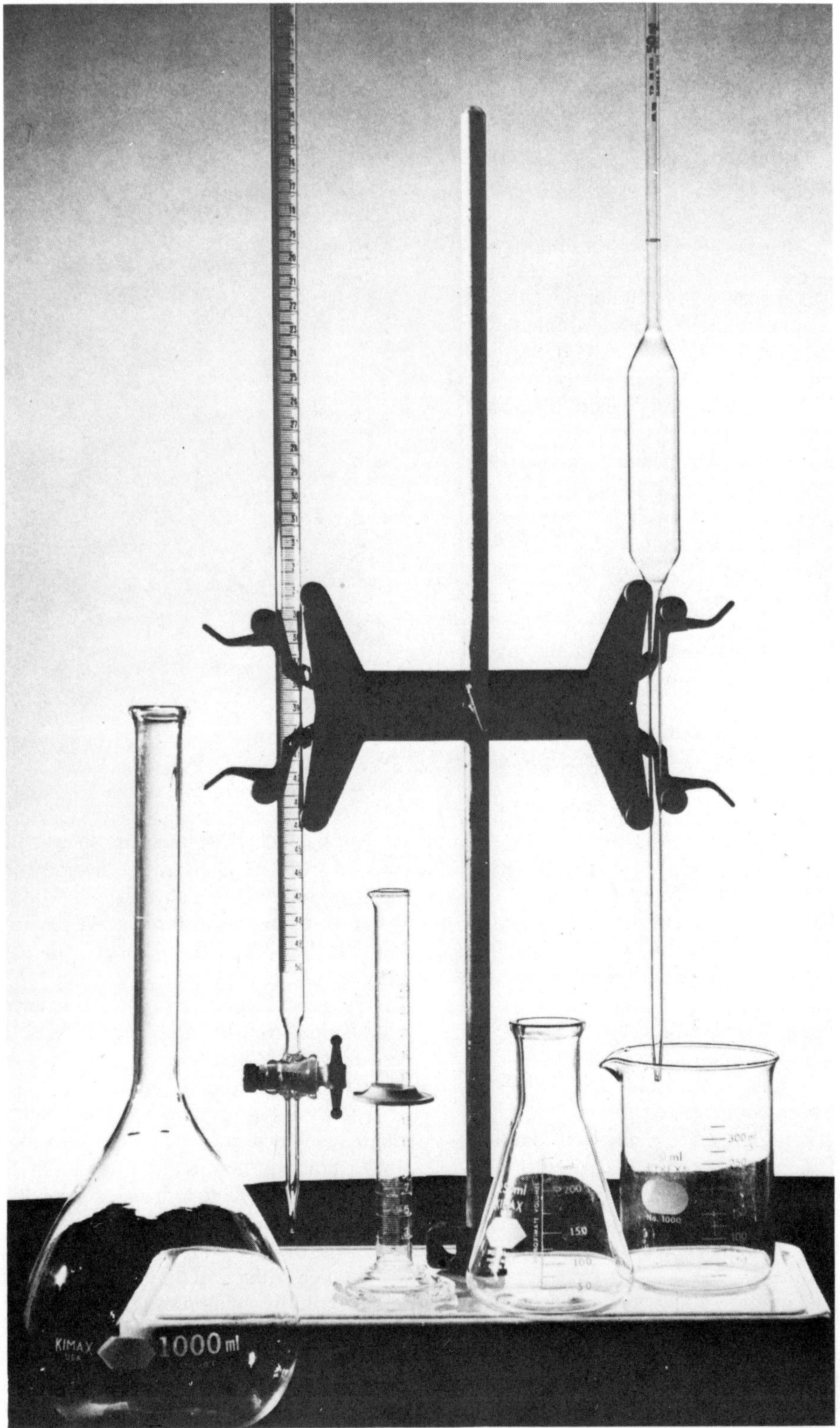

Fig. 4-1. Glassware. *Left to right,* Volumetric flask, buret, graduated cylinder, Erlenmeyer flask, pipet, and beaker.

must be determined, are conveniently performed by use of a buret. The buret, being graduated, allows a direct reading of the volume used in reaching the end point, the point at which the added titrant has reacted with the entire quantity of substrate present in the sample.

Instrumentation

Just as certain types of glassware are important to the laboratory, so also are several instruments. All radiopharmacy or radioassay laboratories must be equipped with a minimum of three instruments: an analytical balance, a centrifuge, and a pH meter.

The analytical balance. The analytical balance (Fig. 4-2) is vital to any laboratory where mass measurements of solids are routinely required, usually in small quantities (<1 g). The balance shown in Fig. 4-2 allows mass measurements accurate to ±0.1 mg. The zero adjust (upper right corner) has both coarse and fine controls for bringing the balance to zero mass. The large outer dial (coarse) is used for rapid approximate zeroing, and the small inner dial (fine) is then used for the precise zero adjustment. In using the balance one should use the following procedure:

1. Turn the pan-release control (bottom center) to the left (full pan release).
2. Adjust the zero controls until all units read zero.
3. Turn the pan release to off (↑) and place the weighing container on the pan.
4. Turn the pan release to the right (partial pan release).
5. Turn the lower left control to *T* (tare).
6. Dial in the weight of the container.
7. As the balance approaches equilibrium (the mobile weight scale in the window starts to move), turn the pan-release lever to the left (full pan release).
8. Turn the lower left control to *I*.
9. Readjust the zero controls until all units again read zero. At this point, the weight of the container has been compensated for.
10. Turn the pan-release lever to the right (partial).
11. Dial in the approximate weight desired; for example, if 3.5 g is required, set the weight dial at 3 g.
12. Add material to the container until the movable scale is activated.
13. Increase the weight setting to the final value.
14. Turn the pan-release lever to the left (full release), and continue adding material until the desired weight is reached.
15. Turn the pan-release lever to the off position and remove the container from the balance pan.
16. Return all weight settings to zero, including the tare weight.

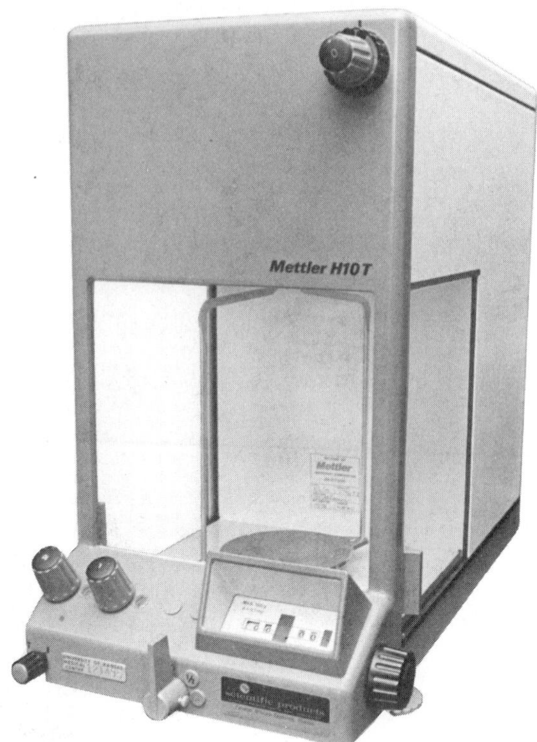

Fig. 4-2. Analytical balance.

The balance is designed so that as the units on the weight dials are changed the instrument automatically adds or removes weights from a knife-edge counterbalance inside the instrument. If the foregoing procedure is followed, the balance will give dependable results with a minimum of service.

The centrifuge. Quite often it is necessary to separate solids from liquids, such as red blood cells from the plasma. When such separations are necessary, a centrifuge is used (Fig. 4-3).

The centrifuge is composed of a balanced motor and shaft on which cups or holders are mounted. A container holding the mixture to be separated is placed in one cup and a counterbalance container (having the same weight as the sample container) is placed in the cup opposite the sample.

The centrifuge exerts a strong centrifugal force on the sample by spinning the material at relatively high speeds (500 to 1500 rpm) and, as in the case of blood, the heavier red blood cells settle to the bottom of the container, leaving the lighter plasma on top. One can then draw off the plasma, thus effecting a separation of the two components.

The use of the pH meter and its description is discussed in a later section devoted to pH.

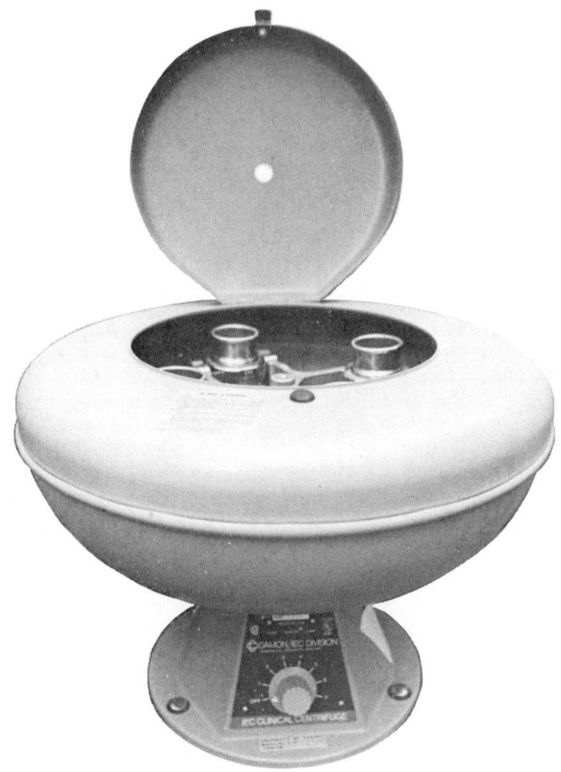

Fig. 4-3. Centrifuge.

ELEMENTS AND COMPOUNDS

In introducing the study of chemistry, as it applies to nuclear medicine and radiopharmacy, as well as any other discipline, it is desirable to define the word "chemistry." Chemistry can best be defined as the study of matter and the changes that matter undergoes.

All matter exists in one of three physical states—solid, liquid, or gas. Each substance differs in physical and chemical properties from all other substances.

Physical properties are the attributes characteristic of a substance, such as odor, color, hardness, luster, density, and structure. These properties depend on the conditions imposed upon the substance and may be affected by a change in temperature, pressure, or radiation. However, a substance, be it an element or a compound, that has undergone a change in physical properties because of a change in conditions, will exhibit the initial properties when the substance is returned to the original condition. For example, sulfur, which is a yellow solid at room temperature, becomes a liquid when heated to 113° C and returns to the yellow solid when allowed to cool. Physical changes are readily reversible.

In contrast to a change in physical properties, chemical change results in a complex and deep-seated change. Chemical change always results in the formation of one or more "new" substances, each of which has chemical and physical properties unique to itself.

Most chemical changes are reversible only with great difficulty, and many, for example, the burning of wood or paper, are irreversible.

Electronic structure

Since each element has unique chemical and physical properties, it is logical to ask why this is so. To answer this question, one must probe the very nature of the elements: their constitution and behavior.

Experimental evidence has shown that all elements are made up of minute particles called atoms and that an atom is the smallest unit of an element that can exist and still maintain the properties of the element. All atoms of a given element are identical in chemical properties, and the atoms of each element differ in properties from the atoms of all other elements. To understand why this is so requires a knowledge of the structure of atoms and the components necessary to their formation.

Structurally, all atoms can be described as a sphere composed of two parts. One part is a small compact nucleus located at the center of the sphere; the second part, a region of space surrounding the nucleus, is populated by small particles called electrons.

The nucleus is composed, mainly, of two types of particles, protons (p^+) and neutrons (n^0). Protons are small particles, each of which has a charge of +1, whereas neutrons, also small particles, have no charge and are therefore neutral. Since it is known that like charges repel, one must wonder what forces hold the protons together in the nucleus. This question cannot be adequately explained in this discussion; suffice it to say that there are other particles within the nucleus that overcome these repulsive forces and act as a "nuclear glue."

The mass of an atom is, for all practical purposes, contained in the nucleus and is equal to the sum of the masses of the protons and neutrons. Each proton and neutron has arbitrarily been given a value of one atomic mass unit (1 a.m.u.), which has been found by experiment to be equal to 1.67×10^{-24} g. By definition, the number of protons in the nucleus of an atom is the same as the atomic number of the element. Since the mass of the neutron is known to be essentially the same as that of the proton, all the mass of the atom is attributed to the protons and neutrons, and the sum of the two is equal to the atomic mass of the atom, expressed in atomic mass units (a.m.u.). Thus, the atomic mass minus the atomic number equals the number of neutrons present in the nucleus.

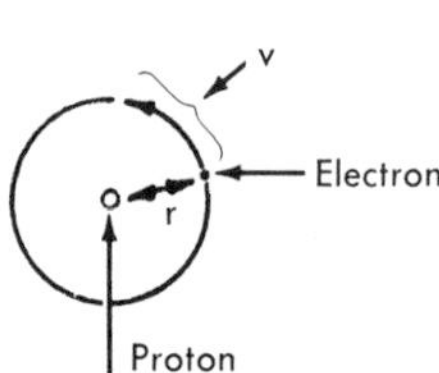

Fig. 4-4. Bohr's model of the hydrogen atom. **v,** Velocity of electron. **r,** Average radius of orbit of electron about nucleus.

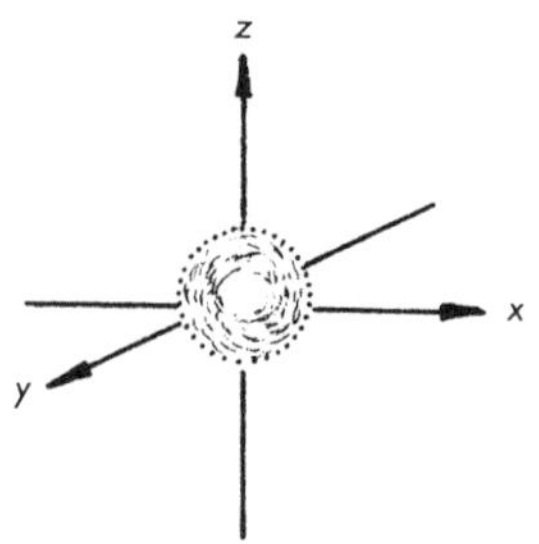

Fig. 4-5. Atomic s orbitals.

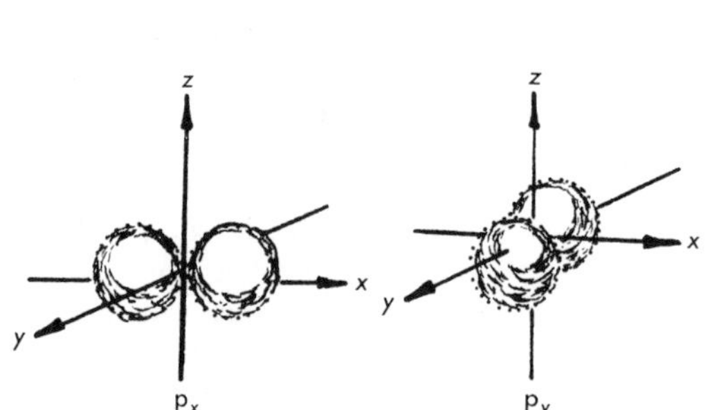

Fig. 4-6. Atomic p orbitals.

The net charge on an atom of an element is zero; that is, it is neutral. Therefore, since we know that protons have a positive charge (+1), there must be one negative charge present for each proton in the nucleus. These negatively charged particles are called electrons (e^-), each of which has a net charge of −1. For most purposes, the mass of the electron is considered to be zero, since, when compared to the mass of the proton and neutron, its mass is negligible (5.5×10^{-4} a.m.u.). The number of electrons present in an atom, being equal to the number of protons, also signifies that the number of electrons is equal to the atomic number.

As noted earlier, electrons are found in the space surrounding the nucleus. However, they are not found at fixed points but are circulating about the nucleus and occupy specific regions with respect to the nucleus and with respect to other electrons (Fig. 4-4). The relative distance of an electron from the nucleus, and the shape and the orientation of the region it occupies, with respect to other regions, has been determined by a combination of spectroscopic evidence and a mathematical treatment known as "quantum mechanics," both of which are discussed in Chapter 2. However, the results of these treatments are useful in that they allow a description of each electron of an atom in terms of its general position, its relative energy, and the shape of the region that it will occupy. Each electron can be described by a set of four quantum numbers (note that lower-cased letters refer to single particles, whereas capital letters would refer to systems):

1. The principle quantum number is designated by the letter n, which can have a positive integral value, with the exception of zero, that is, 1, 2, 3, and so on. This quantum number indicates the relative distance from the nucleus at which the electron is found, and also its relative energy. These are major energy levels and are often called "shells."
2. The secondary quantum number is designated by ℓ. The values of ℓ have a range of positive, integral numbers from zero to $n - 1$; that is, if $n = 3$, then $\ell = 0$, 1, and 2. This quantum number describes the geometric shape of the subenergy level in which the electron is found. These subenergy levels are found within a major energy level and are usually referred to as "orbitals."
3. The magnetic quantum number is designated by m. The numerical value of m can vary from negative ℓ to positive ℓ, that is, if $\ell = 1$, then $m = -1, 0, +1$. This quantum number defines the orientation of the orbital in space; that is, an s orbital being spherically symmetric (Fig. 4-5) has no discernible orientation. However, orientations of the three p orbitals are mutually perpendicular along the x, y, and z axes (Fig. 4-6).

Table 4-1. Relationship of quantum numbers

Shell *(n)*	**1**	**2**				**3**								
Subshell (ℓ)	**0**	**0**	**1**			**0**	**1**			**2**				
m value	0	0	−1	0	+1	0	−1	0	+1	−2	−1	0	+1	+2
s value	±½	±½	±½	±½	±½	±½	±½	±½	±½	±½	±½	±½	±½	±½
Number of electron*	↑↓	↑↓	↑↓	↑↓	↑↓	↑↓	↑↓	↑↓	↑↓	↑↓	↑↓	↑↓	↑↓	↑↓

*↑ denotes e^- with +½ spin; ↓ denotes e^- with −½ spin.

4. The spin quantum number is designated *s*. This quantum number can have only one of two numberical values, +½ or −½. This is so because only two electrons may occupy the same orbital (the Pauli exclusion principle) and must have opposite spins. Electrons, being negatively charged, are mutually repulsive. However, evidence has shown that electrons are not simply charged particles moving in space, but are also spinning about an axis while undergoing translational motion. The spin of the electron gives rise to a magnetic field, and the fields arising (as north and south poles of a magnet are attracting) consequently reduce the degree of repulsion from like charges. This permits two electrons having common *n*, *ℓ*, and *m* quantum numbers to occupy the same orbital.

The quantum numbers used to identify an electron do not describe the energy of the electron quantitatively. However, the larger the *n* and *ℓ* values for the electron, the further the electron will be from the nucleus, and consequently these electrons will have a greater energy than those electrons of lower *n* and *ℓ* values. Also, the number of orbitals of equivalent energy contained within a major energy level is given by $m = -\ell$ to $+\ell$. For example, the second major energy level, $n = 2$, contains two types of subenergy levels. When $\ell = 0$, $m = 0$, indicating that only one orbital of this type is present, which is termed an "s orbital." However, when $\ell = 1$ and $m = -1$, 0, and +1, indicating that there are three orbitals of this type, each of equivalent energy, they are called "p orbitals." Thus the second energy level is composed of a total of four subenergy levels or orbitals. For higher values of *n*, in addition to s and p orbitals, there are also d and f orbitals.

From the foregoing discussion it follows that no two electrons can have the same set of quantum numbers; this is known as the *Pauli exclusion principle* (Table 4-1).

An examination of Table 4-1 indicates that the total number of electrons that a given shell *(n)* can accommodate is equal to $2n^2$.

At this point it is necessary to describe the order in which the major and subenergy levels will be filled by electrons. An electron will always enter the lowest energy level available, and obviously the greater the attraction between an electron and the nucleus, the lower the energy of the electron will be. Thus the first electron will enter the 1s orbital of the first energy level, and the second electron, differing in quantum number from the first electron only in the sign of the spin quantum number, will also enter the 1s orbital; these electrons will be paired. Recalling that a given shell can accommodate $2n^2$ electrons, in this case $n = 1$ and $2n^2 = 2$, we find that the first energy level is filled.

The next electron must now enter the second energy level, $n = 2$, and will occupy the 2s orbital, the same will be true for the next electron. The 2s orbital now containing two electrons, whose spins are paired, is filled, and the next electron must enter one of the three 2p orbitals. One might expect the next electron to enter the same p orbital to give paired electrons; however, spectroscopic evidence indicates that this electron enters one of the two remaining empty p orbitals and has the same spin number as the first p electron. This behavior is summarized by Hund's rule, which states that for an atom where orbitals of equal energies are being filled, the electrons will remain unpaired until each orbital is half filled, that is, one electron in each of the orbitals.

To facilitate the assignment of electrons to the lowest energy orbital available, the sequence indicated below is helpful:

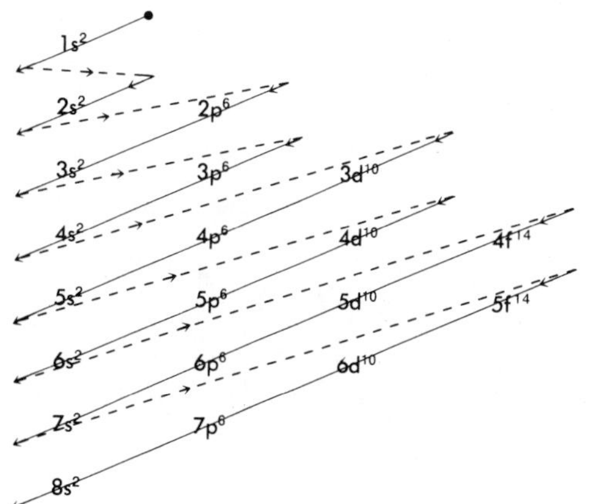

TRANSITION ELEMENTS

Group IA	IIA	IIIB	IVB	VB	VIB	VIIB	VIIIB	VIIIB	VIIIB	IB	IIB	IIIA	IVA	VA	VIA	VIIA	0
1 H 1.00797																	2 He 4.0026
3 Li 6.939	4 Be 9.0122											5 B 10.811	6 C 12.01115	7 N 14.0067	8 O 15.9994	9 F 18.9984	10 Ne 20.183
11 Na 22.9898	12 Mg 24.312											13 Al 26.9815	14 Si 28.086	15 P 30.9738	16 S 32.064	17 Cl 35.453	18 Ar 39.948
19 K 39.102	20 Ca 40.08	21 Sc 44.956	22 Ti 47.90	23 V 50.942	24 Cr 51.996	25 Mn 54.9380	26 Fe 55.847	27 Co 58.9332	28 Ni 58.71	29 Cu 63.54	30 Zn 65.37	31 Ga 69.72	32 Ge 72.59	33 As 74.9216	34 Se 78.96	35 Br 79.909	36 Kr 83.80
37 Rb 85.47	38 Sr 87.62	39 Y 88.905	40 Zr 91.22	41 Nb 92.906	42 Mo 95.94	43 Tc (99)	44 Ru 101.07	45 Rh 102.905	46 Pd 106.4	47 Ag 107.870	48 Cd 112.40	49 In 114.82	50 Sn 118.69	51 Sb 121.75	52 Te 127.60	53 I 126.9044	54 Xe 131.30
55 Cs 132.905	56 Ba 137.34	57 La* 138.91	72 Hf 178.49	73 Ta 180.948	74 W 183.85	75 Re 186.2	76 Os 190.2	77 Ir 192.2	78 Pt 195.09	79 Au 196.967	80 Hg 200.59	81 Tl 204.37	82 Pb 207.19	83 Bi 208.980	84 Po (210)	85 At (210)	86 Rn (222)
87 Fr (223)	88 Ra (226)	89 Ac** (227)	104 Rf (261)	105 Ha (260)													

*Lanthanum series

58 Ce 140.12	59 Pr 140.907	60 Nd 144.24	61 Pm (145)	62 Sm 150.35	63 Eu 151.96	64 Gd 157.25	65 Tb 158.924	66 Dy 162.50	67 Ho 164.930	68 Er 167.26	69 Tm 168.934	70 Yb 173.04	71 Lu 174.97

**Actinium series

90 Th 232.038	91 Pa (231)	92 U 238.03	93 Np (237)	94 Pu (242)	95 Am (243)	96 Cm (247)	97 Bk (247)	98 Cf (251)	99 Es (254)	100 Fm (253)	101 Md (256)	102 No (254)	103 Lw (257)

Metals
Nonmetals
Rare gases

Fig. 4-7. Periodic table of elements. (Courtesy Sheehan, D. C., and Hrapchak, B. B.: Theory and practice of histotechnology, St. Louis, 1980, The C. V. Mosby Co.)

The arrows and broken lines indicate the proper order of filling. The symbols and their significance are as follows:

EXAMPLE: Given the term $4p^3$ indicate the n, ℓ, m, and s values.

1. $n = 4$, the fourth energy level.
2. Since p electrons are involved, $\ell = 1$.
3. With ℓ being 1, $m = -1, 0, +1$ (the three p orbitals), each of which can accommodate 2 electrons for a total of 6.
4. The superscript 3 denotes the presence of 3 electrons in the p orbitals. Following Hund's rule, each orbital (p_x, p_y, p_z) will each contain 1 electron, all of which will have parallel spins ($s = +\frac{1}{2}$).

Had the electrons cited in the above example been the electrons of highest energy in a neutral atom, the element to which they belong would be known. These being the highest energy electrons would indicate that all orbitals of lower energy had been filled. Thus, by counting the number of electrons (using the diagram above) and recalling that the number of electrons is equal to the atomic number of the element, we find that the element corresponding to the atom has an atomic mass of 33. The periodic chart (Fig. 4-7) shows element number 33 to be arsenic (As).

Periodic chart of the elements

Early in the nineteenth century chemists had noted a relationship between atomic weight and properties of the elements. Even though many of the elements had not yet been discovered, chemists were able to recognize those elements having similar properties and group them into families. Later in the century, about 1870, several chemists had segregated the known elements into groups (families) and had shown that properties were a function of atomic number rather than atomic weight and that the properties of a given element, both physical and chemical, were similar to those elements having an atomic number differing by 8, 18, 32, and so on. For example, lithium (atomic number 3), sodium (atomic number 11), potassium (atomic number 19), and rubidium (atomic number 37) exhibited similar physical properties in being shiny, ductile, malleable, and good conductors of electrical current. Chemically these elements are similar in that they form compounds with other elements in the same proportions. Thus *one* atom of Li or Na reacts with *one* atom of fluorine, forming lithium fluoride (LiF) or sodium fluoride (NaF), but *two* atoms of Li or Na react with *one* atom of oxygen to form lithium oxide (Li_2O) or sodium oxide (Na_2O). Other families such as fluorine, chlorine, bromine, iodine, and astatine, or oxygen, sulfur, selenium, tellurium, and polonium are groups of elements exhibiting similar chemical and physical properties.

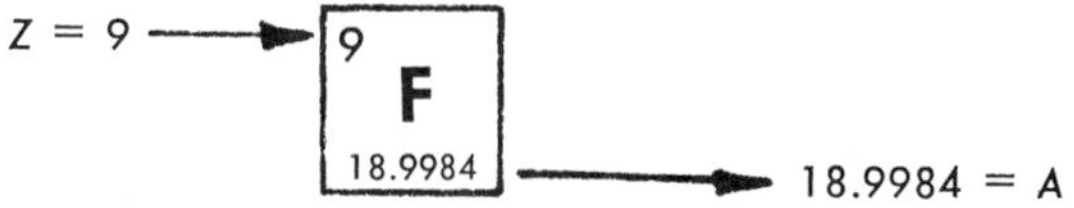

Fig. 4-8. Periodic-chart representation of fluorine.

The periodic chart contains the elements known at this time (Fig. 4-7). Elements of similar properties, as discussed above, are grouped together in columns (placed vertically) to form a family having the same electron configuration in the outermost shell; for example, Li, Na, and so on, each contain *one* electron in the outer shell, whereas F, Cl, and so on, each contain *seven* electrons in the outer shell. However, the elements in a row (placed horizontally) differ from each other in chemical and most physical properties. From a consideration of the electron configuration of the elements as discussed earlier it is apparent that the elements in a given row differ in electron configuration from all other elements contained in that row. Thus sodium (Na), having one electron in the 3s atomic orbital, differs from the element of next higher atomic number, magnesium (Mg), which has two electrons in the 3s atomic orbital, and so on.

The information contained in the periodic chart is not restricted to electron configuration of the outer shell but also indicates the complete electronic structure and the relative atomic mass of each element. Each element is identified by its chemical symbol, as shown in Fig. 4-7. The number above the chemical symbol is the atomic number (Z number) of the element and the number below the symbol is the average atomic mass (A number) of the element. For example, the element fluorine (Fig. 4-8) has an atomic number, or Z number, of 9, which indicates the number of protons and electrons present in the atom. The number 18.9984 shown below the symbol indicates the average atomic mass, or A number, of the element. Recalling that the atomic mass number minus the atomic number gives the number of neutrons present in the nucleus and that the mass of the neutron and proton are essentially identical, one would expect the atomic mass of an element to be an integer. Obviously, the value for fluorine or any other element is not integral and indicates that all atoms of an element are not identical. The nonintegral atomic mass arises from the fact that all atoms of a given element do not contain the same number of neutrons. If some atoms contain a greater or lesser number of neutrons in the nucleus than do other atoms, the average atomic mass of a collection of such atoms will not be integral. Atoms that differ only in the number of neutrons present in the nucleus are called "isotopes."

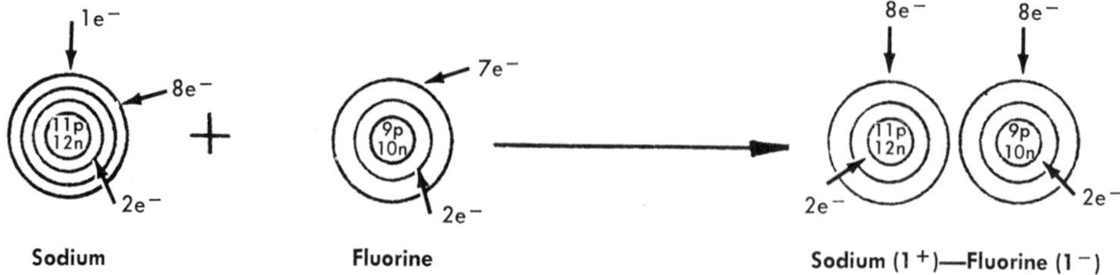

Fig. 4-9. Reaction of sodium atom and fluorine atom to produce ionic compound.

Stable electron configurations—the noble gases

Chemists of the nineteenth century had also noted that certain elements were unreactive and would not combine with other elements to give compounds. It is now known that these elements are all members of the eighth group shown in the periodic chart and constitute a family of elements. These elements all exist in the gaseous state under normal conditions and, being inert, are commonly referred to as the "noble gases." Referring to the periodic chart (Fig. 4-7), note that each of the noble gases contain eight electrons in the outer shell, indicating that for these elements the s and p orbitals within the outer shell are completely filled.

Elements other than the noble gases combine with other elements and do so in such a way that the resulting electron configuration of the elements undergoing reaction is changed to an electron configuration of the noble gases. *This gives a stable electron configuration to each element, one that all elements strive to attain.* For this to be true, the reacting elements must either donate electrons to, or accept electrons from, another element. For example, sodium, having an electron configuration of $1s^22s^22p^63s^1$, differs in electron configuration from the noble gas neon (Ne) (in which the second energy level is completely filled, $1s^22s^22p^6$) by one electron; that is, sodium contains one more electron, $3s^1$. Therefore, for sodium to attain an electron configuration identical with neon it must donate (transfer) the 3s electron to another element.

Assuming that sodium is undergoing a reaction with fluorine (F), $1s^22s^22p^5$, we note that the electron configuration of fluorine differs from that of the noble gas neon by one electron. However, fluorine needs to acquire one electron to attain noble-gas configuration, *whereas sodium had only to donate one electron to achieve the same electron structure.* We may now write an equation for the reaction of one atom of sodium with one atom of fluorine (Fig. 4-9).

Upon comparing the electron structures of sodium (1+), fluorine, (1−) and neon (neutral) we see that they are identical; that is, *each* has an electron structure of $1s^22s^22p^6$. Note, at this point, that only electrons were involved in this reaction and that the sodium atom in transferring an electron to the fluorine atom acquires a net charge of 1+ and the fluorine atom in accepting the electron from sodium acquires a net charge of 1− (compare the number of protons in the nucleus to the total number of electrons present for sodium and fluorine in the products).

Although the foregoing was a rather simple example, an understanding of the chemistry of most elements can be explained in the same manner. *Most elements undergo reaction by donating or accepting electrons so as to attain the electron configuration of a noble gas.* The transition metals are an exception to this rule.

Ionic compounds

The reaction of sodium with fluorine, discussed in the preceding section, involved a complete transfer of electrons and resulted in the formation of charged particles called "ions." In those reactions involving a complete transfer of electrons, the ion resulting from the element donating electrons is called a "cation," in this case a sodium ion (Na^{1+}), and the element accepting electrons is called an "anion" (fluoride ion, F^{1-}). The elements occupying the left-hand part of the periodic chart are known as metals and tend to undergo chemical reaction by donating electrons. Conversely, the nonmetals, occupying the right-hand part of the periodic chart, tend to undergo chemical reaction by accepting electrons. Each metallic element differs from the other metals in its ability to donate electrons, and the nonmetallic elements differ from each other in their ability to accept electrons. The ability of an element to accept electrons is known as its *electronegativity,* with the element having the greatest ability to accept electrons (fluorine) arbitrarily being assigned a value of 4. This is the Pauling scale; others exist and are in common use. The ability of all other elements to accept electrons is compared numerically to fluorine. These values are shown in Table 4-2.

Thus, in the foregoing reaction between sodium and fluorine, the fluorine atom (electronegativity 4.0) readily acquires an electron from sodium (electronegativ-

Table 4-2. Electronegativity values of selected elements

						H 2.1
Li 1.0	Be 1.5	B 2	C 2.5	N 3.0	O 3.5	F 4.0
Na 0.9	Mg 1.2	Al 1.5	Si 1.8	P 2.1	S 2.5	Cl 3.0
K 0.8	Ca 1.0	Sc 1.3	Ge 1.8	As 2.0	Se 2.4	Br 2.8
Rb 0.8	Sr 1.0	Y 1.2	Sn 1.8	Sb 1.9	Te 2.1	I 2.5

ity 0.9), resulting in ions, both of which are isoelectronic with neon. Elements that tend to react by transfer of electrons must differ in electronegativity by approximately 2.5 electronegativity units.

At this point we must note that the sodium and fluorine ion produced in this reaction, though having an electron configuration identical with that of neon, differ from the noble gas in that sodium still contains 11 protons in its nucleus and fluorine retains its nine protons. The sodium ion produced now possesses one more proton in its nucleus than it has electrons in the energy levels surrounding it; therefore sodium in this state must have a net charge of 1+. Similarly, fluorine now containing one additional electron must have a net charge of 1−. Since opposite charges attract each other, it should not be surprising that the resulting ions approach each other and are held together by these electrostatic attractions to form an ionic compound. *All elements that undergo reactions to form ions result in the formation of ionic compounds.*

Covalent compounds

Elements whose electronegativities differ by less than 2.5 also undergo reaction in order to attain electron configurations identical with one of the noble gases. However, in this case neither element is sufficiently electronegative to completely acquire the electrons of the second element, the result being that they react in a manner so as to share the electrons in their valence shell (valence electrons are those in the outermost shell). For example, in the reaction of carbon (electronegativity 2.5) with chlorine (electronegativity 3.0), the compound formed *has no charge*. Letting circles (○) and crosses (x) indicate the electrons involved in the reaction, and understanding that the electrons of lower energy (in shells closer to the nucleus) are still present, we can represent the reaction as follows:

$$\overset{\circ}{\underset{\circ}{\circ C \circ}} + 4\,\overset{xx}{\underset{xx}{{}^{x}Cl\,{}^{x}_{x}}} \rightarrow \begin{matrix} & \overset{xx}{{}^{x}_{x}Cl^{x}_{x}} & \\ \overset{xx}{\underset{xx}{{}^{x}_{x}Cl^{x}_{\circ}}} & C & \overset{xx}{\underset{xx}{{}^{x}_{\circ}Cl^{x}_{x}}} \\ & \underset{xx}{{}^{x}_{x}Cl^{x}_{x}} & \end{matrix}$$

Even though the chlorine and the carbon atoms have not reacted by electron transfer, each of the atoms has attained the electron configuration of a noble gas by sharing their valence electrons. Unlike sodium fluoride (NaF), the compound carbon tetrachloride (CCl_4), formed in this reaction, is a molecule in which the four chlorine atoms and the carbon atom are bonded to each other and function as one unit. The product CCl_4 is called a "molecule." The bond, in this case, rather than being ionic as that of NaF, is "covalent." *All compounds that are formed by the sharing of electrons rather than the transfer of electrons are said to have covalent bonds.*

Even though these bonds are described as being covalent, it is apparent that the electronegativities of the two elements (Table 4-2) are not the same; therefore the electrons used in forming the bonds between the carbon atom and the four chlorine atoms cannot be shared equally. This leads to the conclusion that the electron pair in each of these bonds is more strongly attracted to chlorine than to carbon. Covalent bonds formed from two different elements of unequal electronegativity must be *polar covalent,* meaning that the electrons forming the bond are more strongly attracted to one atom than to the other.

Those elements of essentially the same electronegativity react to form bonds that are completely covalent; that is, the electrons of the bond are shared equally between the two atoms. For example oxygen, which composes 20% of the earth's atmosphere, exists as the molecule O_2. It is apparent that the electronegativity of each oxygen atom in the molecule is the same; therefore the electrons that bond these atoms cannot be attracted more strongly by one atom than by the other. This results in an equal sharing of electrons, *and the bond is completely covalent.* Other examples of nonpolar covalent bonds are nitrogen (N_2, which is 80% of the earth's atmosphere), hydrogen (H_2), and the halogens (F_2, Cl_2, Br_2, I_2). As we shall find in a subsequent discussion, the carbon-hydrogen bond in organic molecules is essentially nonpolar covalent because both carbon and hydrogen have electronegativity values of approximately 2.5.

Coordinate covalent bonds

Those compounds containing coordinate covalent bonds are similar to those compounds containing covalent bonds in that the bonding electrons are shared by two atoms. However, the electrons used in forming these bonds are donated by *one atom only*. As an example, let us consider the reaction in which a molecule of sulfuric acid is formed from the following elements:

$$2\,H\square + {}^{\circ}_{\circ}S{}^{\circ}_{\circ} + 4\,{}^{xx}_{x}O^{x}_{xx} \longrightarrow H{}^{x}_{\square}O{}^{\circ}_{x}S{}^{\circ}_{x}O{}^{x}_{\square}H \text{ (with } {}^{x}_{x}O^{x}_{x} \text{ above and below S)}$$

$$\text{or}\quad H—O—\underset{\underset{O}{\downarrow}}{\overset{\overset{O}{\uparrow}}{S}}—O—H$$

The symbol "—" represents a covalent bond, and "↑" represents a coordinate covalent bond in which the arrow points toward the atom that did not contribute any electrons to bond formation.

Considering each bond in the sulfuric acid molecule, and the electrons used in forming each bond, it is apparent that the hydrogen-oxygen bonds and two of the sulfur-oxygen bonds are polar covalent, whereas the remaining two sulfur-oxygen bonds are coordinate covalent bonds, in that the electrons used in forming these bonds were contributed by the sulfur atom only.

Complex ions and chelates

The formation of coordinate covalent bonds need not occur by reaction of neutral elements as shown in the preceding section. There are many reactions in which a coordinate covalent bond is formed by the interaction of a neutral molecule with an ion. In reactions of this type the driving force, or reason for reaction, is that an atom contained within the neutral molecule has not attained the electron configuration of a noble gas. In previous discussions, the metals were assumed to react by transfer of their electrons to form ionic compounds. However, elements such as aluminum (Al) have been found to form compounds in which the bonds are largely polar covalent. This being true, it is apparent that the aluminum atom needs three electrons to attain the noble-gas configuration of argon (Ar). Consequently, aluminum chloride ($AlCl_3$), in a nonpolar solvent, reacts with anhydrous chlorine gas (Cl_2) according to the following equation:

$$\left[{}^{xx}_{xx}Cl{}^{x}_{x}Cl{}^{xx}_{xx}\right]^{-} + Al{}^{\circ}_{\circ}Cl\ (\text{with } Cl \text{ above and below Al}) \rightarrow \left[Cl{}^{x}_{x}Al{}^{\circ}_{\circ}Cl\ (\text{with } Cl \text{ above and below Al})\right]^{-} + {}^{xx}_{xx}Cl^{+}$$

The electrons used in forming the fourth chlorine-aluminum bond are donated by the chloride ion, resulting in the formation of a coordinate covalent bond. The ions that provide the bonding electrons are called "ligands."

A second example of coordinate covalent bond formation is that in which a positive ion undergoes reaction with a neutral molecule, as illustrated in the following reaction:

$$H^{+} + {}^{\circ}_{\circ}N{}^{\circ}_{x}H\ (\text{with } H \text{ above and below N}) \rightarrow \left[H{}^{\circ}_{\circ}N{}^{\circ}_{x}H\ (\text{with } H \text{ above and below N})\right]^{+}$$

The product resulting from reactions of neutral molecules with either a cation or an anion are called "complex ions."

Although elements such as aluminum and nitrogen can share one pair of electrons with simple ions to form complex ions, other elements, especially the transition elements, must accept two or more pairs of electrons to attain a noble-gas electron configuration. These complexes are especially important in nuclear medicine and in many cases involve the formation of chelates in which the electron pairs (two or more pairs) are donated by functional groups present in the ligand molecule. The term "chelate" from the Greek word *chēlē*, 'claw,' is reserved for these ligands. The complex ytterbium–pentetic acid (Yb-DTPA) (Fig. 4-10), used as a cisternographic scanning agent, is an excellent example of a chelate. In this case the electrons used in forming the coordinate covalent bonds are donated by the functional groups present in the pentetic acid molecule (see below).

$$\begin{array}{l} {}^{-}\,{}^{xx}_{x}O—C(=O)—CH_2 \diagdown \qquad\qquad\qquad\qquad\qquad\qquad \diagup CH_2—C(=O)—O^{-} \\ \qquad {}^{\circ}_{\circ}N—CH_2—CH_2—\overset{\circ\circ}{N}—CH_2—CH_2—N{}^{\circ}_{\circ} \\ {}^{-}\,{}^{xx}_{x}O—C(=O)—H_2C \diagup \qquad\qquad |\ CH_2—C(=O)—O^{-} \qquad \diagdown CH_2—C(=O)—O^{-} \end{array}$$

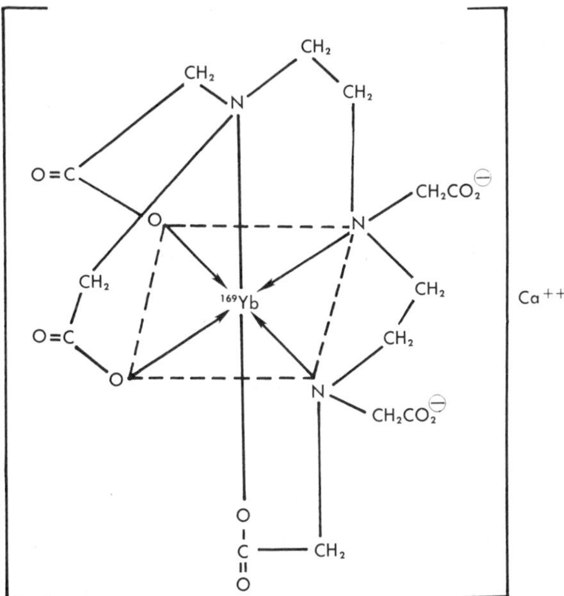

Fig. 4-10. Ytterbium–pentetic acid (Yb-DTPA) complex. *Arrows,* Coordinate covalent bonds; *dotted line,* plane through these atoms.

Although the structure of many complex ions of technetium are still under investigation, it is reasonable to assume that their structures are similar to those formed by ytterbium.

LAWS OF CONSTANT COMPOSITION AND MULTIPLE PROPORTION

The fact that elements generally react with other elements to attain a noble-gas electron configuration leads to the conclusion that any two elements that undergo reaction must do so in a definite ratio of atoms, that is, one Na to one F and one C to four Cl. It then follows that the elements must also react in definite ratios by weight. This is stated by the *law of constant composition:* A compound, regardless of its origin or method of preparation, always contains the same elements in the same proportions by weight.

In some cases, depending on reaction conditions, an element will combine with another to give products that differ in the ratio of atoms of the two elements. For example, sodium usually reacts with oxygen to form sodium oxide (Na_2O), but under other conditions they react to form sodium peroxide (Na_2O_2). However, in each case the ratio of sodium to oxygen is definite. This is stated by the *law of multiple proportions:* when two elements combine to form two or more different compounds, the ratio of the mass of one element that combines with a fixed mass of a second element is a simple ratio of whole numbers, for example, 2:1 or 3:2.

Sample problems

EXAMPLE 1: When subjected to quantitative elemental analysis, two samples of a compound containing only carbon and oxygen give the following data:

	Weight of sample	Weight of C found	Weight of O found
Sample 1:	0.7335 g	0.2002 g	0.5333 g
Sample 2:	0.6162 g	0.1682 g	0.4480 g

Do these data uphold the law of constant composition? If the law is upheld, the percentage of carbon and oxygen must be the same in each sample. To determine this, the ratio of the weight of each element to the total weight of the sample must be equal to the ratio of the percent of the element to 100%.

Sample 1:

$$\text{Percent carbon} = \frac{0.2002}{0.7335} = \frac{\%\ \text{C}}{100\%} \qquad \%\ \text{C} = 27.29$$

$$\text{Percent oxygen} = \frac{0.5333}{0.7335} = \frac{\%\ \text{O}}{100\%} \qquad \%\ \text{O} = 72.71$$

Sample 2:

$$\text{Percent carbon} = \frac{0.1682}{0.6162} = \frac{x\%\ \text{C}}{100\%} \qquad \%\ \text{C} = 27.29$$

$$\text{Percent oxygen} = \frac{0.4480}{0.6162} = \frac{x\%\ \text{O}}{100\%} \qquad \%\ \text{O} = 72.71$$

The percentage of carbon and oxygen being the same for both samples indicates that they are of identical composition and thus support the law of constant composition.

EXAMPLE 2: A third sample, obtained from a different source, was also found to contain only carbon and oxygen and gave the following data upon analysis:

	Weight of sample	Weight of C found	Weight of O found
Sample 3:	0.3599 g	0.1543 g	0.2056 g

Show that these data illustrate the law of multiple proportions. Following the procedure used in example 1:

Sample 3:

$$\text{Percent carbon} = \frac{0.1543}{0.3599} = \frac{\%\ \text{C}}{100\%} \qquad \%\ \text{C} = 42.87$$

$$\text{Percent oxygen} = \frac{0.2056}{0.3599} = \frac{\%\ \text{O}}{100\%} \qquad \%\ \text{O} = 57.13$$

Obviously this composition indicates that sample 3 was obtained from a compound different from that of samples 1 and 2. Though the samples differ in composition, the law of multiple proportions states that the ratios of the masses of the elements in each compound should be related as simple whole numbers. Thus:

$$\text{For sample 1: } \frac{\%\ O}{\%\ C} = \frac{72.71}{27.49} = 2.66$$

$$\text{For sample 3: } \frac{\%\ O}{\%\ C} = \frac{57.13}{42.87} = 1.33$$

Therefore the ratio of oxygen to carbon in sample 1 and sample 3 are related by the ratio of 2.66:1.33 or 2:1.

GRAM ATOMIC WEIGHTS, GRAM MOLECULAR WEIGHTS, AND THE MOLE CONCEPT

The chemistry discussed thus far has been based on the interactions of individual atoms. Although this description is a valid one, the isolation and use of single atoms in the laboratory is neither practical nor possible. The smallest sample that can be accurately measured in the laboratory will contain 10^{15} to 10^{17} atoms or molecules.

In order for a reaction to be accurately described by a chemical equation, it is only necessary that the number of atoms or molecules of the reactants be present in the *ratio* given by the coefficients for these substances. In the following reaction, the ratio of hydrogen (H_2) molecules to oxygen (O_2) molecules must be 2:1.

$$2H_2 + 1O_2 \rightarrow 2H_2O$$

The chemist, being unable to count the number of atoms or molecules necessary for a given reaction, must resort to an indirect method to achieve this ratio. The fact that each element possesses a unique atomic mass (Fig. 4-7) indicates that even though equal weights of hydrogen and oxygen could be measured, the number of molecules of hydrogen present in the sample would be 16 times that of the oxygen molecules; that is, one hydrogen molecule has a weight of 2 relative to a weight of 32 for one oxygen molecule. A convenient method that allows the measurement of the required quantities of the reactants by accurate weighing of each substance is based directly upon their gram atomic weight (g.a.w.) or gram molecular weight (g.m.w.). By definition, these are the weights in grams that are numerically equal to the atomic weights (a.m.u.) or molecular weights (the sum of the atomic weights of all atoms present in the molecule) of the elements or compounds involved. From this definition, it is apparent that 1 g.m.w. of any two substances will contain the same number of atoms or molecules. The number of atoms or molecules in 1 g.a.w. or g.m.w. has been shown by experiment to be 6.02×10^{23}. This number is called *Avogadro's number,* and 1 g.a.w. or g.m.w. of any substance is commonly referred to as 1 *mole*.

These concepts are illustrated in the following examples:

EXAMPLE 1: How many moles (gram atomic weights) of chromium (Cr) are contained in 28 g? From the periodic chart, the atomic weight of chromium is found to be 52 a.m.u.; therefore the weight of Cr contained in 1 mole (g.a.w.) is 52 g.

$$\frac{1\ \text{mole}}{52\ \text{g}} = \frac{x\ \text{mole}}{28\ \text{g}}$$

$$x = \frac{(28\ \text{g})\ (1\ \text{mole})}{52\ \text{g}}$$

$$x = \frac{28}{52}\ \text{mole}$$

$$x = 0.538\ \text{mole}$$

EXAMPLE 2: How many grams are contained in 0.59 moles (gram molecular weights) of sulfuric acid? Sulfuric acid, H_2SO_4, being a molecule, requires that we first determine its molecular weight.

$$\begin{aligned} 2\ \text{H} \times 1\ \text{a.m.u.} &= 2\ \text{a.m.u.} \\ 1\ \text{S} \times 32\ \text{a.m.u.} &= 32\ \text{a.m.u.} \\ 4\ \text{O} \times 16\ \text{a.m.u.} &= 64\ \text{a.m.u.} \\ \hline \text{Molecular weight} &= 98\ \text{a.m.u.} \end{aligned}$$

Therefore 1 mole (g.m.w.) would contain 98 g of sulfuric acid, and

$$\frac{98\ \text{g}}{1\ \text{mole}} = \frac{x\ \text{g}}{0.59\ \text{mole}}$$

$$x = \frac{(98\ \text{g})\ (0.59\ \text{mole})}{1\ \text{mole}}$$

$$x = (98\ \text{g})\ (0.59)$$

$$x = 57.82\ \text{g}$$

EXAMPLE 3: How many molecules are contained in 0.50 mole of nitrogen (N_2)? One mole (g.m.w.) of N_2 (28 g) would contain Avogadro's number of molecules (6.02×10^{23}), therefore:

$$\frac{6.02 \times 10^{23}\ \text{molecules}}{1\ \text{mole}} = \frac{x\ \text{molecules}}{0.50\ \text{mole}}$$

$$x = \frac{(0.50\ \text{mole})\ (6.02 \times 10^{23}\ \text{molecules})}{1\ \text{mole}}$$

$$x = (0.50)\ (6.02 \times 10^{23})\ \text{molecules}$$

$$x = 3.01 \times 10^{23}\ \text{molecules}$$

EXAMPLE 4: How many moles of water (H_2O) are present in a sample containing 5×10^{12} molecules? One mole of H_2O contains 6.02×10^{23} molecules, therefore:

$$\frac{1\ \text{mole}}{6.02 \times 10^{23}\ \text{molecules}} = \frac{x\ \textit{mole}}{5.0 \times 10^{12}\ \text{molecules}}$$

$$x = \frac{(1 \text{ mole})(5.0 \times 10^{12} \text{ molecules})}{6.02 \times 10^{23} \text{ molecules}}$$

$$x = \frac{(5.0 \times 10^{12}) \text{ mole}}{6.02 \times 10^{23}}$$

$$x = 0.83 \times 10^{-11} \text{ mole}$$
$$x = 8.3 \times 10^{-12} \text{ mole}$$

EMPIRICAL AND MOLECULAR FORMULAS

All substances presently known were initially obtained from natural sources or chemical reactions, and in many cases their elemental composition and structures were unknown. The elements present in such compounds must be determined by *qualitative chemical analysis,* and the relative amount of each element by *quantitative chemical analysis.* The information obtained in these analyses is useful in determining the empirical formula of a substance.

The ratio of the elements contained in a substance (the relative number of each kind of atom present) is indicated by the empirical formula. However, the empirical formula may not truly reflect the molecular formula of the substance, which may be a whole number multiple of the empirical formula. For instance, the organic substance, oxalic acid, which is a constituent of some plants, has an empirical formula of CHO_2, but a molecular formula of $C_2H_2O_4$.

EXAMPLE: A compound, upon analysis, was found to have the following composition by weight:

Carbon (C) = 50.7%
Hydrogen (H) = 4.25%
Oxygen (O) = 45.1%

What is the empirical formula of the compound?

Since percentage is based upon 100, it may be assumed that a 100 g sample of the compound would contain:

50.7 g C
4.25 g H
45.1 g O

Also knowing that a definite atomic weight (and gram atomic weight) is a unique property of each element, the relative abundance of each element is obtained by the following:

Carbon: $$\frac{50.7 \text{ g}}{12 \text{ g}} = \frac{x \text{ g.a.w.}}{1 \text{ g.a.w.}}$$

$$x = \frac{50.7 \text{ g}}{12 \text{ g}} (1 \text{ g.a.w.})$$

$$x = 4.23 \text{ g.a.w.}$$

Hydrogen: $$\frac{4.25 \text{ g}}{1 \text{ g}} = \frac{x \text{ g.a.w.}}{1 \text{ g.a.w.}}$$

$$x = \frac{(4.25 \text{ g})(1 \text{ g.a.w.})}{1 \text{ g}}$$

$$x = 4.25 \text{ g.a.w.}$$

Oxygen: $$\frac{45.1 \text{ g}}{16 \text{ g}} = \frac{x \text{ g.a.w.}}{1 \text{ g.a.w.}}$$

$$x = \frac{(45.1 \text{ g})(1 \text{ g.a.w.})}{16 \text{ g}}$$

$$x = \frac{45.1}{16} \text{ g.a.w.}$$

$$x = 2.82 \text{ g.a.w.}$$

However, each element must be present in in integral value of its atomic weight, or gram atomic weight. To obtain integral values for each element, one must divide the above values of the gram atomic weight by the smallest value obtained. Thus:

Oxygen: $$\frac{2.82 \text{ g.a.w.}}{2.82 \text{ g.a.w.}} = 1$$

Carbon: $$\frac{4.23 \text{ g.a.w.}}{2.82 \text{ g.a.w.}} = 1.5$$

Hydrogen: $$\frac{4.25 \text{ g.a.w.}}{2.82 \text{ g.a.w.}} = 1.5$$

These values indicate that the empirical formula of the compound is $C_{1.5}H_{1.5}O_1$. Obviously, these values are not integral and the actual number of atoms present in the molecule must be a multiple of these. Multiplying the value for each element by 2 results in an empirical formula of $C_3H_3O_2$, indicating an integral or whole number value for each element.

Further analysis of the above substance indicated its molecular weight to be 142. What is the molecular formula of the compound?

The molecular weight of the compound is derived from the following empirical formula:

Carbon	(3) (12) = 36
Hydrogen	(3) (1) = 3
Oxygen	(2) (16) = 32
Empirical weight	= 71

Inasmuch as the molecular formula must be a multiple of the empirical formula, that is, $\frac{142}{71} = 2$, the molecular formula is $C_6H_6O_4$.

Empirical or molecular formulas may be characteristic of several different compounds and provide no information pertinent to the structure of the molecule.

SOLUTIONS AND COLLOIDS

Much of the chemistry encountered in nuclear medicine involves solutions. A solution is a homogeneous mixture of two substances, one of which is called the *solute,* which can be a gas, liquid, or solid, and the second substance, generally a liquid, is called the *solvent*. One must choose a solvent that will dissolve the solute and yet not undergo chemical reaction with the solute.

In working with solutions one must know the concentration of solute in a given volume of solution and therefore must be familiar with the methods and units used in defining concentrations.

Molarity

Molarity expresses the number of moles of solute contained in 1 liter of solution.

$$\text{Molarity (M)} = \frac{\text{Number of moles of solute}}{\text{Number of liters of solution}}$$

Sample problems

EXAMPLE 1: What is the molarity of a solution prepared by dissolving 16 g of barium chloride ($BaCl_2$) in sufficient water to give a total volume of 450 ml?

Step 1: How many moles of $BaCl_2$ are in the 16 g sample?

$$1 \text{ mole } (BaCl_2) = 137.5 \text{ g} + 2(35.5 \text{ g})$$
$$1 \text{ mole } (BaCl_2) = 208.5 \text{ g}$$

$$\frac{1 \text{ mole}}{208.5 \text{ g}} = \frac{x \text{ mole}}{16.0 \text{ g}}$$

$$x = \frac{(16.0 \text{ g})(1 \text{ mole})}{208.5 \text{ g}}$$

$$x = \frac{16.0 \text{ mole}}{208.5}$$

$$x = 0.077 \text{ mole}$$

Step 2: Molarity (M) = mole/liter

$$\text{M} = \frac{0.077 \text{ mole}}{0.450 \text{ liters}}$$

$$\text{M} = 0.171 \text{ mole/liter (molar)}$$

EXAMPLE 2: How would 20 liters of 6.0 M sodium hydroxide (NaOH) solution be prepared from solid NaOH?

Step 1: How many grams of NaOH are in 6.0 moles?

$$1 \text{ mole (NaOH)} = 23 \text{ g} + 16 \text{ g} + 1 \text{ g}$$
$$1 \text{ mole (NaOH)} = 40 \text{ g}$$

$$\frac{x \text{ g}}{6.0 \text{ moles}} = \frac{40 \text{ g}}{1 \text{ mole}}$$

$$x = \frac{(40 \text{ g})(6.0 \text{ moles})}{1 \text{ mole}}$$

$$x = (40)(6.0) \text{ g}$$
$$x = 240 \text{ g in } 6.0 \text{ moles of NaOH}$$

Step 2: One liter of 6.0 molar (M) solution requires 240 g of NaOH. Therefore for 20 liters of 6.0 M solution, (20) (240 g) = 4800 g of NaOH dissolved in sufficient water to give a total volume of 20 liters.

EXAMPLE 3: How could the solution prepared in example 2 be used to obtain 1.0 liter of 0.50 M NaOH solution?

Step 1: The 6.0 M NaOH must be diluted with additional water. What volume of the 6.0 M solution contains 0.50 moles of NaOH?

$$\frac{1.0 \text{ liter}}{\underset{\text{(NaOH)}}{6.0 \text{ mole}}} = \frac{x \text{ liter}}{\underset{\text{(NaOH)}}{0.50 \text{ mole}}}$$

$$x = \frac{(1.0 \text{ liter})(0.50 \text{ M})}{(6.0 \text{ M})}$$

$$x = \frac{0.50 \text{ liter}}{6.0}$$

$$x = 0.083 \text{ liter}$$

Step 2: If 0.083 liter of 6.0 M NaOH contains 0.50 moles of NaOH, then to obtain a 0.50 M solution, one must add enough water to bring the volume to exactly 1.0 liter.

Molality

A *molal* solution differs from a *molar* solution in that a molal solution is defined as the number of moles of solute contained in 1 kilogram (kg) of solvent.

$$\text{Molality } (m) = \frac{\text{Number of moles of solute}}{\text{Number of kilograms of solvent}}$$

Whereas 1 liter of a *molar* solution is prepared by the addition of sufficient solvent to the solute to give a total volume of 1 liter, a *molal* solution is prepared when the solute is dissolved in 1 kg (in the case of water, 1 liter) of solvent. The total volume of a 1 molal solution will generally be greater than that of a 1 molar solution.

EXAMPLE: Calculate the molality of a solution prepared by dissolving 20.4 g of sodium chloride (NaCl) in 192 g of H_2O.

Step 1: How many grams are contained in 1 mole of NaCl?

$$1 \text{ mole (NaCl)} = 23 \text{ g} + 35.5 \text{ g}$$
$$1 \text{ mole (NaCl)} = 58.5 \text{ g}$$

Step 2: How many moles are contained in 20.4 g of NaCl?

$$\frac{1 \text{ mole}}{58.5 \text{ g}} = \frac{x \text{ mole}}{20.4 \text{ g}}$$

$$x = \frac{(20.4 \text{ g})(1 \text{ mole})}{58.5 \text{ g}}$$

$$x = \frac{(20.4)}{58.5} \text{mole}$$

$$x = 0.349 \text{ mole}$$

Step 3: From the definition of molality:

$$m = \frac{0.349 \text{ mole}}{0.192 \text{ kg}}$$

$$m = 1.82 \text{ molal solution}$$

It should be noted that most solutions are usually expressed in terms of molarity rather than molality.

Normality

A third method of expressing concentration, and one that is in general more useful than that of molarity or molality, is in terms of normality (N). Normality is defined as the number of equivalents (Eq) of solute per liter of solution. The number of equivalents present in a solution, rather than being defined as the number of moles of solute per liter, is defined as the number of moles of reactant species that is contained in 1 mole of the solute. For example, as we have discussed earlier, in the reaction $H^+ + {}^-OH \rightarrow H_2O$ the reactants must arise from two different substances, one of which provides H^+ and another that provides ^-OH (conventionally OH^-, also ionically $\bar{O}H$). Those compounds that give H^+ ions are called acids, as we shall discuss later. Two of the most common acids are hydrochloric acid (HCl) and sulfuric acid (H_2SO_4). Both of these acids may be considered to be completely ionized in aqueous solution to give the H^+ ion and the corresponding anions. It should be apparent that ionization of 1 mole of HCl will give rise to 1 mole of H^+ ion, whereas the ionization of 1 mole of H_2SO_4 will give rise to 2 moles of H^+ ion. Thus, in comparing HCl with H_2SO_4, we note that 0.5 mole of H_2SO_4 will provide the same number of H^+ ions that would be provided by 1 mole of HCl. Therefore the weight of H_2SO_4 that will provide one equivalent of H^+ ion (1 mole) is one half of its molecular weight: $\frac{98 \text{ g}}{2} = 49$ g whereas the weight of HCl required to produce one equivalent (1 mole) of H^+ is equal to its molecular weight (36.5 g). Similarly, the substances that provide OH^- ion (called bases) will have equivalent weights dictated by the number of moles of OH^- that will be provided by 1 mole of the base. Thus:

$$\text{Normality (N)} = \frac{\text{Number of equivalents}}{\text{Number of liters of solvent}}$$

and

$$\text{Normality (N)} = \frac{\text{(Moles of solute) (``Moles'' of reactant provided)}}{\text{1 liter of solution}} = \frac{\text{Equivalents}}{\text{Liter}} = \frac{\text{Eq}}{\text{Liter}}$$

A second type of reaction to utilize *normal* solutions is that in which an oxidation-reduction is involved. This type is yet to be discussed, and suffice it to say at this point that the equivalent weight of a reagent in an oxidation-reduction reaction is determined by the number of electrons that it accepts or donates.

How are equivalent weights calculated? The equivalent weight, in grams, of an acid is calculated when the gram molecular weight of the acid is divided by the number of potential hydrogen ions contained in the molecule, and for a base the gram molecular weight is divided by the number of hydroxide ions.

Problems

EXAMPLE 1: What is the equivalent weight of HCl?

$$\text{Equivalent weight (normality)} = \frac{\text{g.m.w.}}{\text{Number of } H^+ \text{ ions}}$$

$$\text{Equivalent weight} = \frac{36.5 \text{ g}}{1} = 36.5 \text{ g}$$

EXAMPLE 2: What is the equivalent weight of H_2SO_4?

$$\text{Equivalent weight} = \frac{\text{g.m.w.}}{\text{Number of } H^+ \text{ ions}}$$

$$\text{Equivalent weight} = \frac{98 \text{ g}}{2}$$

$$\text{Equivalent weight} = 49 \text{ g}$$

EXAMPLE 3: What is the equivalent weight of 1 mole of calcium hydroxide, $Ca(OH)_2$?

$$\text{Equivalent weight} = \frac{\text{g.m.w.}}{\text{Number of } OH^- \text{ ions}}$$

$$\text{Equivalent weight} = \frac{74 \text{ g}}{2}$$

$$\text{Equivalent weight} = 37 \text{ g}$$

From the foregoing discussion it is evident that the normality of a solution must be a whole-number multiple of a corresponding molar solution.

Problems

EXAMPLE 1: What is the normality of a 90 ml sample of a solution that contains 10 g of NaOH?

Step 1:

$$\text{1 equivalent weight of NaOH} = \frac{\text{1 g.m.w. of NaOH}}{1\ OH^- \text{ ion}}$$

$$\text{1 equivalent weight} = \frac{40 \text{ g}}{1} = 40 \text{ g of NaOH}$$

Step 2: The number of equivalents of NaOH in solutions:

$$\frac{1 \text{ Eq}}{40 \text{ g}} = \frac{x \text{ Eq}}{10 \text{ g}}$$

$$x = \frac{(1 \text{ Eq})(10 \text{ g})}{40 \text{ g}}$$

$$x = \frac{10}{40} \text{ Eq} = 0.25 \text{ Eq of NaOH}$$

Step 3: Normality equals equivalents/liter, therefore:

$$N = \frac{Eq}{Liter} = \frac{0.25}{0.09}$$

N = 2.78 normal

Note: Since normality equals molarity for NaOH, this solution is both 2.78 N and 2.78 M.

EXAMPLE 2: What is the normality and molarity of 100 ml of an aqueous solution containing 50.0 g of phosphoric acid (H_3PO_4)?

Step 1: How many grams of H_3PO_4 are contained in 1 g.e.w. (gram equivalent weight)?

$$1 \text{ g.e.w.} = \frac{1 \text{ g.m.w.}}{\text{Number of } H^+ \text{ ions}}$$

$$1 \text{ g.e.w.} = \frac{98.0 \text{ g}}{3} = 32.7 \text{ g of } H_3PO_4$$

Step 2: What is the number of equivalents in 50 g of H_3PO_4?

$$Eq = \frac{50.0 \text{ g}}{32.7 \text{ g}}$$

$$Eq = 1.53 \text{ Eq of } H_3PO_4$$

Step 3: Normality, by definition:

$$N = \frac{1.53 \text{ Eq}}{0.100 \text{ liter}}$$

$$N = 15.3 \text{ normal}$$

Step 4: Since H_3PO_4 is triprotic (3 H^+ ions), the molarity of this solution will be:

$$M = \frac{N}{3} = \frac{15.3}{3}$$

$$M = 5.10 \text{ molar } H_3PO_4$$

Colloids

A second type of mixture, one that is of importance in nuclear medicine, is the *colloid*. Unlike true solutions, colloids consist of minute particles that are suspended in a dispersing medium. Colloid particles vary in shape and range in size from 10^{-9} to 10^{-7} meters in diameter. Although several important types of colloids exist, we shall restrict our discussion to the colloid in which a solid is dispersed in a liquid, this colloid being called a *sol*.

Although one might expect the particles to settle out on standing, the dispersed colloid particles remain suspended in the dispersing medium indefinitely. This behavior is attributed to a constant bombardment of the dispersed particles by the molecules of the dispersing medium; thus the colloid particles are in constant motion. This phenomenon is called *brownian movement* and may be observed with the proper type of microscope.

Unlike true solutions, colloids exhibit an optical effect characterized by the scattering of light when a narrow beam of light is passed through the colloid. The scattering of light is attributable to the deflection of light by the colloid particles and is called the *Tyndall effect*.

A third property characteristic of colloids is an electrical charge effect in which charged particles such as ions are bound or adsorbed on the surface of the colloid particle. An important example, probably involving this effect, is the ^{99m}Tc-labeled sulfur-colloid used for liver scanning.

CHEMICAL REACTIONS AND CHEMICAL EQUATIONS

The ability to predict chemical reactions and to correctly write and understand the chemical equations describing the reactions is of utmost theoretical and practical importance. The basis for one type of chemical reaction, the combination reaction, in which two elements react to produce one substance, and the chemical equations describing this reaction are discussed previously in this chapter. In addition to combination reactions, several other types of chemical reactions must be considered, which are as follows:

1. Metathesis or double decomposition
2. Oxidation-reduction
   a. Replacement
   b. Electrochemical

Since all reactions are described by a chemical equation, it is necessary that the terms and symbols used in writing equations be learned. The symbols indicating the physical state of substances involved in a reaction are as follows:

A gas is indicated by "(g)" and may alternatively be indicated by the symbol "(↑)," for example, O_2(g) or O_2(↑).

A liquid is designated by "(l)," for example, H_2O (l).

A solid is indicated by "(s)" or, if there is a product precipitating from solution, by the symbol "(↓)," for example, $BaSO_4$(↓).

The symbol "→" separates the reactants from the products of the reaction.

A correct chemical equation also requires that the equation be balanced; that is, the number of atoms of each element appearing as reactants must be found in equal number in the products. The steps as one proceeds in completing and balancing an equation are as follows:

1. Determine the correct formulas for those compounds obtained as products from a knowledge of the valence or oxidation numbers of the elements or the charge on ions involved in the reaction. The valence or oxidation number of monatomic ions is equal to the net charge of the cation or anion. The charge of many complex ions is not readily discernible and should be committed to

Table 4-3. Common ions, their symbols and charge

Ion	Chemical symbol	Charge
Hydroxide	OH^-	1−
Nitrate	NO_3^-	1−
Nitrite	NO_2^-	1−
Phosphate	PO_4^{3-}	3−
Carbonate	CO_3^{2-}	2−
Bicarbonate	HCO_3^-	1−
Sulfite	SO_3^{2-}	2−
Sulfate	SO_4^{2-}	2−
Bisulfate	HSO_4^-	1−
Ammonium	NH_4^+	1+
Stannous or tin (II)	Sn^{2+}	2+
Stannic or tin (IV)	Sn^{4+}	4+
Ferrous or iron (II)	Fe^{2+} (FeO)	2+
Ferric or iron (III)	Fe^{3+} (Fe_2O_3)	3+
Cuprous or copper (I)	Cu^+ (Cu_2O)	1+
Cupric or copper (II)	Cu^{2+} (CuO)	2+
Permanganate	MnO_4^-	1−
Manganese (IV)	Mn^{4+} (MnO_2)	4+
Manganese (II)	Mn^{2+} (MnO)	2+
Pertechnetate	TcO_4^-	1−
Technetium (IV)	Tc^{4+} (TcO_2)	4+
Chromate	CrO_4^{2-}	2−
Chromium (III)	Cr^{3+}	3+
Mercurous	Hg^+	1+
Mercuric	Hg^{2+}	2+
Cyanide	CN^-	1−
Thiocyanate	SCN^-	1−

memory. Once determined, the formula of a compound cannot be changed in subsequent balancing operations. (See Table 4-3.)

2. Balance those ions of elements other than hydrogen, oxygen, or polyatomic ions.
3. *Then* balance the hydrogen and oxygen atoms.
4. The correct coefficients for reactants and products must be the smallest whole numbers possible, for example:

$$2H_2 + O_2 \rightarrow 2H_2O$$

not

$$4H_2 + 2O_2 \rightarrow 4H_2O$$

5. Finally, the sum of the charges of the reactants must equal the sum of the charges of products.

The balanced equation specifies the ratio or quantity of reactants required and the ratio or quantity of products produced. This is called the *stoichiometry* ('element-equality') of the reaction. The following example illustrates the foregoing steps and the stoichiometry of a reaction:

Complete and balance the following equation:

$$Fe(OH)_3 + H_2SO_4 \rightarrow$$

Step 1: From Table 4-3, the hydroxide ion has a charge of 1−. Therefore the iron present in $Fe(OH)_3$ must have a charge of 3+. Similarly, for H_2SO_4 each hydrogen has a charge of 1+ and so the sulfate anion must have a charge of 2−. Products formed in this reaction must involve an interchange of cations and anions by the two reactants. Therefore ferric ion combines with sulfate ion and hydrogen ion combines with hydroxide ion. *All products formed must be neutral, that is, have no charge.* Iron having a 3+ charge and sulfate having a 2− charge dictates that the correct formula for this product must be $Fe_2(SO_4)_3$. The remaining product is H_2O, and the equation showing both reactants and products is as follows:

$$Fe(OH)_3 + H_2SO_4 \rightarrow Fe_2(SO_4)_3 + H_2O \text{ (unbalanced)}$$

Step 2: Since each reactant and product contains hydrogen or oxygen or both, those compounds containing iron may be used in starting the balancing procedure.
Reactant: 1 Fe^{3+}
Product: 2 Fe^{3+}
Therefore:

$$2\ Fe(OH)_3 + H_2SO_4 \rightarrow Fe_2(SO_4)_3 + H_2O \text{ (unbalanced)}$$

It is now convenient to balance the polyatomic sulfate ion.
Reactant: 1 SO_4^{2-}
Product: 3 SO_4^{2-}
Therefore:

$$2\ Fe(OH)_3 + 3\ H_2SO_4 \rightarrow Fe_2(SO_4)_3 + H_2O \text{ (unbalanced)}$$

Step 3: Complete the balancing of elements, considering hydrogen and oxygen.
Reactants: 12 H^+
Product: 2 H^+
Therefore:

$$2\ Fe(OH)_3 + 3\ H_2SO_4 \rightarrow Fe_2(SO_4)_3 + 6\ H_2O \text{ (balanced)}$$

Check the oxygen, other than those contained in sulfate ions.
Reactant: 6 O^{2-}
Product: 6 O^{2-}

Step 4: The coefficients of reactants and products cannot be reduced to smaller whole numbers; therefore they are correct as written in step 3.

Step 5: Since all compounds, reactants, and products are electrically neutral, the sum of the charges of the reactants equals that of the products and the equation, complete and balanced, is that shown in step 3.

The stoichiometry of the balanced equation states that 2 molecules or moles of $Fe(OH)_3$ react with 3 molecules or moles of H_2SO_4 to yield 1 molecule or mole of $Fe_2(SO_4)_3$ and 6 molecules or moles of H_2O.

All balanced equations give the information shown in the foregoing example. The value of the chemical equation lies in the fact that it is the basis for calculating the amount of product produced from a given quantity of reactants and, conversely, allows calculation of the quantities of reactants required to produce a desired quantity of products.

Metathesis reactions

The term "metathesis" means mutual exchange and is often referred to as double decomposition. When two compounds undergo metathesis, both compounds are decomposed and two new compounds are formed. The positive ions of each compound react with the negative ions of the other compound, as shown in the following equation:

$$A^+B^- + C^+D^- \rightarrow A^+D^- + C^+B^-$$

These reactions generally involve ionic compounds as reactants and nearly always give ionic products, one of which is usually a solid.

EXAMPLES: Predict the products obtained in the following reactions and balance the equations:

1. $CdSO_4 + KOH \rightarrow$
2. $Pb(NO_3)_2 + H_2S \rightarrow$

(See Table 4-3 for ionic charges.)
Double decomposition would give:

1. $CdSO_4 + KOH \rightarrow Cd(OH)_2\downarrow + K_2SO_4$ (unbalanced)
2. $Pb(NO_3)_2 + H_2S \rightarrow PbS\downarrow + HNO_3$ (unbalanced)

Balance equation 1:
Reactant: 1 Cd^{2+}
Product: 1 Cd^{2+}; therefore the reactant KOH must be multiplied by 2 to balance K^+ ions.

$$CdSO_4 + 2KOH \rightarrow Cd(OH)_2\downarrow + K_2SO_4$$

Inspection of this equation shows that both SO_4^{2-} and OH^- ions occur in equal numbers in both the reactants and the products, and the equation as shown is balanced.

Balance equation 2:
Reactant: 1 Pb^{2+}
Product: 1 Pb^{2+}; therefore Pb^{2+} ions are balanced. Then:
Reactant: 1 S^{2-}
Product: 1 S^{2-}; therefore S^{2-} ions are balanced. Then:
Reactant: 2 NO_3^{1-}
Product: 1 NO_3^{1-}; therefore the product HNO_3 must be multiplied by 2 to balance NO_3^{1-} ions.

$$Pb(NO_3)_2 + H_2S \rightarrow PbS\downarrow + 2HNO_3$$

Inspection shows that the H^+ ions occur in equal numbers in both the reactants and products, and the equation as shown is balanced.

Oxidation-reduction reactions

Oxidation-reduction reactions, commonly called *redox* reactions, are those reactions in which certain atoms gain or lose electrons and thus undergo a change of oxidation number. The oxidation number of a monatomic ion is its charge. For example, the oxidation number of F^- ion is -1 (or it can be expressed $1-$). If the oxidation number changed during a reaction ($2F^- \rightarrow F_2 + 2e^-$), an oxidation or reduction has occurred (F^-, oxidation number -1, has undergone oxidation to give neutral F_2). The process of oxidation always involves the loss of electrons, and consequently the oxidation number of the element involved changes in a positive direction. For example, the ion Fe^{2+} readily undergoes oxidation by loss of an electron to give Fe^{3+}. For each reactant undergoing oxidation there must be a second reactant that undergoes reduction. The reactant undergoing reduction must gain one or more electrons, and thus its oxidation number changes in a negative direction. For example, if the foregoing reaction, in which Fe^{2+} was oxidized to Fe^{3+}, is reversed so that $Fe^{3+} + 1e^- = Fe^{2+}$, then a reduction has occurred. Changes in oxidation number generally occur within the limits of ±5 as indicated below.

Oxidation →

$-5\ -4\ -3\ -2\ -1\ 0\ +1\ +2\ +3\ +4\ +5$

← Reduction

Confusing as it may seem, an oxidizing agent is a reactant that, by acquiring electrons from a second reactant, causes an increase in oxidation number of the second reactant. Conversely, a reducing agent is the reactant that donates electrons and brings about a reduction of the oxidation number of the other reactant (the oxidizing agent). This change is illustrated in the equation at the top of the opposite page.

In all redox reactions the total number of electrons lost by the reducing agent must equal the total number of electrons gained by the oxidizing agent.

The oxidation states of substances involved in redox reactions are undergoing change, many equations cannot be balanced by simple inspection. However, the total ionic charge of the reactants must be equal to that of the products, and the number of atoms of each element in the reactants must equal the number of atoms of the same elements in the products. In balancing

Oxidation number = 0		Oxidation number = 0		Oxidation number = +2 (or ++)		Oxidation number = −2 (or =)
Ca	+	S	→	Ca^{++}	+	$S^{=}$
Reducing agent		**Oxidizing agent**		**Oxidized**		**Reduced**

redox equations, one must observe several definitions and rules.

Rules for balancing redox equations

1. The oxidation state of all elements is zero; that is, the number of electrons and protons are equal and the charge is zero.
2. The oxidation state of a monatomic ion is equal to the charge of that ion. Some elements maintain the same oxidation number in the majority of compounds in which they are found, as shown in Table 4-4.
3. The sum of all oxidation numbers of the atoms of a compound must equal zero.

Those elements generally exhibiting only one oxidation state are shown in Table 4-4.

For example, chlorine in the compound $HClO_3$ (chloric acid) has an oxidation number of +5. In determining the oxidation number of chlorine from the formula one must make use of Table 4-4, which states that oxygen "always" has an oxidation number of −2 and that hydrogen, in most compounds, has an oxidation number of +1. Since there are three oxygens in the $HClO_3$ molecule, the sum of the oxidation numbers for oxygen are required to be 3(−2), or −6, and hydrogen has an oxidation number of +1. Since rule 3 states that the sum of all oxidation numbers for each compound must equal zero, and the sum of the oxidation numbers of hydrogen and oxygen (+1 + [−6]) equals −5, the oxidation number of chlorine must be +5. Note that the oxidation number of the atoms involved in a compound are determined by their electronegativity and the electronegativity of the elements to which they are bonded.

Having established the rules for balancing redox equations, let us consider the use of these rules in the following examples. The most convenient method of balancing charge is by use of half-reactions. Half-reactions involve only the ions undergoing a change in oxidation number during reaction.

EXAMPLE 1: Balance the equation:

$$HNO_3 + H_2S \rightarrow NO + S + H_2O \text{ (unbalanced)}$$

By inspection of the equation, determine the oxidation state of each atom on both sides of the equation to determine which atoms have undergone a change of oxidation number.

Consider each compound separately:

$$\overset{+1}{H}\ \overset{+5}{N}\ \overset{3(-2)}{O_3} + \overset{2(+1)}{H_2}\ \overset{-2}{S} \rightarrow$$

$$\overset{+2}{N}\ \overset{-2}{O} + \overset{0}{S} + \overset{2(+1)}{H_2}\ \overset{-2}{O} \text{ (unbalanced)}$$

In arriving at these oxidation numbers the use of the foregoing rules and Table 4-4 tell us that hydrogen "always" has an oxidation number of +1 and oxygen −2. The sum of the oxidation numbers of hydrogen atoms in HNO_3 is +1 and, since there are three oxygen atoms in this substance, the sum for oxygen atoms is 3(−2) = −6. Rule 3 states that the sum of the oxidation numbers for the HNO_3 molecule must be zero; therefore nitrogen must have an oxidation number of +5; that is, the equation (hydrogen +1, plus oxygen −6 equals −5) requires that the oxidation number of nitrogen be +5.

$$H(+1)\ \ N(+5)\ \ O_3(-6)\ \ \text{or}\ \ (+1) + (+5) + (-6) = 0$$

The equation states that the product containing nitrogen is NO and, using the procedure just described, we

Table 4-4. Elements generally exhibiting one oxidation state

Element	Common oxidation numbers	Rare oxidation number
Hydrogen	+1 (H^+)	−1 (H^-)
Alkali metals (Na, K, and so on)	+1 (Na^+)	
Alkaline earth metals (Mg, Ca, and so on)	+2 (Mg^{++})	
Oxygen	−2 ($O^{=}$)	−1 (O^-), +2 (O^{++})
Fluorine	−1 (F^-)	
Chlorine, bromine, and iodine	−1 (Cl^-)	Cl: +1, +3, +5, +7 Br: +1, +3, +5 I: +1, +5, +7

find that nitrogen in the product has an oxidation number of +2.

$$\overset{+2}{N}\ \overset{-2}{O} \quad \text{or} \quad (+2) + (-2) = 0$$

Therefore the half-reaction in which nitrogen is involved is as follows:

$$N^{5+} + 3e^- \rightarrow N^{2+}$$

Similarly, it is found that sulfur occurs as a reactant in H_2S, having an oxidation number of −2.

$$\overset{2(+1)}{H_2}\ \overset{-2}{S} \quad \text{or} \quad (+2) + (-2) = 0$$

Sulfur occurs in the product in the elemental form, and by rule 1 it must have an oxidation number of zero. The half-reaction involving sulfur is:

$$S^{2-} - 2e^- \rightarrow S^0$$

Inspection of the equation shows that the oxidation numbers of hydrogen and oxygen remain the same in both the reactants and products; that is, they do not change.

Considering the half-reactions and recalling that the number of electrons acquired by the oxidizing agent must equal the number of electrons donated by the reducing agent, we may readily note that the half-reaction involving nitrogen must be multiplied by 2 and the half-reaction involving sulfur be multiplied by 3. The six electrons donated by sulfur must equal the six electrons accepted by nitrogen.

$$2(N^{5+} + 3e^- \rightarrow N^{2+})$$
$$3(S^{2-} - 2e^- \rightarrow S^0)$$

Applying the coefficients of the half-reactions, the full equation in which nitrogen and sulfur are balanced must be written as:

$$2HNO_3 + 3H_2S \rightarrow 2NO + 3S + H_2O \text{ (unbalanced)}$$

The atoms of the remaining elements must now be balanced, and balancing may be done by inspection.

Nitrogens are balanced.
Sulfurs are balanced.
Reactant: 8 H's
Product: 2 H's

Multiplying H_2O (the product) by 4 balances H's and gives the equation:

$$2HNO_3 + 3H_2S \rightarrow 2NO + 3S + 4H_2O$$

Inspection shows that the oxygens are also balanced and the equation has been balanced by a simple inspection process. Let us consider a second example of a redox reaction.

EXAMPLE 2:

$$K_2Cr_2O_7 + HCl \rightarrow KCl + CrCl_3 + H_2O + Cl_2 \text{ (unbalanced)}$$

Following the process outlined in the preceding example, we find that the elements undergoing oxidation and reduction are as follows:

$$2(Cr^{6+} + 3e^- \rightarrow Cr^{3+}) \text{ reduction (oxidizing agent)}$$
$$3(Cl^- - 2e^- \rightarrow Cl_2^0) \text{ oxidation (reducing agent)}$$

Note that all the Cl^- ion in the reaction does not undergo oxidation, as some is used in forming the products KCl and $CrCl_3$ in which the oxidation number of −1 is retained.

Multiplying, to balance changes in oxidation number, gives:

$$K_2Cr_2O_7 + 6HCl \rightarrow KCl + 2CrCl_3 + H_2O + 3Cl_2 \text{ (unbalanced)}$$

Balancing the remaining elements gives:

$$K_2Cr_2O_7 + 14\ HCl \rightarrow 2KCl + 2CrCl_3 + 7H_2O + 3Cl_2 \text{ (balanced)}$$

Electrolytic reactions

A special type of oxidation-reduction is that involving use of an electric current supplied by an external source and makes use of an electrolytic cell (Fig. 4-11).

The anode is highly electron deficient and may be thought of as being positive in charge, while the cathode is rich in electrons and therefore has a large negative charge. This being the case, positive ions (cations) in solution or in the liquid state migrate to the cathode and are reduced by a transfer of electrons from the cathode to the cation. Conversely, the anions, being negatively charged, migrate to the anode and in transferring electrons to the anode undergo oxidation. These processes are summarized as follows:

Cathode: $A^+ + 1e^- \rightarrow A^0$ (reduction)
Anode: $B^- - 1e^- \rightarrow B^0$ (oxidation)

Electrolysis is utilized primarily in the industrial production of certain elements such as elemental sodium and chlorine. A second important process involving electrolysis is that of electroplating, in which elemental chromium, nickel, or silver is deposited or plated on the surface of other metals as a protective or decorative coating.

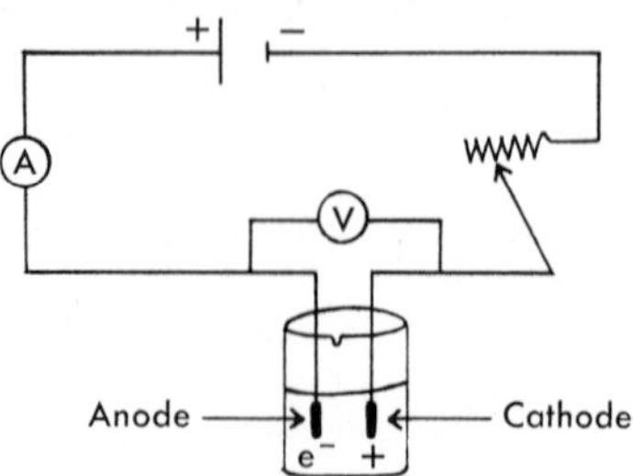

Fig. 4-11. Oxidation-reduction involving use of electric current. *A*, Amperage; *V*, voltage.

An important application of electrolytic reduction in the area of nuclear medicine is involved in the process of labeling human serum albumin (HSA) with technetium (Tc^{4+}); thus, at the cathode:

$$^{99m}Tc^{7+} + 3e^- \rightarrow {}^{99m}Tc^{4+} \text{ (reduction)}$$
$$^{99m}Tc^{4+} + HSA \rightarrow {}^{99m}Tc\text{-}HSA$$

ACIDS AND BASES

An understanding of the chemistry and theory of acids and bases is vital to the practice of nuclear medicine, since the acidity of the body fluids must remain essentially constant. All compounds and, more importantly, solutions of the compounds are acidic, basic, or neutral. The properties of acids and bases are given below.

Acids	Bases
1. Taste sour	1. Taste bitter
2. Cause certain organic dyes, called indicators, to change color; for example, blue litmus paper in the presence of an acid changes to red.	2. Cause certain organic dyes, called indicators, to change color; for example, red litmus paper in the presence of a base changes to blue.
3. Release CO_2 from carbonate salts.	3. Feel slick (slimy).
4. Common acidic materials: vinegar, citrus juices, soda (seltzer and all carbonated beverages).	4. Common bases: aqueous ammonia solution, soap, and lye (NaOH).

Concepts of acids and bases

Acids and bases have been defined in the historic evolution of chemistry by the Arrhenius (1884), Brönsted-Lowry (1923), and Lewis (1923) concepts. Each of these concepts remains useful in the current understanding of acid-base chemistry.

Arrhenius defined an acid as a substance that yields hydrogen ion (H^+) or hydronium ion (H_3^+O) when dissolved in water, and bases as those substances that yield hydroxide ions (OH^-) when dissolved in water.

The Brönsted-Lowry concept provides a more general definition of acids and bases. It defines an acid as a substance that can provide (or donate) a proton (H^+) to a second substance, which, by definition is a base. For example, acetic acid can donate a proton directly to a base such as ammonia:

$$\underset{\textbf{Acid}}{CH_3COOH} + \underset{\textbf{Base}}{NH_3} \rightarrow \underset{\textbf{Acetate ion}}{CH_3COO^-} + \underset{\textbf{Ammonium ion}}{NH_4^+}$$

Brönsted-Lowry acids and bases are not restricted to aqueous solutions, as are Arrhenius's acids and bases; therefore this concept is valid for any solvent system. Thus the following reaction can occur:

$$\underset{\textbf{Acid}}{H_2SO_4} + \underset{\textbf{Base}}{NaCl} \rightarrow \underset{\textbf{Acid}}{HCl} + \underset{\textbf{Base}}{HSO_4^-}$$

Sulfuric acid is used as both a reactant and a solvent.

Lewis, in 1923, proposed a still more general definition of acids and bases. The Lewis concept defines an acid as any compound that can *accept* an *electron pair* and a base as any compound that can *donate* an *electron pair*. Acid-base reactions of this type often involve the formation of a coordinate covalent bond and are illustrated by the reaction of boron trifluoride with ammonia:

```
   F       H            F   H
   |       |            |   |
F—B  +  :N—H  ——→  F—B⁻—N⁺—H
   |       |            |   |
   F       H            F   H
 Acid    Base
```

Boron trifluoride, having an empty orbital, can accept the 2 nonbonding electrons of the nitrogen in ammonia (recall that the second energy level can accommodate 8 electrons).

Neutralization reactions

The majority of reactions that have been discussed previously cannot be classified as neutralization reactions. The process of neutralization involves the reaction of acids with bases as defined by the Arrhenius concept, H^+ or H_3^+O and OH^-. The products of neutralization are invariably a salt and water. If equal quantities, as defined by normality of an acid and base, are mixed, the resulting solution is neither acidic nor basic. The discipline of medicine makes use of acids and bases, not only in clinical diagnostic procedures, but also as agents in treating certain injuries and disorders. Antacids, containing aluminum and magnesium hydroxides, are commonly used to neutralize excess stomach acid (HCl). Sodium bicarbonate (a base) finds use as a neutralizing agent in the treatment of acid burns, and picric acid is often used to accelerate the rate of mitosis.

A general equation describing the neutralization process may be written as:

$$HA + BOH \rightarrow AB + H_2O$$
$$\text{Acid} + \text{Base} \rightarrow \text{A salt} + \text{Water}$$

The driving force for all neutralization reactions is the formation of the stable water molecule, and equations for these reactions can be balanced by simple inspection.

$$H_2SO_4 + NaOH \rightarrow Na_2SO_4 + H_2O \text{ (unbalanced)}$$

By inspection:

1. SO_4^{2-} ions are balanced
2. *Reactant:* 1 Na^+
   Product: 2 Na^+
3. Multiplying the reactant NaOH by 2 gives:

$$H_2SO_4 + 2NaOH \rightarrow Na_2SO_4 + H_2O \text{ (unbalanced)}$$

4. Multiplying the product H_2O by 2 to balance hydrogen gives:

$$H_2SO_4 + 2NaOH \rightarrow Na_2SO_4 + 2H_2O$$

Inspection shows that the oxygen atoms are balanced; therefore the equation is balanced.

Calculations

Laboratory procedures using neutralization reactions are quite common and are generally used in determining unknown quantities of acids or bases present in biologic or chemical samples. A useful relationship for calculation of the quantity of an acid or base in a given sample is:

$$V_1N_1 = V_2N_2$$

V_1 = Volume of the standard solution (prepared in the laboratory)
N_1 = Normality of the standard solution
V_2 = Volume of the unknown solution
N_2 = Normality of the unknown solution

The usefulness of this equation becomes readily apparent when one applies it to the evaluation of results of neutralization reactions obtained by titrimetric procedures. Since the normality of the standardized solution of acid or base (equivalents per liter or equivalents per milliliter) is known, one can titrate a known volume or weight of a sample containing an unknown quantity of acid or base and, by the use of the volume-normality relationship given above, ascertain the quantity of acid or base present in the sample.

Titrations are performed by taking an aliquot (V_2, a precisely measured volume) of the solution containing an unknown quantity (N_2 in the foregoing equation) of acid or base and placing it in a titration vessel, usually an Erlenmeyer flask. A standard solution of acid or base whose concentration is precisely known is then carefully delivered into the titration flask by use of a buret. The point at which neutralization occurs, the end point, is detected by use of an organic indicator that changes color when neutralization occurs. The volume, V_1, of standard acid or base required to exactly neutralize the substance in the "unknown" is read from the buret. At this point the values of V_1, N_1, and V_2 are known, and by use of the relationship $V_1N_1 = V_2N_2$, the number of equivalents (N_2) of the substance contained in the "unknown" can be calculated. The following examples illustrate the usefulness of titrimetric procedures as analytical tools.

EXAMPLE 1: What is the normality of a hydrochloric acid solution, 25 ml of which requires 37 ml of 0.30 N NaOH solution for neutralization?

V_1 (NaOH) = 37 ml
N_1 (NaOH) = 0.30 N
V_2 (HCl) = 25 ml
N_2 (HCl) = ?

Using $V_1N_1 = V_2N_2$, solve for N_2:

$$(37 \text{ ml})\ (0.30 \text{ N}) = (25 \text{ ml})\ (N_2)$$

$$N_2 = \frac{(37 \text{ ml})\ (0.30 \text{ N})}{25 \text{ ml}}$$

$$N_2 = \frac{11.1}{25} \text{ N}$$

$$N_2 = 0.44 \text{ N}$$

EXAMPLE 2: Given 30.0 ml of 0.25 M H_3PO_4 (phosphoric acid) solution, what volume of 0.25 M $Ca(OH)_2$ (calcium hydroxide) solution would be required for neutralization?

Step 1: Since the equation is valid only when concentrations are expressed as normalities, we must first find the normality of both the H_3PO_4 and $Ca(OH)_2$ solutions. H_3PO_4 is a triprotic acid (3 H^+ ions), therefore:

$$\text{Normality} = 3\ (\text{Molarity})$$

or

$$\text{N} = 3\ (0.25 \text{ M})$$
$$\text{N} = 0.75 \text{ for } H_3PO_4$$

$Ca(OH)_2$ is a dibasic (2 OH^- ions) base; therefore:

$$\text{Normality} = 2\ (\text{Molarity})$$

or

$$\text{N} = 2\ (0.25 \text{ M})$$
$$\text{N} = 0.50 \text{ for } Ca(OH)_2$$

Step 2: Using $V_1N_1 = V_2N_2$

V_1 (H_3PO_4) = 30.0 ml
N_1 (H_3PO_4) = 0.75 N
V_2 (Ca[OH]$_2$) = ?
N_2 (Ca[OH]$_2$) = 0.50 N
(30.0 ml) (0.75 N) = (V_2) (0.50 N)

$$V_2 = \frac{(30.0 \text{ ml})\ (0.75 \text{ N})}{0.50 \text{ N}}$$

$$V_2 = \frac{22.5}{0.50} \text{ ml}$$

$$V_2 = 45.0 \text{ ml of } Ca(OH)_2$$

Strong versus weak acids and bases

The foregoing discussion of acids and bases implied that all acids and bases dissociate completely in aqueous medium giving either a H_3O^+ ion or a OH^- ion. In reality, only *strong acids* such as HCl, HBr, HI, H_2SO_4, and HNO_3 may be considered to be completely ionized in aqueous solutions; that is:

$$H_2SO_4 + 2H_2O \rightarrow 2H_3O^+ + SO_4^{2-}$$

The common bases NaOH and KOH are *strong bases*

and dissociate completely when dissolved in water; that is:

$$NaOH + H_2O \rightarrow Na^+ + OH^-$$

Many acids are defined as being *weak,* in that they do not completely dissociate in water because the conjugate base of the acid is of nearly the same base strength as water. Some of the common weak acids are acetic acid, carbonic acid, phenol, water, and boric acid. For example, less than 0.5% of the acetic acid molecules in a 1 M solution undergo reaction with water to produce H_3O^+ ion, the remaining 99.5% of the molecules remain undissociated. Equations for such reactions are written as follows:

$$CH_3COOH + H_2O \rightleftharpoons CH_3COO^- + H_3O^+$$

The double arrow separating reactants and products indicates that a dynamic equilibrium is established in which the rate of the reverse reaction, that is:

$$H_3O^+ + CH_3COO^- \rightarrow CH_3COOH + H_2O$$

is equal to the rate of the forward reaction:

$$CH_3COOH + H_2O \rightarrow CH_3COO^- + H_3O^+$$

Thus at equilibrium the concentration of each species in the solution remains constant. The disproportionate length of the arrows in the equation simply indicates that the acetic acid remains largely undissociated.

A similar situation exists for aqueous solutions of *weak bases,* for example, NH_3, Na_2CO_3, and H_2O. Thus a 0.1 M solution of NH_3 in water undergoes reaction to the extent of 0.5%:

$$NH_3 + H_2O \rightleftharpoons NH_4^+ + OH^-$$

EQUILIBRIUMS AND EQUILIBRIUM CONSTANTS

The extent of dissociation of weak acids and bases and the resulting equilibriums have been studied exhaustively. These studies have resulted in a mathematical statement that allows calculation of the degree of dissociation. The mathematical expression describing the general equilibrium reaction

$$HY + H_2O \rightleftharpoons Y^- + H_3O^+$$

is expressed as follows:

$$K_{HY} = \frac{[Y^-][H_3O^+]}{[HY][H_2O]}$$

Note: The brackets "[ ]" indicate concentration of the species in moles per liter.

This equation states that the mathematical product of the concentrations of the reaction products divided by the mathematical product of the concentrations of the reactants is a constant (this is valid only at a given temperature). For example, the equilibrium expression for

$$NH_3 + H_2O \rightleftharpoons NH_4^+ + OH^-$$

is expressed as follows:

$$K_{NH_3} = \frac{[NH_4^+][OH^-]}{[NH_3][H_2O]}$$

Inasmuch as water is present in large excess in most solutions, its concentration remains essentially constant; therefore the term for the concentration of water is incorporated with the equilibrium constant and the mathematical expression is normally given as:

$$K_{NH_3} = \frac{[NH_4^+][OH^-]}{[NH_3]}$$

Experiment has shown that K_{NH_3} is equal to 1.8×10^{-5} at 25° C. In general, the larger the numerical value of K, the stronger the acid or base, depending on whether H_3O^+ or OH^- ion is one of the products.

A most important equilibrium reaction is that involving pure water because reactions involving acids and bases are normally conducted in aqueous medium. Even though water is neutral, it was classified as both a weak acid and a weak base in the preceding section.

Experiment has shown that water undergoes autoionization, in which one molecule of water functions as an acid and a second molecule functions as a base, giving the equation:

$$H_2O + H_2O \rightleftharpoons H_3O^+ + OH^-$$

It is apparent that, even though autoionization is occurring, water is neutral because the concentration of H_3O^+ ion is exactly equal to the concentration of OH^- ion. The equilibrium expression for water is:

$$K = \frac{[OH^-][H_3O^+]}{[H_2O]}$$

or

$$K_W = [H_2O]K = [OH^-][H_3O^+]$$

The concentration of water being constant gives:

$$K_W = [OH^-][H_3O^+]$$

K_W has been determined experimentally to be 1×10^{-14}. For pure water

$$[H_3O^+] = [OH^-] = \sqrt{1 \times 10^{-14}} = 1 \times 10^{-7}$$

THE pH CONCEPT

Following the logic of the preceding discussion, an aqueous solution, no matter whether acidic, basic, or neutral, must have a concentration of H_3O^+ and OH^- ions, the product of which must equal 1×10^{-14}; for example:

$$K_W = [H_3O^+][OH^-] = 1 \times 10^{-14}\ M^2/l^2$$

Any solution in which $[H_3O^+]$ is equal to $[OH^-]$ must be neutral, and any solution in which $[OH^-]$ and $[H_3O^+]$ are unequal must be either basic or acidic. However, at all times $[H_3O^+] \times [OH^-]$ equals 1×10^{-14}. As with the solutions discussed previously, the concentration of H_3O^+ is expressed as moles/liter. This has been further simplified, and is commonly expressed in terms of pH, from the French *puissance d'hydrogène* meaning "power of hydrogen," or "hydrogen power," as a number between zero and 14.

The pH of a solution is defined as being equal to the negative log of the $[H_3O^+]$; that is:

$$pH = -\log [H_3O^+]$$

Thus a neutral solution having a concentration of H_3O^+ equal to 10^{-7} has a pH of 7:

$$pH = -\log [H_3O^+] = -\log 10^{-7}$$

For those solutions in which $[H_3O^+]$ is larger than 10^{-7}, the solution will contain a concentration of H_3O^+ ions greater than that of OH^- ions and will therefore be acidic. Whenever the $[H_3O^+]$ is greater than $[OH^-]$, the pH will be less than 7, and for those solutions in which the $[H_3O^+]$ is less than $[OH^-]$, the pH will be greater than 7 and the solution will be basic.

Values of pH

1, 2, 3, 4, 5, 6 **7** 8, 9, 10, 11, 12, 13, 14
Acidic *Neutral* *Basic*

In an analogous manner, the pOH of a solution is the negative log of $[OH^-]$; therefore, knowing that pH is equal to $-\log [H_3O^+]$ and that K_W is equal to 1×10^{-14}, we find that pOH must equal 14 − pH. For example, if a solution is found to have a $[H_3O^+]$ of 1×10^{-3}, the pH of the solution will be $-\log (1 \times 10^{-3})$, or 3, and the pOH therefore must be 14 − 3, or 11.

EXAMPLE 1: What is the pH of a solution that has a $[H_3O^+]$ of 2.3×10^{-5} M? Using the relationship $pH = -\log [H_3O^+]$, we proceed as follows:

$$pH = -\log (2.3 \times 10^{-5})$$
$$pH = -(\log 2.3 + \log 10^{-5})$$
$$pH = -(0.36 + [-5] \log 10)$$
$$pH = -(0.36 - 5)$$
$$pH = -(-4.64)$$
$$pH = 4.64 \text{ (The solution is acidic.)}$$

EXAMPLE 2: A solution is found to have a concentration of OH^- equaling 3.0×10^{-8} M. What is its pH?

a. Using $pOH = -\log [OH^-]$, find pOH:

$$pOH = -\log (3.0 \times 10^{-8})$$
$$pOH = -(\log 3.0 + [-8] \log 10)$$
$$pOH = -(0.477 + [-8])$$
$$pOH = -(-7.523)$$
$$pOH = 7.52$$

b. Using pH + pOH = 14:

$$pH + 7.52 = 14$$
$$pH = 14 - 7.52$$
$$pH = 6.48 \text{ (The solution is acidic.)}$$

EXAMPLE 3: Find the $[H_3O^+]$ of a solution that has a pH of 9.8 using $pH = -\log [H_3O^+]$.

$$9.8 = -\log [H_3O^+]$$
$$\log [H_3O^+] = -10 + 0.2$$

Using antilogs:

$$[H_3O^+] = (\text{antilog } 0.2)(\text{antilog } -10)$$
$$[H_3O^+] = 1.58 \times 10^{-10} \text{ M}$$

EXAMPLE 4: Given the following information for a solution of acetic acid:

$$K_a = 1.8 \times 10^{-5}$$
$$[HOAc] = 0.5 \text{ M (``HOAc'' is acetic acid.)}$$

Find the pH of the solution.

a. The equilibrium reaction is:

$$\begin{array}{lcl} HOAc & \rightleftharpoons & H^+ + OAc^- \\ 0.5\text{ M} & & x\text{ M} + x\text{ M} \end{array}$$

We know that

$$K_a = \frac{[H^+][OAc^-]}{[HOAc]}$$

Therefore:

$$1.8 \times 10^{-5} = \frac{x^2}{5 \times 10^{-1} - x} = \frac{x^2}{5 \times 10^{-1}}$$

HOAc, being a weak acid, is largely undissociated, and x, compared to 5.0×10^{-1}, is very small and may be eliminated from the denominator without seriously affecting the value calculated for x.

$$x^2 = (1.8 \times 10^{-5})(5 \times 10^{-1})$$
$$x^2 = 9 \times 10^{-6}$$
$$x = 3 \times 10^{-3} \text{ M} = [H^+] = [OAc^-]$$

b. Using $pH = -\log [H_3O^+]$, proceed as follows:

$$pH = -\log (3 \times 10^{-3})$$
$$pH = -(\log 3 + [-3] \log 10)$$
$$pH = -(-2.52)$$
$$pH = 2.52 \text{ (The solution is acidic.)}$$

Determination of pH. The measurement of pH is generally accomplished by two methods, one of which provides reasonably accurate values and the other, more precise values. The less sensitive method makes use of a paper containing a universal indicator. The universal indicator is a mixture of organic dyes, which themselves are acids and bases, and it undergoes changes in color upon being converted from one form

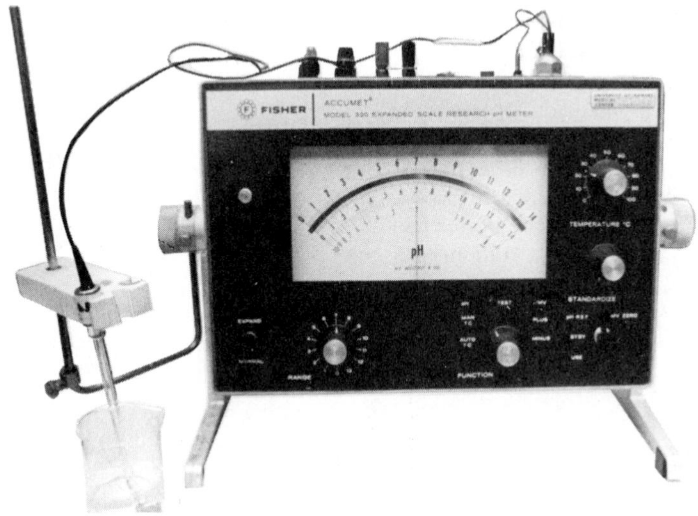

Fig. 4-12. pH meter.

to the other, that is, acid to base or base to acid. These color changes occur at specific pH values.

Accurate determination of pH values, which are usually necessary in radioimmunoassay analysis or the preparation of radiopharmaceuticals, are determined by use of a pH meter (Fig. 4-12).

A pH meter has two electrodes. Note that the one in Fig. 4-12 contains both electrodes in a single probe. One electrode of known potential (a calomel electrode) serves as a reference and involves the following electrode reaction:

$$2Hg + 2Cl^- \rightleftharpoons Hg_2Cl_2 + 2e^-$$

This reaction has a constant potential of −0.27 volts. The second electrode (a glass electrode) consists of a metal wire dipping into a solution of known pH, and this solution is separated by a thin glass membrane from the solution whose pH is to be determined. The potential across the glass membrane, and thus the half-cell voltage of this electrode is a function of the pH of the solution outside the membrane. A third component of a pH meter is a voltmeter or potentiometer capable of measuring voltages accurate to at least ±0.01 volt. The voltmeter or potentiometer is designed, based upon the potential difference of the two electrodes, to give a reading in pH units.

BUFFER SOLUTIONS

All biologic systems are dependent on fluids that are maintained within very narrow limits of pH. For example, human blood must be maintained within a pH range of 7.3 to 7.5 and therefore requires a means by which these pH limits can be maintained. The mechanism by which this is achieved is referred to as *buffering* and involves a solution that contains a mixture of substances, some that are acidic and others that are basic. Again, with blood being used as an example, the substances involved in the buffering effect are carbonates, bicarbonates, carbonic acid, the phosphates (PO_4^{3-}, HPO_4^{2-}, and $H_2PO_4^-$), and certain proteins that function by maintaining the pH of blood in the range of 7.3 to 7.5.

A relatively simple buffer system is one consisting of a mixture of acetic acid and its conjugate base acetate ion. To understand how this system can function to maintain a pH within a small range, we must recall that acetic acid, being a weak acid, is described by an equilibrium expression. Let us examine what occurs when a "foreign" acid or base is introduced into the acetic acid–acetate ion buffer system.

$$HOAc \rightleftharpoons H^+ + OAc^-$$

$$K_a = 1.8 \times 10^{-5} = \frac{[H^+][OAc^-]}{[HOAc]}$$

The above equation shows that undissociated acetic acid is present and is available to react with any base entering the system. For example, if a small quantity of sodium hydroxide is added to the system ($HOAc + NaOH \rightarrow NaOAc + H_2O$), the concentration of acetic acid will decrease while the concentration of acetate ion will increase. Conversely, when an acid, such as HCl, is added to the system ($NaOAc + HCl \rightarrow HOAc + NaCl$), the concentration of acetic acid increases while the concentration of acetate ion is decreased. The concentration of the buffer-system components will undergo change, but the expression governing the equilibrium will still be valid.

Although buffer solutions will not maintain a fairly constant pH if large quantities of acids or bases are added to them, it is remarkable how much they can accommodate without an appreciable change in pH. This is illustrated in the following example:

EXAMPLE: Consider 1 liter of the acetate buffer that is 0.1 M in acetic acid and 0.1 M in sodium acetate.

$$\begin{array}{llll} HOAc \rightleftharpoons & H^+ & + OAc^- & K_a = 1.8 \times 10^{-5} \\ 0.1\ M & x\ M & + x\ M & \\ NaOAc \rightarrow & Na^+ & + OAc^- & (100\%\ \text{ionized}) \\ 0.1\ M & 0.1\ M & 0.1\ M & \end{array}$$

a. Calculate the pH of this buffer solution:

$$K_a = \frac{[H^+][OAc^-]}{[HOAc]} = \frac{[H^+](1 \times 10^{-1} + x)}{(1 \times 10^{-1} - x)} = 1.8 \times 10^{-5}$$

Since the acetic acid contributes a negligible amount of the total quantity of OAc^-, the $[OAc^- + x]$ may be assumed to be 0.1 M. Similarly the $[HOAc - x]$ may be assumed to be 0.1 M; therefore:

$$1.8 \times 10^{-5} = \frac{[H^+](1 \times 10^{-1})}{(1 \times 10^{-1})}$$

and

$$[H^+] = 1.8 \times 10^{-5}\ M$$

The pH of the solution will be, to a first approximation:

$$\begin{aligned} pH = -\log[H^+] &= -\log(1.8 \times 10^{-5}) \\ pH &= -(\log 1.8 + [-5]\log 10) \\ pH &= -(0.26 - 5) \\ pH &= 4.74 \end{aligned}$$

b. Calculate the pH of the solution after addition of 0.01 mole of HCl, assuming that the increase in total volume of the buffer solution will be negligible.

$$\begin{array}{llll} HCl & + NaOAc \rightarrow & NaCl & + HOAc \\ 0.01\ M & 0.01\ M & 0.01\ M & 0.01\ M \end{array}$$

The reaction states that for each equivalent of HCl added, 1 equivalent of OAc^- will be consumed, thus forming an equivalent of HOAc. The concentrations now become:

$$\begin{array}{ll} HOAc & \rightleftharpoons H^+ + OAc^- \\ (0.1\ M + 0.01\ M) & x\ M + (0.1 - 0.01\ M) \end{array}$$

Following the same rationale as used in part (a), calculate the $[H^+]$.

$$K_a = \frac{[H^+][OAc^-]}{[HOAc]} = \frac{[H^+](0.09)}{(0.11)} = 1.8 \times 10^{-5}$$

$$[H^+] = \frac{(1.1 \times 10^{-1})(1.8 \times 10^{-5})}{(9 \times 10^{-2})}$$

$$[H^+] = 0.22 \times 10^{-4} = 2.2 \times 10^{-5}\ M$$

Therefore:

$$\begin{aligned} pH &= -\log[H^+] = -\log(2.2 \times 10^{-5}) \\ pH &= -(\log 2.2 + [-5]\log 10) \\ pH &= -(0.34 - 5) \\ pH &= 4.66 \end{aligned}$$

Comparing the pH of the original buffer solution, 4.74, with the pH of the solution after addition of 0.01 mole of HCl, 4.66, we see that the pH has changed by only 0.08. As a problem to solve, what change in pH would be expected if 0.01 mole of NaOH had been added to the original solution?

Similarly the buffer systems involved in maintaining a narrow pH range for blood involve simple acid-base reactions such as those just described.

ORGANIC COMPOUNDS

The chemistry that has been discussed in the preceding sections has involved, with the exception of acetic acid, substances that are referred to as being inorganic. Inorganic substances comprise all those elements and compounds derived from elements other than carbon, the number of which can be counted in the thousands. Organic chemistry is best defined as the chemistry of carbon, and the number of organic compounds recorded in the literature are numbered in the millions. Carbon differs from all other elements in its unique ability to form strong covalent bonds to other carbon atoms, thus resulting in myriads of compounds ranging from those of low molecular weight to highly complex molecules containing thousands of carbon atoms. Obviously, a thorough discussion of organic chemistry is beyond the scope of this chapter; however, the importance of organic chemistry, as applied to nuclear medicine specifically and all living systems generally, requires some foundation in this subject.

Historically, organic chemistry as a discipline is relatively young, since philosophical and theologic thought held that organic substances, being found primarily in living systems, required a vital force for their creation and that man would never accomplish the creation or synthesis of these substances. In 1828 the German chemist, Friedrich Wöhler, while working with the inorganic substance ammonium cyanate ($NH_4^+CNO^-$), found that when it was heated it was converted to the nonionic organic substance urea

$\left(H_2N-\overset{\overset{\displaystyle O}{\|}}{C}-NH_2\right)$, which is a metabolic product excreted in the urine. This discovery gave rise to great controversy in the scientific community, and serious investigation in organic chemistry did not occur until the mid 1800s.

Types of organic compounds and nomenclature

Organic compounds are divided into families or homologous series in which all members of a given family exhibit essentially the same type of chemical reactivity. Each family of simple organic compounds is characterized by a *functional group,* the most reactive site of the molecule, which determines the chemical reactions that all members of the family will undergo. The main families of organic compounds and their characteristic functional groups are given in Table 4-5.

As we have previously noted, each compound possesses a name unique to itself; this is also the case with organic compounds. Although many organic compounds, especially those isolated as naturally occurring

Table 4-5. Families of organic compounds and their functional groups

Family	Structure	IUPAC name	Suffix	Functional group
Alkanes	H | H—C—H | H	Methane	*-ane*	(None)
Alkenes	H H \ / C=C / \ H H	Ethene	*-ene*	\ / C=C / \
Alkynes	H—C≡C—H	Ethyne	*-yne*	—C≡C—
Arenes (aromatic compounds)	H | C // \ H—C C—H | ‖ H—C C—H \\ / C | H	Benzene	*-ene*	| —C—H |
Alcohols	H H | | H—C—C—H | | H O—H	Ethanol	*-ol*	—O—H
Phenols	O—H | C // \ H—C C—H | ‖ H—C C—H \\ / C | H	Phenol	*-ol*	—O—H

Continued.

Table 4-5. Families of organic compounds and their functional groups—cont'd

Family	Structure	IUPAC name	Suffix	Functional group
Ethers	$\begin{array}{ccccccccccccc} & & H & & H & & & & H & & H & & \\ & & \mid & & \mid & & & & \mid & & \mid & & \\ H & - & C & - & C & - & O & - & C & - & C & - & H \\ & & \mid & & \mid & & & & \mid & & \mid & & \\ & & H & & H & & & & H & & H & & \end{array}$	Diethylether	*-ether*	$-O-$
Halides	$\begin{array}{ccccc} & & H & & \\ & & \mid & & \\ H & - & C & - & Br \\ & & \mid & & \\ & & H & & \end{array}$	Bromomethane	The substituents *chloro-*, *fluoro-*, etc. are prefixed to parent alkane.	—*X*(F, Cl, Br, I)
Aldehydes	$\begin{array}{ccccccc} & & H & & O & & \\ & & \mid & & \Vert & & \\ H & - & C & - & C & - & H \\ & & \mid & & & & \\ & & H & & & & \end{array}$	Ethanal	*-al*	$\begin{array}{cccc} & O & & \\ & \Vert & & \\ - & C & - & H \end{array}$
Ketones	$\begin{array}{ccccccccc} & & H & & O & & H & & \\ & & \mid & & \Vert & & \mid & & \\ H & - & C & - & C & - & C & - & H \\ & & \mid & & & & \mid & & \\ & & H & & & & H & & \end{array}$	2-Propanone	*-one*	$\begin{array}{ccc} & O & \\ & \Vert & \\ - & C & - \end{array}$
Carboxylic acids	$\begin{array}{ccccccc} & & H & & O & & \\ & & \mid & & \Vert & & \\ H & - & C & - & C & - & OH \\ & & \mid & & & & \\ & & H & & & & \end{array}$	Ethanoic acid	*-oic*	$\begin{array}{cccc} & O & & \\ & \Vert & & \\ - & C & - & OH \end{array}$
Esters	$\begin{array}{ccccccccccccc} & & H & & O & & & & H & & H & & \\ & & \mid & & \Vert & & & & \mid & & \mid & & \\ H & - & C & - & C & - & O & - & C & - & C & - & H \\ & & \mid & & & & & & \mid & & \mid & & \\ & & H & & & & & & H & & H & & \end{array}$	Ethyl ethanoate	*-oate*	$\begin{array}{ccccccc} & O & & & & & \\ & \Vert & & & & \mid & \\ - & C & - & O & - & C & - \\ & & & & & \mid & \end{array}$
Amides	$\begin{array}{ccccccc} & & H & & O & & \\ & & \mid & & \Vert & & \\ H & - & C & - & C & - & NH_2 \\ & & \mid & & & & \\ & & H & & & & \end{array}$	Ethanamide	*-amide*	$\begin{array}{ccccc} & O & & & \\ & \Vert & & & / \\ - & C & - & N & \\ & & & & \backslash \end{array}$
Amines	$\begin{array}{ccccc} & & H & & \\ & & \mid & & \\ H & - & C & - & NH_2 \\ & & \mid & & \\ & & H & & \end{array}$	Methamine	*-amine*	$\begin{array}{ccccc} & \mid & & & / \\ - & C & - & N & \\ & \mid & & & \backslash \end{array}$
Thiols	$\begin{array}{ccccccc} & & H & & H & & \\ & & \mid & & \mid & & \\ H & - & C & - & C & - & SH \\ & & \mid & & \mid & & \\ & & H & & H & & \end{array}$	Ethanethiol	*-thiol*	$\begin{array}{ccccc} & \mid & & & \\ - & C & - & S & - \\ & \mid & & & \end{array}$

products in the early years of organic chemistry, are still referred to by the names (common or trivial names) given them by their discoverers, the multitude of organic compounds now known requires a systematic method of naming them. Currently, the generally accepted rules for naming organic compounds are those set down by the International Union of Pure and Applied Chemistry (IUPAC). Using alkanes as an example, the IUPAC rules are as follows.

Those molecules in which all the carbon atoms are bonded so as to form a continuous chain are called "normal" alkanes, Table 4-6.

All other alkanes are named as though they had been derived from the hydrocarbon with the longest continuous chain, this being the parent compound (rule 1).

EXAMPLE:

```
                  CH3
                   |
   CH3   CH3      CH2
    |     |        |
CH3—CH — CH — CH — CH3
```

Rule 1: The longest chain consists of six carbon atoms; therefore the parent hydrocarbon is *hex-*

Table 4-6. Normal alkanes (C_nH_{2n+2})

Number of carbons	Name	Expanded formula	Condensed formula
1	Methane	$H-\overset{\displaystyle H}{\underset{\displaystyle H}{C}}-H$	CH_4
2	Ethane	$H-\overset{\displaystyle H}{\underset{\displaystyle H}{C}}-\overset{\displaystyle H}{\underset{\displaystyle H}{C}}-H$	CH_3-CH_3
3	Propane	$H-\overset{\displaystyle H}{\underset{\displaystyle H}{C}}-\overset{\displaystyle H}{\underset{\displaystyle H}{C}}-\overset{\displaystyle H}{\underset{\displaystyle H}{C}}-H$	$CH_3-CH_2-CH_3$
4	Butane	$H-\overset{\displaystyle H}{\underset{\displaystyle H}{C}}-\overset{\displaystyle H}{\underset{\displaystyle H}{C}}-\overset{\displaystyle H}{\underset{\displaystyle H}{C}}-\overset{\displaystyle H}{\underset{\displaystyle H}{C}}-H$	$CH_3-(CH_2)_2-CH_3$
5	Pentane	$H-\overset{\displaystyle H}{\underset{\displaystyle H}{C}}-\overset{\displaystyle H}{\underset{\displaystyle H}{C}}-\overset{\displaystyle H}{\underset{\displaystyle H}{C}}-\overset{\displaystyle H}{\underset{\displaystyle H}{C}}-\overset{\displaystyle H}{\underset{\displaystyle H}{C}}-H$	$CH_3-(CH_2)_3-CH_3$
6	Hexane	$H-\overset{\displaystyle H}{\underset{\displaystyle H}{C}}-\overset{\displaystyle H}{\underset{\displaystyle H}{C}}-\overset{\displaystyle H}{\underset{\displaystyle H}{C}}-\overset{\displaystyle H}{\underset{\displaystyle H}{C}}-\overset{\displaystyle H}{\underset{\displaystyle H}{C}}-\overset{\displaystyle H}{\underset{\displaystyle H}{C}}-H$	$CH_3-(CH_2)_4-CH_3$

Starting with pentane, the alkanes are named systematically with a numerical prefix indicating the number of carbon atoms, that is, pent-, hex-, hept-, oct-, non-, dec-, undec-, dodec-, tridec-, tetradec-, pentadec-, hexadec-, heptadec-, octadec-, nonadec-, eicos- (20), heneicos- (21), docos-, tricos-, tetracos-, and so on.

Table 4-7. Alkyl groups derived from the alkanes by removal of one hydrogen

Common alkyl groups		Derived from
Methyl	$CH_3—$	Methane
Ethyl	$CH_3—CH_2—$	Ethane
Propyl	$CH_3—CH_2—CH_2—$	Propane
Isopropyl	$CH_3—\underset{\mid}{CH}—CH_3$	Propane
Butyl	$CH_3—CH_2—CH_2—CH_2—$	Butane
sec-Butyl	$CH_3—\underset{\mid}{CH}—CH_2—CH_3$	Butane
Isobutyl	$(CH_3)_2CH—CH_2—$	—
tert-Butyl	$CH_3—\underset{CH_3}{\overset{CH_3}{C}}—$	—

ane; however, unlike hexane, there are three branches in the above molecule in which CH_3 groups have been substituted for hydrogens of the parent compound. The CH_3 groups belong to a family of "alkyl" groups, which are derived from the alkanes by removal of one hydrogen. These are named by replacement of the "-ane" ending of the alkane by "-yl" (Table 4-7).

Rule 2: The carbon atoms of the parent structure are numbered from the end that will give the *lowest numbers* to those carbons to which the alkyl groups are attached.

```
                         CH3 6
                          |
          CH3   CH3      CH2 5
           |     |        |
    CH3 — CH  —  CH  —   CH  4
     1     2     3        |
                         CH3
```

Number as above and *not* as follows:

```
                         CH3 1
                          |
          CH3   CH3      CH2 2
           |     |        |
    CH3 — CH  —  CH  —   CH  3
     6     5     4        |
                         CH3
```

Rule 3: The groups attached to the parent structure are given both a name and a number to indicate their point of attachment. If the same group occurs as a substituent in the molecule more than once, then the prefixes di-, tri, tetra-, and so on, are used to specify the number of times this group appears. If more than one type of group is attached to the parent compound, these groups are named in alphabetical order. Therefore, the correct name for the above compound is "2,3,4-trimethylhexane."

Note that a comma (with no space) is used between numbers and a hyphen between the number and the name of the substituent.

Note in Table 4-7 that the isobutyl and *tert*-butyl groups were not shown to be derived from one of the normal alkanes. The names given these groups arise from an older nomenclature in which both of the alkanes containing four carbon atoms were called butanes. This pair of structural isomers consists of the normal butane and a second compound having the structure

```
    CH3
       \H
        C — CH3
       /
    CH3
```

which is called isobutane. Inspection of the structure of isobutane shows that two alkyl groups can be derived, depending on the hydrogen that is removed. The prefixes "secondary" and "tertiary" are used to indicate the carbon through which the alkyl substituent is attached. If the carbon of the alkyl group, at the point of attachment, is bonded to only one other carbon, the alkyl group is designated as "primary"; if bonded to two other carbons, the alkyl group is "secondary"; and it is "tertiary" if bonded to three other carbons, for example, the *sec*-butyl and *tert*-butyl groups.

The IUPAC rules for naming all organic compounds follow, in general, the above rules with the following modifications: (1) the ending (suffix) of the name is dictated by the main functional group present in the compound, (2) the longest continuous chain (parent compound) must contain the main functional group, and (3) the chain is numbered so that the main functional group receives the lowest possible number.

EXAMPLE:

```
                         CH3 6
                          |
          CH3    OH      CH2 5
           |     |        |
    CH3 — CH  —  CH  —   CH  4    2,4-Dimethyl-3-hexanol
     1     2     3        |
                         CH3
```

Alkanes. This family of compounds, also called "saturated hydrocarbons," is important in that these compounds are a major source of energy but are of little importance in nuclear medicine. Perhaps the greatest utility in nuclear medicine would be their use as solvents; however, as a point of interest the saturated hydrocarbon cyclopropane

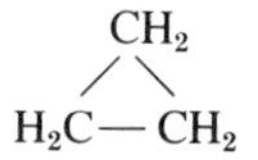

$$\begin{array}{c} CH_2 \\ / \quad \backslash \\ H_2C - CH_2 \end{array}$$

(with the prefix "cyclo-" indicating a ring or cyclic system) has found use as a general anesthetic.

Alkenes. This family of hydrocarbons, which contains a carbon-carbon double bond (C=C) is potentially useful as a substrate in labeling procedures. Although several substances are currently under investigation, their usefulness as scanning agents has yet to be proved. Potential agents may arise through addition of radioactive reagents to the carbon-carbon double bond.

$$R-HC=CH-R' + HI \rightarrow R-\overset{H}{\underset{H}{C}}-\overset{H}{\underset{I}{C}}-R'$$

The alkynes, having chemical properties similar to the alkenes, are also of interest as potential sources of radiopharmaceuticals.

Arenes and aromatic compounds. This family of compounds contains at least one aromatic ring, which is characterized by benzene, the simplest of the aromatic compounds.

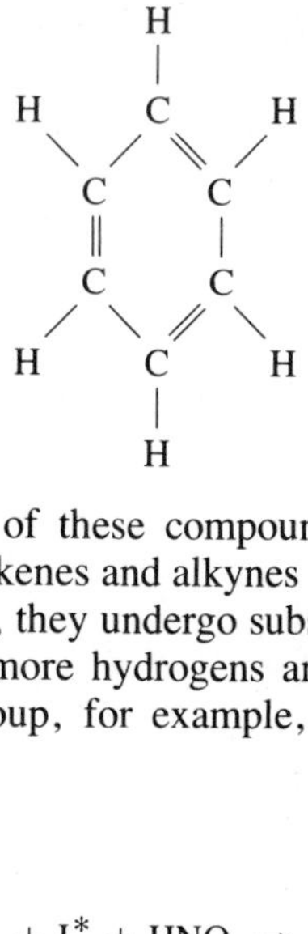

H C H C C C C H C H H H (benzene structure)

The chemistry of these compounds differs greatly from that of the alkenes and alkynes in that, rather than addition reactions, they undergo substitution reactions, in which one or more hydrogens are replaced by another atom or group, for example, the iodination of benzene:

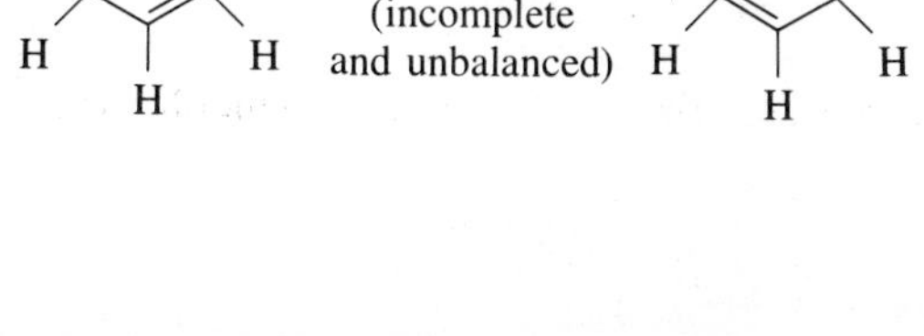

$$C_6H_6 + I_2^* + HNO_3 \rightarrow C_6H_5I^*$$
(incomplete and unbalanced)

This reaction is found to be especially useful in the preparation of *ortho*-iodohippuric acid, which has found use as a renal function agent.

The substance rose bengal, a molecule of complex structure that contains aromatic rings, which when labeled with radioactive iodine atoms as substituents, is very useful as an imaging agent in the determination of liver function. Among other aromatic substances containing a radioactive halogen are the brominated estrogens, which have been approved for experimental imaging procedures in humans.

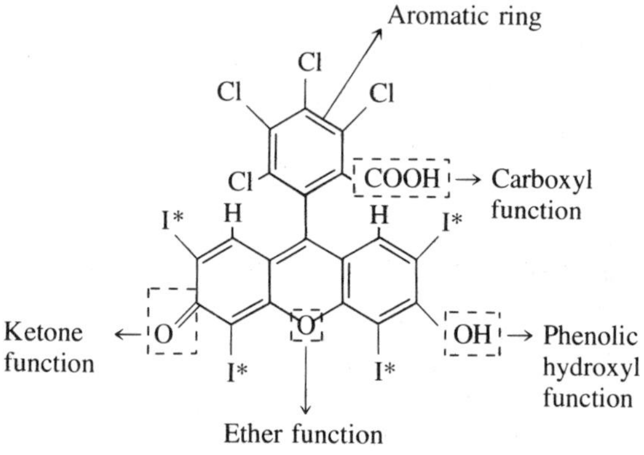

Aromatic ring; Cl; Cl; Cl; Cl; COOH → Carboxyl function; I*; H; H; I*; Ketone function ← O; O; OH → Phenolic hydroxyl function; I*; I*; Ether function

I*–rose bengal

An especially important radiolabeled aromatic compound used for determination of thyroid function is T_3:

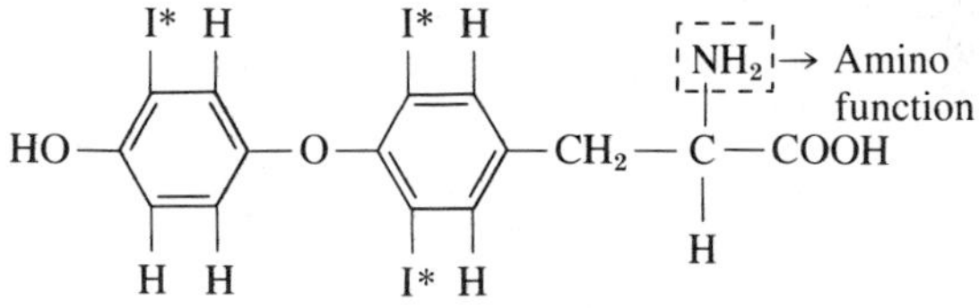

I* H; I* H; NH$_2$ → Amino function; HO–(ring)–O–(ring)–CH$_2$–C–COOH; H; H H; I* H

3,5,3′-Triiodothyronine (T_3)

Alcohols and phenols. Alcohols and phenols contain the functional group —OH. Inspection of the structures of rose bengal and T_3 shows that each contains a phenolic hydroxyl (—OH) function as a part of the molecule. Likewise, brominated estrone, mentioned in the preceding section, also contains this functional group.

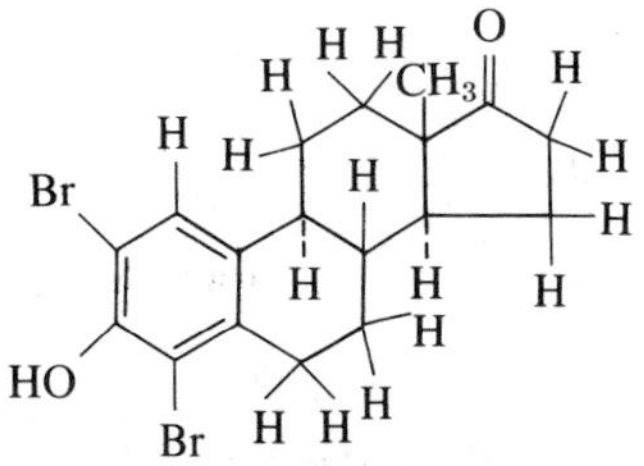

Br; HO; Br; CH_3; O; H (multiple)

2,4-Dibromoestrone

Molecules containing this structural feature are highly important in preparation of radiopharmaceuticals.

Ethers. The ether linkage, R—O—R, also occurs in rose bengal and T_3, and its importance as a structural feature, as with the phenolic —OH function, lies in its ability to facilitate substitution reactions in which radioactive halogens are introduced into the aromatic ring.

Halides. Radiopharmaceuticals that contain halogen, especially those containing radioactive bromine or iodine, again for example, rose bengal, T_3, and brominated estrogen, are of utmost importance and have great effectiveness in the practice of nuclear medicine solely because of the presence of the radioactive halogen in these molecules. However, the functional and structural features contained in the rest of these molecules are of equal importance in that they determine the organ or site in which the total radioactive substance is localized.

Aldehydes and ketones. The carbonyl function

$$(-\overset{\overset{\displaystyle O}{\|}}{C}-)$$

is common to both aldehydes and ketones. The presence of this functional group is not especially important to the labeling of organic molecules, but, as noted in the preceding section, its presence is vital in determining the biodistribution of the radioactive substance.

Carboxylic acids. Several compounds containing the carboxyl function have been noted in previous sections. In addition, pentetic acid (DTPA) forms a complex with ^{169}ytterbium to give ^{169}Yb–pentetic acid (^{169}Yb-DTPA), a cisternographic imaging agent.

$$C_6H_4(I^*)-\overset{\overset{\displaystyle O}{\|}}{C}-\underset{\underset{\displaystyle H}{|}}{N}-CH_2-\overset{\overset{\displaystyle O}{\|}}{C}-OH \xrightarrow{NaOH}$$

***o*-Iodohippuric acid**

$$C_6H_4(I^*)-\overset{\overset{\displaystyle O}{\|}}{C}-\underset{\underset{\displaystyle H}{|}}{N}-CH_2-\overset{\overset{\displaystyle O}{\|}}{C}-O^-\ {}^+Na$$

Hippuran

The sodium salt of *o*-iodohippuric acid, hippuran, in filtering through the glomeruli of the kidneys, provides an effective means of evaluating kidney function, especially important in patients who have received a kidney transplant.

Esters, functioning as derivatives of carboxylic acids, are formed by means of an acid-catalyzed condensation reaction between a carboxylic acid and an alcohol. These substances have not as yet been found to be useful as precursors to radiopharmaceuticals.

$$R-\overset{\overset{\displaystyle O}{\|}}{C}-OH + R'-OH \xrightarrow{H^+} R-\overset{\overset{\displaystyle O}{\|}}{C}-O-R' + H_2O$$

Amides. Hippuran (previous section), in addition to the carboxylate group, also contains an amide function.

$$C_6H_4(I^*)-\overset{\overset{\displaystyle O}{\|}}{C}-\underset{\underset{\displaystyle H}{|}}{N}-CH_2-\overset{\overset{\displaystyle O}{\|}}{C}-O^-\ {}^+Na$$

Hippuran, showing the amide function

Components of all biologic tissues have amide functions, which usually are referred to as "peptide linkages." The protein human serum albumin (HSA), whose structure is not completely known, when labeled with ^{99m}Tc, is used as a blood pool–scanning agent.

Amines and thiols. Amines and thiols are the nitrogen and sulfur analogs of the alcohols. Substances in which the amino group ($-NH_2$) is an important structural component are the proteins and amino acids from which they are derived.

$$H_2N-\underset{\underset{\displaystyle H}{|}}{\overset{\overset{\displaystyle R}{|}}{C}}-\overset{\overset{\displaystyle O}{\|}}{C}-OH \xrightarrow{Enzymes}$$

Amino acid

$$\boxed{H_2N}\left[\underset{\underset{\displaystyle H}{|}}{\overset{\overset{\displaystyle R}{|}}{C}}-\overset{\overset{\displaystyle O}{\|}}{C}-\underset{\underset{\displaystyle H}{|}}{N}-\underset{\underset{\displaystyle H}{|}}{\overset{\overset{\displaystyle R}{|}}{C}}\right]_x \overset{\overset{\displaystyle O}{\|}}{C}-OH + xH_2O$$

Protein

Of the compounds useful in nuclear medicine, two of the most important are pentetic acid (DTPA; see the previous carboxylic acids) and penicillamine.

$$\begin{array}{c} \quad\quad CH_3\ NH_2\ O \\ \quad\quad |\quad\ |\quad\ \| \\ H_3C-C-C-C-OH \\ \quad |\quad\ | \\ \quad SH\ \ H \end{array}$$

Penicillamine

Penicillamine contains a carboxyl, an amino, and a thiol function. Labeling with ^{99m}Tc provides the most effective kidney-imaging agent currently available. The way in which ^{99m}Tc interacts with this molecule is still under investigation.

CONCLUSION

The foregoing comments, in which the significance of the various organic functional groups to nuclear medicine have been noted, should not be considered by the student to be a complete knowledge of the chemistry of these compounds. A thorough understanding of each of the radiopharmaceutical compounds requires not only a knowledge of their structure and biologic fate, but also ultimately a knowledge of the chemical processes by which they are prepared. A discussion of the procedures used in preparing these substances is contained in Chapter 5. Of course, a thorough understanding of the theoretical and preparative techniques of organic chemistry as related to nuclear medicine and to an insight into the chemical basis of life, is an unending quest.

SUGGESTED READINGS

Boyd, R. W., and Morrison, R. T.: Organic chemistry, ed. 3, Boston, 1973, Allyn & Bacon, Inc.

Daub, G. H., and Seese, W. S.: Basic chemistry, ed. 2, Englewood Cliffs, N.J., 1977, Prentice-Hall, Inc.

Masterton, W. L., and Slowinski, E. J.: Chemical principles, ed. 3, Philadelphia, 1973, W. B. Saunders Co.

Miller, G. H.: Principles of college chemistry, San Francisco, 1972, Canfield Press.

Roberts, J. D., and Caserio, M. C.: Basic principles of organic chemistry, ed. 2, Menlo Park, Cal., 1977, W. A. Benjamin, Inc.

Skoog, D. A., and West, D. M.: Fundamentals of analytical chemistry, ed. 3, New York, 1976, Holt, Rinehart & Winston.

Chapter 5

RADIOCHEMISTRY AND RADIOPHARMACOLOGY

Karen D. McElvany, Sally J. Wagner, and Michael J. Welch

PRODUCTION OF RADIONUCLIDES

Nuclear stability

When a radionuclide is being produced, it is of importance to be able to predict its mode of decay. If the radionuclide is being considered for use in nuclear medicine, it should of course decay by gamma (γ) or positron (β^+) emission, rather than by beta (β^-) emission. Certain combinations of neutrons and protons produce stable nuclei, whereas others do not. Fig. 5-1 shows an approximate plot of neutron-proton ratios; the solid line indicates the neutron-proton ratio of stable elements and the dotted line represents a ratio of one. It is evident from this figure that as elements become heavier, the ratio of neutrons to protons in the stable isotopes increases. Unstable (radioactive) nuclides possess numbers of neutrons and protons such that they do not lie on this line of stability. When radionuclides decay, they do so in such a manner as to form stable isotopes.

If a nuclide is too rich in neutrons (a nuclide below the line of stability shown in Fig. 5-1), it will tend to decay by conversion of a neutron into a proton within the atomic nucleus:

$$\underset{\text{(energy)}}{n \rightarrow p + e^- + \nu} \qquad (\beta^- \text{ decay})$$

This will, of course, result in β^--particle decay, and the radionuclide will not be of potential use for in vivo detection. A nuclide that is rich in protons (a nuclide above the line of stability) is also unstable; stability is achieved when the neutron-to-proton ratio is increased. Two possible ways of achieving this are as follows:

$$p \rightarrow n + e^+ + \nu \qquad (\beta^+ \text{ decay})$$

$$p + e^- \rightarrow n + \nu \qquad (\text{electron capture})$$

It is seen that above the line of stability we tend to find positron- or gamma ray–emitting isotopes, and below the line, β^- particle–emitting radionuclides. There are, of course, exceptions to these generalities, and these particularly occur when an element has several stable isotopes (for example, xenon, which has stable isotopes of atomic mass 124, 126, 128, 129, 130, 131, 132, 134, and 136).

Radionuclides can be produced in two types of nuclear devices: nuclear reactors or charged-particle accelerators. These two modes of production are discussed separately.

Reactor-produced radionuclides

The core of a nuclear reactor consists of material (usually uranium) undergoing nuclear fission. Because of the many fission events in the volume surrounding this core, there is a very high neutron flux. It is possible to produce radionuclides by two means: first, by simple irradiation of material within this neutron flux and, second, by separation of the products produced by the nuclear fission event.

The neutrons around the core of a nuclear reactor are low-energy (thermal) neutrons and typical nuclear reactions induced are of the type:

$$^{Y}_{Z}A + n \rightarrow {}^{Y+1}_{Z}A + \gamma \qquad (1)$$

$$^{Y}_{Z}A + n \rightarrow {}_{Z-1}^{Y}B + p \qquad (2)$$

In a reaction of the first type, the target atom $^{Y}_{Z}A$, with atomic number Z and atomic mass Y, absorbs a neutron, and energy is emitted in the form of γ rays. This is written as an (n,γ) type of reaction and the following are examples:

$$^{98}Mo(n,\gamma)^{99}Mo$$

$$^{112}Sn(n,\gamma)^{113}Sn$$

$$^{197}Au(n,\gamma)^{198}Au$$

In the second type of reaction, after absorption of a neutron, a proton is emitted. Since this changes the atomic number of the nucleus, an isotope of a different element, B, is formed. Examples of this type of nuclear reaction are as follows:

$$^{14}N(n,p)^{14}C$$

$$^{3}He(n,p)^{3}H$$

Note that the first type of reaction forms a radioisotope from a stable isotope of the same element, and so

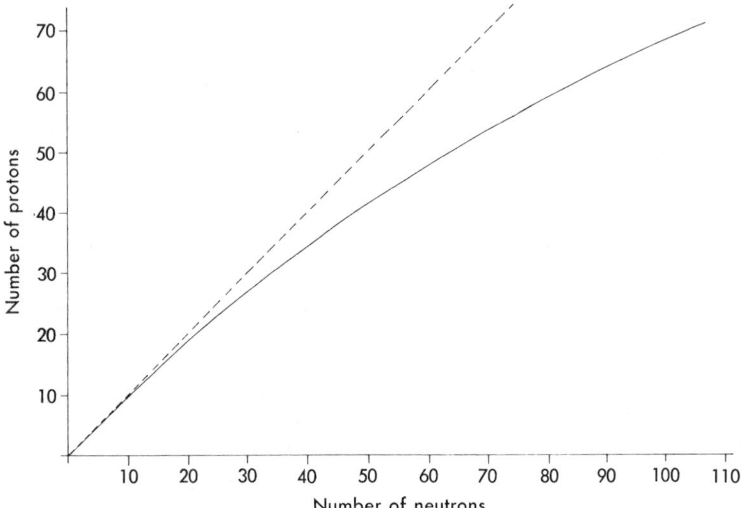

Fig. 5-1. *Solid line,* Number of neutrons and protons in stable isotopes. *Broken line,* Neutron/proton ratios of 1.

high specific-activity products cannot be produced. In the second type of reaction, the product nuclide is an isotope of a different element, and so high specific-activity, carrier-free (that is, with no stable isotope of the same element) radioisotopes are produced.

In reactions of type (1) we are simply adding a neutron to a stable isotope; in reaction (2) the *overall* effect of the reaction is simply to convert a proton to a neutron. Both of these types of reactions will produce neutron-rich products that will most likely decay by β^- emission. The main application of (n,γ) reactions in producing isotopes for nuclear medicine has been to produce the parent of a daughter radionuclide that will actually be utilized, as in the following examples:

$$^{98}Mo(n,\gamma)^{99}Mo \xrightarrow{\text{67-hour half-life}} {}^{99m}Tc \text{ (isotope used)}$$

$$^{112}Sn(n,\gamma)^{113}Sn \xrightarrow{\text{115-day half-life}} {}^{113m}In \text{ (isotope used)}$$

$$^{124}Xe(n,\gamma)^{125}Xe \xrightarrow{\text{17-hour half-life}} {}^{125}I \text{ (isotope used)}$$

The second way in which nuclear reactors can be used to produce radionuclides is by separation of the products formed from nuclear fission. Fission is the process by which the isotopes of some heavy elements decompose into isotopes of two lighter elements. Nuclides that undergo fission include ^{233}U, ^{235}U, ^{239}Pu, and ^{241}Am. In controlled fission of the type occurring in a nuclear reactor, the following type of reaction sequence occurs:

$$n + {}^{235}_{92}U \rightarrow {}^{236}_{92}U \rightarrow {}^{89}_{36}Kr + {}^{144}_{56}Ba + 3n$$

The neutron interacts with the ^{235}U nucleus to form unstable ^{236}U, which decomposes into the two smaller

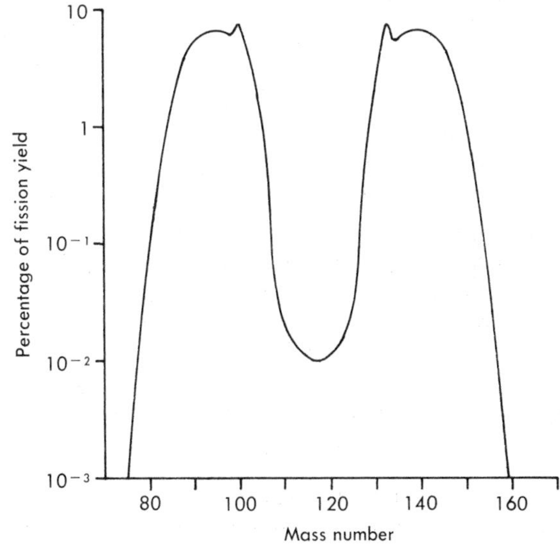

Fig. 5-2. Relative yields of fission products of various masses formed after uranium fission.

atoms. Fission does not always form krypton and barium; these are simply given as examples. A whole range of fission products (Fig. 5-2) is formed ranging in mass from about 70 to 165 and including many radioisotopes of the elements in the center of the periodic table. Note that fission usually gives products of unequal mass and that high yields of nuclides that are of interest in nuclear medicine (^{99}Mo, ^{131}I, ^{133}Xe) are formed. During the fission process, two isotopes of intermediate mass are formed from one of high mass. As shown in Fig. 5-1, heavier elements have greater neutron-to-proton ratios; thus fission initially forms products far from the line of stability on the neutron-rich side of that line. As with products of (n,γ) reactions, fission products tend to decay by β^- emission, and so only a limited number have found use in nuclear medicine. Unlike products from (n,γ) reactions, fission products are carrier free. As an example, although ^{99}Mo is formed in the presence of many other radionuclides, it is formed from uranium, not from molybdenum. The problem associated with the application of fission products is that it is necessary to separate the product of interest from all the others formed.

Accelerator-produced radionuclides

Accelerators are devices that accelerate charged particles (ions). Although accelerators of heavy ions have been developed, those used for isotope production are generally cyclotrons, which produce beams of protons (p or $^1_1H^+$), deuterons (d or $^2_1H^+$), helium-3 ions ($^3_2He^{2+}$), and α particles (α or $^4_2He^{2+}$) or electron accelerators, which produce beams of high-energy electrons. Cyclotrons can be used to produce radionuclides by a series of nuclear reactions, including the following:

(p,n)	(d,n)	(^{3}He,n)	(α,n)
(p,pn)	(d,p)	(^{3}He,2n)	(α,2n)
(p,d)	(d,α)	(^{3}He,α)	(α,pn)
(p,α)			

Since the bombarding particle always includes at least one proton, most of the reactions form nuclides on the proton-rich side of the line of stability; thus most accelerator-produced nuclides decay by photon (γ-ray) emission. In nearly all the examples given, the product nuclide is an isotope of a element different from the target element; consequently, carrier-free nuclides can be produced.

Electron accelerators can also be used to form proton-rich radionuclides by (γ,n) reactions using bremsstrahlung, produced by electron interaction with a target, as the γ source. One problem with this mode of nuclide formation is that only low specific-activity products can be prepared.

There is one major difference between the use of the cyclotron and the reactor to produce radionuclides. In a reactor there are many positions where a sample can be irradiated by thermal neutrons, and the irradiation may not be the main use of the reactor. The price of radionuclides produced by reactor irradiation is low; the price of fission products is largely associated with the separation process. In the case of an accelerator the whole machine is being utilized in producing a single radionuclide. There are nine commercial cyclotrons producing (or being constructed to produce) nuclides for nuclear medicine in the United States, whereas only one reactor is dedicated to that task. This means that cyclotron-produced radionuclides are very expensive and tend only to be used when they are far superior to any other agent. Cyclotron radiopharmaceuticals available at present (or in the final stages of approval) include ^{67}Ga, ^{201}Tl, ^{111}In, ^{127}Xe, ^{123}I, and the generator ^{81}Rb $\rightarrow$ ^{81m}Kr. Cyclotron-produced radionuclides are used only where there exists no competitive (albeit inferior) reactor-produced radiopharmaceuticals. Consider, for example, the use of iodine radionuclides. Iodine 131 and iodine 125 are both reactor-produced isotopes, with ^{131}I usually being fission produced, and ^{125}I being prepared from ^{125}Xe, as discussed above. Neither of these nuclides have ideal decay characteristics based on either half-life or decay mode. Iodine 123, with a 13.3-hour half-life and 159 keV γ ray, is suitable for visualization with an Anger camera. Also, for an equal number of millicuries, ^{123}I gives much less absorbed dose than does either ^{125}I or ^{131}I. It is, however, very expensive, since it has to be produced with a cyclotron by one of the following nuclear reactions:

$$^{122}\text{Te(d,n)}^{123}\text{I}$$
$$^{123}\text{Te(p,n)}^{123}\text{I}$$
$$\left.\begin{array}{l} ^{122}\text{Te}(^{3}\text{He,2n})^{123}\text{Xe} \\ ^{122}\text{Te}(\alpha\text{,3n})^{123}\text{Xe} \\ ^{123}\text{Te}(^{3}\text{He,3n})^{123}\text{Xe} \\ ^{127}\text{I(p,5n)}^{123}\text{Xe} \end{array}\right\} \xrightarrow{\text{2-hour half-life}} {}^{123}\text{I}$$

Consequently the use of ^{123}I has been limited by its price.

GENERATOR SYSTEMS

We have just discussed a parent-daughter system (^{123}Xe $\rightarrow$ ^{123}I) where the daughter half-life is longer than the parent half-life. The opposite situation, where the parent half-life is longer than the daughter, is of more general interest in nuclear medicine. There are actually only a very limited number of generator systems that can even be considered for use in nuclear medicine, and some of these systems are listed in Table 5-1.

There are two general types of parent-daughter systems that we need to consider; these are when the parent half-life is very much greater than the daughter half-life, or when it is just slightly greater than the daughter half-life. When the parent half-life is very much greater than that of the daughter, the radionuclides are said to be in "secular equilibrium." The generator system tin 113 (118-day half-life)/indium 113m (1.7-hour half-life) is an example where the nuclides are in secular equilibrium. When the parent half-life is just greater than that of the daughter, the radionuclides are said to be in "transient equilibrium."

Table 5-1. Important decay properties for several generators of short-lived radionuclides

Generator	Parent $T_{\frac{1}{2}}$	Daughter $T_{\frac{1}{2}}$	Daughter E_{γ}(%)
^{99}Mo-^{99m}Tc	2.78 days	6 hours	140 keV (90)
^{68}Ge-^{68}Ga	275 days	68 minutes	511 keV (176)
^{81}Rb-^{81m}Kr	4.7 hours	13 seconds	190 keV (65)
^{82}Sr-^{82}Rb	25 days	1.3 min	511 keV (192)
^{87}Y-^{87m}Sr	3.3 days	2.8 hours	388 keV (80)
^{113}Sn-^{113m}In	115 days	1.7 hours	393 keV (64)
^{132}Te-^{132}I	3.2 days	2.3 hours	Many
^{137}Cs-^{137m}Ba	30 years	2.6 minutes	662 keV (89)
^{191}Os-^{191m}Ir	15 days	4.9 seconds	129 keV (25)

The generator system molybdenum 99 (67-hour half-life)/technetium 99m (6-hour half-life) is an example of radionuclides in transient equilibrium.

Equations governing generator systems

If initially there is no daughter activity present in a generator, the daughter activity can be calculated from the equation

$$A_2 = \frac{\lambda_2}{\lambda_2 - \lambda_1} \cdot A_1^0 \, (e^{-\lambda_1 t} - e^{-\lambda_2 t})$$

where A_1^0 is parent activity at zero time, A_2 is daughter activity at time t, and λ_1 and λ_2 are the decay constants for the parent and daughter, respectively. This general equation can be simplified for the special cases of secular and transient equilibrium.

In the case of secular equilibrium, λ_2 will be very much greater than λ_1, and so

$$\lambda_2 - \lambda_1 \simeq \lambda_2$$

and the equation is simplified to

$$A_2 = A_1^0 \, (e^{-\lambda_1 t} - e^{-\lambda_2 t})$$

If we consider the growth of the daughter for a time, t, where t is much less than the half-life, $T_{\frac{1}{2}}$, of the parent but less than 7 times the $T_{\frac{1}{2}}$ of the daughter, our equation becomes simplified even more, and

$$A_2 = A_1^0$$

At equilibrium the amount of daughter activity present equals that of the parent. The growth of the daughter can be simplified to

$$A_2 = A_1^0 \, (1 - e^{-\lambda_2 t})$$

and this equation describes the growth of the daughter activity with time (Fig. 5-3).

In the case of the transient equilibrium, however, the time to reach equilibrium is not negligible compared to the parent half-life. In this case at equilibrium:

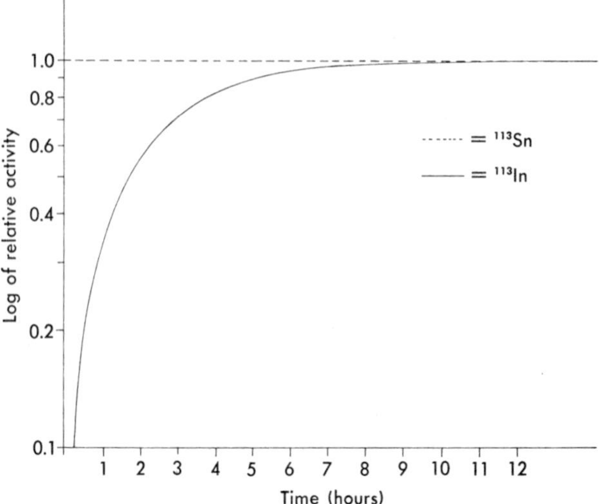

Fig. 5-3. Growth of ^{133m}In activity in a ^{113m}Sn → ^{113m}In generator.

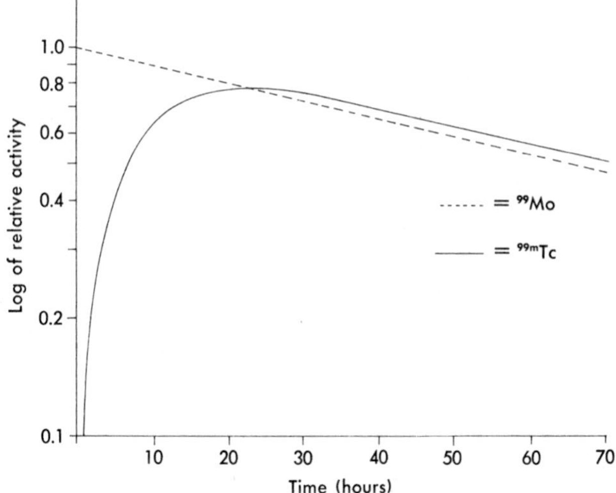

Fig. 5-4. Growth of ^{99m}Tc activity in a ^{99}Mo → ^{99m}Tc generator.

$$A_2 = \frac{\lambda_2 A_1}{\lambda_2 - \lambda_1}$$

The ratio of daughter activity to parent activity is given by the ratio

$$\frac{\lambda_2}{\lambda_2 - \lambda_1}$$

showing that the daughter activity is greater than the parent activity. The growth and decay of the parent and daughter for the ^{99}Mo-^{99m}Tc system is shown in Fig. 5-4; notice that the maximum ^{99m}Tc activity is present in approximately 24 hours (actually 22.83 hours).

Separation of daughter radionuclides

The most common method of separating daughter nuclides from their parents is by chromatography. In this discussion we consider the ^{99m}Tc generator, where the separation technique is based on the relative differences in the distribution coefficient values of aluminum oxide for the anions molybdate and pertechnetate. The passage of physiologic saline through an alumina column containing molybdate and pertechnetate will result in the elution of the pertechnetate. Commercial generators are designed to permit this separation to take place simply, reliably, efficiently, and with a very low risk of bacterial contamination. An ideal generator will have a good elution concentration profile, high ^{99m}Tc-elution efficiency, and low contamination with other radionuclides or aluminum. Since fission-produced ^{99}Mo is carrier free, generators made with this material can use smaller columns than are possible with ^{99}Mo produced by irradiation of ^{98}Mo. In the case of the former, the $^{99m}TcO_4^-$ is produced at a greater concentration than in the latter. The more ^{99}Mo present in a generator, the greater the radiation dose to the $^{99}MoO_4^{2-}$, and the lower the elution efficiency of the $^{99m}TcO_4^-$. Large commercial generators have an added oxidizing agent (such as potassium dichromate) which increases the elution yield of large generators by converting reduced molybdenum and technetium species formed by radiolysis back into the original compounds. Because of this radiation effect, there is a limit to the size (in curies) of a column that a generator may have.

The other type of system used to separate $^{99m}TcO_4^-$ from $^{99}MoO_4^{2-}$ is solvent extraction. Using this technique, one can separate the two species because one of them (TcO_4^-) is highly soluble in an organic solvent, whereas the other (MoO_4^{2-}) is only slightly soluble. In the solvent-extraction generator, molybdate dissolved in 5 N sodium hydroxide is extracted with methyl ethyl ketone. The methyl ethyl ketone is separated from the aqueous layer, passed through a small alumina column for removal of traces of molybdate extracted in the organic layer, and evaporated to dryness. The residue is then redissolved in saline prior to use. Advantages of the solvent-extraction generator are that larger amounts of ^{99}Mo can be extracted than are possible with chromatographic generators, and the final dissolution can be made in any amount of solvent; thus very high concentrations of pertechnetate can be obtained. The main disadvantage is that, with a complicated extractor, highly trained personnel are required. One of the major uses of solvent-extraction generators is to provide pertechnetate for the preparation of commercial instant technetium radiopharmaceuticals.

Since technetium 99m decays with a 6-hour half-life to the long-lived daughter technetium 99, trace amounts of carrier technetium 99 are always present in the generator eluate. This problem only becomes significant when the generator has not been eluted for a long period of time, and thus larger amounts of carrier technetium 99 have been allowed to accumulate.

Technetium radiopharmaceuticals

Technetium was introduced into nuclear medicine in 1957. This isotope, which was discovered in the late 1930s during neutron and deuteron bombardment of naturally occurring ^{98}Mo, heralded a new era for clinical nuclear medicine. The widespread acceptance of ^{99m}Tc as the radionuclide of choice for a variety of nuclear medicine imaging procedures has been based largely on its physical properties. These properties include the absence of beta decay, a half-life of 6 hours, and a 140 keV photon, which provides good penetration from deep-seated body organs and is easily imaged with both cameras and rectilinear scanners.

Technetium is eluted from a column generator with physiologic sodium chloride as the pertechnetate ion, a singly charged anion with oxygens at the corners of a tetrahedron. In this form, it is very similar in size to the iodide ion (Fig. 5-5) and its biologic distribution is similar. It concentrates primarily in the thyroid and salivary glands, gastric mucosa, and choroid plexus. Technetium will cross the placental barrier; thus one must consider the radiation dose that will be delivered to the fetus when determining the efficacy of such an examination on a pregnant woman.

Pretreatment of a patient with sodium or potassium perchlorate, or with Lugol's solution (a solution of 5% iodine [I_2] and 10% potassium iodide), influences the distribution of technetium. Perchlorate is approximately the same size as pertechnetate, and it competitively inhibits the uptake of the ^{99m}Tc-pertechnetate into the thyroid and salivary glands, choroid plexus, and gastric mucosa. Stable iodine 127 is also taken up by the thyroid gland and blocks the uptake of pertechnetate. Since the activity in the choroid plexus presents a problem in brain imaging, the advantages of per-

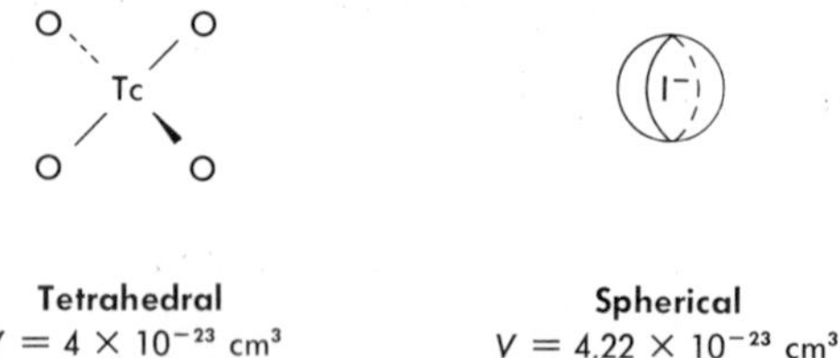

Fig. 5-5. Comparison of sizes of TcO_4^- and I^- ions. *V*, Volume.

chlorate or Lugol's pretreatment are readily appreciated.

Pertechnetate ($^{99m}TcO_4^-$) is excreted through both the kidneys and gastrointestinal tract. The colon is the critical organ in terms of radiation exposure and receives 1 to 2 rads per 10 mCi of ^{99m}Tc-pertechnetate.

In $^{99m}TcO_4^-$, technetium is in the +7 valence state and has all seven of the outer electrons involved in covalent bonding. It is by far the most stable of all valence states of technetium in aqueous solution.

Other than pertechnetate, the only radiopharmaceutical with a +7 valence state is technetium-sulfur colloid. Originally, sulfur colloid was prepared by acidification of the pertechnetate solution with hydrochloric acid to form the ionic technetium hexachloride ($TcCl_6^+$) species. Hydrogen sulfide gas was then bubbled into the solution (Fig. 5-6), and air oxidation of dissolved H_2S produced the carrier sulfur colloid. ^{99m}Technetium-sulfur colloid probably exists as the ^{99m}Tc heptasulfide coprecipitated with the colloidal sulfur particles, stabilized with gelatin. The final suspension is maintained at a pH of 5.5 to 6.0 to avoid conversion of the heptasulfide back to pertechnetate. In more recent kit preparations the technetium heptasulfide and the colloidal sulfur particles are generated by the decomposition of sodium thiosulfate.

Upon injection, technetium-sulfur colloid is rapidly cleared from the blood. The reticuloendothelial cells phagocytize the colloid particles. In normal subjects, approximately 90% of the ^{99m}Tc-sulfur colloid activity localizes in the liver, with the remainder taken up by the spleen and bone marrow. Metabolism of the colloid occurs only to a limited extent. Approximately 85% of the liver radiopharmaceutical is permanently localized within the liver. In a normal person the radiation dose is 400 mR/mCi to the liver.

Reduced technetium complexes

To prolong the intravascular biologic half-life of technetium, one can attach it to carriers that have a reasonably long life in plasma. First, chemical reduction of pertechnetate is necessary from the +7 valence state to a lower state where it will be a more reactive species capable of combining with a large number of compounds. This has been accomplished by use of a variety of reducing systems, for example, iron ascorbate, stannous chloride, and electrolytic methods. One such complex is technetium-labeled human serum albumin, which has been employed as a blood pool–scanning agent. The most common method of producing ^{99m}Tc-albumin involves the use of the stannous chloride–reducing system.

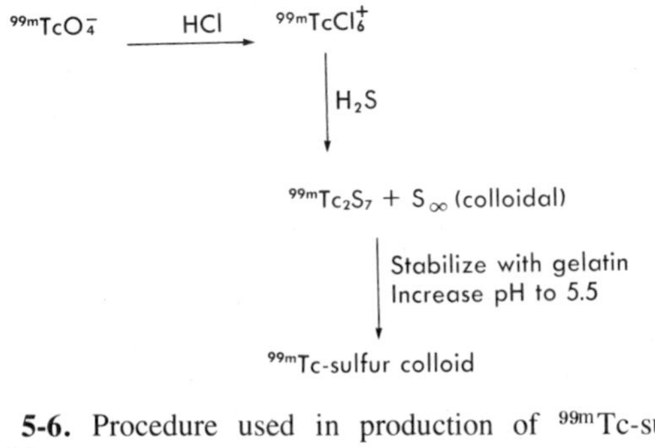

$$^{99m}TcO_4^- \xrightarrow{HCl} {}^{99m}TcCl_6^+ \xrightarrow{H_2S} {}^{99m}Tc_2S_7 + S_\infty \text{ (colloidal)}$$

Fig. 5-6. Procedure used in production of ^{99m}Tc-sulfur colloid.

Lung scanning with ^{99m}Tc requires aggregation of the ^{99m}Tc-labeled albumin (human serum albumin, HSA) using heat and a reducing agent in order to form particles of a size sufficient to be trapped in the capillaries of the lung. Since the smallest vessels in the vasculature range from 7 to 10 micrometers (μm) in diameter, labeled macroaggregates greater than 10 μm are readily trapped, a process that allows for lung visualization through capillary blockade.

Albumin microspheres are also used for lung imaging. The microspheres are prepared when an aqueous suspension of human serum albumin is dropped into hot oil; they are isolated by filtration and then mechanically sieved to sort out particles 10 to 45 μm in size. The albumin microspheres are treated with stannous chloride, which will reduce and bind technetium 99m. A suspending agent and ultrasound are used to assure a nonclumped suspension.

Another intravascular tracer is technetium-labeled red blood cells. One method of labeling is incubation of the red cells with the pertechnetate followed by the addition of stannous chloride (Fig. 5-7). Presumably the $^{99m}TcO_4^-$ crosses the cell membrane and is then reduced intracellularly by stannous chloride. Extracellular technetium is removed when the cells are washed with saline. Another method of labeling red blood cells, known as the pretinning method, involves the addition of stannous ion to the red blood cells before addition of the pertechnetate. This can be done either in vitro or in vivo. One procedure for pretinning involves the addition of stannous citrate to the red blood cells. The remaining extracellular tin is removed by use of the metal chelating agent EDTA. The cells are washed with saline to remove the stannous chelate and the pertechnetate is then added to the cells.

The effects of stannous ion (Sn [II]) on ^{99m}Tc-pertechnetate is not limited to an in vitro reaction. Alteration in the tissue distribution of ^{99m}Tc-pertechnetate in rats previously treated with stannous chloride has been noted. Even at a dose of 0.02 mg of Sn (II) per kilogram, an altered distribution of ^{99m}Tc-pertechnetate is observed up to 2 weeks after Sn (II) injection. The altered distribution is most likely attribut-

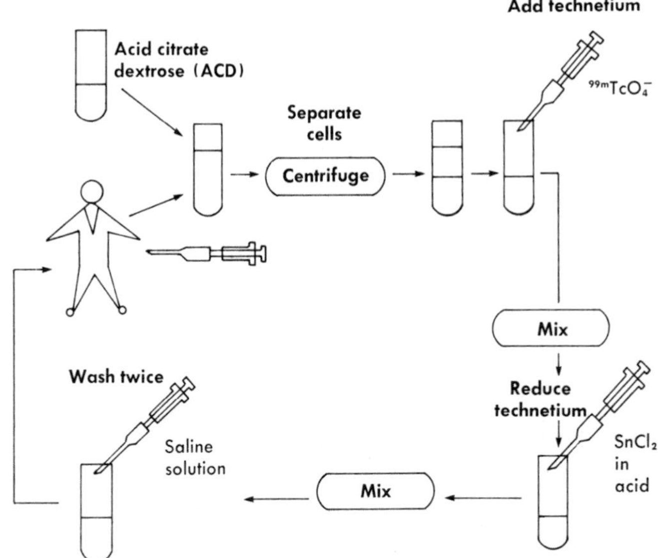

Fig. 5-7. Procedure used for in vitro labeling of red blood cells with ^{99m}Tc.

able to chemical reduction and fixation of ^{99m}Tc-pertechnetate to red cells.

This technique is presently being used in several institutions to label red blood cells in vivo by injection of $SnCl_2$ and then subsequent injection of ^{99m}Tc-pertechnetate. ^{99m}Tc–red blood cells can be used to image major blood pools and large peripheral vessels, and also for red blood cell–volume calculations. Technetium-labeled red blood cells can be damaged by either heat or chemical denaturation and can be used to image the spleen, which removes damaged cells from the circulation.

The group of technetium chelates that revolutionized nuclear medicine in 1972 were the phosphate derivatives for skeletal scintigraphy. Prior to this, one was forced to deal with the undesirable nuclear characteristics for the Anger camera of fluorine 18, strontium 85, or strontium 87m for bone imaging (Table 5-2). It has been suggested that localization of these Tc-phosphate complexes is dependent primarily on their pharmacologic activity. Bone mineral appears as hydroxyapatite, $3Ca_3(PO_4)_2 \cdot Ca(OH)_2$, in a lattice arrangement. The mechanism of uptake of the polyphosphates has not yet been clearly defined and may very well be associated with phosphate ion replacement in the hydroxyapatite crystal.

There are two basic types of phosphate compounds (Fig. 5-8). First, the inorganic phosphate derivatives, which have phosphorus-oxygen bonds (P—O—P), and, second, the organic phosphates, which contain a carbon atom bonded to two phosphorus atoms (P—C—P).

Table 5-2. Radionuclides used for skeletal imaging

Radionuclide	$T_{\frac{1}{2}}$	Energy
^{99m}Tc	6 hours	140 keV
^{18}F	110 minutes	511 keV
^{85}Sr	64 days	514 keV
^{87m}Sr	2.8 hours	388 keV

The inorganic phosphates are composed of differing lengths of the basic POP unit ($[—P—O—P—]_n$). When there is only one POP unit, the phosphate is pyrophosphate; when there is more than one POP unit, it is a polyphosphate. The polyphosphates undergo hydrolysis in vivo by alkaline phosphatases, which degrade them to the basic —P—O—P— unit, pyrophosphate. Since the bonds in the —P—O—P— moiety are subject to hydrolysis, the PCP bond of the organic phosphates, which are not degraded enzymatically, make organic phosphates more stable in vivo. Labeling of a phosphate with technetium is achieved first by reaction of the phosphate with stannous chloride to form a stannous phosphate chelate, followed by addition of technetium, which is reduced and complexes with the phosphate.

^{99m}Technetium-pentetic acid (^{99m}Tc-DTPA) and ^{99m}Tc-glucoheptonate are two chelates used for kidney studies. They are low molecular weight, water-soluble compounds that are rapidly excreted by glomerular filtration; hence images of the kidneys are obtained. (Pentetic acid and glucoheptonate are also used for brain imaging, since they remain in the circulation

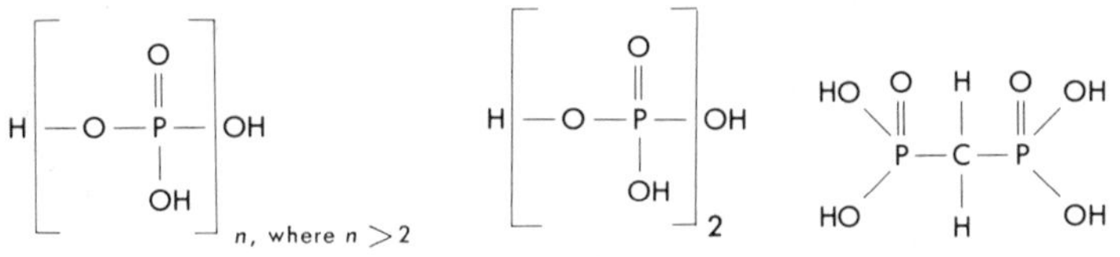

$$\left[H-O-\overset{\overset{\displaystyle O}{\|}}{\underset{\underset{\displaystyle OH}{|}}{P}}-OH \right]_n, \text{ where } n > 2$$

Polyphosphate

$$\left[H-O-\overset{\overset{\displaystyle O}{\|}}{\underset{\underset{\displaystyle OH}{|}}{P}}-OH \right]_2$$

Pyrophosphate

$$(HO)_2\overset{\overset{\displaystyle O}{\|}}{P}-\overset{\overset{\displaystyle H}{|}}{\underset{\underset{\displaystyle H}{|}}{C}}-\overset{\overset{\displaystyle O}{\|}}{P}(OH)_2$$

Methylene-diphosphonate (MDP)

Fig. 5-8. Phosphorus-containing compounds used in radiopharmaceuticals for skeletal scintigraphy.

until they are excreted by the kidneys.) DMSA (2,3-dimercaptosuccinic acid) is another chelating molecule that has been labeled with ^{99m}Tc and used for renal imaging. The cortical retention of this agent appears to be superior to other currently available agents, with 50% of the injected activity being retained in the renal cortex 1 hour after administration.

The chelating group iminodiacetic acid, capable of binding technetium, has been attached to biologically active molecules. These substituted iminodiacetic acids provide the basis for a new class of radiopharmaceuticals based on bifunctional drug and biochemical analogs. One of these analogs, the proposed technetium-99m gallbladder-scanning agent, is ^{99m}Tc-HIDA (*N,N'*-[2,6-dimethylphenylcarbamoylmethyl]iminodiacetic acid). In animal studies, 85% of the administered dose was cleared by the liver within 1 hour after injection and excreted through the biliary system into the gastrointestinal tract in a manner similar to ^{131}I–rose bengal.

GALLIUM AND INDIUM RADIONUCLIDES

Gallium and indium are both in group IIIA of the periodic table, which contains boron, aluminum, gallium, indium, and thallium. The two metals gallium and indium have similar chemical properties, and the production of their various radiopharmaceuticals are very similar; thus they are discussed together in this chapter.

Four radionuclides of indium and gallium have been used in nuclear medicine: ^{111}In, ^{113m}In, ^{67}Ga, and ^{68}Ga. Indium 113m and gallium 68 are short-lived, generator-produced radionuclides, as shown below:

$$^{113}Sn \xrightarrow[T_{\frac{1}{2}} = 118 \text{ days}]{} {}^{113m}In \xrightarrow[T_{\frac{1}{2}} = 1.7 \text{ hours}]{\text{I.T. (390 keV)}} {}^{113}In$$

$$^{68}Ge \xrightarrow[T_{\frac{1}{2}} = 275 \text{ days}]{} {}^{68}Ga \xrightarrow[T_{\frac{1}{2}} = 68 \text{ minutes}]{88\%\ \beta^+ \quad 12\% \text{ electron capture}} {}^{68}Zn$$

For the manufacture of the indium generators, ^{112}In is neutron irradiated to produce ^{113}Sn; the tin is then adsorbed onto a solid support, often zirconium oxide, and the indium is eluted with dilute (0.05 M) hydrochloric acid.

The germanium 68 used in the germanium-68/gallium-68 generator is cyclotron produced, often by the $^{69}Ga(p,2n)^{68}Ge$ nuclear reaction. In commercially available generators, the germanium 68 is eluted with a dilute solution of EDTA (ethylenediaminetetraacetic acid) to give gallium-EDTA.

Gallium 67 and indium 111 are both cyclotron-produced radionuclides, gallium 67 having a half-life of 78 hours and indium 111 a half-life of 67 hours. There are several nuclear reactions that can be used to produce the radionuclides, examples of which follow:

$$^{67}Zn(p,n)^{67}Ga$$
$$^{68}Zn(p,2n)^{67}Ga$$
$$^{111}Cd(p,n)^{111}In$$
$$^{109}Ag(\alpha,2n)^{111}In$$

As discussed earlier, these radionuclides are cyclotron produced and are therefore expensive. It is important to note that in the decay schemes of gallium 67 and indium 111, the abundances of γ rays for ^{67}Ga are 93 keV (40%), 184 keV (24%), 296 keV (22%), and 388 keV (7%) and for ^{111}In are 173 keV (89%) and 247 keV (94%). So, for the same number of millicuries injected, ^{111}In emits more countable photons.

Chemistry of gallium and indium

Gallium and indium have only one valence state (+3), which is stable in an aqueous solution; thus all the radiopharmaceuticals prepared from these nuclides contain the metal in the +3 oxidation state. This, of course, makes the chemistry of radiopharmaceutical production with indium and gallium simpler than that for technetium. The chemistry of both indium and gallium is similar to that of iron, and, like iron, both indium and gallium form very strong complexes with the plasma protein transferrin. This means that if a gallium or indium radiopharmaceutical is made with a weak chelate, the metal will simply exchange in vivo and form indium or gallium transferrin. Gallium and indium both form insoluble hydroxides, and this is of great importance in the understanding of gallium and indium radiopharmaceuticals. Since indium and gallium are trivalent, the hydroxide is formed by the reaction of 1 metal ion with 3 hydroxide ions:

$$In^{3+} + 3OH^- \rightarrow In(OH)_3 \quad \text{(solid)}$$

The equilibrium constant for the dissociation of the hydroxide

$$In(OH)_3 \rightarrow In^{3+} + 3OH^-$$

is given as follows:

$$K_{eq} = \frac{[In^{3+}][OH^-]^3}{[In(OH)_3]_{(solid)}}$$

Since the denominator is the concentration of a solid, which is constant, the equilibrium constant times the concentration of $In(OH)_3$ is called the "solubility product":

$$K_{sp} = [In^{3+}][OH^-]^3 = 10^{-33}$$

The solubility of indium hydroxide varies with the pH, and the exact relationship is shown in Fig. 5-9. It is seen that at a pH higher than around 4.5, indium hydroxide is very insoluble; thus at neutral pH it will precipitate or coprecipitate with other hydroxides such as iron hydroxide.

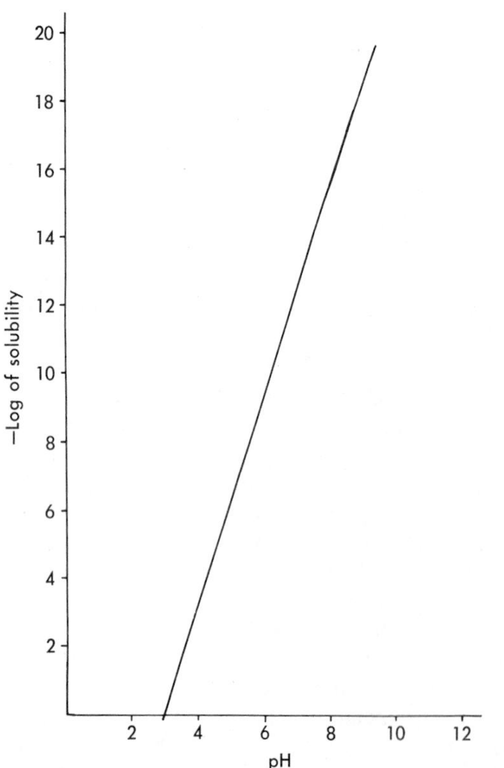

Fig. 5-9. Variation in solubility of indium hydroxide as a function of pH.

Insoluble hydroxides are formed by a simple increase in the pH of the eluate of a tin-indium generator, which contains 6% $In(H_2O)_6^{3+}$, 80.5% $InCl(H_2O)_5^{2+}$, 11.5% $InCl_2(H_2O)_4^{+}$, 2% $InCl_3(H_2O)_3$, or gallium in dilute HCl (which will have a similar composition).

Gallium and indium form weak complexes (that is, ones that will exchange rapidly with transferrin) that are soluble at neutral pH with lactate, citrate, and acetate. Both metals will also form very stable chelates with EDTA and DTPA (pentetic acid) that will only exchange slowly with transferrin.

Gallium and indium radiopharmaceuticals

We can now discuss the production of radiopharmaceuticals labeled with gallium and indium. With the exception of the eluate of the commercial germanium-68 generator, all the procedures are simple. The germanium-68/gallium-68 case is complicated by the fact that it is necessary to break down the strong ^{68}Ga-EDTA complex before the production of other radiopharmaceuticals is attempted. Although this can be broken down to gallium chloride by a number of procedures, it adds two or three steps to any radiopharmaceutical production.

Of all the gallium and indium radiopharmaceuticals, the most widely used is gallium citrate as an agent for imaging tumors and sites of inflammation. Upon injection of the citrate, greater than 90% of the gallium is bound to plasma proteins (largely transferrin), and the activity clears slowly from the plasma. The clearance of the activity from the plasma is enhanced if the plasma is saturated with gallium (or iron). Since the gallium binds to transferrin, gallium chloride has a very similar in vivo distribution to the citrate; however, the chloride must be injected at acid pH.

Gallium and indium colloids can be prepared very easily and conveniently, since the hydroxides are insoluble. Adding a small amount of ferric chloride, increasing the pH, and adding gelatin as carrier, allows the formation of colloids that can be used as liver- and spleen-scanning agents. Larger particles prepared in a similar manner can be used as lung-scanning agents. One can prepare strong gallium and indium chelates with DTPA or EDTA by simply mixing the gallium or indium chloride with the complexing agent and increasing the pH with a buffer. These chelates are rapidly cleared through the kidney and have been used for kidney and brain scanning, as well as for cisternography.

Because of the great stability of indium and gallium with transferrin, only very strong chelates can be used in vivo. A series of phosphonic acids with similar structures to DTPA and EDTA, but with phosphate groups instead of acetate moieties, can be used for bone or myocardial infarct imaging. Several research groups have developed bifunctional chelates where DTPA or EDTA is modified so that either one will not only bind indium or gallium, but also be covalently attached to a molecule of biomedical interest. For example, both DTPA and EDTA have been attached to proteins to form stable gallium and indium proteins other than labeled transferrin.

The final complex of gallium and indium of interest in nuclear medicine is the complex with 8-hydroxyquinoline (oxine). The complexes with oxine will exchange with transferrin, but in the absence of plasma they will label blood cells. Techniques have been developed to label red blood cells, leukocytes, lymphocytes, and platelets with indium 111, and erythrocytes and platelets with gallium 68. These agents remain stable in vivo for several days, since the metal is bound inside the cell. Labeled leukocytes have been used for abscess localization, and labeled platelets have been used to visualize both venous and arterial thrombi.

HALOGENATED RADIOPHARMACEUTICALS

Halogens are those elements in group VII of the periodic table; they include fluorine, chlorine, bromine, and iodine. Iodinated T_3 is used in thyroid function studies; however, the most widely used halogenated radiopharmaceuticals in both in vitro and in vivo nuclear medicine are halogenated proteins to measure plasma volume (iodinated albumin) or detect thrombi (iodinated fibrinogen), or for radioimmoassay (labeled antibodies). For applications in radioimmunoassay, ^{125}I-labeled proteins are generally used, whereas for in vivo studies, ^{125}I, ^{131}I, and ^{123}I have been used. Over the past few years there has been interest in the use of brominated compounds labeled with ^{75}Br or ^{77}Br for nuclear medical applications.

For the labeling of proteins, it is important to use "mild" iodination agents that do not denature the protein. Iodination of proteins involves the formation of positively charged iodine species that iodinate various groups in the protein. Under the conditions used for protein iodination, the tyrosine residues in the protein are iodinated to the greatest extent to give monoiodotyrosine and diiodotyrosine.

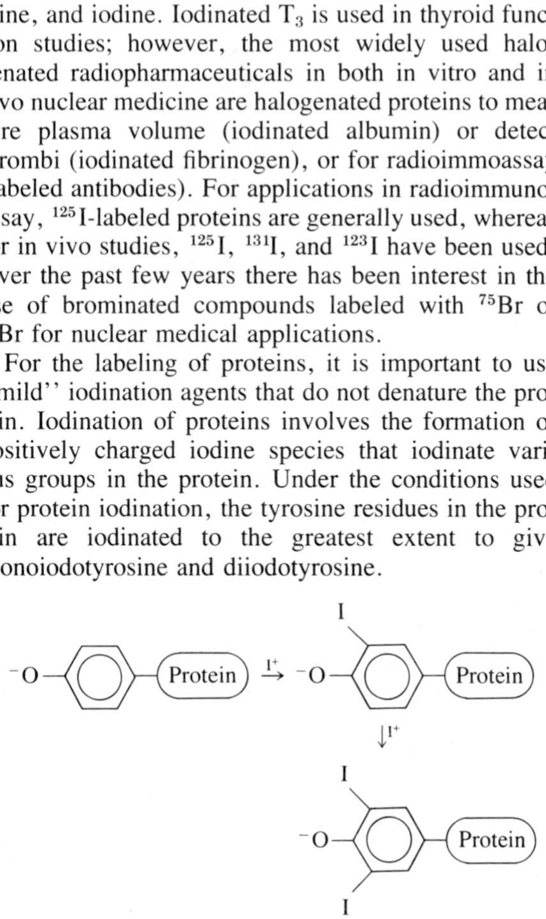

$^{-}$O–(phenyl)–(Protein) $\xrightarrow{I^+}$ $^{-}$O–(iodophenyl, I)–(Protein) $\xrightarrow{I^+}$ $^{-}$O–(diiodophenyl, I, I)–(Protein)

Histidyl and cysteinyl residues can also be iodinated, but to a lesser extent than the tyrosyl residues.

The various methods used for iodination include elemental iodine (I_2), iodine monochloride, chloramine-T, enzymes (peroxidases), and indirect methods. They are as follows:

1. I_2 iodination ("δ" indicates partial charge).

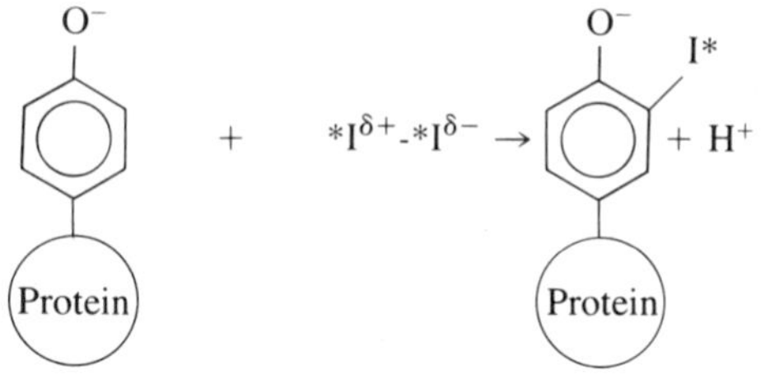

   O$^-$–(phenyl)–(Protein) + $*I^{\delta+}$-$*I^{\delta-}$ → O$^-$–(phenyl, I*)–(Protein) + H^+

2. Iodine monochloride iodination.

   $ICl + *I^- \xrightarrow{pH\ 4} *ICl \xrightarrow{pH\ 8}$ $HO^{\delta-}$-$*I^{\delta+}$ → O$^-$–(phenyl)–(Protein) → O$^-$–(phenyl, I*)–(Protein)

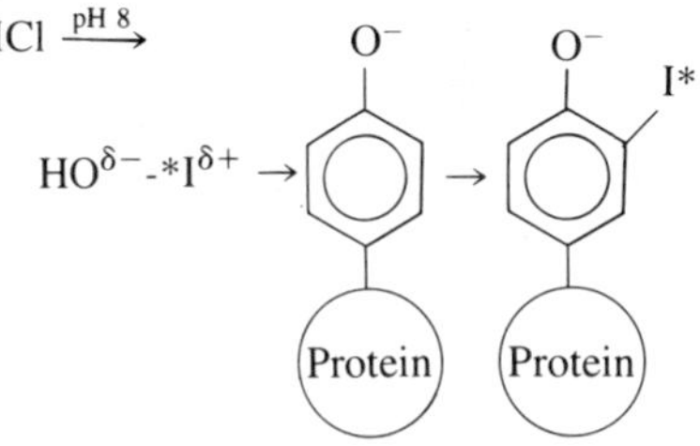

3. Chloramine-T iodination. Chloramine-T, which has the following structure:

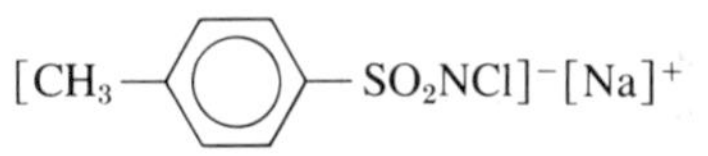

   $[CH_3$–(phenyl)–$SO_2NCl]^-[Na]^+$

   is a strong oxidizing agent that converts iodide ion to an iodinating species (possibly HOI). The exact mechanism of chloramine-T iodination is unknown.
4. Enzymatic iodination. Various peroxidases have been found to catalyze the iodination of proteins. Lactoperoxidase is commonly used, although chloroperoxidase, myeloperoxidase, and bromoperoxidase have also been used to halogenate with both iodine and bromine. In a typical iodination, the protein, enzyme, radioiodine, and a small amount of hydrogen peroxide are mixed to effect the labeling.
5. Indirect iodination. Most methods of direct iodination involve the addition of an oxidizing agent to the protein. One can avoid this by first iodinating a molecule with a structure similar to tyrosine, which can then be attached to the protein. *N*-succinimidyl-3-(4-hydroxyphenyl)propionate (SHPP) is the molecule that has been used for this application. The SHPP is initially iodinated, usually by the chloramine-T technique, sep-

Table 5-3. Comparison of methods used for halogenation of proteins

Method of iodination	Specific activity	Maximum labeling yield	Retention of biologic activity	Comments
I_2	Low	50%	Good	—
Iodine monochloride (ICl)	Low	100%	Good	—
Chloramine-T	Very high	100%	Poor	Highest activity per milligram of protein of all labeling methods
Enzymatic	High	100%	Good	Labeling of enzyme occurs; must separate from labeled protein
Indirect	High	≃80%	Variable, depends on role of site of iodination in biologic process	Involves attachment of a large group to protein

arated from the iodinating solution, and then mixed with the protein at pH 5.

Table 5-3 compares these various methods of iodination; the method of choice depends on the application. For in vivo studies, retention of biologic activity of the protein is probably the most important criterion in the choice of a labeling technique.

Other iodinated compounds used in nuclear medicine are iodohippuran and iodinated rose bengal. These are often labeled by exchange of radioiodine with stable iodine in the nonradioactive iodinated compounds. It is important to test for free iodine prior to use of any radioiodinated compounds.

OTHER USEFUL RADIONUCLIDES

Two other radionuclides in use at the present time are krypton 81m (from the rubidium-81/krypton-81m generator) and thallium 201. Rubidium 81 decays primarily by electron capture with a half-life of 4.7 hours. Its gamma emissions are at 450 and 511 keV, and its 13-second half-life daughter decays with the emission of 190 keV photons. Rubidium 81 can be prepared by the (α,2n) nuclear reaction on bromine 79, irradiated as potassium or sodium bromide. Preparations produced in this manner contain ^{82m}Rb. Pure ^{81}Rb can be prepared by the ^{80}Kr(^{3}He,pn)^{81}Rb or ^{80}Kr(d,n)^{81}Rb reactions by irradiation of enriched ^{80}Kr. For preparation of the rubidium-krypton generator, the rubidium is adsorbed onto either zirconium phosphate or an ion-exchange column.

Thallium 201 is prepared when natural thallium metal is bombarded with protons to produce 9.3-hour half-lived lead 201 by the (p,3n) nuclear reaction. The lead is separated from the thallium target and allowed to decay to thallium 201, which is isolated in carrier-free form.

Table 5-4. Tests for quality assurance

Test	Method
Radionuclidic purity	Gamma-ray spectroscopy
Radionuclidic purity (^{99}Mo breakthrough)	Differential photon absorption
Radiochemical purity	Chromatography
Chemical purity	Spectroscopy-colorimetry
Particle sizing	Microscopy
Sterility	Microbiologic testing
Pyrogenicity	Biologic testing

RADIOPHARMACY QUALITY CONTROL

Quality control can be divided into two categories: (1) manufacturer controls and (2) user quality controls applicable to "in-house" radiopharmaceutical preparations (Table 5-4). Manufacturers impose a large number of quality controls on their radiopharmaceuticals; each of these are described briefly.

Radionuclidic purity is the proportion of the total radioactivity present as the stated radionuclide. As well as determining the presence of other sources of radioactivity that are present, one must define the identity and amount of each radionuclide. This is essential for estimation of the overall radiation dose to the patient. For example, the radionuclide impurities found in ^{99m}Tc depend on the method of producing the ^{99}Mo; that is, is it obtained from neutron bombardment or fission-product separation? It also depends on the method of extracting the ^{99m}Tc from ^{99}Mo; that is, is it separated by use of methyl ethyl ketone extraction or column chromatography? The requirements for radionuclidic purity as listed by the *United States Pharmacopeia* for sodium ^{99m}Tc-pertechnetate solution are listed in Table 5-5.

Table 5-5. Allowable radionuclidic impurities in sodium ^{99m}Tc-pertechnetate solution expressed per millicuries of ^{99m}Tc administered

^{99}Mo → ^{99m}Tc generator containing neutron bombardment–produced ^{99}Mo		^{99}Mo → ^{99m}Tc generator containing fission-produced ^{99}Mo	
^{99}Mo	1 μCi (5 μCi per dose)	^{99}Mo	1 μCi (5 μCi per dose)
Other gamma ray–emitting nuclides	0.5 μCi (2.5 μCi per dose)	^{131}I	0.05 μCi
		^{103}Ru	0.05 μCi
		^{89}Sr	0.0006 μCi
		^{90}Sr	0.00006 μCi
		Other gamma ray–emitting nuclides	0.1 μCi
		Alpha particle–emitting nuclides	0.001 nCi

It is necessary to use a multichannel analyzer to assay for any gamma-emitting radiocontaminants that may be present. The manufacturer usually performs this type of quality control. In the case of ^{99m}Tc, one radiocontaminant that would be expected is ^{99}Mo. It is possible to assay routinely for ^{99}Mo breakthrough using most gamma-ionization dose calibrators and a lead vial holder of sufficient thickness to absorb the 140 keV gamma ray of ^{99m}Tc, but allow for penetration of the 740 keV gamma ray of ^{99}Mo. The U.S.P. allowable ^{99}Mo contamination is less than 1 μCi/mCi of ^{99m}Tc and less than 5 μCi per patient dose.

Radiochemical purity is the proportion of the stated radionuclide in the stated chemical form. The biologic distribution (and thus the quality of the image) and the radiation-absorbed dose are directly related to this purity. There are several chromatographic methods used to determine the radiochemical purity; some of these are gel-permeation chromatography, gas-liquid chromatography, and paper chromatography. The method applicable to routine in-house quality control of technetium radiopharmaceuticals is paper or instant thin-layer chromatography.

Chromatography involves the separation of a chemical mixture into its components along the stationary phase (adsorbent) because of different velocities in the mobile phase (migrating solvent). Radiochromatography differs from regular chromatography only in that the presence of the component is determined by the location of its radioactivity rather than by some other physical or chemical property. The R_f of a compound is defined as the measure of its migration distance.

$$R_f = \frac{\text{Distance of center of spot from origin}}{\text{Distance of solvent front from origin}}$$

R_f = "1," meaning that the component migrates with the solvent front

R_f = "0," meaning that the component remains at the point of application

The ideal separation of a component in a solvent system gives an R_f value greater than zero but less than one, to indicate a true chemical separation. A component that migrates at the solvent front or remains at the origin is not truly separated. However, for routine rapid quality control of technetium radiopharmaceuticals and the separation of known impurities (free pertechnetate, $^{99m}TcO_4^-$, and free reduced technetium, $^{99m}TcO_2$) from the labeled radiopharmaceuticals, R_f values of 1 and 0 are acceptable.

A typical paper radiochromatogram of ^{99m}Tc-sulfur colloid with $^{99m}TcO_4^-$ contaminant is shown in Fig. 5-10. The radioactivity in these peaks may be measured in several ways. One method involves the use of a commercial radiochromatogram scanner. In this system, the paper chromatography strip is moved across one or two detectors. Most commercial scanners were not designed for nuclear medicine application but for ^{14}C and ^{3}H detection; thus gas-flow detectors are commonly used. A rate meter indicates the count rate, and the counts are also graphically printed out by a strip chart recorder. A simplified scanner can be made by use of a strip chart recorder. In this system, the chromatogram is mechanically moved across a Geiger-Müller tube (covered by a lead sleeve with a slit opening) by a movement of the recorder. A manual counting system can also be employed, where the chromatogram is cut into strips and each strip is counted with a well counter.

Radiochemical purity of a radiopharmaceutical preparation can be calculated with the following expression:

$$\text{Percentage of radiochemical purity} = \frac{\text{Area } R}{\text{Area } R + \text{Area } I}$$

$$= \frac{\text{Counts in strip } R}{\text{Counts in strip } R + \text{Counts in strip } I \text{ (Total counts)}}$$

where R refers to the radiopharmaceutical and I refers to the impurity.

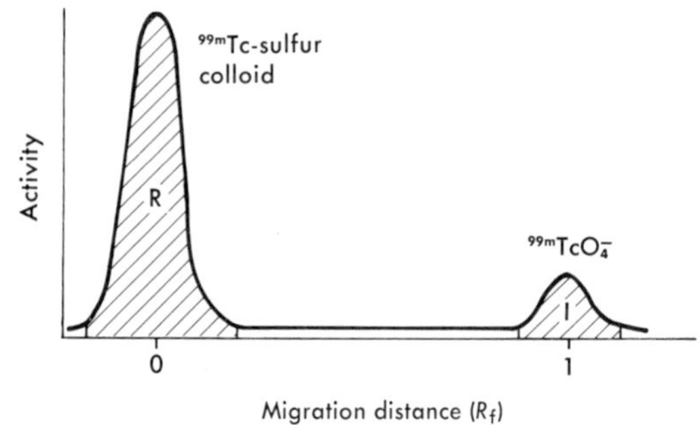

Fig. 5-10. Paper radiochromatogram showing separation of ^{99m}Tc-sulfur colloid from $^{99m}TcO_4^-$. *R*, Technetium-sulfur colloid; *I*, pertechnetate.

Chromatography of technetium-99m radiopharmaceuticals allows the determination of (1) the presence of free reduced technetium, (2) the presence of free pertechnetate, and (3) the amount of activity attached to the desired radiopharmaceutical.

There are three groups of ^{99m}Tc radiopharmaceuticals for chromatographic purposes:

1. The first group contains sulfur colloid. With this compound, the presence of free reduced ^{99m}Tc is not a problem, since technetium is bound in the +7 valence state. Sulfur colloid is a colloidal ^{99m}Tc radiopharmaceutical, and the chromatographic system for it involves a single solvent (acetone) and chromatographic paper to allow for determination of free pertechnetate.
2. Macroaggregated albumin (MAA) is a reduced radiopharmaceutical but is also particulate; thus the use of rapid quality control can only allow for the determination of free pertechnetate. Separation of free reduced ^{99m}Tc (which is a colloid at physiologic pH) and ^{99m}Tc bound to MAA is impossible with this system. Use of a Millipore filter with a 1 μm diameter allows separation of the colloidal reduced technetium and the technetium-labeled MAA. After the macroparticles have been removed, chromatography (with saline as the solvent) on the filtrate will determine the percentage of free $^{99m}TcO_4^-$ and the percentage of $^{99m}TcO_2$.
3. The third group contains pentetic acid (DTPA), glucoheptonate, methylene diphosphonate, pyrophosphate, polyphosphate, DMSA, and albumin. The chromatographic procedure for this group involves two solvents (acetone and saline solution) to determine the percentage of free pertechnetate, the percentage of free reduced technetium and the percentage of labeled radiopharmaceutical.

Table 5-6 shows the R_f values of technetium radiopharmaceuticals. The steps in a typical chromatographic procedure are as follows:

1. Place 1 ml of appropriate solvent in a 10 ml glass vial.
2. Mark the 1 × 6 cm chromatography strips into 1 cm segments with a pencil.
3. Spot the radiopharmaceutical using a tuberculin syringe in the center of the strip (near the first pencil mark located 1 cm from the bottom of the strip).
4. Place the strip into the solvent before the spot has air-dried to avoid air oxidation of the radiopharmaceutical. Allow the solvent front to move up to the strip until it has reached a height of 5 cm.
5. Cut the strips at the pencil markings and count each strip for activity, or use a scanner to measure the amount of activity along the strip.
6. Calculate the percentage of free $^{99m}TcO_4^-$, that of $^{99m}TcO_2$, and that of ^{99m}Tc bound to the radiopharmaceutical.

Chemical impurities are all the substances that either adversely affect the labeling or directly cause adverse bioeffects. In microgram concentrations, aluminum can adversely affect the formation of radiopharmaceuticals. Its concentration should not exceed 20 μg/ml in the neutron bombardment generator and 10 μg/ml in the fission generator. Aluminum can be detected by a spectrophotometric method. The absorbance of aluminum solutions of known concentrations after reaction with aluminum reagent is measured by the absorbance in the visible region of the spectrum; a standard curve is then prepared by a plot of the absorbance of solutions containing known concentrations of aluminum mixed with an aluminum reagent versus the aluminum concentration. This curve allows the determination of unknown aluminum concentrations. A more convenient method of aluminum determination is the use of an indicator paper impregnated with aluminon reagent (the ammonium salt of aurintricarboxylic acid) that yields a red color because of the chelate $Al(C_{22}H_{13}O_9)_3$ when Al^{3+} is present in a spot of the eluate solution. A solution of known Al^{3+} concentration (10 or 20 μg/ml) is used to provide a color comparison.

The presence of excess Al^{3+} can cause formation of colloidal Tc-Al particles by coprecipitation and therefore results in liver uptake, aggregation of sulfur colloid to larger particles with resultant capillary blockade (lung visualization), and labeled red blood cell aggregation with concomitant uptake of the damaged cells.

Most of the commercially available technetium kits contain stannous ion as the reducing agent. In most cases, more stannous ion is contained in each kit than is required to reduce and bind the technetium that is added; this excess of stannous ion has been found to

Table 5-6. Chromatographic systems used for quality control of ^{99m}Tc radiopharmaceuticals

Radiopharmaceutical	Solvent	Solid support	R_f		
			Free $^{99m}TcO_4^-$	Free $^{99m}TcO_2$	^{99m}Tc-labeled radiopharmaceutical
Sulfur colloid	Acetone	ITLC-SG*	1	—	0
Macroaggregated albumin (MAA)	Acetone	ITLC-SG	1	—	0
Pyrophosphate, Diphosphonate, Pentetic acid (DTPA), Glucoheptonate, 2,3-Dimercaptosuccinic acid (DMSA), Albumin	Acetone	ITLC-SG	1	0	0
	Saline	ITLC-SG	1	0	1

*Instant thin-layer-chromatography silica gel–impregnated glass-fiber sheets, Gelman Instrument Company, Ann Arbor, Michigan.

cause some problems. For example, liver uptake has been noted on an otherwise normal bone scan. This may be attributable to the formation of technetium-tin colloids, which tend to localize in the liver. Another problem that can occur with excess stannous ion is inadvertent red blood cell labeling. Since only a small percentage of the stannous ion present in some kit formulations is used to reduce and bind the technetium, a certain amount of free stannous ion is injected into the patient. This stannous ion will remain in the bloodstream for approximately 1 week. Upon injection of pertechnetate, such as for a brain scan, in vivo reduction of the technetium by the stannous ion can occur to cause red blood cell labeling. This would result in increased blood-pool activity.

Particle sizing of macroaggregated albumin (MAA) or human albumin microspheres (HAM) is another important quality control test. This microscopic test is conveniently conducted on a hemocytometer grid on which 100 to 200 particles are sized, and the entire field is scanned for unacceptably large MAA particles or clumping of human albumin microspheres.

The final series of quality control procedures is microbiologic testing. The objective of *sterility testing* is to provide assurance that the sterilization process was conducted properly. The sterility test required by the *United States Pharmacopeia* (U.S.P.) involves inoculation of the product in both fluid thioglycollate and soybean-casein digest media. Fluid thioglycollate provides conditions for growth of aerobic and anaerobic bacteria. Soybean-casein digest medium supports growth of fungi and molds. The official sterility test requires 14 days, but because of the short half-life of technetium, the U.S.P. allows for the release of these radiopharmaceuticals prior to the completion of the tests.

The U.S.P. also requires *pyrogen testing*. Pyrogens are any agents that cause a rise in temperature; they are generally considered to be heat-stable by-products of the growth of bacteria, yeasts, and molds. The word "pyrogen" is often used to mean bacterial endotoxin. To test for the presence of pyrogens, the U.S.P. requires the monitoring of three healthy rabbits for 3 hours after intravenous injection of the test sample. The test is positive if any rabbit shows an increase of 0.6° C or more above the base-line temperature, or if the sum of the three temperature increases exceeds 1.4° C.

Limulus amebocyte lysate (LAL), which has been isolated from the horseshoe crab *(Limulus),* reacts with gram-negative bacterial endotoxins in nanogram or greater concentrations to form an opaque gel. Gram-negative endotoxins are recognized as the most important source of pyrogen contamination. So, although this is not an official pyrogen test, it is possible that this in vitro test can be used as an initial screening procedure for pyrogens when a radiopharmaceutical is suspected as the cause of a pyrogen reaction.

The short half-life of ^{99m}Tc-labeled injectable drugs necessitates an emphasis on aseptic technique. The use of laminar–air flow enclosures to improve the environment for radiopharmaceutical formation helps to maintain sterility and apyrogenicity. A laminar–air flow work space provides a clean environment for radiopharmaceutical formulation and processing. HEPA (high-efficiency particulate air) filters remove particles of 0.3 μm and larger with an efficiency of 99.97%. Vertical laminar–air flow hoods are preferred in a radiopharmacy; horizontal flow presents a potentially serious contamination hazard to personnel, because it forces radioactivity out into the room. If the laminar–air flow cabinet is reinforced, it can support a leaded glass shield to provide protection for the technologist while the radiopharmaceuticals are prepared.

The practical approach in the nuclear medicine lab is the establishment of a continuous program of selective sterility testing in order to monitor the effectiveness of personnel aseptic technique. One technetium preparation should be saved each week, allowed to decay for a week, and then taken to the lab for bacteriologic testing. If aseptic technique has been correctly followed, there will be no bacterial contamination.

ACKNOWLEDGMENT

This chapter is based on a series of lectures presented by the authors and their colleagues to the nuclear medicine technologist trainees at the Mallinckrodt Institute of Radiology. The help of these colleagues, especially Maria G. Straatman, is appreciated.

SUGGESTED READINGS

Subramanian, G., Rhodes, R. A., Cooper, J. F., and Sodd, V. J., editors: Radiopharmaceuticals. New York, 1975, The Society of Nuclear Medicine, Inc.

Welch, M. J., editor: Radiopharmaceuticals and other compounds labelled with short half-lived radionuclides, Oxford, 1977, Pergamon Press.

Chapter 6

RADIATION SAFETY AND PROTECTION

Lisa B. Goldworm and Richard A. Goldworm

The Occupational Safety and Health Administration (OSHA) governs the use of all ionizing radiation. By-product material is controlled by the Nuclear Regulatory Commission (NRC). OSHA's authority is identical to that of the NRC, and in general the regulations of the NRC are used when one deals with any radioactive material. These are published in Title 10 of the Code of Federal Regulations (10CFR). OSHA Regulations are published in Title 29, Part 1910 of the Code of Federal Regulations (29CFR, Part 1910).

To use radioactive material, an individual or institution must have a license from the NRC or the state where the material is used.[2] If a state has the authority to issue a license, it is referred to as an agreement state. To be an agreement state, it must pass legislation that governs the use of radioactive material in the same manner as the NRC. It must also establish its own regulating agency and inspection program.

The type of license obtained depends on the scope and size of nuclear medicine practice and research capabilities of the institution. Regardless of the type of license, each institution must have an individual designated as a radiation safety officer,[2] who is trained in radiation safety and who is responsible for meeting the requirements of the NRC or agreement state.

CLASSIFICATION OF AREAS[2]

Unrestricted area means any area whose access is not controlled by the licensee for purpose of protection of individuals from exposure to radiation and radioactive materials, and any area used for residential quarters. It is further defined as an area in which, if an individual were continuously present, could not receive a dose in excess of 2 millirems in any one hour or 100 millirems in any 7 consecutive days.

Restricted area means any area whose access is controlled by the licensee for purposes of protection of individuals from exposure to radiation and radioactive materials. Permissible dose levels for individuals with access to restricted areas are considerably higher than for those in unrestricted areas and can be found in 10CFR, Part 20.

Posting of signs means that each radiation area shall be conspicuously posted with a sign or signs bearing the conventional three-bladed radiation caution symbol and the words: "Caution radiation area" or "Caution high radiation area." A "radiation area" is defined as any area accessible to personnel, in which there exists radiation, originating in whole or in part within licensed material, at such levels that a major portion of the body could receive in any one hour a dose in excess of 5 millirems, or in any 5 consecutive days a dose in excess of 100 millirems. A "high radiation area" defines the dose delivered in any one hour to be in excess of 100 millirems.

PERSONNEL MONITORING[2]

The regulations of the NRC are designed to help ensure the health and safety of everyone involved with radioactivity. Since radioactivity is generally considered harmful to humans, dose limitations are placed on each individual. These limitations are referred to as the "maximum permissible dose" (MPD), established in 1958 by the National Council on Radiation Protection and Measurement. It allows the *radiation worker,* whose minimum age must be 18, to receive a maximum dose to the *whole body* of 5 rems per year.

The dose to the whole body, when added to the accumulated occupational whole body dose, shall not exceed 5 ($N - 18$) rems, where N equals the individual's age in years at his last birthday. For the general public, those persons 18 years of age or older, the MPD is 0.5 rem per year. For a pregnant woman, the MPD is 0.5 rem in the gestation period.

Exposure received by radiation workers is usually calculated by calendar quarter. A calendar quarter is any 13 complete consecutive weeks, starting with a date in January. The following is the MPD per calendar quarter:

1. Whole body; head and trunk; active blood-forming organs; lenses of eyes; gonads	1.25 rem
2. Hands and forearms; feet and ankles	18.75 rem
3. Skin of whole body	7.5 rem

A licensee may permit a radiation worker to exceed the limitations of (1) above if during any calendar quarter the total occupational dose to the whole body does not exceed 3 rems *and* the dose to the whole body, when added to the accumulated occupational whole body dose, does not exceed 5 $(N - 18)$ rems. The licensee must assure that no individual exceeds these limits. If exceeded, form NRC-3 must be filed and corrective steps must be taken to ensure that there is no recurrence. Depending on the exposure, the individual might be assigned either temporarily or permanently to a position not involving exposure to radiation.

The NRC maintains the philosophy that radiation exposures should be kept "as low as is reasonably achievable" (ALARA). Implementation of the ALARA concepts should maintain internal and external radiation exposure to personnel below 10% MPD. NRC regulatory guides 8.10 and 8.18 give information relevant to ensuring ALARA exposures.

Monitoring of personnel is accomplished by the use of either film badges or thermoluminescent dosimeters (TLD). In nuclear medicine both hand and body monitoring should be done. The film badge is in common use for body monitoring, and the TLD devices are primarily used for extremity exposure.

Internal radioactivity is monitored by bioassay. A typical bioassay for ^{125}I or ^{131}I is the measurement of radioactivity in the thyroid gland. This may be accomplished in the same way as the thyroid uptake measurement if one knows the efficiency of the instrument for the radioisotope in question using the following equation:

$$\frac{\left(\begin{array}{c}\text{Individual's}\\ \text{counts per}\\ \text{minute}\end{array}\right) - \left(\begin{array}{c}\text{Background}\\ \text{counts per}\\ \text{minute}\end{array}\right) \times \text{Efficiency}}{2.22 \times 10^{6} \text{ disintegrations per minute}} = \text{Microcuries in gland}$$

Bioassays for other isotopes may require urine, fecal, or sweat samples. If an accident occurs with unknown amounts and types of radionuclides, a whole body count may be warranted, but this is rare.

Instructions to workers[2]

Training sessions with all persons handling licensed materials are necessary at least annually. All licensees are required to inform individuals working in or frequenting restricted areas of the following:

1. Proper storage, transfer, or use of radioactive materials or radiation in such portions of that area
2. Health-protection problems associated with exposure to such materials or radiation
3. Precautions or procedures to minimize exposure
4. Purposes and functions of protective devices employed

Additionally, the licensee shall instruct such individuals in:

1. The applicable provisions of the NRC regulations concerning exposure to personnel
2. Their responsibility to report promptly to the licensee any condition that may lead to or cause a violation of NRC regulations or to unnecessary exposure to radiation or radioactive material
3. The appropriate response to warnings in the event of any unusual occurrence or malfunction that may involve exposure

The licensee shall also advise workers concerning radiation exposure reports pursuant to Part 19.13 of 10CFR.

All radiation workers should be aware and understand special precautions relating to exposure during pregnancy. Federal guidelines state the occupational exposure for the expectant mother should not exceed 0.5 rem. Information relating to this is found in USNRC Regulatory Guide 8.13.

LABORATORY SAFETY

To help ensure a safe laboratory the following regulations must be adhered to by *all* personnel:

1. Never eat, drink, smoke, or apply cosmetics in areas where radioactive materials are used or stored.
2. Food and drink are never stored in areas where radioactive materials are used or stored.
3. Wear laboratory coat, gloves, or other protective garments at all times while handling radioactive materials.
4. Wear the appropriate monitoring device at all times while in areas where radioactive materials are used or stored.
5. Never pipet radioactive material by mouth.
6. Dispose of radioactive waste in designated containers.
7. Do not dispose of nonradioactive waste in designated radioactive waste containers.
8. Monitor hands, feet, and clothing before leaving the area and after each procedure.
9. Use absorbent pads on work surfaces and trays.
10. Work surfaces and trays should be smooth and nonporous.
11. Laboratory should be kept free of dust and dirt; floors should be double waxed.
12. Label all radioactive material containers with the chemical form and quantity of radionuclide, date of assay, and radiation symbol.
13. All equipment from a procedure using radioactive material should be segregated, monitored, and labeled if contaminated.
14. Radioactive material should be handled with

tongs or handling devices if appropriate to the procedure.

15. Appropriate equipment, for example, syringe shields, fume hoods, and glove boxes, should be employed to reduce personnel exposure.
16. Fume hoods used for procedures where volatile radioactive materials are employed should have a linear velocity of 150 feet per minute at the hood face.
17. The laboratory must be surveyed regularly and the results recorded.

AREA MONITORING

Monitoring of an area will detect radioactive contamination and allow evaluation of shielding of stored radioactive materials. The guidelines for laboratory surveys are as follows:

1. All elution, preparation, and injection areas will be surveyed daily with a low-range thin-window G-M survey meter and decontaminated if necessary.
2. Laboratory areas where only small quantities of radioactive material are used (less than 100 μCi) will be surveyed monthly.
3. All other laboratory areas will be surveyed weekly.
4. The weekly and monthly survey will consist of:
   a. A measurement of radiation levels with a survey meter sufficiently sensitive to detect 0.1 mRem/hour.
   b. A series of wipe tests to measure contamination levels. The method for performing wipe tests will be sufficiently sensitive to detect 100 dpm/100 cm^2 for the contaminant involved.
5. A permanent record will be kept of all survey reresults, including negative results. The record will include:
   a. Location, date, and type of equipment used.
   b. Name of person conducting the survey.
   c. Drawing of area surveyed, identifying relevant features such as active storage areas and active waste areas.
   d. Measured exposure rates, keyed to location on the drawing (point out rates that require corrective action).
   e. Detected contamination levels, keyed to locations on drawing.
   f. Corrective action taken in the case of contamination or excessive exposure rates, reduced contamination levels or exposure rates after corrective action, and any appropriate comments.
6. Area will be cleaned if the contamination level exceeds 100 dpm/100 cm^2.

Note: For daily surveys where no abnormal exposures are found, only the date, the identification of the person performing the survey, and the survey reports will be recorded.

DECONTAMINATION

Absorbent padding with an impervious backing is used to cover work surfaces to make decontamination easier. Many times the padding can be disposed of leaving no contamination on the work surface. Follow these rules if contamination occurs:

1. Use an absorbent material to remove liquid spills and to prevent spread.
2. Collect all materials involved, for example, absorbent material, bed sheets, clothes, and equipment, handling them with gloves and tongs if possible. These will later be disposed of or decontaminated. Avoid further contamination.
3. Use soap and water or designated commercial decontaminating solution until acceptable radiation levels are reached. If it cannot be decontaminated or monitored immediately, cover the area with an impervious-backed absorbent padding, absorbent side down, and tape it with "caution radioactive material" tape.
4. Always notify the radiation safety officer immediately.

PERSONNEL DECONTAMINATION

Any person who has become contaminated by radioactive material must be decontaminated quickly. This prevents absorption through the skin, ingestion, and spread of the radioactivity. These steps should be followed:

1. Remove all contaminated clothing.
2. If bleeding occurs, run water over the cut to encourage bleeding and thereby force out any foreign material.
3. If the chemical form of the radioactive material is corrosive in nature, follow procedures to neutralize the chemical and then decontaminate.
4. If lifesaving measures are necessary, for example, tourniquet for heavy bleeding, use first-aid procedures before decontaminating.
5. Use soap and water or designated commercial decontaminant for skin contamination.
6. Always notify the radiation safety officer and the physician in charge immediately.

STORAGE

Proper storage of any radioactive material is important to reduce personnel exposures, prevent accidental spills, and prevent material loss. For proper storage these rules should be followed:

1. All radioactive material should be stored behind or within lead shielding. The lead shielding should be thick enough to reduce activity to back-

ground levels. If this is impossible, a sign must be posted stating the exposure rate at the surface.
2. Do not store radioactive material in breakable containers unless the containers are placed in a second unbreakable container. The original container should be capped.
3. Do not store radioactivity in any unsecured area unless it is within a locked immovable container, for example, a locked refrigerator or freezer.
4. Never store radioactive material without a label stating type and amount of radionuclide, date of assay, and a radiation symbol.

RECEIVING SHIPMENTS[2]

According to the regulations of the NRC, packages must be monitored for surface contamination and external exposure. The following must be done and recorded.

1. Visually inspect package for any sign of damage.
2. Measure the exposure rate at 3 feet from the surface. It must be less than 10 mR/hour.
3. Measure surface exposure rate. It must be less than 200 mR/hour.
4. Put on gloves.
5. Open outer package following manufacturer's directions.
6. Open inner package and check final container for breakage or discoloration.
7. Verify the contents by comparing the requisition, packing slip, and bottle label.
8. Wipe external surface of final container using moistened cotton swab or filter paper held with forceps, and then assay and record.
9. Monitor the package and packing material:
   a. If they are contaminated, treat as radioactive waste.
   b. If they are not contaminated, obliterate labels and discard in regular trash.
10. If at any point in the procedure there is damage or the measured levels exceed those stated, notify the radiation safety officer. These records must be maintained for 2 years after disposal or transfer.

ACCOUNTABILITY AND DISPOSITION[2]

A running inventory and disposal record of radioactive materials must be maintained by all licensees. In the practice of nuclear medicine where radiopharmaceuticals are administered to patients it is extremely important that these records be complete, accurate, and well maintained. As a rule, records of receipt, storage, use, and disposition are kept in the "hot lab," or radiopharmacy. Typical examples of these records are shown in Figs. 6-1 and 6-2.

Fig. 6-1 is an example of a receipt and kit-preparation log sheet. Note that the lot number in column 10 is one assigned by the radiopharmacy and appears on the dispensing sheet (Fig. 6-2) and its label (Fig. 6-3) as well.

Fig. 6-2, the dispensing sheet, is an all-purpose record, in that it is used for purchased radiopharmaceuticals and technetium-99m compounds that are prepared from kits. The top left side of the form may be used for recording data from the manufacturer's label, and items 1 to 4 serve as a quality assurance check that the label information is correct.

Each time that a radiopharmaceutical is used, an entry is made on the dispensing sheet. When the radiopharmaceutical has expired or decayed to a point where it is no longer useful, or has been completely used, dispose of the container and contents if any remain.

As a general rule, technetium waste is best disposed of by allowing it to decay in an area that is adequately shielded for 10 half-lives or more. If, after monitoring, the waste is at background levels, it may be disposed of with the nonradioactive trash. If a laboratory has an adequate amount of storage space, other short-lived radionuclides, that is, thallium 201, gallium 67, or indium 111, may be disposed of in this manner.

In most institutions this is not usually the case, and so disposal must be by other means. Some radiopharmaceutical manufacturers will accept waste from their customers, but, in general, commercial disposal firms are employed to dispose of waste products. The firms provide containers for the waste and transport them to burial sites. Recently several states have closed burial sites within their borders, and the problem of waste disposal may become more severe.

Other types of disposal include release into the sanitary sewerage system, burial in soil, or incineration. For further information on these methods of waste disposal, the reader is referred to 10CFR, Part 20.301 to 20.305. The only exception to the waste-disposal requirements of the NRC is excreta from individuals being medically diagnosed or undergoing therapy with radioactive material that may be released into the sanitary sewer in any amount.

At the time a radionuclide is disposed of, a record must be generated indicating what form it was in and what quantity was disposed of. These records must be maintained until the NRC authorizes their disposition. This may present a problem particularly for those institutions using a large amount of radioactive material. 10CFR, Part 20.401 (c)(4) states: "Records which must be maintained pursuant to this part may be the original or a reproduced copy or microform if such reproduced copy or microform is duly authenticated by authorized personnel and the microform is capable of

RADIOPHARMACY RECEIPT AND KIT PREPARATION LOG									
Date	Radio-pharmaceutical	Surface reading (mR/hour)	3-foot reading (mR/hour)	Wipe test (net counts per minute)	Assay (mCi/ml)	Assay date	Assay time	Manufacturer	Lot number

Fig. 6-1. Radiopharmacy receipt and kit preparation log.

RADIOPHARMACEUTICAL DISPENSING LOG

Radiopharmaceutical__________

Date received__________

Institution lot number__________

Total activity__________ μCi or mCi (Cross out one:)

Total volume__________ ml

Concentration__________ μCi/ml or mCi/ml

Assay (hour/date)__________

Manufacturer lot number__________

Expiration date__________

Comments__________

1. Dose calibrator assay

   Whole vial__________mCi

   Total volume__________

   Hour/date__________

   1 ml aliquot__________mCi/ml

2. pH__________
3. Clarity__________
4. Particle size__________

Date	Time	Patient	Test	Decay factor	Activity	Dose calibrator	Milliliters removed	Milliliters left	Initials

Disposal: Date__________Total activity__________Total volume__________

Disposed by (initials)__________

Fig. 6-2. Radiopharmaceutical dispensing log.

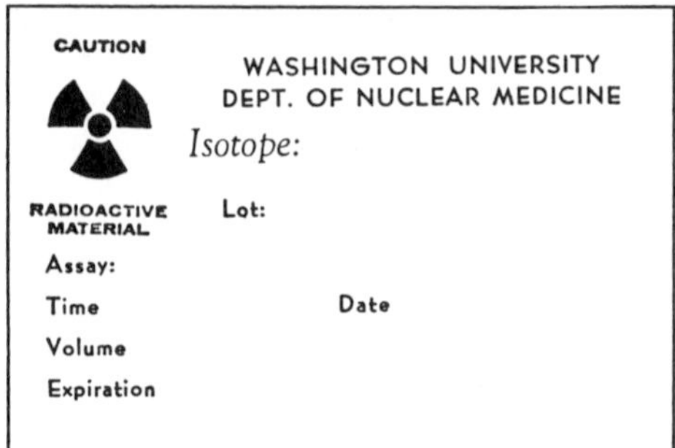

Fig. 6-3. Label.

producing a clear and legible copy after storage for the period specified by Commission regulations."

UNITS OF RADIATION MEASUREMENTS

Roentgen (R). The roentgen is the unit that is used in the measurement of total radiation exposure. One roentgen is defined as the amount of x or gamma radiation that produces 1 electrostatic unit (esu) of charge in 1 cc of dry air. Mathematically, this translates to the following:

$$1 \text{ roentgen} = 2.58 \times 10^{-4} \text{ coulombs per kilogram of air}$$

There are limitations inherent in the use of the roentgen as a unit. First, the roentgen is a measure of the total radiation exposure, but it has no relationship to the exposure rate. Second, the roentgen is defined only for x and gamma radiation. A basic use of the roentgen in the laboratory is with the survey meter, which measures the radiation level in units of milliroentgens per hour (mR/hour).

Radiation absorbed dose (rad). The rad is used in the measurement of the radiation energy absorption (dose) in matter. The rad is defined as the amount of radiation required for absorption of 100 ergs per gram of irradiated material. Recently, a new unit, the gray (Gy), has been proposed to replace the rad as the basic unit of radiation absorption. The gray is defined as the amount of ionizing radiation required for absorption of 1 joule per kilogram of irradiated material. Therefore, the gray would be equal to 100 rads. The rad, being the basic unit for absorbed dose, has many uses in the laboratory. One basic use is the measurement of exposure of the organ(s) of interest from the injection of a radiopharmaceutical.

Relative biologic effectiveness (RBE). This factor was postulated when it was realized that different types of ionizing radiation have different effects in biologic material. By definition the RBE is the rate of the absorbed dose of x or gamma radiation required to have the same biologic effect as the absorbed dose of the type of radiation of interest.

$$\text{RBE} = \frac{\text{Dose, in rads, of x or gamma radiation}}{\text{Dose, in rads, of radiation of interest that gives the same effect}}$$

For example, it has been found that 0.05 rad of 1 meV alpha radiation gives the same biologic response as 1 rad of x or gamma radiation; therefore, the RBE value for 1 meV of alpha radiation is 20.

Obviously, all ionizing radiation gives rise to the same types of biologic response, but different types of ionizing radiation give rise to different degrees of biologic response. Therefore, different types of radiation cause different amounts of ionization and consequently different RBE values.

Roentgen equivalent man (rem). The RBE concept makes it possible to express the amount of radiation absorption by a biologic system. The unit involved in this respect is called the "rem." The rem measures the biologically effective dose resulting from exposure to ionizing radiation. The rem equals the dose, in rads, multiplied by the RBE.

$$\text{rem} = \text{rad} \times \text{RBE}$$

Currently the tabulated lists of permissible exposure of humans to ionizing radiation are given in rem units.

There is a major limitation associated with the use of the RBE and consequently the rem. Although it is true that different types of ionizing radiation cause different amounts of biologic damage per rad, it is also true that the same type of ionizing radiation will cause different amounts of biologic damage per rad in *different* biologic tissues. This is true because there are many other factors, such as pH and oxygen content in tissue, that affect the amount of biologic response to the ionizing radiation. There the use of a single-valued RBE for a specific type of ionizing radiation is erroneous.

The concept of the RBE (rem dose) as a unit is now limited to radiation biology. A unit, the quality factor (QF), is currently in use instead of the RBE. QF is another means for expressing the linear energy transfer–dependent response of a biologic system to ionizing radiation. If two different types of ionizing radiation invoke the same degree of biologic response per rad absorption, their QF values will be the same. The QF is an empirically determined unit usually resulting from analysis of animal experiments.

Another factor arises in determination of biologic effectiveness of radiation. This factor is the distribution of the radionuclide within the body. The biologic response would depend on the distribution. Therefore the distribution factor (DF) must be taken into account. This relationship is expressed as:

Radiation protection dose in rem = Dose in rad × QF × DF

Specific ionization (SI). This unit is a measurement of the average number of ions pairs produced per unit of path traveled by the incident radiation.

Linear energy transfer (LET). The LET and the SI are closely related. The SI deals with the number of events, whereas the LET deals with the energy expended over the SI events. The LET is the average loss of energy per unit of path traveled by the incident radiation.

METHODS OF RADIATION PROTECTION

The only completely safe method of avoiding exposure to all radiation, outside of cosmic-ray bombardment, is never to work with or come near *any* radioactive materials. This complete shielding is somewhat impossible if one is to live these days.

For anyone who plans to work in nuclear medicine or in any related field, some exposure to ionizing radiation is an inescapable hazard because you will usually be working with or near radioactive materials. Therefore you must be aware of the necessity of methods for radiation protection. The three basic methods for radiation protection are distance, shielding, and time. The careful use of a combination of these three methods will minimize your radiation exposure.

Distance

This method of radiation protection is obvious for particulate radiation in which the range in air is measured in centimeters (or less!). If you were to stand about 3 feet (1 meter) from an alpha or beta source, your exposure rate is effectively zero. Remember that x and gamma radiation often accompany alpha and beta decay and that their respective ranges in air are much greater than 3 feet.

How does distance provide protection from x and gamma radiation? As you might expect, the farther you are from a radiation source, the lower your exposure rate. At first you might assume that the decrease in exposure rate is a linear function; however, the decrease is quadratic in nature. If the distance between the source and the detector (or object of interest) is doubled, then the exposure rate is decreased by a *factor of 4*. This rule is known as the "inverse square law." It applies to all types of radiation, including light waves, sound waves, microwaves, and of course x and gamma radiation. A formal statement of the inverse square law is as follows:

The amount of radiation (that is, *intensity* of radiation) at a given distance from a source is inversely proportional to the square of the distance.

Symbolically the inverse square law would read:

$$I_1D_1^2 = I_2D_2^2$$

whereby I_1 is intensity (exposure rate) at distance (D_1) from a point source, and I_2 is intensity (exposure rate) at distance (D_2) from the same point source.

Problem: A point source registers 400 mR/hour at a distance of 3 cm. Answer the following:

1. What does the point source register at 6 cm?
2. What does the point source register at 1 cm?
3. At what distance does the point source register 800 mR/hour?
4. At what distance does the point source register 6.25 mR/hour?

SOLUTION: Use the equation with the following values:

$$I_1 = 400 \text{ mR/hour}$$
$$D_1 = 3 \text{ cm}$$

1. $D_2 = 6$ cm; solve for I_2:

$$I_1D_1^2 = I_2D_2^2$$
$$(400 \text{ mR/hour})\ (3 \text{ cm})^2 = I_2\ (6 \text{ cm})^2$$
$$\frac{(400 \text{ mR/hour})\ (3 \text{ cm})^2}{(6 \text{ cm})^2} = I_2 = 100 \text{ mR/hour}$$

2. $D_2 = 1$ cm; solve for I_2:

$$I_1D_1^2 = I_2D_2^2$$
$$(400 \text{ mR/hour})\ (3 \text{ cm})^2 = I_2\ (1 \text{ cm})^2$$
$$\frac{(400 \text{ mR/hour})\ (3 \text{ cm})^2}{(1 \text{ cm})^2} = I_2 = 3600 \text{ mR/hour} = 3.6 \text{ R/hour}$$

3. $I_2 = 800$ mR/hour; solve for D_2:

$$I_1D_1^2 = I_2D_2^2$$
$$(400 \text{ mR/hour})\ (3 \text{ cm})^2 = (800 \text{ mR/hour})\ (D_2)^2$$
$$\frac{(400 \text{ mR/hour})\ (3 \text{ cm})^2}{800 \text{ mR/hour}} = D_2^2 = 4.5 \text{ cm}^2$$
$$D_2 = 2.12 \text{ cm}$$

4. $I_2 = 6.25$ mR/hour; solve for D_2:

$$I_1D_1^2 = I_2D_2^2$$
$$(400 \text{ mR/hour})\ (3 \text{ cm})^2 = (6.25 \text{ mR/hour})\ (D_2)^2$$
$$\frac{(400 \text{ mR/hour})\ (3 \text{ cm})^2}{(6.25 \text{ mR/hour})} = D_2^2 = 576 \text{ cm}^2$$
$$D_2 = 24 \text{ cm}$$

As you can see, distance is a simple, effective method of minimizing the radioactive exposure rate and is used generally in conjunction with shielding for radiation protection.

Shielding

Shielding is another method of radiation protection. For photonic radiation (x and gamma radiation), shielding is a practical method of minimizing exposure. How does shielding work as a method of radiation protection? One must first consider how photonic radiation is attenuated and what do we mean by attenuation? Attenuation is the process of decreasing the intensity and energy of gamma radiation or x radiation by nuclear and electronic interactions. Photonic radiation is attenuated in four ways:

1. Photoelectric effect
2. Compton scattering
3. Pair production
4. Nuclear absorption of the photons resulting in nuclear reactions

These four methods of photonic attenuation are discussed in detail in Chapter 2. We are only concerned with the total attenuation of photonic radiation, which is the sum of these four methods.

Lead is considered a good shielding material. Why? The density and thickness of the shielding material are interrelated in respect to radiation attenuation. Density of the shielding material is directly proportional to its stopping power (effectiveness in attenuation of photonic radiation). The thickness of the shielding material follows the same relationship. Therefore shielding is usually measured in terms of density thickness, which is given by the following:

$$\text{Density} \times \text{Thickness} = \text{Density thickness}$$

$$\frac{\text{g}}{\text{cm}^3} \times \text{cm} = \text{g/cm}^2$$

Usually these concepts are reliable; however, in actual calculations they do not always hold true. Lead is a very good shielding material because of its high density (11.84 g/cm^3 at 25° C).

From this discussion one might expect that attenuation of photonic radiation is linearly related to density thickness of the shielding material, but this is not the case. It is a logarithmic function with respect to thickness (linear attenuation) or density thickness (mass attenuation). Quantitatively, these relationships depend on attenuation coefficients μ and μ/ρ, the linear coefficient and the mass coefficient, respectively. The linear attenuation coefficient, μ, is defined as the fraction of the amount of photonic radiation removed from the initial amount per centimeter of absorbing (shielding) material. The formula for linear attenuation is:

$$I_2 = I_1 e^{-\mu t}$$

where I_2 is the amount of gamma radiation per unit area (intensity) that emerges from the shielding material; I_1 is the amount of radiation per unit area before absorption (initial intensity); μ is the linear attenuation coefficient; and t is the thickness in centimeters of shielding material.

Problem: A point source has an initial intensity of 200 mR/hour. What is the intensity of the source after it passes through 3 cm of an absorber, which has a linear coefficient of 0.15 cm^{-1}?

SOLUTION:

$$\begin{aligned} I_2 &= I_1 e^{-\mu t} \\ I_1 &= 200 \text{ mR/hour} \\ t &= 3 \text{ cm} \\ \mu &= 0.15 \text{ cm}^{-1} \end{aligned}$$

$$\begin{aligned} I_2 &= (200 \text{ mR/hour})\, e^{-(0.15 \text{ cm}^{-1})(3 \text{ cm})} \\ I_2 &= (200 \text{ mR/hour})\, e^{-0.45} \\ I_2 &= (200 \text{ mR/hour})(0.638) \\ I_2 &= 127.6 \text{ mR/hour} \end{aligned}$$

The mass attenuation coefficient, μ/ρ, is defined as the fraction of the photonic intensity removed from the initial photonic intensity per gram/cm^2 of absorbing (shielding) material. The formula for mass attenuation is

$$I_2 = I_1 e^{-(\mu/\rho)(\rho t)}$$

where I_2 is the intensity of gamma radiation that emerges from the shielding material; I_1 is the initial intensity of the gamma radiation; ρ is the density of the shielding material (g/m^3); t is the thickness in centimeters of shielding material; and μ/ρ is the mass attenuation coefficient (cm^2/g).

Problem: What is the measured intensity of gamma radiation from a source that had an initial intensity of 300 mR/hour after it passes through 2 cm of a shielding material that has a density of 7.1 g/cm^3 and a mass attenuation coefficient of 0.07 cm^2/g.

SOLUTION:

$$\begin{aligned} I_2 &= I_1 e^{-(\mu/\rho)(\rho t)} \\ I_1 &= 300 \text{ mR/hour} \\ t &= 2 \text{ cm} \\ \rho &= 7.1 \text{ g/cm}^3 \\ \mu/\rho &= 0.07 \text{ cm}^2\text{/g} \end{aligned}$$

$$\begin{aligned} I_2 &= (300 \text{ mR/hour})\, e^{-(0.07 \text{ cm}^2/\text{g})(7.1 \text{ g/cm}^3)(2 \text{ cm})} \\ I_2 &= (300 \text{ mR/hour})\, e^{-(0.994)} \\ I_2 &= (300 \text{ mR/hour})(0.369) \\ I_2 &= 110.7 \text{ mR/hour} \end{aligned}$$

Usually one is not concerned with calculating attenuation of photonic radiation, but you will be dealing with shielding and its effect on radiation. These formulas show that attenuation of photonic radiation is predictable. You will be more concerned with a unit known as the half-value layer (HVL). This unit is defined as the thickness of any shielding material necessary to reduce the intensity of the radiation by a factor of two. This relationship is shown in the following manner:

$$I_2 = I_1 \, (\tfrac{1}{2}) \text{ number of HVLs}$$

Problem: The *final intensity* of a gamma emitter is to be 25 mR/hour, and its initial intensity is 800 mR/hour. How many HVLs of absorber must be placed in front of this gamma emitter?

SOLUTION:

$$I_2 = I_1 \, (\tfrac{1}{2})^{\text{number of HVLs}}$$
$$I_2 = 25 \text{ mR/hour}$$
$$I_1 = 800 \text{ mR/hour}$$
$$25 = 800 \, (\tfrac{1}{2})^{\text{number of HVLs}}$$
$$\frac{25}{800} = (\tfrac{1}{2})^{\text{number of HVLs}}$$
$$\frac{1}{32} = (\tfrac{1}{2})^{\text{number of HVLs}}$$
$$(\tfrac{1}{2})^5 = (\tfrac{1}{2})^{\text{number of HVLs}}$$

5 HVLs necessary

Problem: The HVL of the absorber is 2.4 cm. How much absorber must be placed in front of the gamma-ray emitter in the last example to fulfill the conditions set?

SOLUTION:

1 HVL = 2.4 cm
5 HVLs = 12 cm

In summary, let's look at the factors involved in the use of shielding as a method of radiation protection.

1. Alpha and beta radiation can be completely absorbed by a minimum amount of shielding, but gamma and x radiation are never completely absorbed.
2. The use of shielding in the case of gamma and x radiation is to reduce the intensity to acceptable levels.
3. Density and thickness of the shielding material is directly related to the effectiveness of the attenuation of gamma and x radiation.
4. Any material regardless of its density or thickness will attenuate some x and gamma radiation.

Time

The third common method of protection from radiation exposure is time. Obviously the longer a person remains in a radiation field, the greater his exposure will be. A simple formula for determining exposure is

$$\text{Exposure (mR)} = \text{Exposure rate (mR/hour)} \times \text{Time (hour)}$$

Milliroentgen (mR) is equivalent to mrem if x or gamma radiation is the source because the RBE value for both is 1.

$$\text{Dose (mrem)} = \text{Dose (rads)} \times \text{RBE}$$

Thus:

$$\text{Dose (mrem)} = \text{Dose (rads)}$$

Nuclear medicine personnel should strive for radiation safety awareness at all times. The ''hot lab,'' or radiopharmacy, is not the place to hold long conversations or conduct meetings.

Many times, intravenous injections are difficult to accomplish and require multiple attempts, which use up *time*. Even when syringe shielding is employed, there is still some exposure for the technologist. An alternative method would be to use a scalp vein infusion set (butterfly needle) to attempt the venipuncture. After successful venipuncture, the shielded syringe is attached and the injection made. This method reduces the length of *time* the technologist must spend in holding the shielded syringe.

By itself the ALARA concept is nothing more than a concept. To make it function requires awareness and a sense of responsibility on the part of the radiation worker—*you*—the nuclear medicine technologist.

REFERENCES

1. Nuclear regulatory medical guide 10.8, Guide for the preparation of applications for medical programs, Washington, D.C., 1979, U.S. Nuclear Regulatory Commission.
2. Code of Federal Regulations, Title 10, Chapter 1, Washington, D.C., 1978, U.S. Government Printing Office.

Chapter 7

COMPUTER SCIENCE

Trevor D. Cradduck

In the early 1970s it might have been difficult to justify the need for a chapter on computer science in a textbook on nuclear medicine technology. The advent of commercially available nuclear-medicine computer systems has precipitated a rapid growth in the number of installations of such devices and there is now a number of nuclear medicine procedures being performed that would otherwise be impossible, or at least inordinately difficult, without the assistance of a computer.

Computers are being used primarily for purposes of image analysis, and it is upon this application that this chapter will tend to concentrate. However, computers are also providing considerable assistance in the area of in vitro nuclear medicine (for curve analysis and statistics) and in administrative applications (for patient scheduling and patient registry). I would like to emphasize that although the same hardware may be used for these applications, the software will differ considerably and as a consequence it is unlikely that one system can fulfill all these functions and certainly not simultaneously.

HISTORY OF COMPUTERS

The development of the computer is unparalleled in the history of mankind. Between the advent of the modern electronic computer in 1949 and 1977 the various performance and cost indices that can be assigned to computers have improved 100,000-fold. On the average, power per dollar has doubled every 2 years, or, conversely, every 2 years computers are halved in price for the same computing power. If the automobile industry had been able to achieve the same record of performance since the invention of the horseless carriage, the energy shortage of the 1980s would not be upon us, since cars would be able to travel 550 miles per gallon.

An example of this technologic advancement is provided by the well-known PDP-8.* When first introduced in 1965, the PDP-8 cost about $18,000, occupied a box about 50 cm on each side, consumed 500 watts, and was capable of 500,000 memory accesses per second. The same computer in 1977 (the PDP-8/A) cost less than $1800, occupied a single printed circuit board about 20 × 20 cm, consumed 50 watts, and was capable of 800,000 memory accesses per second. This remarkable development is attributable to the phenomenal changes that have taken place in the world of electronics.

Computing, as such, in ancient times in the Mediterranean countries was done much earlier than 450 B.C. by the Greeks and Egyptians with a counter abacus. In the Orient bamboo rods placed on a board as an abacus were used in China about 600 B.C. spreading to Japan about A.D. 600. But the true Chinese abacus *(suan-pan),* having one more bead per section than the Roman abacus, arose in the twelfth century and as a modification called the *soroban* entered Japan in the sixteenth century. A third type is in use in the Soviet Union. But despite this background, modern-day computers stem from the development of punched-card equipment and that in itself dates from the Jacquard loom—a device using large punched cards to control the pattern of a weave in a loom.

Two early mathematicians, Pascal in 1642 and Leibnitz in 1671, designed and built mechanical calculators. These, however, were the early forerunners of the more familiar hand-cranked calculators of the 1950s and 1960s. Modern computers derive their power from their storage capability and programmability.

It was this latter concept that was embodied in the "analytical engines" that Charles Babbage designed in the early half of the nineteenth century. Charles Babbage is often regarded as the father of modern computing. However, he never did get one of his "engines" to work because he kept on getting better ideas for a new machine before the old one worked. His greatest contribution was to the field of mechanical engineering where he solved a number of problems,

*Digital Equipment Corporation, Maynard, Mass.

such as making gears more accurately than they had ever been made before.

The next major advance was the use of punched cards and the development of associated equipment by Hollerith in connection with the U.S. census in the nineteenth century.

An electromechanical version of the computer was developed by Aiken in the late 1930s, and this became the starting point for the IBM Corporation, whose Mark I was unveiled in 1944 after a period of wartime duties.

Another computer, which was not disclosed until after the war, was the ballistics calculator ENIAC, which was the first electronic machine. This resulted in the design of the more general purpose digital calculator known as EDVAC. ENIAC was the brainchild of Eckert, and Mauchly at the University of Pennsylvania and EDVAC, embodying the concept of a stored program, was conceived by von Neumann and built at the Institute of Advanced Study at Princeton, New Jersey in 1952. Despite its size, this computer embodied less computing power than the present-day programmable hand-held calculators. Nevertheless, it was naívely considered at that time (1950) that five such computers would fulfill the complete computational needs of the whole world!

The compactness and power of the present fourth generation computers is attributable to the development of large-scale integrated circuits. "Large scale" does not imply "large-size"; rather the converse is true. It means that a large number of electronic circuits are concentrated on a small chip of silicon about 5 mm square. This concentration of many hundreds (even thousands) of circuits on such a small piece of silicon results in a considerable reduction in cost as well as a reduction of power requirements. Microcomputers are in effect "computers on a chip" though they usually require a large amount of ancilliary circuitry in order to become operable. Most minicomputers embody similar "computers on a chip" in the central processor unit but are more powerful than their smaller microcomputer brothers. This is primarily attributable to the power of the peripherals, many of which embody microcomputers in their own circuitry.

The rest of this chapter describes the component parts of a computer and the various peripherals that might be found in a nuclear medicine system. The necessary software is also described, along with an example of a computer program.

WHAT IS A COMPUTER?

There are two types of computers—analog and digital. An analog computer depends on continuously variable voltages or currents. In contrast to this, the digital computer depends on discrete voltages or current levels. Like an electric switch, the voltage is either on or off. It is the ability of the transistor to act as a switch that enables it to be used with such facility in a computer. Analog computers do not find any significant application in nuclear medicine, and it will be only the digital computer with which we are concerned.

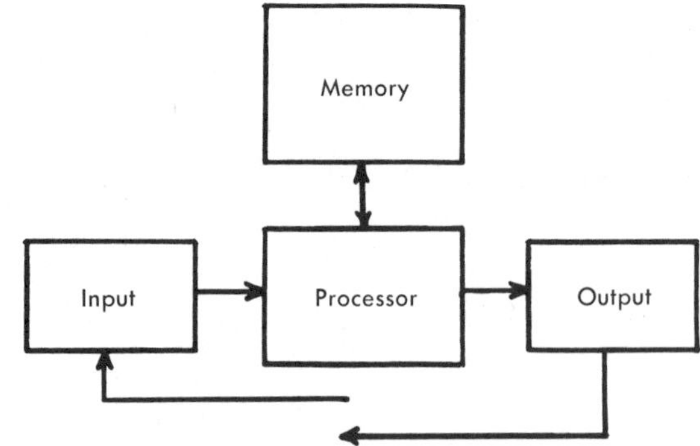

Fig. 7-1. Block schematic indicating the four major components of a computer. Output may be linked back to input in cases where further processing is required or where computer is controlling some external events. In nuclear medicine, operator often issues commands to input that are dependent on some output criteria.

In simple terms a computer is a machine that accepts data from the outside world, processes the data, perhaps places them in a temporary storage, and finally gives the processed data or results of the processing in forms of hard copy, displays, or commands to other devices it may be controlling.

To fulfill these four major functions (input, processing, storage, and output), a computer has four major components as indicated in Fig. 7-1.

The functions of input, processing, storage, and output can be compared to the procedures that we follow when solving a problem, particularly an arithmetic problem. The data are input to our thought processes by either visual or auditory senses. The problem is organized in our minds, and we may need to store interim results by remembering them or by writing them down before reaching the final result and outputting by the process of writing or speaking. There is one major contrast. The computer is a very dumb, but very rapid idiot. It must be given absolutely explicit instructions to fulfill its role. Even a child is capable of reaching the correct conclusion when instructed to put on his or her "shoes and socks." A computer would perform the task in logical progression and therefore finish up with the socks over the top of the shoes.

Let us look at the component parts of a computer in a little more detail.

Storage

A store (as opposed to a shop) is a place to keep things for a while. Storage in a computer holds either data or instructions—each is indistinguishable from the other in a computer. The two basic types of computer storage are *memory* and *registers* (sometimes called *accumulators*).

Memory, which is often referred to as main storage, is analogous to a large chest of drawers. Just as each drawer can store something, so can each unit of memory. In this case, each unit of memory is called a location and can store one computer word. These locations are referenced by number. Just as one could look for something in the third drawer from the top, so too can the processor be instructed to look for a word in location 3. The numbers of these locations are the addresses. Address numbers begin with zero and may extend to several tens or hundreds of thousands. Thus the address of a location is analogous to the position of a drawer and the word in that address is analogous to the contents of the drawer.

Each location in a computer memory is partitioned into smaller subdivisions called bits. Bits are subdivisions that can contain only one item, either a 1 or a 0. "Bit" stands for *bi*nary digi*t*. Locations subdivided into bits are like drawers partitioned into smaller slots. Just as one must first pull out the entire drawer to look into a slot, so too must one look at an entire location when wishing to examine a bit within a word.

Some computers have subdivisions within locations containing a number of bits. These subdivisions are called bytes and usually consist of eight bits. It is frequently possible to examine these subdivisions or bytes individually without looking at the whole location. This implies that the memory is addressable at the byte level as well as at the word level.

The bits in a location or byte are also numbered beginning with zero but these numbers are not generally referred to as addresses. So one may imagine memory as a chest of numbered drawers (like a filing cabinet) each containing a number of slots, or one may simplify the model and imagine a matrix of numbered locations, each containing numbered bits as shown in Fig. 7-2. In the case of most nuclear medicine computers, one might expect to find more than 32,000 locations each having a word length of 16 bits or 2 bytes of 8 bits each.

Registers (or accumulators) are similar to a single location in memory, but they are physically located very close to the processor, since they fulfill the function of a temporary store for easy and quick reference purposes. Also, whereas memory is generally made of either magnetic core or semiconductor memory cells, registers invariably consist of the latter.

Registers, like memory locations, are subdivided into bits. They are also numbered or named, or both, and these numbers or names are referred to as register addresses.

	0	1	2	3	4	5	6	7	8	9	10	11	12	13	14	15
0	1	0	0	1	1	1	1	0	1	0	1	1	0	0	1	1
1	0	1	0	1	1	0	1	0	1	0	0	0	1	1	0	1
2	1	0	0	0	0	0	1	1	1	1	0	1	1	0	0	1
3	0	0	0	0	0	0	0	1	1	1	0	1	0	0	0	0
'																
'																
'																
'																
500	0	0	1	1	0	0	0	1	1	1	1	0	0	0	1	1
'																
'																
'																
4095	1	1	0	0	0	1	1	1	1	1	0	0	0	1	0	0

Fig. 7-2. Memory consists of many computer words (0 to 4095 in this case) where each word contains a number of bits (16 in this case). Each bit can assume only one of two values: 0 or 1.

The key words associated with storage in a computer are as follows:

bit One *bi*nary digi*t*; it is the smallest subdivision of a register or memory location.

word The standard-sized group of bits referred to and used as a group together in a computer. A word usually occupies one memory location, but sometimes equals 2 or 4 memory locations. Most nuclear medicine computers have a word length of 16 bits. Some have word lengths of 12 bits, others 10 bits. A few have 18-bit words.

byte Some number of bits, usually 8 or 6, depending on the computer, but typically one half or one fourth of a word; the smallest usable group of bits that is larger than a bit.

address That number assigned to uniquely define a memory location or register.

register (accumulator) A temporary store equivalent to one memory location and closely associated with the processor.

Processor

The processor, or as it is better known, the CPU (central processor unit), is the brains behind a computer. Under the direction of a program, it acts as a giant electronic switching yard and controls the actions of the computer. Processors have two major components: the instruction control unit (ICU) and the arithmetic and logical unit (ALU) (Fig. 7-3).

The instruction control unit selects and interprets instructions. This unit contains two major registers: the program counter (PC) and the instruction register (IR). The program counter always contains the address in

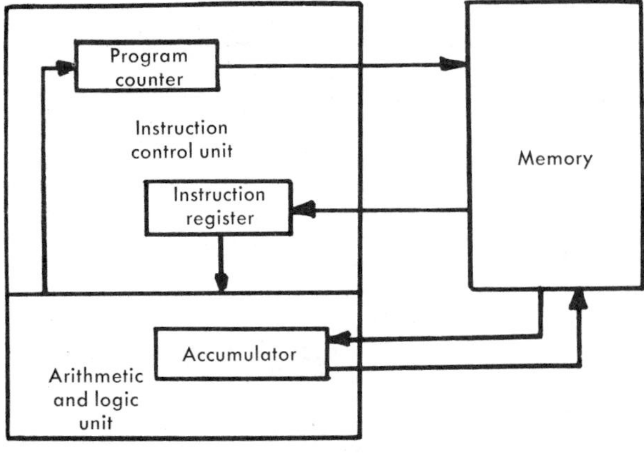

Fig. 7-3. Block schematic of central processor (CPU). Program counter indicates memory location from which next instruction is to be fetched. Instruction is decoded by instruction register and controls actions of arithmetic and logic unit. Data are transferred to and from memory and to and from input/output devices through accumulator. When a program branch is made, arithmetic and logic unit can modify contents of program counter, thereby changing the address from which next instruction will be fetched.

memory from which the next instruction is to be fetched. The processor fetches the next instruction from the location in memory "pointed to" by the program counter and copies that instruction into the instruction register. The instruction control unit then decodes the contents of the instruction register to determine what instruction is to be performed on what operands or data. The instruction control unit then directs the arithmetic and logical unit to execute or perform the indicated operations. At the same time it increments the program counter so that it now holds the address of the next instruction location.

The arithmetic and logical unit contains electronic circuits that execute the instructions. The major register in the arithmetic and logical unit is called an accumulator (AC), and this acts in a manner similar to the accumulator of an adding machine. The accumulator holds the operands used in arithmetic and logical operations, sets the results of operations, and holds data being read from or written into storage. One of the important features of a computer is the ability to modify a program based on a decision. This is called a branching operation, and one way in which this may be achieved is by the arithmetic and logical unit modifying the contents of the program counter as a result of a comparison operation. Thus the next instruction is fetched from a location that depends on the result of a previous computation.

Input/output (I/O)

Input and output functions link the computer to the outside world. This link is necessary to make the computer useful in just the same way as our senses are important to us for purposes of communication. Although they are lumped together here, it is important to appreciate that input and output are separate functions. We cannot speak with our ears; we cannot smell with our eyes. Speaking is output; hearing is input.

Input and output devices carry raw data and instructions into and out of the processor and storage. In some cases the device must transform the signal or data into a form compatible with the computer. There are many kinds of I/O devices: teletypewriters (note that "Teletype" is a registered trademark of Teletype Corporation but "teletypewriter" is the generic name) embody keyboards for input and printers for output, whereas line printers are output devices only; magnetic tape units may be used for both functions; CRT (cathode-ray tube) displays are output devices only and analog-to-digital converters are used to convert scintillation camera pulses into digital information for input purposes. All I/O devices require a buffer.

A buffer is a piece of temporary storage, either a register or a portion of memory, that makes it possible for devices that run at different speeds to work together. Fast devices and the processor move information in and out of a buffer very rapidly. The buffer holds the information while slow devices take the information out or put it into the buffer slowly. This allows the fast device to do other things and see the information from the buffer when it is ready, rather than wait around for the slow device to finish.

For example, pulses from a scintillation camera arrive at the analog-to-digital converter randomly in time. A buffer is established in memory, and the locations corresponding to the position of the scintillation are incremented each time a count is converted. The contents of the buffer are then written out to a disk storage device at the completion of the study in the case of static images, or at the completion of each time frame in the case of dynamic studies.

INFORMATION REPRESENTATION

Binary representation

As we have seen, a computer consists of a large number of electronic switches that have just two modes—on or off. Memory locations have subdivisions, called bits, that can contain either a 1 or a 0. Because of this on/off or 1/0 configuration, all numbers in a computer are represented internally in binary form.

Positive integers are treated as positive binary integers. The decimal values 0 through 10 are represented as follows:

Decimal	Binary	Powers of 2
0	0	0×2^0
1	1	1×2^0
2	10	$1 \times 2^1 + 0 \times 2^0$
3	11	$1 \times 2^1 + 1 \times 2^0$
4	100	$1 \times 2^2 + 0 \times 2^1 + 0 \times 2^0$
5	101	$1 \times 2^2 + 0 \times 2^1 + 1 \times 2^0$
6	110	$1 \times 2^2 + 1 \times 2^1 + 0 \times 2^0$
7	111	$1 \times 2^2 + 1 \times 2^1 + 1 \times 2^0$
8	1000	$1 \times 2^3 + 0 \times 2^2 + 0 \times 2^1 + 0 \times 2^0$
9	1001	$1 \times 2^3 + 0 \times 2^2 + 0 \times 2^1 + 1 \times 2^0$
10	1010	$1 \times 2^3 + 0 \times 2^2 + 1 \times 2^1 + 0 \times 2^0$

Thus the number 5 is represented by

000000000101

in a 12-bit computer and the number 7 is represented by

000000000111

In this notation the rightmost bit represents the coefficient of 2 raised to the power 0, the second right bit represents the coefficient of 2 to the power 1, and so on to 2 to the power 11. Thus 5 is represented by one 2 to the power 2 plus zero 2 to the power 1 plus one 2 to the power 0, which equals 5, and 7 is represented by one 2 to the power 2 plus one 2 to the power 1 plus one 2 to the power 0, which equals 7. The decimal value 132 is represented by one 2 to the power 7 plus one 2 to the power 2 and in binary form is written as:

000010000100

Negative integers may be represented in either 1's complement or 2's complement form. In 2's complement form, −5 is represented by

111111111011

and −2 is represented by

111111111110

To obtain the two's complement negative of a number, one first takes the positive representation, that is, 5 = 000000000101, complements each bit, in other words replaces 1's by 0's and 0's by 1's to obtain the one's complement, that is:

111111111010

and then adds 1 to this complement as though it were a binary integer

$$\begin{array}{r} 111111111010 \\ +\ 1 \\ \hline 111111111101 \end{array}$$

The result is the two's complement of the positive integer. It can be seen that this method of representing a negative number does not leave any ambiguity about zero, but if one uses the one's complement representation, the result is a positive zero—000000000000—and a negative zero—111111111111.

When binary numbers are added, there are only three rules to follow:

$$\begin{array}{ll} 0 + 0 = 0 & \\ 0 + 1 = 1 & \\ 1 + 1 = 0 & \text{Carry 1} \end{array}$$

For example:

$$\begin{array}{r} 1 \\ +0 \\ \hline 1 \end{array} \qquad \begin{array}{r} 1 \\ +1 \\ \hline 10 \end{array} \qquad \text{and} \qquad \begin{array}{r} 110 \\ +011 \\ \hline 1001 \end{array}$$

If we take two larger values such as decimal 7 and decimal 132, which are represented in binary form above, we would have the following:

$$\begin{array}{r} 7 \\ +132 \\ \hline 139 \end{array} \qquad \begin{array}{r} 000000000111 \\ +000010000100 \\ \hline 000010001011 \end{array}$$

which is the binary equivalent of decimal 139. Subtraction is really the addition of one positive number and one negative number.

For an example of binary subtraction let us perform the sum

7 − 2

The binary representations of each of these numbers is given above. If a binary addition is performed and the odd "carry" bit at the end is disregarded, we will obtain the binary representation for the number 5:

$$\begin{array}{rr} & 7 \quad 000000000111 \\ + & -2 \quad 111111111110 \\ \hline & 5 \quad 000000000101 \end{array} \qquad \text{Carry 1}$$

Octal representation

It is immediately obvious that it is tedious to write all of the 1's and 0's of a binary number; one very quickly loses count of how many have already been written down. To overcome this problem and to facilitate the manipulation of binary numbers, one can divide them into groups of three digits and each group is represented by its octal equivalent.

For example, if we take decimal 132, it would be represented in the following manner:

Decimal		Binary		Octal
132	=	000 010 000 100	=	0204

Using the example of binary subtraction from above we have the following:

	Decimal		Binary		Octal
	7	=	000 000 000 111	=	0007
+	−2	=	111 111 111 110	=	7776
	5		000 000 000 101		0005

Notice that just as in binary representation (base 2) where only two numbers, 0 and 1, exist, so too in octal representation (base 8) only the numbers 0 through 7 exist.

In very large computers and some of the 4 and 8 bit-based microcomputers, it is convenient to divide the binary word into groups of 4 rather than 3. In this case, the resulting numbers are represented in hexadecimal (base 16) format and the letters A through F are used to represent the digits 10 through 15.

Fortunately, one need not be able to perform binary or octal arithmetic in order to use a computer. The representation of numbers in octal format must be understood, however, if the operation is to be better understood.

Data versus instructions

We mentioned earlier that the computer is quite unable to differentiate between data and instructions. Both exist as strings of binary digits. It is possible for a computer to attempt to decode a piece of data and act upon the resulting instructions with disastrous consequences. How then does the processor know which is which?

The answer is that if the processor goes to a storage location expecting to find a piece of data, it treats it as data. If it goes to the same location expecting to find an instruction, it will put the contents of that location into the instruction register and treat it as an instruction. It is up to the programmer to be certain that the computer does not go to a memory location looking for the wrong thing.

WHAT DOES A COMPUTER INSTRUCTION LOOK LIKE?

Computer programs can be written in a number of different languages. The most basic of these is machine language. This means that the instructions are in a form that do not have to be translated for the computer to understand them. This most basic machine-language instruction is in binary code and has two parts: an *operation code* (op code), which identifies the instruction to be performed (ADD, JUMP, SKIP, COMPARE, and so on), and a *pointer,* which points to the location of the operand that the processor is to use when executing the instruction. The pointer is the address. If the computer word is sufficiently long, it may contain two pointers, known as source (where the operand is to be found) and destination (where the result is to be placed).

OP CODE	OPERAND

OP CODE	SOURCE	DESTINATION

Let us make up a simple set of instructions and utilize them to create a simple machine-language program. Rather than using the full binary notation, we shall use octal notation and will assume that the three leftmost bits (high-order group) of the instruction represents the op code. Note that this provides for an extremely limited instruction set of only eight possible instructions:

Op code	Instruction and its meaning
0	ADD to the accumulator (AC) the data that is to be found at the address pointed to by the pointer.
1	SKIP the next instruction if the contents of the accumulator (AC) is equal to the contents of the location whose address is in the pointer field.
2	JUMP and take the next instruction from the address pointed to by the pointer.
3	LOAD the contents of the location pointed to by the pointer into the AC.
4	STORE the contents of the AC into the location pointed to by the pointer. (This is the converse of the LOAD operation.)
5	INPUT a word from the buffer of the device whose code is in the pointer field and put the word into the AC.
6	OUTPUT the contents of the AC to the buffer of the device whose code is in the pointer field.
7	HALT and wait for further instructions.

An example of a single instruction might be 3011, which would be interpreted by the instruction control unit as "LOAD the contents of address 011 into the accumulator." By placing a set of such instructions into the memory, loading the address of the first instruction into the program counter (PC), and starting the computer, we can run the program.

What is a program?

A program is a logical sequence of instructions fetched from storage and executed one at a time.

One analogy might be the instructions we are given to go from one place to another. Suppose we are told to do the following:

> Go south on Leslie Street to Highway 401.
> Along 401 to the Yonge Street exit.
> North on Yonge Street to Cummer Avenue.
> Turn right and go east on Cummer Avenue.
> Turn left at the second traffic light.
> Turn right into North York General Hospital.
> Halt.

As we drive along, each instruction is fetched in turn until we arrive at our destination. An instruction executed out of turn would result in our getting lost. The sequence is important.

In executing a program, a computer must also execute each instruction in sequence. The execution of each individual instruction involves a number of intermediate steps:

1. Get address of next instruction from program counter (PC).
2. Fetch instruction (from storage) and put it into instruction resister (IR).
3. Increment program counter (PC) by 1.
4. Interpret the instruction in the instruction register (IR).
5. Get address of operand from pointer field.
6. Fetch operand.
7. Execute instruction.
8. Get destination of result.
9. Put result in destination.
10. Go to step 1.

Fig. 7-4 shows a program listing starting at location 0 of the computer memory. Some routes within the computer have been traced out in order to facilitate the understanding of what the program accomplishes. The input device (perhaps a paper tape reader) has been assigned a device code or address of 777, and the output device (perhaps a CRT display) has a device code of 776.

Let us trace the program, which starts at location 0.

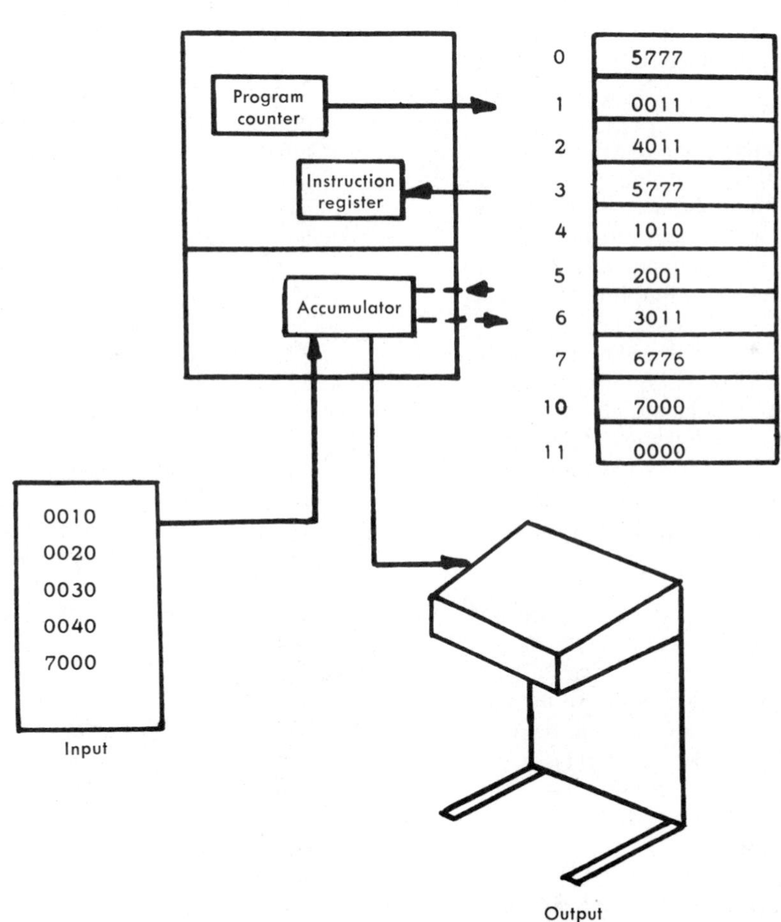

Fig. 7-4. Example of very simple machine language program that reads data from an input device, checks to see if end of list has been reached, and either adds number and reads in next or outputs total to output device. Memory locations 0 through 10 contain program. Location 11 is used as temporary store for sum.

Step by step through a program execution

The program counter (PC) contains 0, which means that location 0 will be accessed for the first instruction, which is then copied into the instruction register (IR) and, momentarily later, the program counter (PC) is incremented by 1 to be ready for the execution of the next cycle.

The contents of memory location 0 is 5777, and this is now in the instruction register (IR); the instruction control unit (ICU) decodes the op code portion (5) as an INPUT command and so the arithmetic and logical unit (ALU) fetches the data from the device represented in the second part of the instruction (that is, device 777) and loads it into the accumulator (AC). The result of this operation is therefore the transfer of the first piece of data (0010) from the input device to the accumulator (AC).

The next cycle commences when the processor fetches the next instruction from the location indicated by the PC, which, because the PC was incremented, is location 1. The instruction in location 1 is 0011. This is copied into the IR, and the PC is incremented again so that it now contains the value 2.

When the ICU decodes the new instruction, the op code portion (0) is interpreted as an ADD and the second portion points to address 011 as the location of the operand. Thus the contents of location 011, which is 0000, is added to the AC (which already contains 0010), leaving the result, 0010, in the AC (that is, the AC has remained unchanged).

The processor fetches the next instruction (4011) from the location indicated by the PC (2), puts it into the IR, and increments the PC to 3.

Op code 4 is a STORE instruction; so the contents of the AC (0010) is now put into the location indicated by the pointer field (011). (Location 011 previously contained 0000, but in any event the original contents would be erased by such a STORE operation.)

The PC now contains 3 and the corresponding instruction (5777) is now loaded into IR and the PC incremented to 4.

Another word is input from device 777; so now the AC contains 0020.

The PC now contains 4; so the instruction 1010 is loaded into the IR and the PC is incremented to 5.

Op code 1 is a SKIP instruction. More specifically, the processor is to skip the next instruction if the AC contains the same value as the location indicated by the pointer. The pointer is 010 and the location 010 contains 7000, but the AC contains 0020, and so the result of the comparison is that the processor will not SKIP, but will fetch the next instruction.

Thus 2001 is loaded into the IR and the PC is incremented to 6.

Op code 2 is a JUMP; so the contents of the pointer field (001) is loaded into the PC thereby resetting it to the second instruction.

This action causes a loop back to the second instruction, which is 0011, and the PC is incremented to 2. In this way a repetitive loop is created.

The op code (0) is decoded (ADD), and the contents of location 11 (0010) is added to the contents of the AC (0020), with the result (0030) remaining in the AC.

The next instruction, 4011, is fetched from location 2, and the contents of the AC (0030) are stored away in location 11.

The next instruction (1010) is fetched, and since, as previously, the contents of the AC are compared to the contents of location 010 and are found to be not equal, there is no SKIP.

The next instruction (2001) is fetched, and 1 is loaded into the PC, causing a JUMP to the start of the loop again.

Once again the instruction 0011 is fetched, thereby ADDing the 0030 in location 11 to the AC and leaving the result (0060) in the AC.

Instruction 4011 is fetched and executed to STORE 0060 from the AC into location 011.

Instruction 5777 is fetched, and 0040 is read from the INPUT device.

Instruction 1010 once again COMPARES 0040 to the contents of location 10, finds that they are not equal, and so does not SKIP.

Instruction 2001 once again loads 1 into the PC, thereby causing a JUMP.

Instruction 0011 ADDS 0060 to the AC (0040), leaving the result (0120) in the AC—remember this is *octal* addition.

Instruction 4011 STORES 0120 into location 11.

Instruction 5777 is another INPUT instruction, and 7000 is read into the AC. At this point the PC has been incremented to 4.

Instruction 1010 is fetched, and the PC is incremented to 5. Op code 1 is decoded, the AC and location 010 are compared, and this time they are found to be equal; so a SKIP is executed by incrementation of the PC from 5 to 6.

The PC contains 6; so 3011 is put into the IR, the PC is incremented to 7, and op code 3 causes the contents of location 11 to be LOADED into the AC.

Instruction 6776 OUTPUTS the contents of the AC to the output device.

Instruction 7000 HALTS the processor.

The overall effect of the program is to repetitively obtain data from an input device, add each element of data to the sum of the data previously input, and, when the input data 7000 is sensed, output the sum to another device. In this case, the sum of four numbers 010, 020, 030, and 040 is output as 120. Remember that this is octal arithmetic!

Two important features should be noted. The ability of a computer to branch as a result of a calculation is demonstrated by instructions 4 and 5. Instruction 4 uses a comparison to cause a SKIP, and instruction 5 causes a JUMP to location 1 in order to create a LOOP in the program. The second point of interest is that the contents of location 10 are used as data by the instruction in location 4 and finally as an instruction itself.

It is obvious that the creation of a program in machine code is difficult and tedious. Few people could even be expected to remember all the numerical op codes for a large instruction set or to keep close track of the addresses of locations in which data are stored.

Fortunately, higher level languages are available to solve these problems. Programs, in whatever language they may be written, are called "software," and we will explore some of the features of computer software, how it can be entered into a computer, and how some software can be used to assist in the creation of other, more sophisticated, software.

SOFTWARE

"Software" is a term that refers to all programs. Programs are "soft" because they are only representations that reside in memory. Except under special circumstances, they can be overwritten, destroyed, or even modified by the processor as it is executing instructions. Hardware cannot be modified by program execution. It is the wires, integrated circuits, and other electronic components that constitute the physical part of the computer. Software is a conceptual expression of a method.

Machine language

A program written in machine language has been analyzed above. Each computer type has its own machine language where the instructions are numerically coded in bits—1's and 0's. As in the example above, machine language is often represented in octal (or hexadecimal) in order to ease the life of the programmer.

It was presumed above that the program was already located in memory before execution was started at location zero. How did the program get there in the first place?

One can load the computer with a program, instruction by instruction, by using the binary switches on the front panel. This might be possible for a simple program like our example above, but it is obviously impossible for a program of any reasonable length.

Loader

The answer is to use another program called a "loader" to load the program of interest. The loader is a short program that merely has the function of reading in sequential words from an input device and depositing them in sequential memory locations. Such a program is obviously a very simple loop, and it is possible to conceive of using the toggle switches for such a short program. Early computers used such a method, but life has been made a great deal simpler by the advent of the "read-only memory" (ROM) or "bootstrap loader."

As the name implies, the contents of a read-only memory cannot be changed by the processor or any input-output device. The read-only memory contains the loader program, and the user simply pushes a switch to have the bootstrap loader program transferred by the hardware to standard memory and started automatically. The loader program then loads the required program from the appropriate device; most present-day bootstrap loaders can load from any one of several devices such as the paper tape reader, a disk, or magnetic tape.

Assembly language

Machine code, or machine language, is numerical, and from our previous example it is obviously difficult to learn and use.

Assembly language is a symbolic form of machine language. In this case the op codes are represented by alphanumeric symbols and the pointer field may be symbol names so that addresses may be referred to by name.

Let us compare our machine language program with the corresponding program written in assembly language:

Location	Machine code	Label	Op code	Operand
0	5777		Input	Device 1
1	0011	Again	Add	Temp
2	4011		Store	Temp
3	5777		Input	Device 1
4	1010		Skip AC EQ	End
5	2001		Jump	Again
6	3011		Load	Temp
7	6776		Output	Device 2
10	7000	End	Halt	
11	0000	Temp	0	

Although assembly language is easier for people to learn and use, the machine does not understand it. It is necessary to translate the assembly language into machine code. This requires another program known as an assembler.

Assembler

The assembler program is loaded into memory, and when it is started, it reads in the user's program written in assembler language. As it does so, it translates the alphanumeric codes into machine language.

Assemblers differ from one machine to another, and it may take up to three passes for the assembler to assemble, check, and list a program. Once assembled, the program can be loaded into memory by the loader and run.

As in the case of loaders, assemblers have become increasingly sophisticated and, whereas original forms would create a paper tape to be read back in after each pass, this action is now transparent to the user, and the assembled program can be written out to the disk immediately.

The assembly-language program has, of course, to be created in some way or another. One technique might be to use a teletypewriter device with a paper tape punch and then enter the paper tape into the computer when the assembler requests input. It is, however, almost impossible to create a paper tape copy of a program without making some errors and, as a consequence, the program needs to be edited. This requirement leads to the development of programs specifically designed for this process.

Editor

A software editor is a program with which a person sitting at the keyboard may interact in order to create, correct, and output any form of text in what is called ASCII format. ASCII is a particular code that represents all the printing (and many of the nonprinting) characters on the keyboard.

The editor does not itself do any error checking. It does, however, allow the operator to enter text and then review it, delete characters, words, or whole lines, and insert corrections. These programs are, in many ways, similar to the more familiar typewriters with magnetic card or tape memory. They rarely have all of the functionality of the more recently available word-processing systems.

Since any form of text may be entered, the operator may use the editor to create a program in any language, not just those written in assembly language, or indeed any text. The manuscript for this chapter was originally created and edited using an editor program on a computer, but a human editor was still a necessary component.

High-level languages

Machine language is very difficult to learn and to use. Assembly language circumvents many of these problems but, as indicated above, it is still necessary to code every step of the program, since each assembly language instruction results in only one machine language instruction. These languages are called low-level languages, since they communicate with the processor at the lowest and most basic level.

In order to facilitate easier communication with the computer, higher level languages have been developed. Examples of such high level languages are FORTRAN, BASIC, FOCAL, COBOL, ALGOL, and PL/1. In high-level languages, one instruction can be used to replace many machine language instructions. For example, in BASIC the single instruction:

LET X = Y + Z

is equivalent to the three instructions that in our simple assembly language would be:

```
LOAD   Y
ADD    Z
STORE  X
```

Thus high-level languages allow the programmer, with one line of code, to instruct the computer to do more than one thing. Since the rate at which programmers can write acceptable programs averages 10 to 15 lines of code per day, no matter what language is used, applications programs can be written much faster in high-level languages and fewer lines of source or original code will be required.

The various high-level languages have been developed to meet different needs. FORTRAN is, for instance, a very sophisticated language for dealing with scientific problems. COBOL, on the other hand, is a business-oriented language and is particularly suited to the production of reports as required in the world of finance.

High-level languages allow users to write programs in a form more natural to their everyday life. This implies that high-level languages require software more sophisticated than assemblers to translate them into machine code so that the computer can execute them. Two types of software exist for this translation process—compilers and interpreters.

Compilers

Compilers translate entire high-level language programs into what is called "object code," which is, in fact, machine code. Like assemblers, they may require more than one pass to accomplish this process and usually it is necessary to link the object code with other object code programs in order to produce the final run-time program.

Compilers usually have at their disposal, library programs and subroutines that can be compiled and linked together with the user program for execution. It makes little sense for the user to have to write the routine for a sine function or logarithmic function each time he needs it. Such routines are written once and included in the library in a form such that they can be linked with the user's program requiring such routines. FORTRAN, PL/1, ALGOL, and COBOL are commonly implemented as compilers.

Languages using compilers result in a faster running program and every effort is made to optimize the machine code, though it can never be reduced to what would do the job in assembly language. There is, however, a major drawback. No program is perfect when first written, and corrections or improvements require the program to be compiled and linked again before it is can be retried. If the program is to remain fixed and be used repeatedly, it is worth going through the repetitive process required to set it in correct form. Languages using interpreters avoid this delay but require more memory and result in lower program run times.

Interpreters

Interpreters perform the same function as compilers but use a different method. A compiler translates the whole program at once and puts it in a machine language form suitable for execution. An interpreter translates only one high-level language instruction (or a small block of instructions) at a time and executes it before translating the next. The sequence is translate, execute, translate, execute, and so on. BASIC and FOCAL are both examples of interpreters, or as they are sometimes called, "incremental compilers."

Interpreters are generally used with interactive timesharing systems in conjunction with their own special editors in situations where programs are to be written and run immediately. Interpreters require additional memory space to accommodate the language processor, source program, and that part of the program that is in machine code at any one point in time. Interpreters also result in slower running programs since the translation process must precede execution every time the program is run. On the other hand, corrections and program modifications are easy and simple to institute, and this can be a decided advantage when the execution time is less critical than program-development time.

Most nuclear-medicine systems embody programs written in both assembly code and a high-level language. The programs that are specific to nuclear medicine and are used for data acquisition and analysis will be used time and again by all users; so it is advantageous to write them in assembly code and supply them to the user in machine-code form.

The user will also want to develop programs specific to his or her own needs. Such a program might be one to calculate cardiac output using a particular protocol. In this case, it is desirable to use a high-level language and FORTRAN or BASIC might well be used in such an instance.

Debugger

No program is error free when first written. If it is, then it is time to celebrate before Murphy's law, If anything can go wrong, it will, is obeyed! Errors are called program "bugs," and it is useful to have a program that can allow the user to run the program in an interactive mode, halt it at will, examine the contents of registers or memory locations, and modify the program while it is in its machine-code form. Interpreters allow this activity at the source or within various levels of high-level language, but programs in machine code require a special debugging program to be entered into memory at the same time. A debugging program must therefore be small enough to fit into memory at the same time as the user's program, and the user must be capable of reading machine code in order to carry out the debugging process. Once the user program has been debugged, the correct version can be output so that it can be reentered and run later as necessary.

Operating systems

Operating systems are programs that automate the use of other software by the user. Of all the component parts of a computer system, the operating system is the most important. A poor operating system means that the system is hard to use, and users will avoid using such a system.

Operating systems embody three major functions: program development control, job control, and data control.

Program development control includes calling the editor from a peripheral storage device, storing user programs in peripheral storage, and calling appropriate assemblers and loaders to load, execute, and link the program with library routines. These operations replace those jobs that would otherwise have to be carried out by a computer operator.

Job control involves handling the transition of the computer from one user to another and from one job to another.

The first forms of operating system completed the job under the direction of a job-control card and then cleared memory and read in the next job-control card to obtain the directions to be followed with the next program in the card-reader hopper. This type of operation is called ''batch mode.''

Batch mode is relatively wasteful of computer time. Much of the time the computer itself might be idle while some input or output routine is performed. This realization led to the development of multi–job operating systems where jobs are swapped out of memory when they are waiting for some peripheral device to respond to an input/output request. When one job is swapped out, the job with the next level of priority is swapped in and execution carried out until it too becomes idle. In this manner the computer is used more efficiently.

An extension of multiprogramming is timesharing. In timesharing-operating systems the computer's time is sliced equally between users. There can be many users connected to the computer, and since the major portion of their time at the terminal is spent in reading, thinking, or typing, the computer appears, to all intents and purposes, to be serving each of them individually as if each is the only user connected.

The operating systems incorporated into nuclear medicine computer systems are real-time operating systems. They are designed especially to respond to external stimuli in the real-time environment. It is possible to have one program operating on a low priority (in the background) and another (in the foreground) that responds to inputs demanding a higher priority, such as pulses from a scintillation camera. Such a system appears to be running two programs simultaneously when, in reality, the foreground program is not making use of the processor all the time but can gain control whenever it is required.

The third function of the operating system, data control, involves transferal of blocks of data from one device to another and handling of the format changes necessary to satisfy the various mechanisms. Data control also involves error detection and correction and sending of messages to the operator requesting tape reels to be mounted, devices to be turned on, and so on.

PERIPHERAL DEVICES

When properly programmed, computers can display a great capacity for solving problems quickly. However, the data for those problems, the programs themselves, and the results must be entered into the computer or written out by the computer to the outside world. All these actions involve the use of peripheral devices. Peripheral devices are those devices that serve the input/output requirements of the computer. With very few exceptions they involve electromechanical action and, compared to the electronic action of the computer itself, these devices are relatively slow.

Let us look at some of the peripheral devices more commonly found on nuclear medicine computers (Fig. 7-5).

Keyboard/printers

The most familiar device is the keyboard/printer, sometimes called the teletypewriter. Note that ''teletype'' is a trade name, but one should use ''teletypewriter'' to describe the typewriter-like devices common to so many computers. Usually the console or operator's control device is such a terminal.

Two common types prevail: the impact printer and the heat-sensitive printer. Impact printers can be quite noisy, but they possess the virtue that no special, and hence more expensive, paper is required; on the other hand, special heat-sensitive paper is needed for the oft-called silent printer.

In any case I must emphasize that the keyboard and printer are two specific entities. The keyboard may be used to input characters without an echo being generated at the printer just as the printer can behave as a stand-alone device.

A

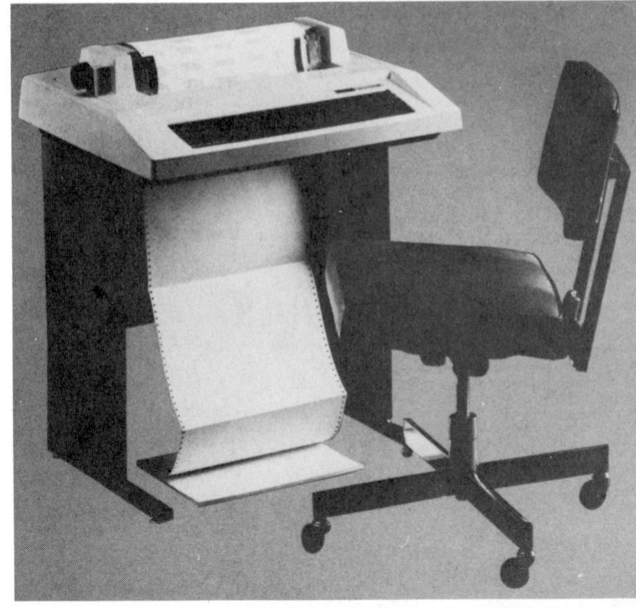

B

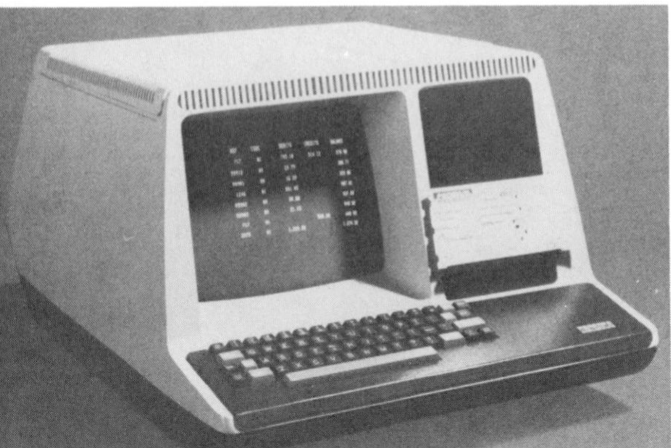

Fig. 7-5. Examples of two terminal devices. **A,** Keyboard/printer that embodies a dot matrix impact printer and, **B,** cathode-ray tube or video terminal that performs same role but does not provide for hard copy. (Courtesy Digital Equipment Corp., Maynard, Massachusetts.)

Video terminals

Video, sometimes called CRT (cathode-ray tube), terminals are frequently used to replace keyboard/printers where a hard-copy record is not required. Just as the keyboard and printer are separate entities, so too the keyboard and screen of a video terminal act as separate input and output devices.

Video terminals are frequently much faster than keyboard/printers because there are no electromechanical components involved and they are truly silent. They can also provide substantial economic savings since paper is an expensive commodity and none is used in this case. The lack of hard copy can, in some circumstances, be a disadvantage, but in this case the system could be equipped with a fast printer of some kind for those occasions when hard copy is required.

Paper tape reader/punch

Early software was frequently distributed in the form of paper tape. The older teletypewriters were often equipped with paper tape reader/punches, but these only operated at 10 characters per second, a rate that resulted in very slow input/output operations. Paper tape readers capable of reading up to 300 characters per second were familiar devices in the late 1960s. Their primary function in a nuclear medicine system would be to read paper tapes from such instruments as multisample well counters or for the convenient and cheap interchange of short programs.

The use of paper tape has largely been superseded by the introduction of floppy disks and cassette tapes.

Card readers

Cards at one time constituted the major form of computer input/output. Programs were punched on cards one line at a time (up to 80 characters long) and a program was made up of a deck of such cards. Woe to the programmer who had the misfortune to drop the deck of cards, and it happened quite frequently, enough for cards to become the bane of a programmer's life. Storage on such an inconvenient medium also presented problems. Card readers and card punches are extremely rare in nuclear medicine systems.

However, punched cards still offer a most convenient medium for credit-card invoicing and mark-sense cards are often used in the hospital environment for standard questionnaires. There is at least one computerized radiology reporting system that utilizes mark-sense forms for the radiologist's input to the system.

Disks

Disks come in two basic forms: floppy disks and hard (cartridge) disks (Fig. 7-6). Floppy disks consist of a ferrous oxide coating on a Mylar base. Hard disks are larger flat platters of aluminum also coated with ferrous oxide. In each case, the purpose of the ferrous oxide coating is that it can be magnetized and thus store information in much the same way as a ferrite-core

A

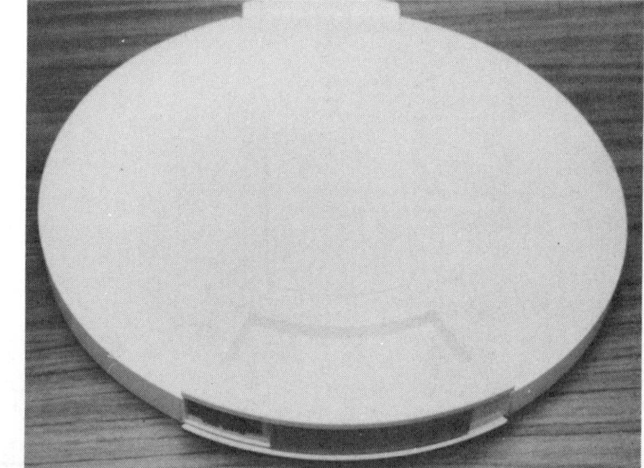

B

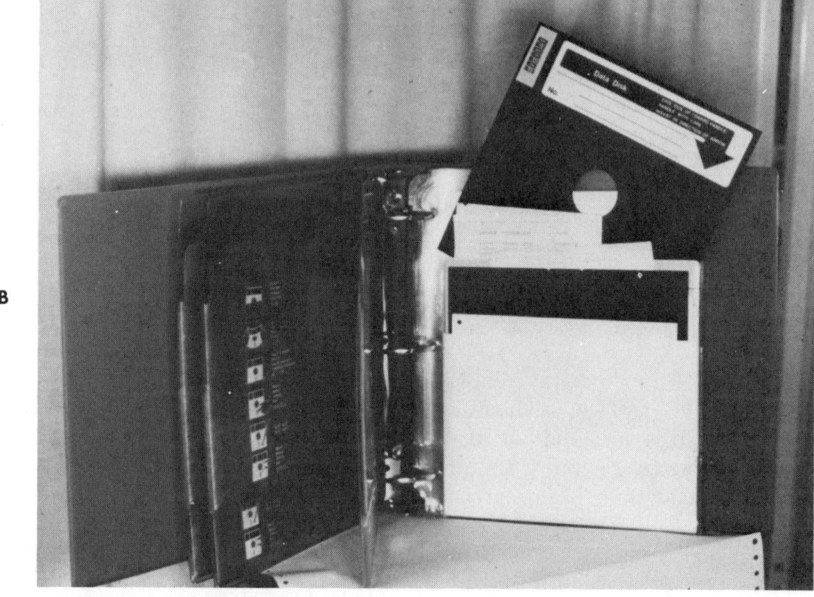

Fig. 7-6. Examples of two types of disks used in typical nuclear medicine systems. **A,** Cartridge disks are relatively fast and may contain up to 5 megabytes of information, but disks themselves cost about $100 each, and drives cost about $12,000. **B,** Floppy disks are very much cheaper ($8 each and $4,000 for drive) but can contain very much less information—only 512 kilobytes and are very much slower.

memory. Disks are similar to phonograph records (floppy disks are about the size of 45 rpm records), but the information is stored on them in a series of concentric tracks rather than one continuous groove.

The data are written on the disk by a read/write head that ''flies'' just above the surface of the disk and causes the ferrous oxide to be magnetized, either one way or the other, depending on the direction of an electric current through the head. In this manner, the computer's 1's and 0's may be simulated by the direction of magnetization. The data are read from the disk by the same head detecting the direction of magnetization through the induced current as the disk rotates beneath it.

Disk systems constitute the major bulk memory device for computer systems almost without exception. The range of disk drives is extremely large—from relatively cheap, low-capacity floppy disks to large, fast, and expensive disk-pack systems.

The major advantage of disk storage is the random nature of disk read/write operations. When reading a paper tape, punched cards, or magnetic tape, one must sequentially examine each item before arriving at the one required. If the data are on a disk, the head can be

Table 7-1. Common disk-drive systems

Disks (for programs and fast retrieval)	Bulk memory: Access time (msec)	Capacity (megabytes)	Cost ($1000)
Floppy	400	0.5	5
Cartridge (single)	65	5.2	9
Cartridge (double)	50	28	15
Small pack	43	67	23
Large pack	37	.176	35
Fixed head	8.5	1	18
Magtape: (backup and archiving)	Several minutes	50	15

moved directly to the appropriate track and one need only wait for the disk to complete the next rotation before the particular data item may be read. The access time for such a disk is the sum of the time taken by the head to reach the correct track and the time for the disk to rotate into the correct position.

In fixed-head systems a read/write head is provided for each track, so that the head movement is eliminated and only the disk rotation need cause any delay. The access time is, on the average, the time for the disk to rotate one half revolution.

Most nuclear medicine systems use disk-cartridge systems. The cartridges are usually removable, and those embodying a single platter can contain up to 10 million bytes of information (or programs). Some double-platter cartridges have become available more recently, and they may have a capacity for as much as 28 million bytes. Some systems use fixed-head disk drives and some use floppy disks. Mobile data-acquisition systems use both cartridge disks and floppy disks, though movement of the former along bumpy corridors must be regarded with some concern. Disk packs containing as many as 20 platters have enormous capacities (197 million bytes) and are used in nuclear medicine systems to provide large nonremovable storage capacity.

Floppy disks provide a very convenient medium for data or program transfer. The access time is, however, long and the capacity is limited. Indeed, though floppy disks are cheap, their cost per byte of stored data is extremely high compared to cartridge disks and is exorbitant when compared to magnetic tape.

At the other end of the scale, disk-pack drives, which contain multiple platters, though the most expensive, have the largest capacity and the fastest access times. They also offer the best cost/byte ratio. Such drives are being installed on large systems being used for cardiac studies where capacity and speed are of prime importance.

Table 7-1 is a list of some more common disk-drive systems and indicates in a very explicit fashion that money buys systems of higher capacity and reduced access time. The obvious anomaly to this general rule is the fixed head disk, which is relatively expensive for its capacity but has a fast access time. Disk technology is advancing very rapidly, and the figures quoted in Table 7-1 may well be improved upon by factors of two or more within the space of a few years.

Note that in the case of all disk drives a controller is needed to interface that disk drive to the computer. Given a particular type of disk drive, one controller can probably handle up to four or eight such drives. However, a mix of disk drives implies a mix of controllers and a concomitant increase in cost. Another point of note is that, despite the similar physical appearances of disk cartridges, they are not interchangeable between drives of different manufacture. The format in which the data are written depends on the software so that, even given the same manufacturer, if the operating system is different it is most likely that disks written on one system cannot be read on another.

Magnetic tape

Of each of the magnetic recording media, magnetic tape is perhaps the most familiar to nuclear medicine departments.

Magnetic tape has enormous storage capacity, but suffers from the strong disadvantage that a whole tape must be read in order to reach the data at the far end. Magnetic tape is a sequentially addressed medium. Disks can be addressed randomly.

Computer compatible tape may be 7 tracks or 9 tracks wide. Nine tracks has now become the industry standard.

However, ''computer compatible'' does not mean that such tapes can be read on any computer. The tape reel may mount on the drive, but there is no guarantee that the format in which the data are written conforms to any set standard. Indeed, just as for disks, it is entirely possible that tapes written under different operating systems, on similar computers, manufactured by the same company may not be interchangeable.

This fact is worth noting, since magnetic disks and tapes have been postulated as the medium for data transfer from mobile scintillation cameras to computers and this transfer may not, in fact, be a simple matter. It may require extra hardware and will unquestionably require extra software.

Magnetic tape drives differ primarily in their speed, which can range from 12½ to 75 inches per second (ips), and in the density with which data can be packed on the tape. The density may be 800 or 1600 bytes per inch (bpi). The former is more common on minicomputer systems. Though, as technology improves, this is changing and more fast 1600 bpi tape drives are becoming economically attractive.

Line printers

When a large amount of hard copy (printed matter) results from an operation, it is desirable to have a fast printer available. Most keyboard/printer terminals operate at 30 characters per second, whereas line printers can print a whole line of output at a time and the more expensive ones can operate as fast as 1200 lines per minute (lpm). This would probably exceed the needs of most nuclear medicine departments, but if a data file such as a patient index or registry is contemplated, then a slower, cheaper printer operating at 300 lpm is almost a necessity. The 30-character-per-second printers are not designed for continuous printing operations.

Some fast character printers are available. They operate on similar principles as the printer terminals in the sense that they print one character at a time, but they can do this at up to 180 characters per second, which can result in line speeds of the order of 100 lpm or more depending on the average length of each printed line. The printers are far more economic than line printers for a small facility.

Cathode-ray tube (CRT) displays

The principle function of any nuclear medicine computer system is image analysis. Therefore a major component of any such system is an image-display system. Several types of output devices have been used to perform this role (Fig. 7-7).

Normal, nonstorage CRT displays similar to the analog scopes of scintillation cameras have been used. In these devices the electron-beam intensity is modulated so that the brightness represents the count intensity of each pixel (picture element). This type of display requires continual refreshing or rewriting and this operation can consume a large portion of computer time. In addition, the beam has a tendency to "bloom" at increasing intensities, causing pixels of varying size to be displayed. Such displays can, however, be used to display a dynamic study in *ciné* mode with fairly rapid framing rates.

Large screen–storage type of CRT displays have also been used. In this case, the electron beam can only be turned on or off. Thus each pixel is represented by a number of individual dots, and the number of dots or dot density corresponds to the pixel-count content.

Once the image is "painted" on the storage screen, the computer is free to perform other functions. It is not needed to refresh the display. However, the time taken to "paint" the image (up to 12 seconds) precludes the use of such a display for the cine playback of dynamic studies.

Video displays

Both nonstorage and storage types of CRT displays fulfilled a need, but neither was entirely satisfactory. The burgeoning of technology in the television or video area led to the economic development of video-output displays for computers such as nuclear medicine systems.

These displays embody a buffer memory unit, which is separate from the computer's memory. The data to be displayed are copied from the computer memory or disk to the display memory, and the latter is used to continually refresh the TV screen. Because a separate buffer memory is used, the display is flicker free (commercial TV displays 30 pictures per second) and takes very little time to be written.

An added advantage is that the use of TV technology can provide a facility for color-coded images. It is frequently useful to be able to display one image in one color range and overlay it with an image displayed in a different color scale. Ventilation-perfusion studies of the lung, liver-pancreas scans, and selective coronary angiography are examples of procedures where this facility is desirable.

Spatial resolution of display systems is important. Video displays are limited to the number of lines per frame on the order of 512, so that a spatial resolution of 512 × 512 elements is the theoretical limit with present technology.

The number of gray scales or color levels to be displayed can always be guaranteed to generate heated discussion among users. Many will claim that the present economic limit of 16 levels is sufficient to meet most needs. Others will claim that 64, 128, or even 256 levels should be used in order to provide a "continuous" tone. The human eye can, at best, distinguish about 20 gray-scale levels and that is in a step wedge where the edges of the step cause the eye itself to perform some contrast enhancement. Thus it would appear that 16 or 32 levels are sufficient in most circumstances. In any case, it should be possible for the user to be able to change to different color scales or black and white under program control, and this facility becomes increasingly difficult as the numbers of color levels is increased.

Analog-digital converters

An important component of any nuclear medicine computer system is the interface to the scintillation camera. This interface will embody two analog-to-digital converters (ADCs).

Two common designs for ADCs exist. The ramp converter causes a capacitor to be charged by the incoming signal, and the time taken for discharge is measured by a clock. This time is recorded as a digital signal (by a count of clock pulses) and is proportional to

A

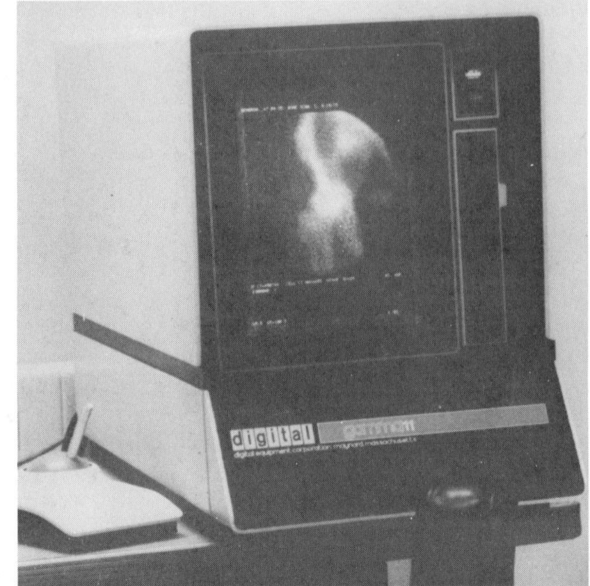

B

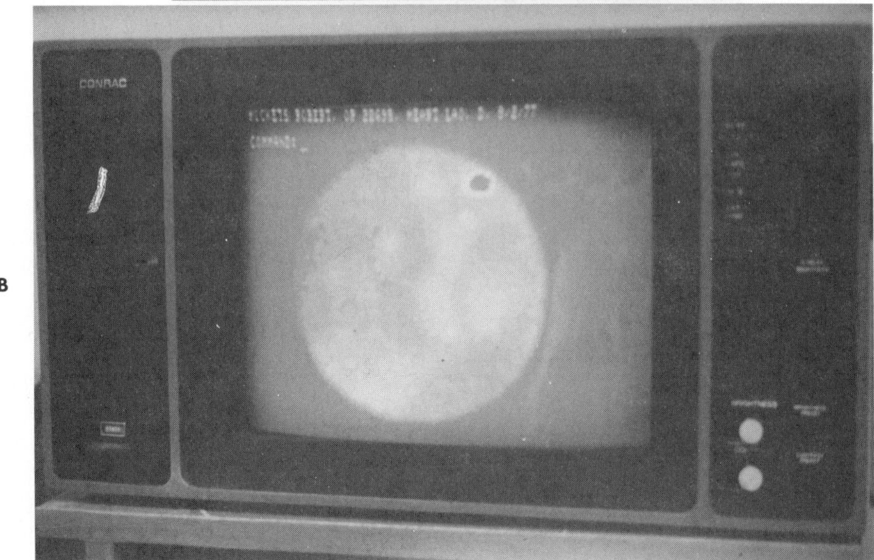

Fig. 7-7. Several methods of image display have been used. **A,** Old-style CRT storage screen display. **B,** More modern video display using TV technology.

the magnitude of the input signal. This type of ADC usually has good differential linearity, so that negligible distortion is introduced during the analog-to-digital process.

Successive approximation converters constitute the second major type. A voltage is compared to the input signal and is either increased or decreased by a feedback mechanism until it matches the input signal. Since the feedback is through a digital-to-analog converter, which is much like a series of binary switches, it is possible to determine the digital value of the voltage that most approximates the input signal. Successive approximation converters are usually faster and cheaper than ramp converters but do not exhibit such good differential linearity. This linearity can be improved by use of a more expensive converter to convert to a larger number of output bits and discard the lower order bits.

ADCs must also be fast if the dead time of the conversion process is to be kept to a minimum.

ADCs will also be required if physiologic signals,

such as those from an electrocardiograph, are to be recorded. In some cases, ADCs will be required to record the outline of regions of interest, depending on the type of transducer used for this function. In both instances, the ADCs can be very much slower, and consequently less expensive, than the ADCs required for the scintillation camera signals.

ADVANCED INPUT/OUTPUT

The input/output operations for a computer may take one of several forms. The protocol that is used is largely dependent on the priority of the transfer and the speed with which it must be performed.

Interrupts

The simplest form of input/output transfer is one that can occur under program control on an interrupt basis. Let us suppose that a program requires data to be entered (from the keyboard, perhaps). In this case, the program can reach the point where it needs information, and it can then interrupt its own operation and look at the buffer of the input device to see if data are waiting. This would normally be indicated by the presence of an electronic "flag" when data reside in the buffer. If no data are present, the program will enter a loop where it continuously keeps looking for the "flag" to be "raised" and, once it has, it jumps out of the loop, reads in the data, and continues operation as before.

This interrupt is one that has taken place under program control.

Another form of interrupt is one in which the peripheral device causes the interrupt. Let us suppose, once again, that a program is running and that in this case data are being printed to a terminal. The printing operation will be under program control as we have described above. But this time the operator wishes to stop the print-out (all the useful data have been printed) and allow the program to run to completion. In one operating system this may be done by typing "control-O" (^O). Under these circumstances, the peripheral device (the keyboard) raises an interrupt flag when the character "^O" is typed, and this causes the computer to complete its present instruction cycle and then respond to that interrupt. The computer will scan the input buffer, find a "^O" (control oh) character and react to this by suspending the print-out operation but allowing the program to run to completion.

I must emphasize that the examples given above are just that. There are many types of input/output operations that take place on an interrupt basis. However, some transfers must, perforce, take place rapidly, and the method of raising an interrupt is too slow under such circumstances. One prime example of such a data transfer is the time when data from a scintillation camera must be input to a computer. The technique used to perform such rapid transfer of data is by direct memory access (DMA).

Direct memory access transfers

When a direct memory access (DMA) transfer takes place, the peripheral device (that is, the analog-digital converter interface) transfers data directly to the memory without interrupting the action of the processor.

When the architecture of the computer is such that each element of the computer can address a common data pathway or bus, it is possible for the peripheral device to address a location in memory without interrupting the program that is running in the central processor. This type of data transfer is very fast, and it is limited primarily by the speed of the memory. It is sometimes known as cycle-stealing, since the device performing the transfer is stealing memory cycles away from the central processor and the transfer is entirely under the control of the external device.

Synchronous/asynchronous transfer

When data are transferred in or out of memory, it is apparent that, quite apart from the method of interrupt, the computer may either accept data and acknowledge that acceptance for each piece of data (say an individual character) at a time, or alternatively it may be assumed that a large amount of data can be transferred in blocks without any acknowledgements taking place.

The first type of transfer takes place between devices that differ in speed of operation, and this is called an "asynchronous transfer." The devices behave asynchronously since their speeds of operation differ.

When devices have similar speeds and data are transferred under the control of clock "ticks," they are said to behave synchronously and the transfer is a synchronous transfer.

Keyboards and printers are asynchronous devices and magnetic disks are usually synchronous devices.

NUCLEAR MEDICINE APPLICATIONS

Computers that are used for nuclear medicine require some specialized hardware and definitely require software to be specifically written to fulfill a specialized need.

HARDWARE REQUIRED

Scintillation-camera interface

Some mention has been made of analog-to-digital converters. Two converters are required when a scintillation camera is interfaced to a computer. One converter is for the x-axis signals, the other for the y-axis signals. The z-signal is used to gate the analog-digital converters so that conversion only takes place for valid energy signals. The result of a conversion will usually be two 7- or 8-bit data elements that are combined to form a single 16-bit word. This 16-bit word represents the address in memory that must be incremented by one count to correspond to the gamma ray that gave rise to the scintillation in the crystal. The incrementation of memory is usually performed using DMA transfer.

The attributes of a good scintillation-camera interface are that the analog to digital converters shall be linear and fast. In addition, it is desirable that the interface have several levels of buffering, so that random high count rates may be accommodated without drastic loss of data.

Some computer systems can accommodate input from multiple scintillation cameras simultaneously. This, however, is bound to impose some limitations, and it is not possible to perform the full range of studies (both static and dynamic) at each of the cameras. The reason is that the computer may be faced with the conflict of having to accept a pulse from each camera at one and the same moment in time. When this happens, one camera must be given priority over the other or others and one or the other of the pulses will be neglected. Even at the high speed at which a computer operates, it is not possible to resolve the conflict between two simultaneous pulses.

When it is necessary to connect more than one camera to a computer that does not have the ability to select the appropriate camera under program control, a mechanical switch must be used. Since a number of signals are involved, the switch must be a multipole switch. In addition, it is necessary to introduce appropriate circuits so that the signals may be matched and each of the scintillation cameras will appear to be similar to the others so far as the computer interface is concerned.

Given the present type of practice existing in most nuclear medicine departments, it is probably more desirable to add another computer to perform data acquisition only than it is to expect one computer to serve multiple scintillation cameras simultaneously because the performance of such a shared system ultimately suffers and is mediocre at best.

Physiologic signal input

In cardiac studies in particular and in some studies involving respiratory motion, it is desirable to record some physiologic signals. This may be the electrocardiogram (ECG) or merely a record of the respiratory level of the patient.

If the full signal is to be recorded, it is necessary to add another analog-digital converter. This converter can be much slower and less sophisticated than the ones used for the scintillation-camera signals. This converter would be sampled on a regular basis under program control, and the complete digitized wave form would be recorded on a temporal basis, together with the scintillation-camera information.

On the other hand, it may only be necessary to record certain definite markers associated with the physiologic wave form. An example is the recording of the R wave of the ECG. In this case an analog-to-digital converter is not necessary, and instead a timing marker or flag is recorded corresponding to the temporal location of the R wave. One may incorporate this flag into the scintillation-camera data by setting one bit of that datum word corresponding most closely to the time of occurrence of the R wave.

Gating

Some of the more sophisticated types of imaging such as cardiac imaging require that the actions of the computer be synchronized with the patient. This synchronization is more uniformly termed "gating."

More specifically, the R wave of the ECG signal is used as a trigger or marker, and data collection is keyed off that temporal marker. The purpose of this type of data collection is to create a series of images that represent a single cardiac cycle but that have been collected over several hundred cardiac cycles in order to fulfill the requirement for good statistics.

The requirement under these circumstances is for an ECG amplifier that can deliver a signal to an R-wave sensor. The R-wave sensor provides a standard logic-signal pulse, coincident with each R wave, and this pulse is applied to an input of the computer such that the computer program can use it as a time marker. It is not necessary to use a sophisticated gating instrument having gates and delays for both end diastole and end systole. A standard ECG machine and a simple R-wave detector will suffice for most needs. The rest of the "gating" can be done by the computer software.

Memory

The amount of memory included in a computer system is critical in terms of the capability of the system. First of all, program space must be available. Then there must be memory available for buffering of the input data.

The amount of memory required for a static image is dependent on the size of the image (32×32, 64×64, or 128×128) and the depth or count capacity of each pixel. When memory is addressed in word mode a 16-bit computer has the capacity for 65,535 counts per pixel. If memory is addressed at the byte level, twice as many pixels can be accommodated in the same amount of memory, but the maximum capacity of each of those pixels is now reduced to 255 counts.

Dynamic mode requires that the data be buffered.

Table 7-2. Memory requirements

Matrix size	Memory required	Maximum counts (per pixel)	Framing rate (per second)
32 × 32 byte	500	255	50
32 × 32 word	1000	65,535	25
64 × 64 byte	2000	255	12
64 × 64 word	4000	65,535	6
128 × 128 byte	8000	255	Static

Note: 1000 words of memory = 1024 locations.

Thus memory is segmented into 2, 4, 8, or 16 portions, and once the time for one frame is expired, data are entered into the next portion of memory while the data collected earlier are written onto the disk. The larger the number of segments into which the memory is divided, the smaller will be the image size and capacity, but, on the other hand, the maximum framing rate available increases.

The amount of memory required for each size of matrix and count content is shown in Table 7-2. The approximate framing rates for a typical system containing 16,000 words of memory and recording data from only one scintillation camera are indicated. Note that it is not possible to collect 128 × 128 arrays in a dynamic mode since at least two buffers are required and two 8000-word buffers would leave no available program space in a 16,000-word memory.

When simultaneous acquisition and analysis is contemplated, it is apparent that more memory must be available for the array under analysis and for the analysis programs. This accounts for the fact that most nuclear medicine computer systems contain about 32,000 words of memory.

To obtain the maximum number of frames per R-R interval in gated studies, it is usual to restrict the computer operation to acquisition only. This gives greater freedom to the memory assigned for analysis so that a typical system having 32,000 words of memory can collect 48 frames of 32 × 32 byte, or 12 frames of 64 × 64 byte, per R-R interval.

SOFTWARE REQUIRED

Apart from the scintillation-camera interface, the software required of nuclear medicine systems is the most specialized component of the whole system. Memory, central processors, disks, and displays are found in all or most computer systems, but the ability to acquire and display data from scintillation camera is specific only to nuclear medicine. Because this is so, the software becomes the most significant component. Without good software, the very best hardware can be extremely difficult, if not impossible, to use.

One component of the software can remain generalized. This is the operating system.

Operating systems

Ultimately the most basic form of program entry is one in which the user keys a program into the computer through the switch console on the front panel, using machine or binary code. This is obviously a totally unacceptable manner of entering programs when they are of any length and must be replaced frequently.

The next level of sophistication involves loading of the programs from punched paper tape. Once again, this is an unacceptable technique when considerable program-swapping is involved. It is therefore necessary to include some form of fairly rapid bulk memory from which the programs can be quickly recalled into memory. This facility is provided by magnetic disks, be they fixed head, cartridge, or floppy.

Thus a disk will contain a whole family of programs, each of which, when read into memory, will perform a specific function. There may, for instance, be a program for collection of scintillation-camera data in a dynamic mode and another for collection in a static mode. Since both programs could not be expected to function simultaneously, there is little purpose in having them both occupy memory space. Instead, each is requested from the disk as required.

The program that answers these requests and supervises the swapping of programs back and forth to the memory constitutes the operating system. In addition to other features, an operating system includes a "monitor," "supervisor," or "executive" routine that is resident in memory the whole time and that interprets commands made to it either by the operator or by the programs themselves (for example, requests for other programs or access to peripheral devices).

As has been discussed previously, operating systems for nuclear medicine computers must be real-time operating systems that respond to requests from the outside world. In the case of nuclear medicine systems the "outside world" is the scintillation camera.

In addition to their function of swapping programs as required, operating systems have other features, including a file directory, assemblers, and linkers for assembly-language programming, compilers or interpreters for high-level language programming, and utility programs for such applications as editing and debugging. A good operating system contains a wide selection of such programs with appropriate documentation, and its activities will be largely transparent to the ordinary nuclear medicine user.

Application programs

Manufacturers now provide what may be described as "general-purpose scintillation-camera" or "nuclear medicine–specific'' programs. These include facilities for data acquisition and the more routine types of analysis that most nuclear medicine departments will require. Sophistication beyond this level is usually supplied by means of user-written programs in a high-level language that can refer to data collected or analyzed by the system software.

Programs supplied by the manufacturer should be simple to run yet sophisticated in nature. Data for each patient should be stored or filed under that patient's name and should be protected from accidental overwriting by other later data collections. System programs should also be protected from such accidental deletion. The operating system itself is usually capable of maintaining the log of patients entered. The operator need not maintain a hand-written log or directory to determine the location of a patient study. Some manufacturers have adopted the branching-menu approach, and others use the command-line approach. Each method has its own advantages and disadvantages. Menu structures are usually easy to follow but are time consuming, whereas command lines are fast but demand that the user be familiar with the command language used.

Acquisition

Programs for use with a scintillation camera should include programs to acquire data in static, dynamic, list, or gated mode. In static mode, one frame is collected at a time, according to a present count or time. A wait occurs while the patient is positioned for the next view, and the computer collection is restarted manually. This mode is analogous to the well-established static analog picture taken from the simple oscilloscope camera.

In the dynamic mode, the computer acts very much like a multiframe recording camera. It may be programmed to collect the scintillation-camera data for a preset period of time before moving to the next frame. Collection time for each frame or group of frames should be variable so that rapid pictures may be taken of a fast phase (such as the vascular phase of a renal study) followed by slower frames for less rapid phases. The images are stored away as a series of pictures, the collection of each having started immediately after the close of the previous one. This is sometimes called the ''histogram mode'' because the counts are blocked into sections on the time axis. In order to avoid count losses, the data from the scintillation camera are stored sequentially into separate memory portions; while storage into one area is going on, data from the other area are being written on the disk. This buffering explains why at least twice as much memory is required for a dynamic study compared to its static counterpart.

The list mode may be compared to recording a dynamic study on magnetic tape for later playback. The position information of each pulse is recorded, together with information relating its time of collection with respect to other pulses collected during the study. This information must be replayed from the disk and framed as in a dynamic study if images and curves of activity versus time are to be generated. Because the data are written serially to the disk, the maximum acceptable count rate in list mode will be much less than in the other modes of data acquisition. This mode is also very consumptive of disk space, since each event in the crystal uses one word of disk space. Normally in the frame mode one word can be used to record 65,535 counts occurring in one location in the crystal, but in the list mode one word can represent only one scintillation event.

Cardiac imaging has stimulated the development of so-called gated acquisition. Gated acquisition is a variant of dynamic mode. A series of frames is collected and stored in the same manner as a dynamic study is collected, but in this case all the frames are stored in memory until the completion of the study and the gating or triggering event causes data to revert to the first frame and add the data to that already collected. As an example, let us assume that the ECG R wave is being used as a triggering signal and that the R-R interval is to be divided into 48 frames. The computer program will first of all divide the R-R interval into 48 equal elements and determine the time interval for each frame (t milliseconds).

All data collected in the first t milliseconds after the R wave will be allocated to frame 1. The data acquired in the second t milliseconds ($t \rightarrow 2t$) will be allocated to frame 2, and so on until either frame 48 is reached or a new R wave causes the data collection to revert to frame 1 (Fig. 7-8).

This method of data collection is used because the number of counts available during one heartbeat is insufficient to provide useful statistics. By collecting the data from as many as 600 heartbeats additively as if they are all from the same heartbeat, one can significantly improve the statistics. There is one major problem associated with gated acquisition. If an R-R interval is longer or shorter than the average (plus and minus an appropriate tolerance), then the program senses this and rejects the incoming data until the R-R interval is once again within limits. However, the data from the long or short beat have already been collected and added to the previous data before the interval is sensed as being outside of limits. Similarly the data from the interval that is sensed as being once again within limits has already been rejected before the interval is sensed as being acceptable. A good-gated study therefore depends on the patient having a relatively stable heart rate, and frequently those patients on whom such stud-

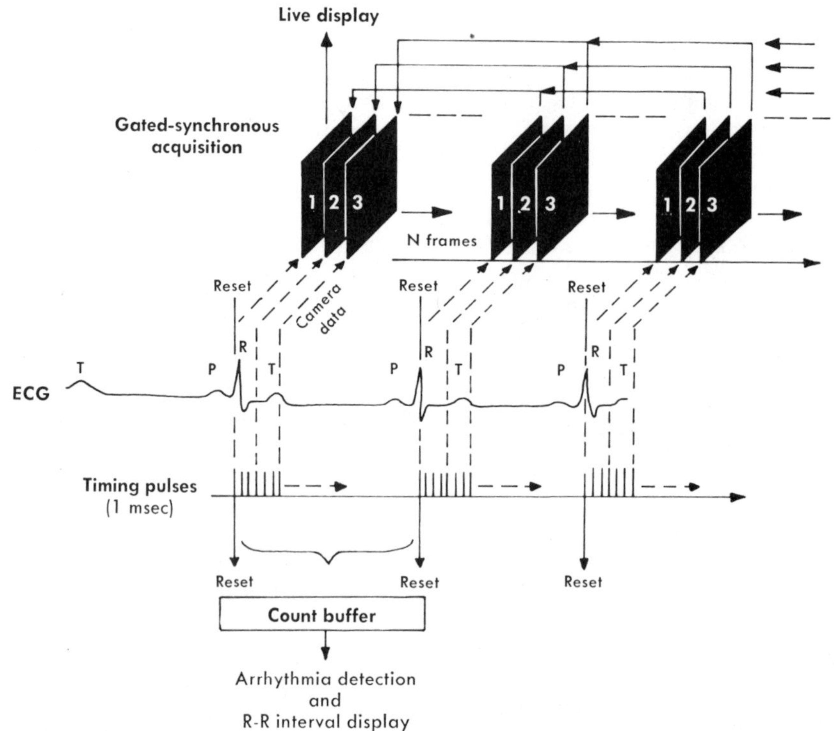

Fig. 7-8. Gated acquisition is programmed in such a manner that as many as 48 frames are stored in memory. Each frame corresponds to a segment of R-R interval and contains information collected over several hundreds of beats. Collection into frame 1 is triggered by R wave of each heartbeat.

ies are to be performed are the very ones who demonstrate premature ventricular contractions. Programs have been written to accommodate the slowly varying heart rate that is evident when a patient falls asleep or overcomes his or her initial apprehension. These programs predict the R-R interval based on a running average of heart rate, but the problem of the intermittent short or long R-R interval still remains. The problem cannot be overcome by buffering the data, since the computer would have to test the R-R interval to determine its acceptability and, while doing this, it could not store further incoming data. It is possible to "correct" a study for data lost during arrhythmic beats, but the results are still subject to some doubt. One may also "gate" a list-mode study.

In addition to the recording of the position and time information, as in normal list mode, gated list mode allows for the recording of a marker corresponding in time to the R wave. In contrast to the gated acquisition previously described, gated list mode allows gating of the study subsequent to data collection. The advantage to be gained is that the R-R intervals may be scanned and only the data corresponding to the chosen interval (with some tolerance) need be accepted. Thus the data collected during unacceptably long or short R-R intervals may be truly rejected. In addition, gating can be performed back from the R wave as well as forward from the R wave. This allows for analysis of the complete heartbeat rather than just that portion from end diastole to end systole (Fig. 7-9).

As with list mode, gated list mode is also limited in terms of the count rates that can be accommodated and uses a good amount of disk space.

For commonly used procedures, the collection parameters for any one of these modes of data collection can usually be predefined so that only the patient's identification need be entered into the computer before it is ready to start acquiring data.

Analyzing data

Provided that data can be collected properly and stored in the correct format, the most important part of any applications software is that devoted to image display and analysis. One should be able to move between images of a study with ease, both forward and backward within an individual study.

It should be possible to control the levels of the upper and lower thresholds that are displayed both with

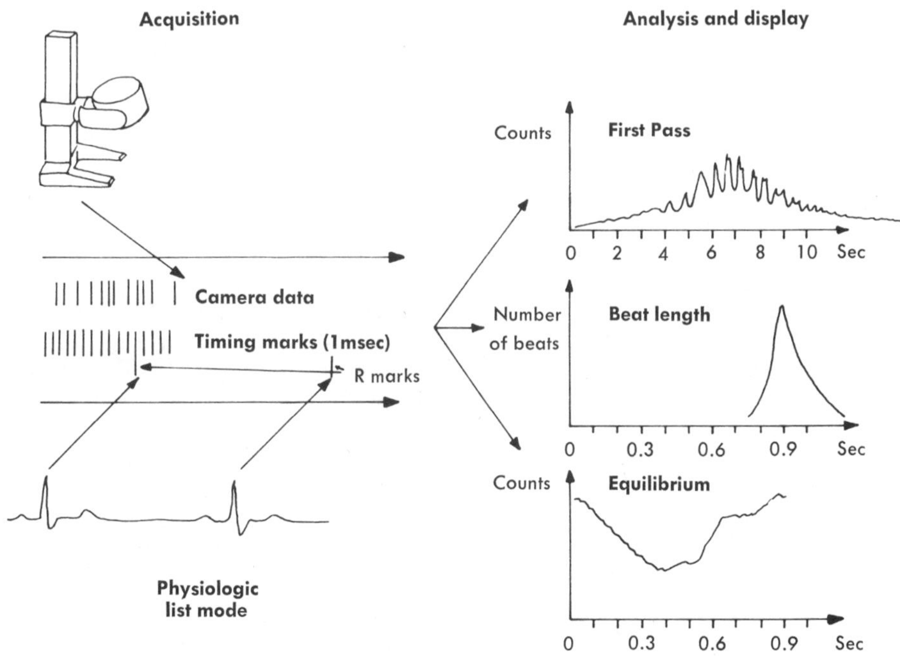

Fig. 7-9. Gated list mode is not truly gated. Data are collected in list mode and occurrences of R wave are also recorded. During analysis one may reject those R-R intervals outside of certain limits and produce a series of frames similar to gated acquisition.

and without enhancement, and to move these thresholds in a well-controlled, easy, and documented manner.

Frame algebra, including addition of a constant or multiplication by a constant, is necessary when several images are to be normalized. Addition and multiplication automatically imply that subtraction and division are available, since the constants can be negative or less than one as well as positive and greater than one. It should also be possible to multiply or divide frames by one another, so that parametric images such as those depicting ventilation-perfusion $(\dot{V}/\dot{Q})$ ratios or regional ejection fractions may be obtained. The ability to shift images horizontally or vertically sometimes facilitates registry of one image with respect to the other before such division is carried out.

Slices or profile cuts of varying width, both horizontal and vertical, are often useful in the establishment of the statistical validity of areas within an image or in the determination of the cross section of some item of interest. Slices are particularly useful for analyzing flood studies from the point of view of quality assurance.

Regions of interest are extremely important. Whatever means is used for defining regions of interest, it should be possible to define both regular (rectangular) and irregular (any-shape) regions. It should also be possible to define these regions by the boundary only, or by marking every cell to be included in the region. This latter facility allows a region with an inner unmarked zone to be defined or for several unique areas to be included as one region of interest. When a large number of regions are being selected—and most systems can accommodate about 10 to 12—it is desirable for the regions to be individually identified, particularly if they overlap. One may assign this identity by associating an alphabetical character or a color (in color displays) with the region.

The programs associated with regions of interest selection usually have the facility for plotting the count-versus-time curves from a dynamic study in a number of different formats: raw or normal, overlaid, averaged for region of interest area, plotted versus frame number or plotted versus time and expanded over chosen time intervals. The axes should be properly labeled in all cases. Another desirable feature enables these curves to be printed or punched out (on paper tape) should the user require a more permanent record.

Playback routines

It is frequently desirable to play back dynamic or gated studies in a cine mode. It is not merely necessary to be able to display the data frame by frame as it was collected, since frequently the data must be modified in some manner to make the playback more meaningful. An example of such a playback might be the beating of the heart within the outline at end diastole or a series of images depicting the regional ejection fraction at each stage of the heartbeat. In order to playback such images at a rapid rate, one first needs to create a file of appropriately modified images and to give the file a format that facilitates rapid recovery of the data from the disk to the display buffer. Programs for the creation and actual playback of playback files should be part of the suite of analysis-and-display software.

Above all, it is necessary for the programs to be simple to use. One should be able to step from one program to another without referring to the command monitor. All commands should be simple one- or two-letter commands that have an obvious meaning, and it should be impossible to corrupt either patient data or programs. If original patient data are to be modified, such as when flood correction is performed or when a study is to be deleted, the program should verify this action so that the user is given an opportunity to abort such action should he have made a typing error or have second thoughts about his request.

User programs

Manufacturers cannot be expected to fulfill all of the program needs of all their users. Very few institutions follow identical protocols for similar procedures; hence a program written for one institution is unlikely to be immediately acceptable in another. Because of this variability of the practice, most manufacturers provide the user with the facility to incorporate his own programs into the software system. In this way, the user can generate programs that are specific to the particular protocols adopted within his own institution, rather than changing the protocols to meet the demands of some more general software.

In order that the task of writing user-specific routines or programs may be made as simple as possible, the manufacturers have incorporated macros and high-level languages into their software. Macros are strings of standard data analysis commands put together in the form of a program and given a name such that the operator no longer needs to enter each of the commands individually but can have them executed by calling the macro by name. These macros can even have loops within them so that repetitive actions such as the creation of playback files can be performed with ease. High-level languages were discussed previously and may consist of either an interpreter or a compiler, which allows the user to create programs in a more easily understood language than assembly code.

Languages

FORTRAN, BASIC, NUTRAN, and FOCAL are all examples of high-level languages provided by some manufacturers. FORTRAN is the most sophisticated of these four programming languages and provides a faster-running program, since it is compiled into a machine language program once and once only. BASIC and FOCAL, on the other hand, are interpreted into machine language line by line every time the program is run. BASIC tends to be faster and have more useful features than FOCAL. The simplicity of these three languages bears an inverse relationship to the sophistication and running time. FOCAL is undoubtedly the simplest of the four languages to learn and FORTRAN the most difficult. NUTRAN is a variant of FORTRAN developed for nuclear medicine activities.

Whichever high-level language is provided by the manufacturer—and it is imperative that some such language be included in the package—it is of paramount importance that the language provide the user with the facility to refer easily to individual elements within images or individual points within dynamic curves. This requirement implies that the manufacturer must add to the language some extra functions, called CALL routines or "hooks," so that reference may be made to data collected and stored under control of the manufacturer's supplied acquisition software.

Exchange of programs

Most manufacturers have user groups, which are most helpful in fostering protocols and in the development of special-interest user programs. It is at this level that some degree of program sharing may be carried out. Several users may find that they use the same protocol for a particular procedure. In this case, sharing of user-written programs makes more sense than the manufacturer spending valuable man-hours developing software that is of limited interest to the majority of the customers. Between users of different systems the best form of exchange is at the level of the algorithm used for a particular procedure. Exchange of programs, even those written in the same languages, is unlikely to be very fruitful, since the programs will usually require considerable modification before they are useful.

ENVIRONMENTAL CONSIDERATIONS

Space requirements

Scintillation-camera signals are analog pulses that can suffer degradation if fed through a coaxial cable of excessive length. Ideally, cables should not exceed 25 feet, though many cameras have been interfaced with computers as far away as 150 feet. Cable runs longer than this will probably require special drivers and pulse-shape restorers to ensure faithful signal reception. Limitations on cable length are imposed by the driving end or scintillation camera, not by the choice of computer or computer interface.

It is therefore desirable to situate the computer within the department in reasonable proximity to the scintillation camera. Locating it in the same room, however, is not desirable. A fair amount of heat is generated, and the fans and printer can also create a disquieting amount of noise. Additionally, placement close to the camera leads to logistics problems in reading and analyzing images when patients are in the room. If possible, a room should be set aside specifically for the computer, so that its futuristic image is not imposed upon an already apprehensive patient and the analysis of studies can be done in relative privacy.

Room size is also important. Although nuclear medicine systems are based on minicomputer and even microcomputer design, they are not too small by the time the necessary peripherals have been added. Each bay or cabinet is 21 inches wide by 25 inches deep. Most nuclear medicine computers use at least two cabinets, requiring floor space of at least 42 × 25 inches. A magnetic tape unit usually adds a third cabinet.

In addition, in order for a serviceman to approach the back of the unit comfortably, the computer must be placed about 3 feet from any wall on any side. The keyboard/printer console and display screen occupy space equivalent to another cabinet and should be placed reasonably close to the computer itself. Cable runs in excess of 25 feet are undesirable unless the display is a remote television monitor.

Storage facilities for disks, magnetic tapes, paper tapes, manuals, and computer supplies must be provided nearby. The physical bulk of manuals and computer-related material always tends to exceed early expectations.

Air conditioning

Systems containing magnetic disk and tape equipment require a well-controlled environment that maintains acceptable temperature, humidity, and cleanliness. Primary planning considerations should include not only adequate electrical power, but also proper lighting and air conditioning.

Optimal conditions for a typical computer system require an ambient temperature of 21° C ± 1° C (70° F ± 2° F) with a noncondensating relative humidity of 45% ± 5%. Magnetic tape will stretch when variations in temperature and humidity occur. A location away from possible steam or water leaks is most desirable because water can cause extensive damage. Condensation on disk surfaces can cause the disk to "crash" and damage the read/write heads. This is the reason, incidentally, why disks should always be allowed to reach the ambient room temperature before being loaded if they have been outdoors.

Since all computers are air cooled, unrestricted air

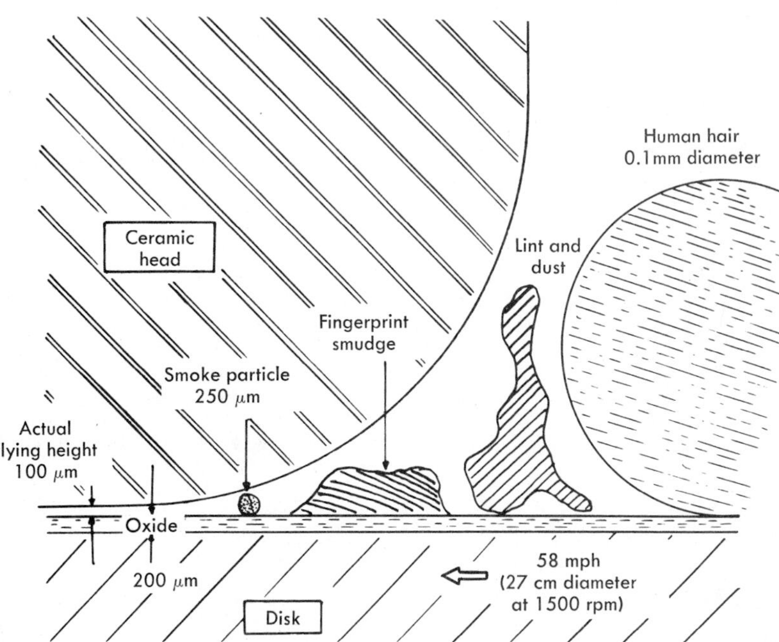

Fig. 7-10. Smoke, dust particles, and human hair can all cause disk "crashes." It is important to store and operate disks in a clean atmosphere.

flow in and around cabinets is necessary. A 30-inch clearance above the cabinet should be allowed.

Heat output from a typical nuclear medicine computer system is of the order of 7000 BTU per hour; with a magnetic tape unit this figure increases to 10,500 BTU per hour, a considerable output. When air-conditioning needs are being assessed, the number of persons who will occupy the room must also be taken into account.

Cleanliness

If temperature and humidity are the computer's nemesis, then dust can be its fatal enemy. Magnetic disks are particularly prone to dust or dirt problems, and magnetic tape can suffer from these problems too, though the results are not likely to be so pronounced or catastrophic.

A disk head literally "flies" above the surface of a disk cartridge, supported there by the boundary layer of air that the disk carries around with it. The flying height is of the order of 1 μm. Fig. 7-10 indicates some comparative sizes of possible dirt particles.

Nuclear medicine departments can be very dusty places. Most dust is lint from sheets and blankets. Disks should be stored in a dust-free cabinet, and if they can be stored on edge, this will help to avoid warping of the platter itself. Several companies provide a service whereby disks can be cleaned and inspected on a regular basis. In some instances this can be done without the cartridge being opened, a method that is certainly more desirable.

Power requirements

Nuclear medicine computers are all made to conform to industrial standards and in North America may be expected to operate on 117 volts AC at 60 Hz. The current rating should be regarded as at least 15 amps per cabinet. Like most nuclear medicine equipment, computers require a reliable power source, and line-voltage disturbances in hospitals can arise from a number of different sources, not least of which are scintillation cameras and scanners.

CONCLUSION

Computers represent a substantial investment in both time and money. They can, used properly, make a significant impact upon the practice of nuclear medicine. To make good use of these instruments, it is important that nuclear medicine personnel become familiar with the terminology adopted by the computer industry and with the various component parts of nuclear medicine computer systems. This is a very rapidly evolving field so that this becomes yet one more body of knowledge that must be assimilated if nuclear medicine itself is to evolve.

SUGGESTED READINGS

1. Coles, E. C.: A guide to medical computing, London, 1973, Butterworth & Co. (Publishers).
2. Cradduck, T. D., and MacIntyre, W. J.: Camera-computer systems for rapid, dynamic imaging studies, Semin. Nucl. Med. **7**:4, 1977.
3. Eckhouse, R. H.: Minicomputer systems: organization and programming (PDP-11), Englewood Cliffs, N.J., 1975, Prentice-Hall, Inc.
4. Hidalgo, J. U., editor: Symposium on computers and scanning, New York, 1974, The Society of Nuclear Medicine, Inc.
5. Hine, G. J., and Sorenson, J. A., editors: Instrumentation in nuclear medicine, vol. 2, New York, 1974, Academic Press, Inc.
6. Katzan, H., Jr.: The human use of computers, New York, 1974, Mason & Lipscomb Publishers, Inc., Petrocelli Books.
7. Larson, K. B., and Cox, J. R., editors: Computer processing of dynamic images from Anger scintillation camera, New York, 1974, The Society of Nuclear Medicine, Inc.
8. Lieberman, D. E.: Digital nuclear medicine, St. Louis, 1977, The C. V. Mosby Co.
9. Proceedings of Symposium on Sharing of Computer Programs and Technology in Nuclear Medicine, Oak Ridge, Tenn., 1971, CONF-710425, Springfield, Va., 1971, U.S. Department of Commerce, Technical Information Center.
10. Proceedings of Second Symposium on Sharing of Computer Programs and Technology in Nuclear Medicine, Oak Ridge, Tenn., 1972, CONF-720430, Springfield, Va., 1972, U.S. Department of Commerce, Technical Information Center.
11. Proceedings of Third Symposium on Sharing of Computer Programs and Technology in Nuclear Medicine, Miami, 1973, CONF-730627, Springfield, Va., 1973, U.S. Department of Commerce, Technical Information Center.
12. Proceedings of Fourth Symposium on Sharing of Computer Programs and Technology in Nuclear Medicine, Oak Ridge, Tenn., 1974, CONF-740531, Springfield, Va., 1974, U.S. Department of Commerce, Technical Information Center.
13. Proceedings of Fifth Symposium on Sharing of Computer Programs and Technology in Nuclear Medicine, Salt Lake City, Utah, 1975, CONF-750124, Springfield, Va., 1975, U.S. Department of Commerce, Technical Information Center.
14. Proceedings of Sixth Symposium on Sharing of Computer Programs and Technology in Nuclear Medicine, Atlanta, Ga., 1976, New York, 1976, Society of Nuclear Medicine.
15. Proceedings of Seventh Symposium on Sharing of Computer Programs and Technology in Nuclear Medicine, Atlanta, Ga., 1977, CONF-770101, Springfield, Va., 1977, U.S. Department of Commerce, Technical Information Center.
16. Rollo, F. D., editor: Nuclear medicine physics, instrumentation, and agents, St. Louis, 1978, The C. V. Mosby Co.
17. Souvek, B.: Minicomputers in data processing and simulation, New York, 1972, John Wiley & Sons, Inc.
18. Spencer, D. D.: Fundamentals of digital computers, New York, 1969, Howard W. Sams & Co., Inc. (subsidiary: The Bobbs-Merrill Co., Inc.).

SECTION TWO

Clinical nuclear medicine

Chapter 8

THE CENTRAL NERVOUS SYSTEM

Karen L. Blondeau, Richard A. Holmes, and Michael M. Mello

Although radionuclide brain imaging has enjoyed phenomenal popularity as a principle method to demonstrate a variety of neuropathologic lesions, the introduction of computerized tomography (CT) has significantly diminished its use in many institutions. Despite this, the prediction that CT will totally replace radionuclide brain imaging has not materialized because of imposed restrictions on the purchase of future CT units and published data that reveals comparable detection accuracy for most types of brain lesions using the two techniques.[11] A resurgence of radionuclide brain imaging is anticipated and is now appearing in many institutions.

HISTORIC FACTORS

The successful detection of a brain tumor with ^{131}I-labeled diiodofluorescein outside of the intact cranium with a Geiger-Müller detector in 1948 heralded the beginning and eventual development of brain imaging.[20] Developments by Cassen and later Kuhl and associates produced the rectilinear scanner that utilized ^{131}I–human serum albumin, introduced by Chou et al., to routinely and noninvasively scan the brain.[3,5,18] The introduction of ^{203}Hg-chlormerodrin for brain scanning by Blau provided a choice but no appreciable improvement in the quality of brain scanning.[2]

The acceptance of the Anger scintillation camera as a clinically useful instrument was accelerated by the discovery and introduction of technetium 99m by Harper and his associates.[1,14] The physical characteristics of $^{99m}TcO_4^-$ (γ photon, 140 keV; half-life, 6 hours) and its labeling ability (preparations for brain, lung, thyroid, liver, kidney, bone, blood-pool imaging) make it ideally suited for the Anger scintillation camera.

ANATOMY AND PHYSIOLOGY

The central nervous system is composed of paired cerebral hemispheres, the cerebellum, and a brainstem, which extends caudally as the spinal cord. The hemispheres are hollow and contain the ventricular system with choroid plexuses, which produce waterlike cerebrospinal fluid (CSF), which bathes the central nervous system (CNS) throughout its extent and provides buoyancy for it in its bony surroundings. Fig. 8-1 is a diagram of the functional lobe topography of the cerebral hemispheres; frontal (memory and motor function), parietal (sensory function), occipital (sight), and temporal (hearing and proprioception function). Although the sylvian fissure separates the temporal from the frontal and parietal lobes, it is indistinguishable as a structure on the brain image. The brain receives approximately 20% of the cardiac output. The blood reaches the brain through the common carotid and vertebrobasilar artery systems. The left common carotid artery originates directly from the aortic arch and the right common carotid from the right subclavian artery. At the level of the upper portion of the thyroid cartilage the common carotid arteries bifurcate into external and internal carotid arteries. The external carotid artery supplies blood to the outer cranium, face, and neck. The internal carotid artery sends blood to the cerebral hemispheres by dividing into anterior and middle cerebral arteries. The vertebral arteries are direct or indirect branches off the aorta and anastomose at the base of the brain (level of the pons) forming the basal artery, which continues anteriorly and ends as the right and left posterior cerebral arteries. Communicating branches from the posterior cerebral arteries connect them to the middle cerebral arteries. The middle cerebral arteries connect to the anterior cerebral arteries as branches of the internal carotid arteries. The anterior cerebral arteries connect through the anterior communicating branches, and all form the Circle of Willis (Fig. 8-2). The three cerebral arteries are regionalized in their distribution with very precise boundaries. Large dural sinuses (that is, superior sagittal, inferior sagittal, and straight transverse) drain the cortex through the internal jugular veins, which pass from the cranium through the jugular foramen (Figs. 8-3 and 8-4).

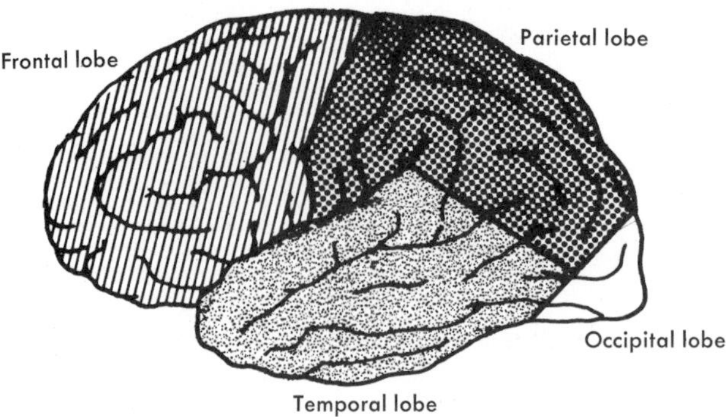

Fig. 8-1. Topographic anatomy of major cortical regions (lobes).

A

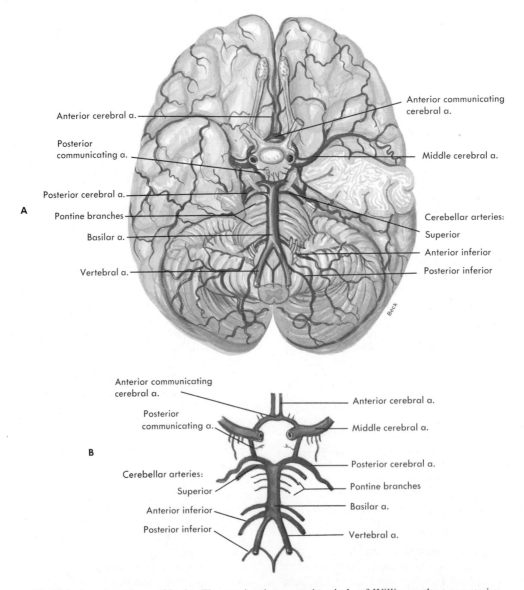

Anterior cerebral a.
Posterior communicating a.
Posterior cerebral a.
Pontine branches
Basilar a.
Vertebral a.
Anterior communicating cerebral a.
Middle cerebral a.
Cerebellar arteries:
Superior
Anterior inferior
Posterior inferior
Beck

B

Anterior communicating cerebral a.
Posterior communicating a.
Cerebellar arteries:
Superior
Anterior inferior
Posterior inferior
Anterior cerebral a.
Middle cerebral a.
Posterior cerebral a.
Pontine branches
Basilar a.
Vertebral a.

Fig. 8-2. Arteries at base of brain. The arteries that comprise circle of Willis are the two anterior cerebral arteries joined to each other by anterior communicating cerebral artery and to posterior communicating arteries. (From Anthony, C. P., and Thibodeau, G. A.: Textbook of anatomy and physiology, ed. 10, St. Louis, 1979, The C. V. Mosby Co.)

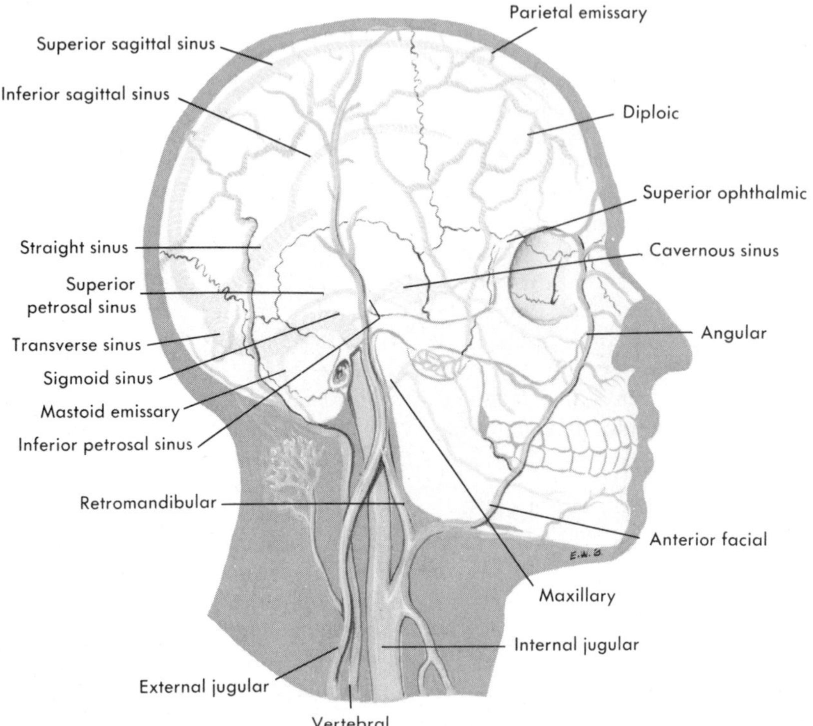

Fig. 8-3. Semischematic projection of large veins of head. Deep veins and dural sinuses are projected on skull. Note connections (emissary veins) between superficial and deep veins. (From Anthony, C. P., and Thibodeau, G. A.: Textbook of anatomy and physiology, ed. 10, St. Louis, 1979, The C. V. Mosby Co.)

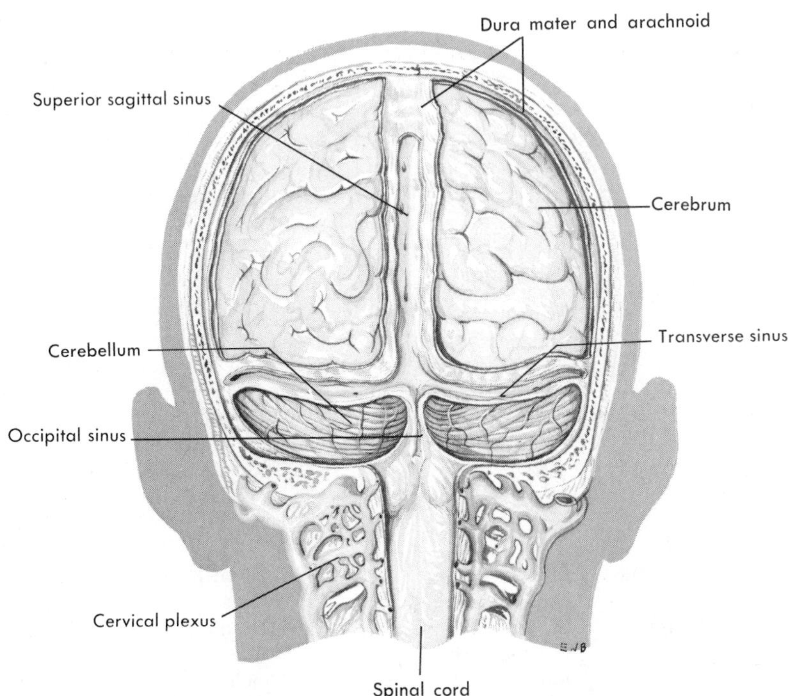

Fig. 8-4. Venous sinuses shown in relation to brain and skull. (From Anthony, C. P., and Thibodeau, G. A.: Textbook of anatomy and physiology, ed. 10, St. Louis, 1979, The C. V. Mosby Co.)

BLOOD-BRAIN BARRIER

The brain possesses the unique ability to limit the passage of all but a few essential compounds into its cells. Shown by electron microscopy to have a microanatomic basis, the barrier is distinct to the central nervous system.[17] Essential nutrients such as glucose, oxygen, electrolytes, and carbon dioxide readily cross into nervous tissue to maintain the brain's integrity. Large metabolic molecules such as urea and most serum proteins normally remain blood borne until diffuse metabolic alterations (that is, tumor, infarction, or abscess) occur.

The following lists the major factors that facilitate the abnormal central nervous system localization of radiopharmaceuticals:

Normal (glucose, oxygen, electrolytes, carbon dioxide)
  Passive diffusion (across capillary membrane)
  Active transport (across neural cell membranes)
Abnormal (urea, serum proteins, antibodies, drugs)
  Pore filtration (across loose endothelial junction)
  Cellular pinocytosis (across basement membrane)

Although the localization of radiopharmaceuticals in brain lesions capitalizes on the deterioration of the blood-brain barrier, the detection of the lesion by imaging does not require an absolute increase in lesion concentration of the radiopharmaceutical. Detection depends on the relative increased concentration in the lesion (target) compared to the lesser background (nontarget) activity. Pertechnetate ($^{99m}TcO_4^-$) and its analogs pentetic acid (DTPA) and glucoheptonate give similar target-to-nontarget ratios of 15 to 25 : 1, and all are excellent brain-imaging radiopharmaceuticals.

THE RADIOPHARMACEUTICALS

A wide choice of radiopharmaceutical agents are available to image the brain (Table 8-1). The most popular are pertechnetate ($^{99m}TcO_4^-$) or its analogs pentetic acid (diethylenetriaminepentaacetic acid, DTPA) and glucoheptonate (GH).[15] An average adult dose (70 kg man) of $^{99m}TcO_4^-$ is 20 mCi (250 to 300 μCi/kg). To eliminate choroid-plexus and salivary-gland uptake that is observed when $^{99m}TcO_4^-$ is used, potassium perchlorate ($KClO_4$) is given orally in an adult dose of 0.75 to 1 g 1 hour or less prior to the injection of the pertechnetate.[22] In children, the $KClO_4$ should be given orally in a dose of 50 mg per year of age. In clinical situations when the patient is unable to swallow, the perchlorate may be administrered rectally.

^{99m}Tc-DTPA and ^{99m}Tc-glucoheptonate require no premedication,[21] and after their administration are rapidly cleared through the kidneys. Unlike $^{99m}TcO_4^-$, they are unaffected in their normal body localization by the prior administration of a ^{99m}Tc-labeled stannous phosphate[21] (that is, pyrophosphate, diphosphonate, and methylene diphosphonate) used to image the skeleton. The excess tin ion in these preparations causes free pertechnetate to bind to circulating red blood cells producing an in vivo blood-pool agent that may degrade the image resolution.[4]

The preference in many laboratories for the ^{99m}Tc-labeled chelates rather than pertechnetate for brain imaging is attributable in part to their apparently more rapid rate of brain lesion uptake. For pertechnetate the optimal time to start the equilibrium image is 3 to 4 hours after injection, whereas the optimal starting time for ^{99m}Tc-DPTA and ^{99m}Tc-glucoheptonate is between 30 to 120 minutes.[21]

Special radiopharmaceuticals such as ^{99m}Tc-labeled human serum albumin and ^{67}Ga citrate are employed to image certain intracranial vascular and inflammatory lesions, but neither possesses lesion specificity, and successful imaging has been erratic.[19] The usual radiogallium dose (adult) is 3 to 6 mCi and the optimal time to start the images is at 48 and 72 hours.

Table 8-1. Radiopharmaceuticals for brain imaging

Radiopharmaceutical	Gamma energy (keV)	Half-life	Critical organ	Whole body	Dose (mCi)	Time to image	Prestudy
^{131}I-labeled human serum albumin	365	8.1 days	*Blood* 2.5 rads/0.4 mCi	750 rads/0.4 mCi	0.20 to 0.40	24 to 48 hours	SSKI
^{99m}Tc-pertechnetate	140	6 hours	*Colon* 0.10 rad/mCi	0.12 rad/10 mCi	15 to 20	1 to 3 hours	Choice of $KClO_4$ or atropine
^{99m}Tc-labeled human serum albumin	140	6 hours	*Blood* 0.15 rad/10 mCi	0.15 rad/10 mCi	15 to 20	2 to 4 hours	None
^{99m}Tc-DTPA (^{99m}Tc-pentetic acid)	140	6 hours	*Bladder* 3 rads/10 mCi	0.06 rad/10 mCi	15 to 20	0.5 to 2 hours	None
^{99m}Tc-glucoheptonate	140	6 hours	*Bladder* 0.5 rad/mCi	0.14 rad/mCi	15 to 20	2 to 3 hours	None

IMAGING

*C*erebral *r*adionuclide *a*ngio*g*ram (CRAG) or "flow" study

The cerebral radionuclide angiogram can be taken from the anterior, posterior, either lateral, or vertex projection.[10] The anterior projection clearly displays and compares both internal carotid arteries, their intracranial branches, and their distribution. The patient's head is positioned against the detector with the chin depressed enough to place the canthomeatal line perpendicular to the collimator face. The median plane of the patient is perpendicular to the detector (Fig. 8-5). A suitably constructed headclamp or masking tape is used to immobilize the head.

For those instances where there is a question of diminished arterial blood flow to the brain, the cervical area is included in the field of view. The patient is positioned in the routine anterior position with the top of the head as close as possible to the edge of the camera's field of view. This allows most of the cervical area to be included in the image.

If the vertex view is chosen, the patient must be positioned so that activity in the great vessels of the thorax will not shine through and cause artifacts in the area of concern. The scintillation camera is inverted and lowered below the level of the stretcher. The patient is placed in the supine position with his head extended off the stretcher and resting on the collimator face. The neck is hyperextended as much as possible to reduce body background (Fig. 8-6). The collimator is angled so that the infraorbital meatal line is parallel to the detector. A lead cape is used to reduce the counts coming from the neck and upper thorax.

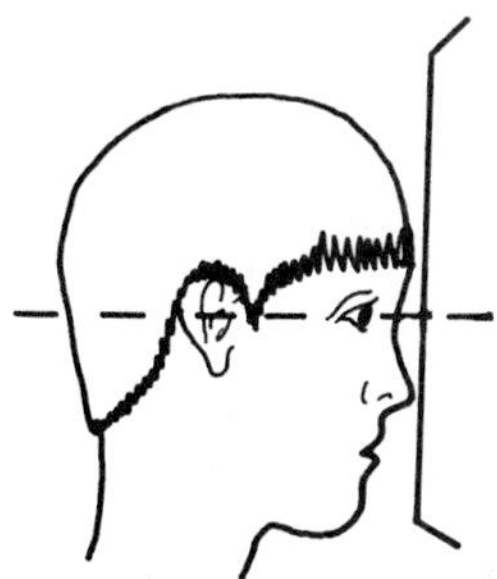

Fig. 8-5. Patient position for anterior CRAG (cerebral radionuclide angiogram).

The dose of radiopharmaceutical should be in a volume not to exceed 2 ml and preferably less than 1 ml. Occluding tourniquets are applied several inches above and below the injection site for 2 to 4 minutes before the injection. Immediately after the injection of the radiopharmaceutical the distal tourniquet is removed followed 10 seconds later by removal of the proximal tourniquet. The scintillation camera, with imaging parameters previously set, is started when activity first appears on the camera's persistence scope or between 6 to 8 seconds after bolus injection, whichever comes first. Serial exposures of 0.5- to 2-second intervals are made for 40 seconds or until the venous structures are identified on the persistence oscilloscope.

Equilibrium (static) images

Routinely, four or five equilibrium images should be taken: the anterior, the posterior, and both laterals. In many laboratories the vertex projection is regarded as a special view and, like oblique views, are reserved for certain clinical situations. The *anterior view* can be taken with the patient supine or sitting. Appropriate camera-head alignment is assured if the canthomeatal line is perpendicular to the detector face (Fig. 8-7).

The *posterior view* is the most difficult routine projection to obtain. It requires positioning of the patient's head to reduce or eliminate the cervical lordo-

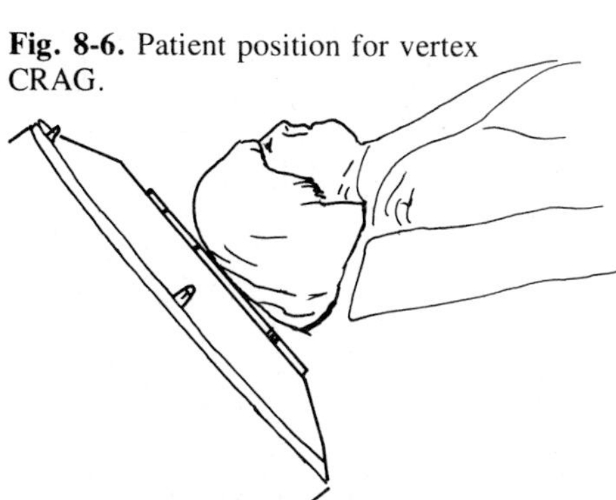

Fig. 8-6. Patient position for vertex CRAG.

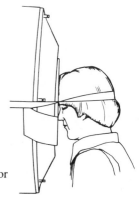

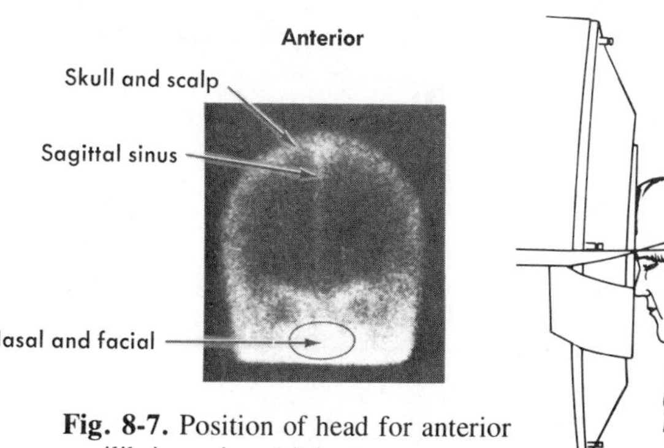

Fig. 8-7. Position of head for anterior equilibrium view (sitting).

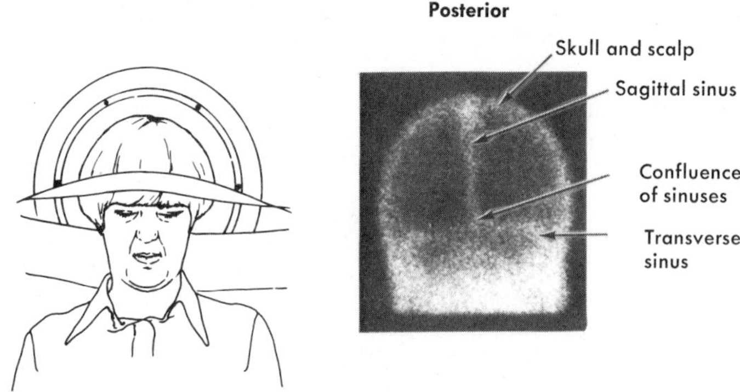

Fig. 8-8. Position of head for posterior flow (CRAG) and equilibrium views (sitting).

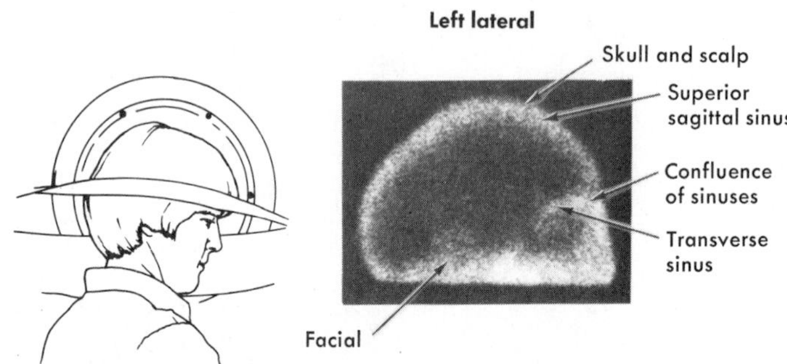

Fig. 8-9. Position of head for lateral equilibrium views (sitting).

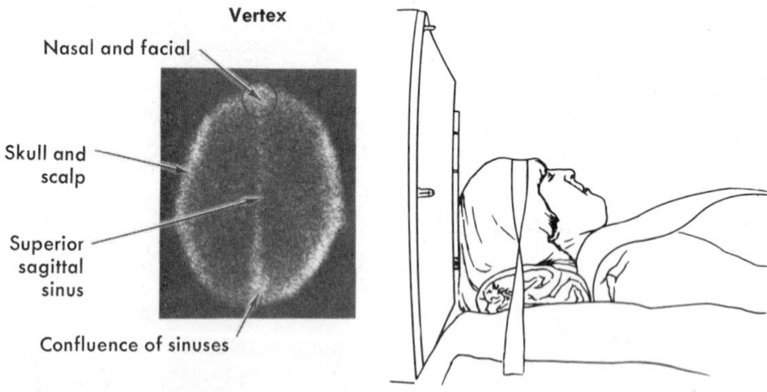

Fig. 8-10. Position of head for vertex equilibrium view (supine).

sis–detector surface angle and center the torcular (confluence of sinuses) so that the posterior fossa is exposed.[17] In the alert and cooperative patient one can best accomplish this by placing the patient's head in a modified *atlas position* where the detector surface is tilted slightly forward with the neck anteroflexed (Fig. 8-8). The median plane is perpendicular to the collimator face. It can also be obtained with the patient supine or prone, but additional care must be taken to assure that the posterior fossa area is seen.

To obtain the optimum *lateral views* requires that the sagittal plane of the head be parallel with the detector surface. One should reduce excessive facial activity resulting from glandular uptake or blood pooling in highly vascular structures by placing a lead shield over the face or aligning the facial activity outside the camera's field of view (Fig. 8-9).

It is essential to shield the camera from shoulder and other body activity when one is obtaining the *vertex view,* regardless of whether the image is taken supine or prone. Appropriate positioning requires parallel alignment of the canthomeatal line with the detector surface to expose both cerebral hemispheres equally and symmetrically (Fig. 8-10).[16]

Special projections may be clinically indicated. The *orbital view* is employed when eye lesions are suspected and are best obtained by abutment of the forehead with the detector surface so that the canthomeatal line is at a 25-degree cephalad angle to the vertical axis of the detector. *Magnified posterior view* images may be required if small posterior fossa lesions are suspected and is accomplished by positioning of the camera's pinhole collimator directly against the skull at the desired site and angle.[17]

NORMAL BRAIN IMAGES

The nuclear medicine technologist must be familiar with what constitutes the normal appearance of a brain image so that when a positioning error occurs, one can repeat the view immediately without being told and avoiding an additional readministration of radioactivity to the patient.

Anterior view

Both cerebral hemispheres appear equal in size and shape with decreased cortical activity surrounded by a halo of increased density produced by scalp, skull, muscle, and meningeal vascular activity. At the apex in the midline the superior sagittal sinus forms a linear density that projects downward but rarely intercepts with the midline cavernous sinus at the base of the brain (Fig. 8-7).

Posterior view

The posterior view simulates the anterior view, except for the crossed activity produced by the intersection of the superior sagittal sinus with the transverse sinuses and the occipital sinus at the centralized torcular (confluence of sinuses). The peripheral activity outlining the occipitoparietal cortex is produced by scalp, skull, and meningeal activity. The transverse sinuses laterally abruptly proceed downward forming the sigmoid sinuses and are the lateral walls of the posterior fossa. The posterior fossa is bound superiorly by the transverse sinuses and inferiorly by the neck musculature activity. At times it may be normally bisected, below the torcular, by linear occipital sinus activity (Fig. 8-8).

Lateral views

The right and left lateral views are mirror images. The superior sagittal sinus begins anteriorly and, as a linear band of activity, increases in width as it proceeds posteriorly along the superior margin ending at the torcular, which appears as a circular intense focus. The transverse sinuses are linear densities with an apical convexity ending in the activity near the auditory canal. They expose the cerebellum as clear round areas. The inferior margin demonstrates numerous irregular impressions related to the pituitary fossa and cavernous sinus, and intense uptake is present in the nasopharynx mucosa, salivary glands, and muscles of mastication (Fig. 8-9).

Vertex view

Symmetric cerebral hemispheres bisected by a straight and ever-widening superior sagittal sinus (SSS) as it proceeds posteriorly to end in the torcular are seen. Scalp, skull, and meningeal activity accounts for a faint border around the hemispheres. An irregular bulge of the SSS in the parietal area is caused by perforating cerebral veins (anastomotic veins of Trolard). When $^{99m}TcO_4^-$ is used, it is concentrated in the salivary glands and is demonstrated as an intense anterior midline activity (oral cavity) and bilateral temporal concentrations (parotid gland). Both can be eliminated with atropine sulfate (1 mg IV with $^{99m}TcO_4^-$) and are not observed if ^{99m}Tc-DTPA or ^{99m}Tc-glucoheptonate are used (Fig. 8-10).

PATHOLOGY

Diseases that are detected by radionuclide brain imaging may occur anywhere from the scalp inward to the cerebral cortex. Changes in the vascularity and factors affecting tissue binding of the radiopharmaceutical (that is, protein binding) are instrumental in the extracortical uptake.

The following is a classification of central nervous system diseases:

Brain tumors
- Gliomas, 45% (glioblastoma multiforme, medulloblastoma)
- Meningiomas, 18%
- Metastatic, 10% (lung, breast)
- Pituitary tumors, 10%
- Others, 17% (acoustic neurinoma, pinealoma)

Vascular lesions
- Congenital
  - Berry aneurysm
  - Arteriovenous malformation

- Traumatic
  - Concussion
  - Epidural hemorrhage
  - Subdural hemorrhage
- Spontaneous
  - Infarction (thrombosis, embolus, hemorrhage)

Inflammatory and degenerative lesions
- Inflammatory
  - Encephalitis
  - Meningitis
  - Abscess
  - Granuloma
- Degenerative
  - Leukodystrophy
  - Multiple sclerosis
  - Phakomatoses (tuberous sclerosis, neurofibromatosis, Sturge-Weber disease)
  - Lipoidoses (Hand-Schüller-Christian disease)

Cystic lesions
- Arachnoid cyst
- Colloid cyst
- Porencephalic cyst
- Dandy-Walker cyst (ventricle IV)
- Hydatid cyst

Extracortical lesions
- Cephalhematoma
- Skull fracture
- Fibrous dysplasia
- Paget's disease
- Metastases

Of the several types of *brain tumors,* grade IV gliomas (glioblastoma multiforme), meningiomas, and metastatic tumors consistently show the most intense concentration of radiopharmaceutical on both the cerebral radionuclide angiogram (CRAG) and the equilibrium images (Fig. 8-11).[11,17] Because of their varied blood supply, delayed imaging may be required for demonstrating certain metastatic tumors. Most low grade (I and II) gliomas, pituitary tumors, and brainstem tumors are difficult to detect by imaging, even if the dynamic study is performed and longer equilibration is allowed. Most brain tumors in children are located in the posterior fossa below the tentorium, and their predilection for the midline (cystic astrocytoma, medulloblastoma) produces a characteristic pattern on the posterior and both lateral brain equilibrium images

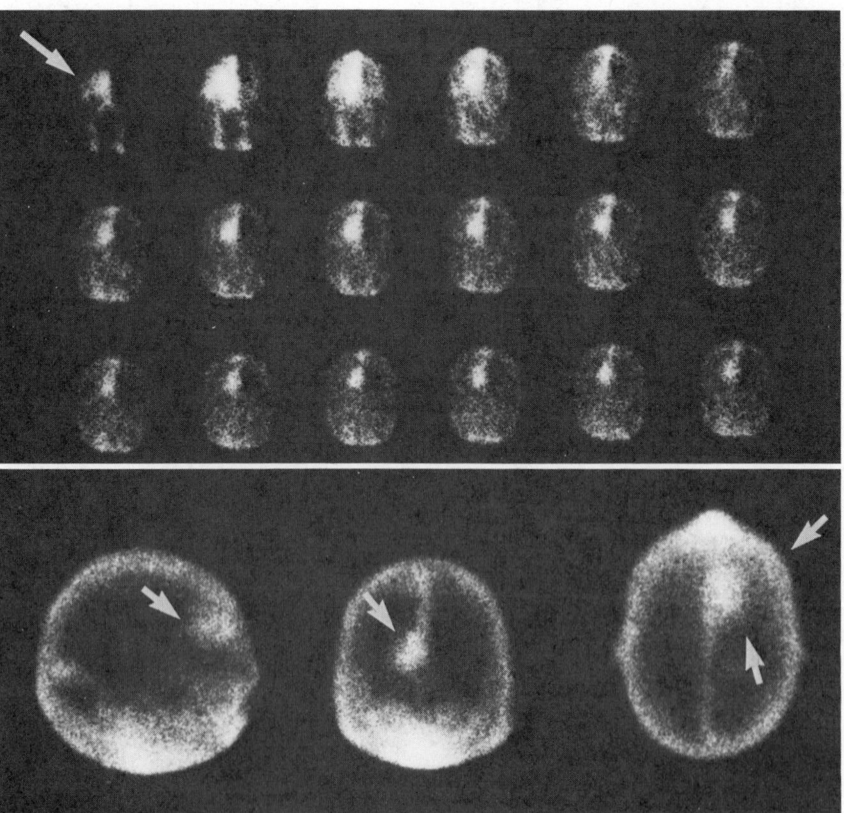

Fig. 8-11. Frontal parasagittal meningioma. *Upper panel,* Progressively increasing tumor uptake with clearing of surrounding background activity. *Lower panel,* Tumor as an intense focal uptake in right parasagittal frontal area.

(Fig. 8-12). A similar, but distinctly asymmetric pattern may be observed in the adult with a large acoustic neurinoma.[17]

Vascular lesions of the central nervous system may be congenital, traumatic, or spontaneous in origin. In the congenital group a berry aneurysm may rupture producing a catastrophic subarachnoid or intracerebral hemorrhage and is rarely demonstrable by brain imaging even if hemorrhaging is active. Arteriovenous malformations (AVM), in contrast, give nearly a pathognomonic pattern on the CRAG.[9,10] The static images may be positive or normal depending on whether the AVM has caused local damage by leaking red cells into the surrounding brain tissue.

Of the traumatic extradural hemorrhages, the chronic (longer than 2 weeks old) subdural hematoma is most amenable to detection by brain imaging (greater than 83% detection accuracy). Development of a neomembrane around the hemorrhage facilitates radiopharmaceutical concentration and may be displayed as a "crescent" abnormality on the anterior and posterior brain image views. Hematomas of sufficient size may also be demonstrated as a photon-deficient peripheral defect on the early CRAG and a crescent deformity on the equilibrium images (Fig. 8-13).

Spontaneous cerebral thrombosis is the most common cause of strokes and usually affects the middle cerebral artery and its branches alone, or in combination with another cerebral artery, in more than 80% of afflicted patients. The discordant finding of regional ischemia on the CRAG and a normal-equilibrium brain image within the first 2 weeks of the insult is characteristic of a "stroke." Conversion of the equilibrium image to abnormal increased cortical uptake confined to a vascular region within 7 days of the insult suggests cerebral embolism as the pathogenesis (Fig. 8-14). Intracortical hematomas are less likely to be demonstrated by conventional imaging and usually require long (4 to 6 hours) equilibration before imaging.

Of the *inflammatory lesions* affecting the brain, the *abscess* is the most consistently detected abnormality.[7] Greater than 90% of brain abscesses are demonstrable by imaging and are more likely to be delineated when one delays the start of the image for 3 hours or longer (Fig. 8-15). A doughnut-like sign (central clearing of the lesion) is not an uncommon finding, and monitoring of the therapeutic course of an abscess with brain imaging shows a lag in image resolution compared to the clinical improvement. Cortical granulomas react like avascular tumors and require histologic evaluation to differentiate from brain tumors.

Degenerative brain lesions such as multiple sclerosis may, during its most acute stage, give a completely normal brain image. On the other hand, the brain image may be grossly abnormal when clinical symptoms are absent and no localizing signs are present. A similar paradox may occur after therapy, and although brain imaging is not contraindicated, its value in these conditions is questionable.

Many *cystic lesions* have been indirectly demonstrated by brain imaging and characteristically produce a "supernormal" defect. Large cysts or cystlike masses may be readily demonstrable on the vertex view.

The introduction of computerized tomography, however, has all but replaced brain imaging for these conditions. In certain circumstances brain imaging may be of special value in children in whom an unusual tenting configuration of the transverse sinuses and torcular ("cyclops" sign) on the routine posterior brain image may indicate a Dandy-Walker cyst of the fourth ventricle.[6]

Of the *extracortical lesions,* those involving the soft

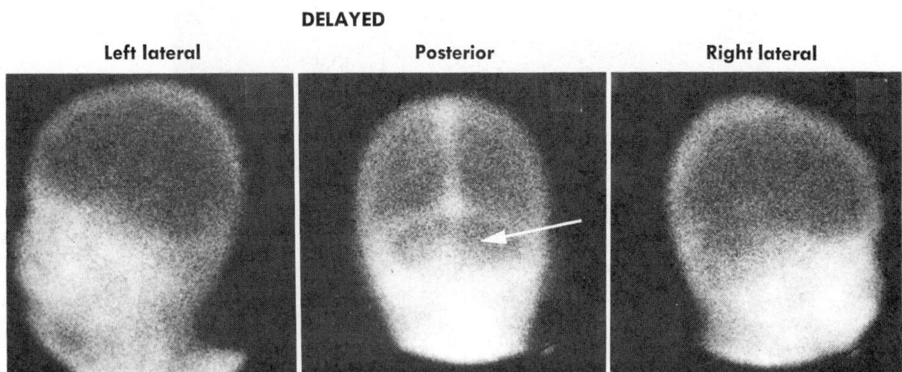

Fig. 8-12. Cystic astrocytoma of cerebellar vermis shown as intense broad infratorcular focus on posterior view that projects symmetrically upward from region of auditory canal on both lateral views.

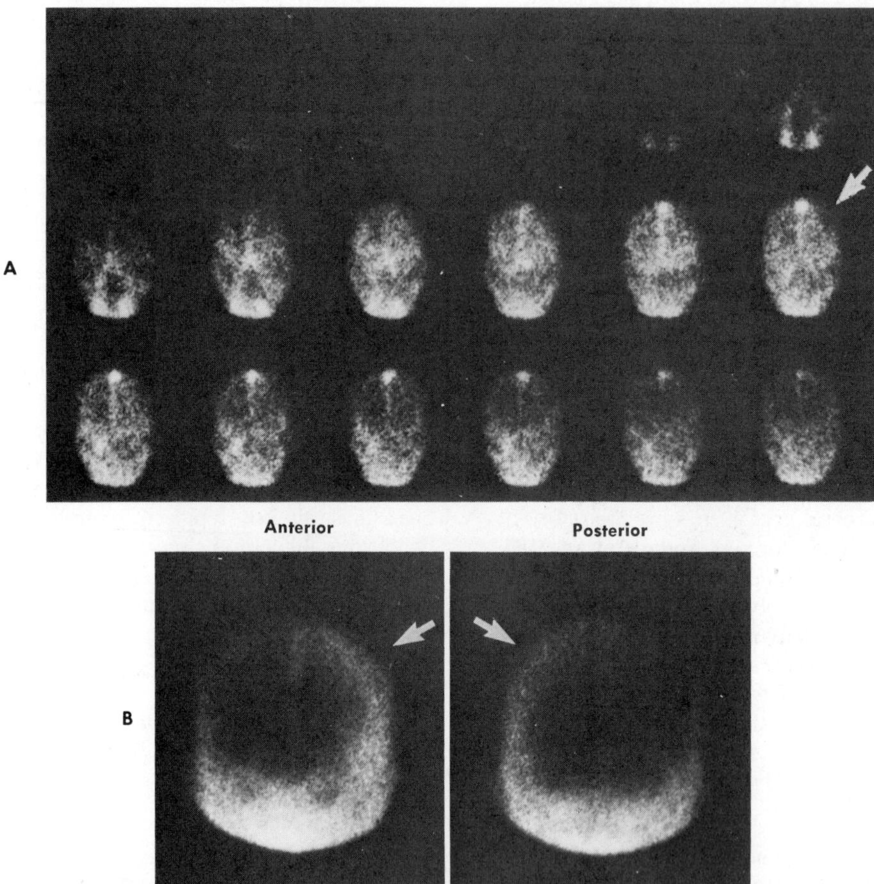

Fig. 8-13. Chronic subdural hematoma showing as large peripheral photon-deficient concavity on CRAG and as well-defined crescent abnormality on equilibrium images.

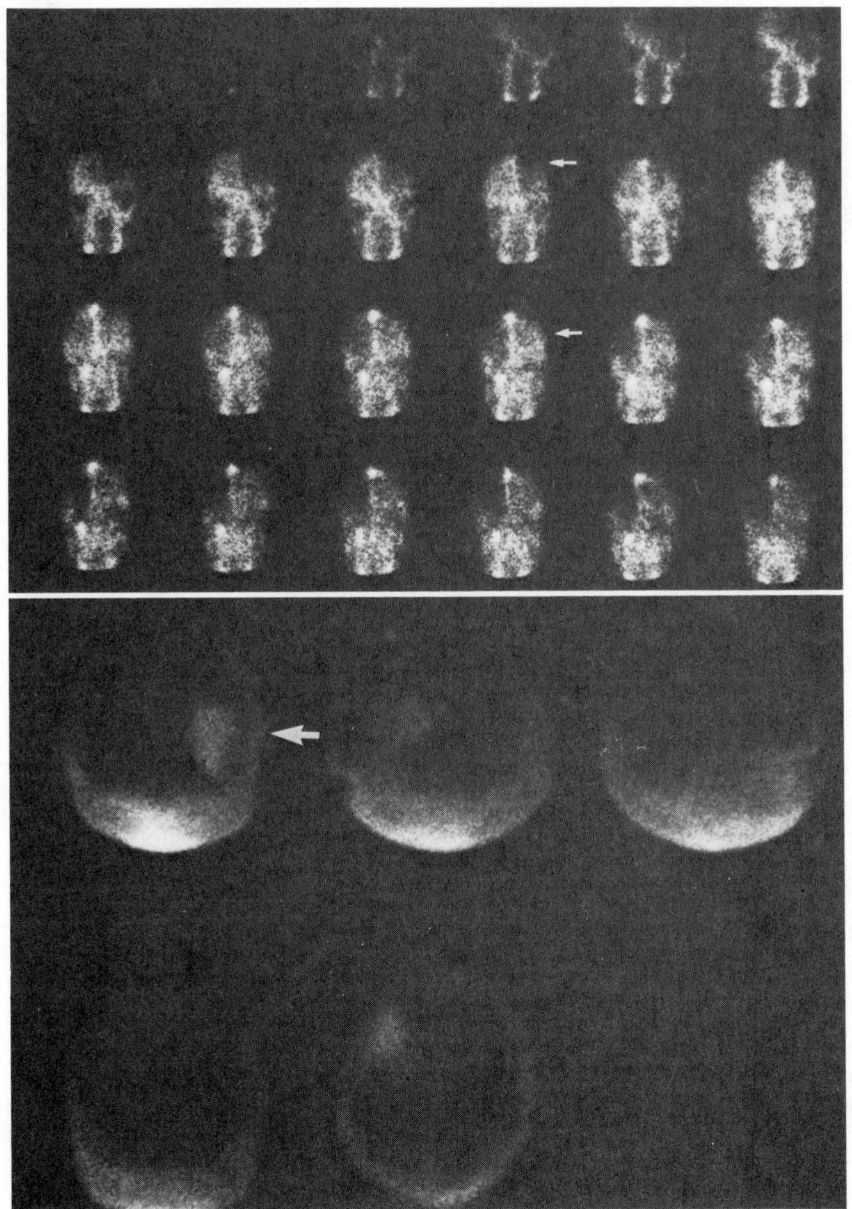

Fig. 8-14. Cerebral infarction showing absent perfusion of left middle cerebral artery and its distribution on CRAG with a "flip-flop" (delayed perfusion of affected side through collaterals) and focal increased uptake in left middle cerebral artery distribution on equilibrium views.

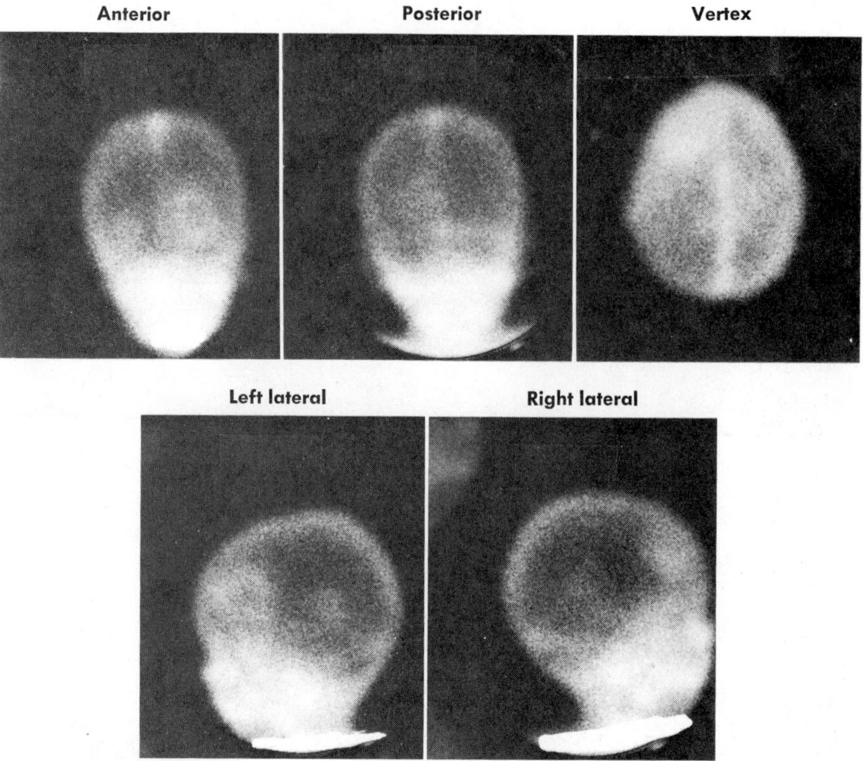

Fig. 8-15. Multiple brain abscesses shown as intense foci of uptake throughout brain on equilibrium images. Doughnut-shaped lesion in left frontal cortex.

tissues are readily diagnosed by observation and palpation and will usually be resolved on the repeat brain image in 10 to 14 days. Diseased cranium such as occurs with bony metastases, fibrous dysplasia, and Paget's disease can be differentiated from superficial cortical lesions by use of imaging with bone-seeking radiopharmaceuticals such as ^{99m}Tc pyrophosphate or ^{99m}Tc methylene diphosphonate.

CISTERNOGRAPHY

Radionuclide cisternography is performed for assessment of the normal and abnormal pathways and the hydrodynamics of cerebrospinal fluid. Cerebrospinal fluid originates as a transudate of blood and is produced primarily from the choroid plexuses located in the lateral, third, and fourth ventricles of the brain (Fig. 8-16). They produce a total of 500 to 700 ml of cerebrospinal fluid each 24 hours, and this drains from the ventricular system through foramina in the roof of the fourth ventricle into the cisterna magna of the subarachnoid space. It then passes down the dorsolateral surface of the spinal cord to the cauda equina, then up over the ventrolateral surface of the cord to the basilar cisterns, then to the superior cisterns, and eventually over the free convexities of the cortex to terminate by excretion into the superior sagittal sinus through the arachnoid villi.[8]

Radiopharmaceuticals

Ideally the optimal radiopharmaceutical for radionuclide cisternography should (1) not be metabolized while in the cerebrospinal fluid, (2) be lipid insoluble so that it will not readily diffuse across tissue membranes, (3) be rapidly cleared from the blood, (4) be primarily excreted by the arachnoid villi, (5) be nonirritating, nonreactive, and nonantigenic when placed intrathecally, (6) be molecularly diffusable throughout the cerebrospinal fluid, (7) be easy to label with a gamma ray–emitting radionuclide, and (8) be nonpyrogenic and easy to sterilize.[17] Although ^{131}I–human serum albumin was dominant as the preferred cisternographic radiopharmaceutical for many years, it met few of these criteria. Except in special situations such as the assessment of ventriculoperitoneal or ventriculoatrial shunt patency or in children in whom ^{99m}Tc–human serum albumin is preferred, either ^{111}In-DTPA or ^{169}Yb-DTPA best meet the listed criteria. Because of its photon abundance (gamma photons, 173 keV and

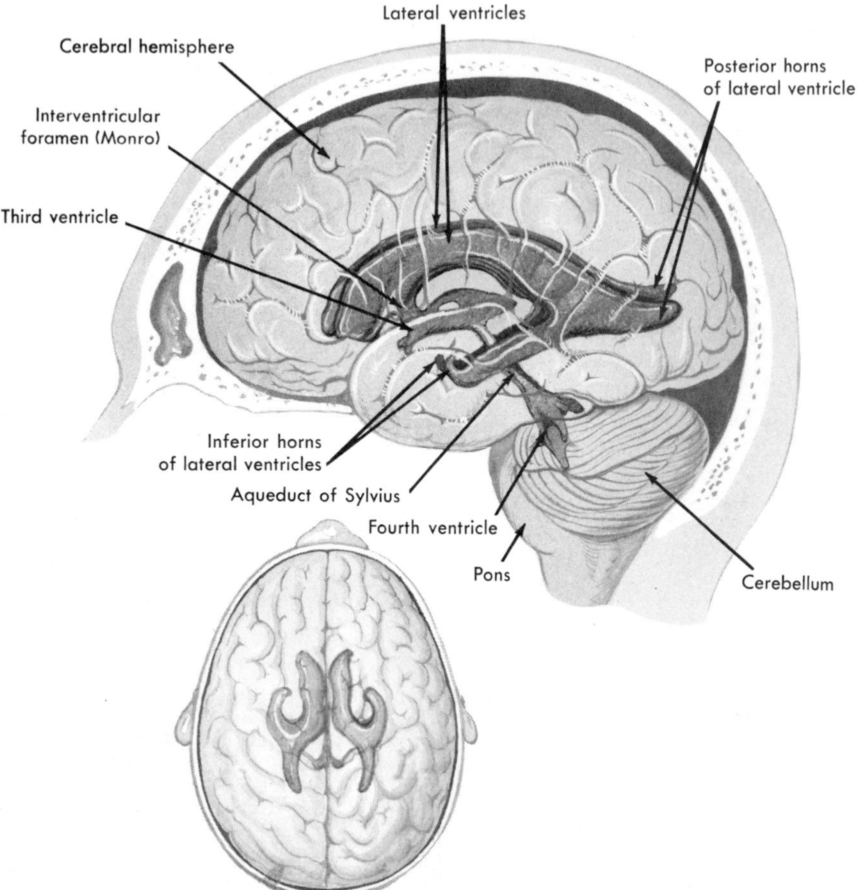

Fig. 8-16. Cerebral ventricles projected on lateral surface of cerebrum. *Smaller drawing,* Ventricles from above. (From Anthony, C. P., and Thibodeau, G. A.: Textbook of anatomy and physiology, ed. 10, St. Louis, 1979, The C. V. Mosby Co.)

247 keV; half-life, 2.8 days), ^{111}In-DTPA is preferred. The shelf life of ^{169}Yb-DTPA (half-life, 31.8 days), however, makes it a reasonable alternative.

Procedure

In most institutions intrathecal injections require signed patient consent. The physician may perform the procedure or directly supervise its performance by qualified personnel. The procedure calls for a sterile field, a sterile spinal tray, and sterile technique to avoid any secondary complications such as infections. A three-way stopcock is attached to the inserted spinal needle to facilitate the administration of the radiopharmaceutical, to monitor the cerebrospinal fluid pressure and to sample the fluid for routine cell and chemical tests.

Immediately after the radiopharmaceutical administration the injection site is imaged to determine whether the instillation was adequate. With the patient remaining recumbent, preferably supine, one positions the head slightly lower than the hips by placing a rolled pillow beneath the upper thighs for the next 1 to 2 hours. In the adult, imaging is performed routinely at 2, 6, 24, and 48 hours. Additional views at other times may be selected by the monitoring physician. Routine images in children are taken between 1 and 2, 4 and 6, at 8, and at 24 hours, with additional times determined by the monitoring physician. When used to evaluate the patency of shunts or cranial leaks, the imaging times and positions will vary with the conditions and the information desired.

Routine cisternographic images are taken from the anterior and one or both lateral projections. Additional vertex views may be taken if indicated. Ideally, each view is taken for 100,000 counts or for a preset time (10 minutes if practical).

Normal cisternogram

The cisternogram *anterior view* is obtained when the face is placed against the detector surface and the neck is flexed dorsally 5 degrees. The 2- and 6-hour images are similar showing a three-pronged activity, the single midline cisterns, and two lateral temporal cisterns, giving the appearance of a ''viking's helmet''. At 24 hours and beyond the radiopharmaceutical moves over the convexities and gives a uniform circumscribed configuration (Fig. 8-17). The two *lateral views* demonstrate the basilar cisterns and subsequently the combined superior and basilar cisterns on the 2- and 6-hour images respectfully. The 24- and 48-hour images describe the entire lateral convexity with ''capping'' along the superior sagittal sinus. The *vertex view* is best considered a modified but more extensive anterior view and symmetrically displays the subarachnoid space as irregular four-edged rectangular activity.

Abnormal cisternogram

A large number of radionuclide cisternographic patterns have been described; they include (1) normal CSF flow, (2) slow CSF flow, (3) ventricular filling (reflux), (4) subarachnoid blocks, (5) asymmetric CSF flow, and (6) CSF pooling. Normal flow has already been described and is symmetric with activity in the basilar cisterns by 2 to 4 hours, over the free convexity by 12 to 24 hours, and capping at the superior sagittal sinus by 24 to 48 hours. Slow cerebrospinal flow is normally encountered with increasing age but is more noticeable with cerebral atrophy. Ventricular filling (reflux) is always abnormal in adults and may be complete or incomplete with no flow (block) or complete or incomplete with slow flow or transient movement. Blocks with subsequent pooling may occur anywhere along the spine or the basal cisterns, or over the cerebral convexities.

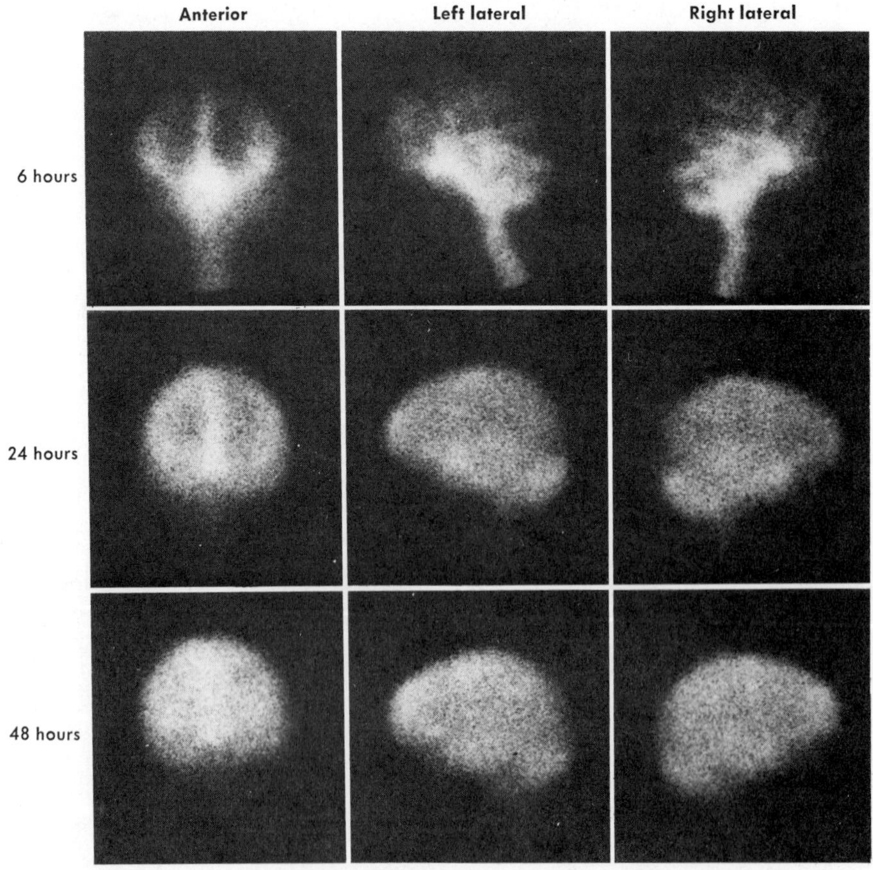

Fig. 8-17. Normal cisternogram showing anterior and both lateral views at 6, 24, and 48 hours after intrathecal administration.

Clinical utility

Hydrocephalus implies a symmetric or asymmetric enlargement of the ventricular system because of a pathologic increase in the volume of intracranial cerebrospinal fluid with or without increased intracranial pressure.

The following is a workable classification of hydrocephalus:

- Hydrocephalus from hypersecretion of cerebrospinal fluid
- Obstructive
  - Noncommunicating (in the ventricular system)
  - Communicating (in the extraventricular system)
- Nonobstructive (hydrocephalus ex vacuo)
  - Generalized
  - Localized

Of particular importance in recent years is the form of obstructive communicating hydrocephalus occurring commonly in middle-aged males with normal cerebrospinal-fluid pressure and the clinical triad of dementia, ataxia, and urinary incontinence. Patients with normal pressure hydrocephalus (NPH) (Hakim-Adams syndrome) may have had previous subarachnoid hemorrhage, infection, head trauma, or neoplasia.[13] In those where the symptoms are recent and the diagnosis is made early, neurosurgical shunting can reverse and eliminate the symptoms.

The pathogenesis of NPH has not precisely emerged and is probably caused from an imbalance of venous and cerebrospinal fluid pressure. Characteristically, ventricular filling (reflux) is found on the radionuclide cisternogram (Fig. 8-18). The rate and completeness of ventricular clearing has been used to predict the use and success of shunting in NPH, but the duration of symptoms appears to be the most reliable prognosticator. Symptoms lasting beyond 1 year are rarely reversed by shunting.

In evaluating shunt patency the radiopharmaceutical may be administered conventionally or be placed at the source of the suspected obstruction or directly into the shunt reservoir. Cerebrospinal fluid leaks through the nose (rhinorrhea) or ear (otorrhea) can be imaged if active draining is present. If the leak is suspected and not actively flowing, absorbent pledgets may be applied at the suspected site and after an appropriate application time (optimally 2 to 4 hours) are removed

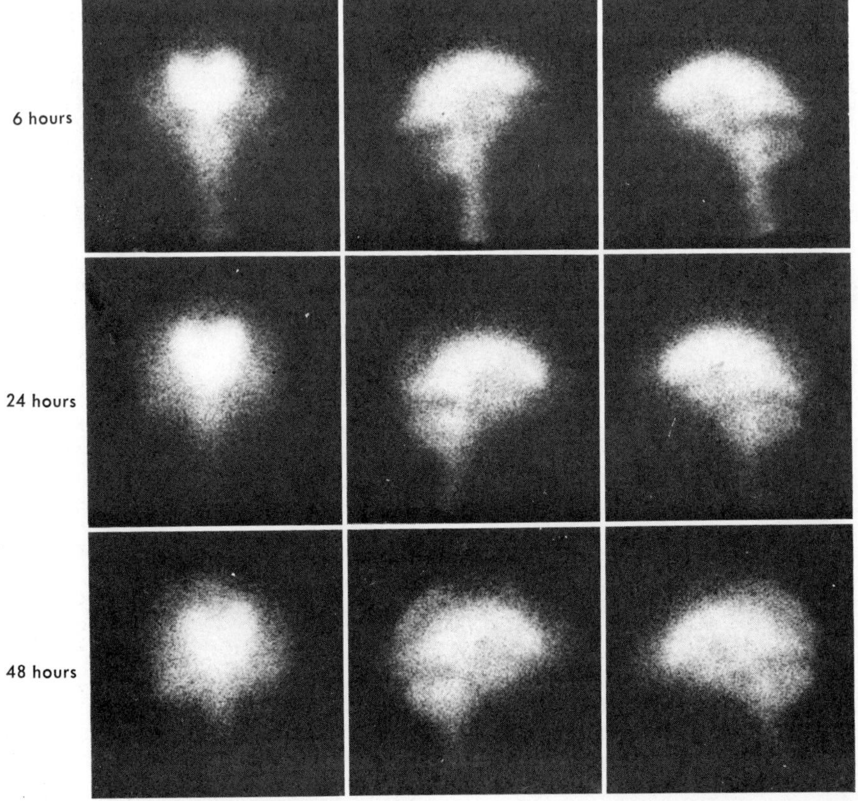

Fig. 8-18. Communicating hydrocephalus (normal pressure hydrocephalus) with lateral ventricular reflux on 6-hour images and no significant ventricular clearing on the 24- and 48-hour images.

and counted. Activity three to four times the background rate is significant for localization.

REFERENCES

1. Anger, H. O.: Scintillation camera, Rev. Sci. Instrum. **29:**27, 1958.
2. Blau, M., and Bender, M. A.: Radiomercury (Hg 203) labeled Neohydrin: a new agent for brain tumor localization, J. Nucl. Med. **3:**83, 1962.
3. Cassen, B., Curtis, L., and Reed, C.: Sensitive directional gamma-ray detector, Nucleonics **6:**78, 1950.
4. Chandler, W. M., and Shuck, L. D.: Abnormal technetium 99m pertechnetate imaging following stannous pyrophosphate bone imaging, 21st Annual Meeting of The Society of Nuclear Medicine, New York, 1975, The Society.
5. Chou, S. N., Anst, J. B., Moore, G. E., and Peyton, W. T.: Radioactive iodinated human serum albumin as a tracer agent for diagnosing and localizing intracranial lesions, Proc. Soc. Exp. Biol. Med. **77:**193, 1951.
6. Conway, J. J., Yarzagaray, L., and Welch, D.: Radionuclide evaluation of Dandy-Walker malformation and congenital arachnoid cyst of the posterior fossa, Am. J. Roentgenol. Radium Ther. Nucl. Med. **112:**306, 1971.
7. Crocker, E. F., McLaughlin, A. F., Morris, J. G., et al.: Technetium brain scanning in the diagnosis and management of cerebral abscess, Am. J. Med. **56:**192, 1974.
8. Darson, H.: Physiology of cerebrospinal fluid, Boston, 1967, Little, Brown & Co.
9. DeLand, F., and Wagner, H. N., Jr.: Atlas of nuclear medicine, vol. 1, The brain, Philadelphia, 1969, W. B. Saunders Co.
10. DeLand, F. H.: Cerebral radionuclide angiography, Philadelphia, 1976, W. B. Saunders Co.
11. Gado, M., Coleman, R. E., and Alderson, P. O.: Clinical comparison of radionuclide brain imaging and computerized transmission tomography I. In DeBlanc, H. J., and Sorenson, J. P., editors: Noninvasive brain imaging: computed tomography and radionuclides, New York, 1975, The Society of Nuclear Medicine, Inc., pp. 147-173.
12. Gonçalves-Rocha, A. F., and Harbert, J. C.: Textbook of nuclear medicine: clinical applications, Philadelphia, 1979, Lea & Febiger, pp. 51-108.
13. Hakim, S., and Adams, R. D.: Special clinical problem of symptomatic hydrocephalus with normal cerebrospinal fluid pressure: observations on cerebrospinal fluid hydrodynamics, J. Neurol. Sci. **2:**307, 1965.
14. Harper, P. V., Beck, R., Charleston, D., and Lathrop, K. A.: Optimization of a scanning method using Tc-99m, Nucleonics **22**(1):50, 1964.
15. Hauser, W., Atkins, H. L., Nelson, K. G., and Richards, P.: Technetium-99m DTPA: a new radiopharmaceutical for brain and kidney scanning, Radiology **94:**679, 1970.
16. Holmes, R. A.: The vertex view in routine brain scanning, Am. J. Roentgenol. **106:**347, 1969.
17. Holmes, R. A., and Staab, E. V.: The central nervous system. In Freeman, M., and Johnson, P. M., editors: Clinical scintillation imaging, New York, 1975, Grune & Stratton, Inc., pp. 247-323.
18. Kuhl, D. E., Chamberlain, R. H., Hale, J., and Garson, R. O.: A high-contrast photographic recorder for scintillation counter scanning, Radiology **66:**730, 1956.
19. Lavender, J. P., Lowe, J., Barker, J. R., Burn, J. I., and Chaudhri, M. A.: Gallium-67 citrate scanning in neoplastic and inflammatory lesions, Br. J. Radiol. **44:**361, 1971.
20. Moore, G. E.: Use of radioactive diiodofluorescein in the diagnosis and localization of brain tumors, Science **107:**569, 1948.
21. Rollo, F. D., Cavalieri, R. R., Born, M., et al.: Comparative evaluation of ^{99m}Tc GH, $^{99m}TcO_4$, and ^{99m}Tc DTPA as brain imaging agents, Radiology **123:**379-383, May 1977.
22. Witcofski, R. L., Janeway, R., Maynard, C. D., Bearden, E. K., and Schultz, J. L.: Visualization of the choroid plexus on the technetium-99m brain scan—clinical significance and blocking by potassium perchlorate, Arch. Neurol. **16:**282, 1967.

Chapter 9

THE ENDOCRINE SYSTEM

Merton A. Quaife, Maria V. Nagel, and Edouard V. Kotlyarov

The historical development of our knowledge in endocrinology has followed a rather traditional approach until the advent of tracer studies at the dawn of the nuclear age.

The endocrine system offers an opportunity for demonstration of the diversity in applications of nuclear medicine technology and techniques. It, more than any other organ system, illustrates the breadth and depth of tracer-technique capability in the diagnostic arena. Applications in categories of dynamic function, volume dilution, visualization, and localization as well as combinations of the foregoing are available. Clinical as well as investigative endocrinology is based on hormones. A significant contribution of nuclear medicine to this area is the explosive advance attributable to the volume-dilution technique application embodied in radioimmunoassay and competitive protein-binding assay procedures. A great advance in sensitivity and specificity occurred with the development of the double-isotope derivative methods of measuring steroids, which permitted reliable measurement in the peripheral blood of normal as well as diseased human subjects. Although this technique was particularly rewarding when applied for investigative purposes, the technique was cumbersome and in some instances more so than the standard bioassay or chemical techniques. In the early 1950s, Berson and Yalow initiated studies of the dynamics of labeled insulin in both in vitro and in vivo systems.[12] These pioneers ushered in the era of in vitro nuclear medicine with the publication of radioimmunoassay methodology for porcine and human insulin.[11,92]

This publication heralded the decade of development and application of radioimmunoassay and subsequent corollary procedures generally referred to as competitive protein-binding assay. Significant advantages over previous hormonal measurements were as follows: (1) decreased cost and greater ease of performance, (2) ability to quantify large numbers of samples at one time, (3) greater sensitivity than bioassays, and (4) ability to quantify hormones in unextracted serum or plasma. The evolution of techniques in competitive protein-binding assays have been reviewed in book form and are suggested as an excellent additional reference source for those interested in pursuing this area further.[59] In general, the technique consists of four basic requirements: (1) a well-characterized specific binding protein, (2) a high-specific-activity, undamaged, labeled hormone, (3) a well-characterized method of separating the protein-bound from the "free," or nonbound, hormone, and (4) a suitable standard preparation for quantitation.

The endocrine system serves as the principal example of nuclear medicine therapy applications in the contemporary practice of nuclear medicine. The endocrine system stands as a unique organ-system that allows correlation of the biologic organizational level information with our classic approach to learning, that is, anatomy, physiology, pathology, and the clinical aspects of endocrinology.

Our desire to better understand the complexities of the endocrine system has led to the following approach to elucidate hormonal production: (1) the definition of the chemical structure and characteristics of each hormone, (2) the chemical details of its biosynthesis, storage, and release, (3) the nature of signals that stimulate release and the reciprocal mechanisms by which the hormone's release may be inhibited, (4) the form in which transport takes place, that is, proteins in the vascular bed that participate in transmitting the hormone from the source to the responsive tissue, (5) the chemical identity of the cellular constituents with which the hormone interacts at the molecular level, (6) the details of the molecular interaction, (7) mechanisms by which the interaction of hormones and the cellular receptor results in either acceleration or deceleration of the metabolic activities of the "target" cell, and finally (8) the ultimate knowledge of how this cellular effect fits into the homeostasis of the total organism in health and disease states for necessary practical application. The application of radioactive-tracer techniques has played a significant role in the evolution of our knowledge and holds promise of even greater value in the future. Its use in the delineation of the intricacies of intermediary metabolism has produced outstanding contributions in understanding the thyroid gland and its hormonal products. As alluded to above, the clinical application of radioimmunoassay and competitive protein-binding techniques supplied by nuclear medicine in the last decade has been a boon to the field of endocrinology.

It is certainly accurate to say that we as yet lack sufficient information to thoroughly understand the totality of the endocrine system and the interaction of its component parts; however, we have acquired significant pieces of the puzzle through the contributions of nuclear medicine.

The evolution of endocrinology from a science of descriptive anatomy through exploration of more dynamic physiologic parameters has been long and arduous. The transition has been assisted in great measure by applications of tracer techniques, both in vivo and in vitro. This chapter explores the applications of radionuclides to diagnosis, treatment, and investigation of human disease processes affecting the endocrine system.

ENDOCRINE SYSTEM AND INTERRELATIONSHIP OF ITS COMPONENT PARTS

Hypothalamus. At the outset, a few comments with respect to specific endocrine interrelationships appear pertinent. The intimate relationship between the central nervous system and the endocrine system has been more firmly established in recent years. Emerging as the neuroendocrine system, the hypothalamus has been shown to exert an all-important controlling influence over the anterior pituitary. The production of neurohormones by the neurons of the hypothalamus and their delivery to the anterior pituitary through the pituitary portal circulation results in stimulation or inhibition of the hormonal elements secreted by the anterior pituitary. Currently, there is evidence for the existence of neurohormones controlling the secretion of adrenocorticotropin (ACTH), thyrotropin (TSH), follicle-stimulating hormone (FSH), luteinizing hormone (LH), and growth hormone (GH). A prolactin-inhibiting factor, which normally holds in check the secretion of prolactin, is also produced by the hypothalamus.

Anterior pituitary. The anterior pituitary hormones represent an area of the endocrine system that is reasonably well understood. ACTH regulates the secretion of cortisol and corticosterone, as well as androgenic and estrogenic hormones from the adrenal cortex. TSH regulates the synthesis and release of thyroid hormones from the thyroid gland, whereas FSH stimulates growth of the graafian follicle and estrogen secretion by the ovary. FSH is responsible for spermatogenesis in the male, but luteinizing hormone (LH), which initiates ovulation and progesterone secretion by the ovary in the female, functions as the interstitial cell–stimulating hormone (ICSH) in males, which is responsible for testerone secretion by the testes. Growth hormone (GH), as the name implies, stimulates the growth of soft tissue and bone and has rather diffuse effects on organic and inorganic metabolism. Prolactin (Pr) is responsible for secretion of milk in the mammalian species.

Posterior pituitary. In the posterior pituitary, hormonal secretions relate to water absorption by the distal portions of the nephron as well as to a general effect on cell-water content embodied in the antidiuretic hormone vasopressin. Oxytoxin affects uterine contractility in the female but has no known physiologic role in the male.

Adrenal cortex. The adrenal cortex is primarily known for the production of the principal glucocorticoid of man—cortisol, or hydrocortisone. This steroid exerts important influences on organ metabolism as well as electrolyte and water balance. The adrenal cortex also secretes aldosterone (a potent sodium-retaining steroid), corticosterone (which has metabolic effects intermediate between cortisol and aldosterone), and substantial amounts of androgenic hormones (which may be clinically significant in females along with small quantities of estrogens). ACTH plays a role in aldosterone secretion; however, the principal influencing factors related to secretion of this steroid are the influence of extracellular fluid volume and serum sodium and potassium concentration. Associated with the aldosterone secretion is the production of angiotensin by the kidney, which exerts a direct action upon adrenocortical secretion of aldosterone.

Adrenal medulla. Epinephrine and norepinephrine (sympathetic amines) represent the principal products of the adrenal medulla. Epinephrine exerts a strong influence on heart rate, metabolic rate, and fat and carbohydrate metabolism, whereas norepinephrine has a pronounced vasoconstrictor-oppressor effect but little metabolic action.

Thyroid gland. Most familiar in the endocrine system is the thyroid gland, secreting thyroxine (T_4) and small quantities of triiodothyronine (T_3), which regulates cell metabolism. More recently it has been shown that the thyroid also secretes thyrocalcitonin, a hormone that lowers serum calcium concentration and inhibits calcium resorption from bone. Thus, through the effect on serum calcium, this hormone indirectly influences parathormone secretion.

Parathyroid glands. The parathyroid glands produce parathormone, which causes calcium mobilization from bone as well as stimulation of calcium absorption from the gut. Simultaneously, parathormone depresses the renal tubular reabsorption of phosphate.

Gonads. The endocrine function of the gonads involves the secretion of estrogens and progesterone from the ovaries in the female. In addition, the ovaries possess the potential to secrete testosterone. The interstitial cells of the testes secrete androstenedione as well as testosterone. In a fashion similar to that described above for the ovaries, there is significant secretion of estrogen by the testes, either by the interstitial cells or the Sertoli cells of the spermatic tubules.

Pancreas. The pancreas, though better known for its exocrine function related to the gastrointestinal system, plays an important role in the endocrine system. The beta cells of the pancreatic islets secrete insulin in response to changes in blood glucose concentration, whereas the alpha cell counterpart, glucagon, exhibits a hyperglycemic influence. In addition, glucagon has been shown to stimulate insulin release independent of its hyperglycemic action.

THE PITUITARY

Anatomic relationships

The pituitary gland lies within a bony cavity, the sella turcica, in the sphenoid bone at the base of the skull (Fig. 9-1). It is a complex histologic structure situated at the end of the pituitary stalk with an abundant blood vessel supply reaching the main body of the gland through a network around this stalk. In terms of size the average pituitary weighs 0.5 g, with dimensions in the order of 10 × 13 × 6 mm. The anterior lobe of the pituitary comprises 75% of the total weight

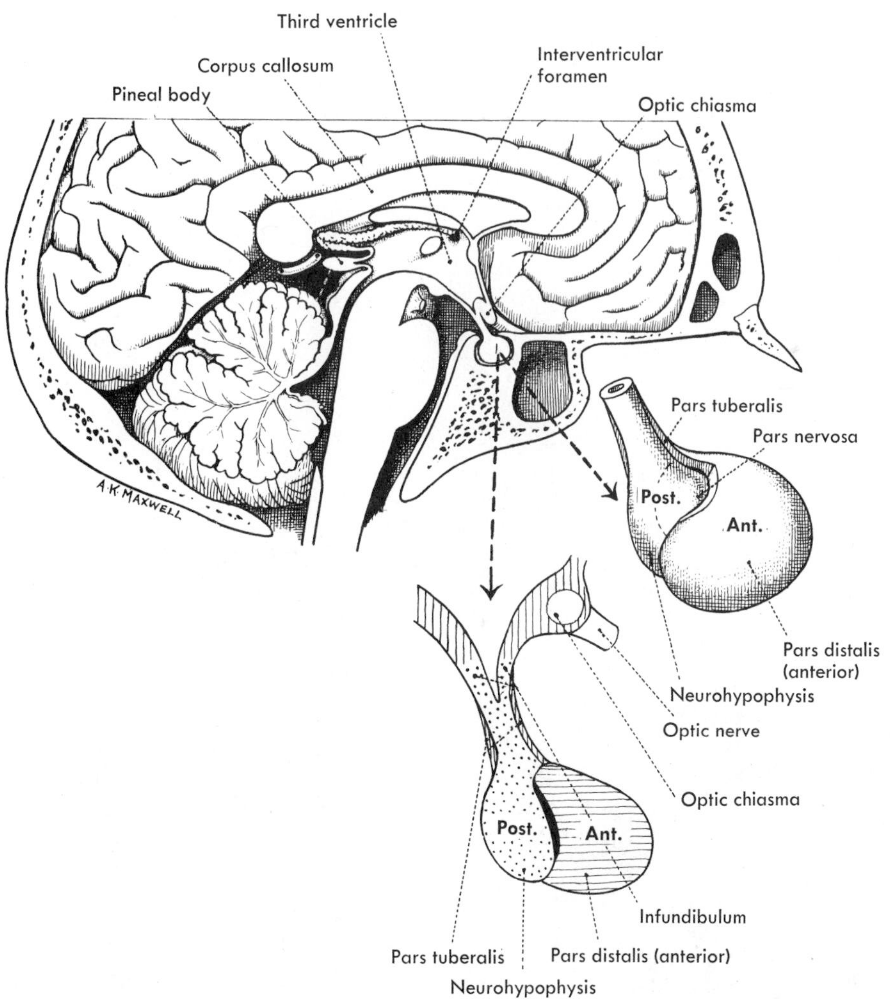

Fig. 9-1. Schemes of relationships of pituitary gland to brain. *Insets,* Exterior and interior of pituitary gland. (From Hamilton, W. J.: Textbook of human anatomy, ed. 2, St. Louis, 1976, The C. V. Mosby Co.; courtesy The Macmillan Press Ltd., Houndsmill Basingstoke, Hampshire, England.)

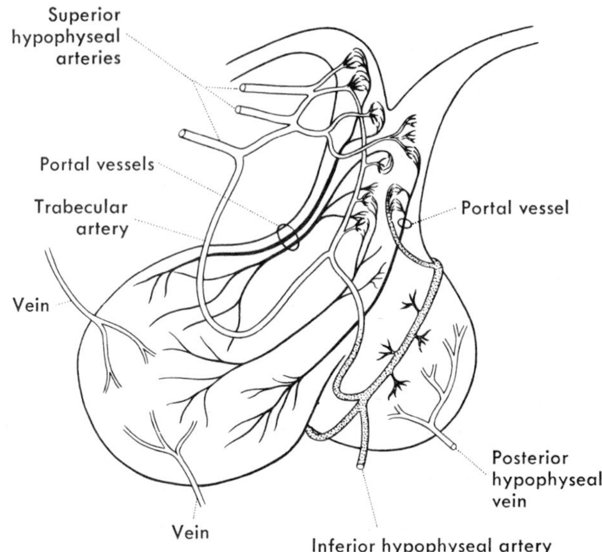

Fig. 9-2. Scheme of arterial blood supply and portal vessels of median eminence and pituitary gland. Principal veins are also shown. (From Hamilton, W. J.: Textbook of human anatomy, ed. 2, St. Louis, 1976, The C. V. Mosby Co.; courtesy The Macmillan Press Ltd., Houndsmill Basingstoke, Hampshire, England.)

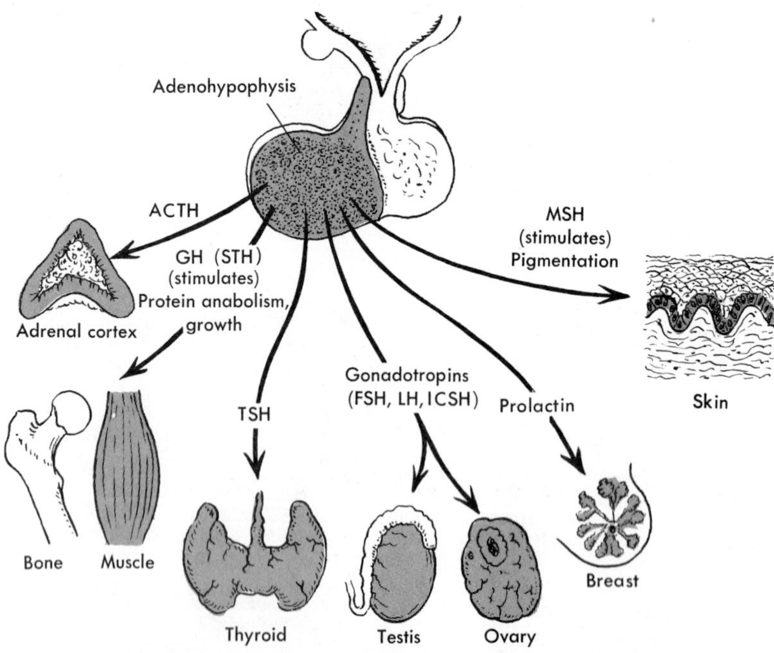

Fig. 9-3. Anterior pituitary hormones and their target organs: adrenocorticotropic hormone (ACTH), thyroid-stimulating hormone (TSH), follicle-stimulating hormone (FSH), luteinizing hormone (LH), male analog of LH (ICSH), and melanocyte-stimulating hormone (MSH). (From Anthony, C. P., and Thibodeau, G. A.: Textbook of anatomy and physiology, ed. 10, St. Louis, 1979, The C. V. Mosby Co.)

of the gland. A unique feature of the pituitary relates to its blood supply (Fig. 9-2). It receives its blood from two sources, first, an arterial supply, which reaches the gland from branches of the superior hypophyseal artery (a branch of the internal carotid artery) and a venous blood supply, which enters the pituitary by a physiologically important portal system that originates in specialized vessels of the median eminence, which are short straight terminal arterials surrounded by dense capillary network. Blood from these capillaries is collected in a series of parallel veins that course down the anterior surface of a pituitary stalk and drain into the sinusoid capillaries of the anterior lobe. In experimental animal models direct observation has confirmed that the direction of the blood flow in the portal veins is from the median eminence to the pituitary. Thus these vessels are the principal transport system for the neurohumeral influence of the hypothalamus upon the adenohypophysis (pituitary). Blood supply to the posterior lobe comes from the inferior hypophyseal arteries and thus is separate from the blood supply to the anterior lobe. The venous supply from both pituitary lobes drains into the cavernous sinus through a number of venous pathways. The nerve supply to the anterior lobe is limited to a fine network derived from the carotid plexus, which accompanies arteriolar branches. The principal function of these nerve pathways appears to be vasomotor in nature.

The histologic characterization of the human pituitary may be described as a consortium of largely independent functional units. Each unit is comprised of a specific cell type, synthesizing and releasing a particular hormone. The historic classification of pituitary cells, that is, acidophilic, basophilic, and chromophobic types, is inadequate to explain the complexities of this gland in light of our current knowledge. Independent secretion of six known hormones and possible secretion of other hormonal peptides of undefined physiologic significance bespeaks the key role of the pituitary as the master gland of the endocrine system (Fig. 9-3). The complexities of the histologic nature of the anterior pituitary have been eludicated by application of histochemical, immunofluorescent, and electron microscopic techniques, along with the nuclear medicine contribution of the physiologic fulcrum, that is, hormonal production and release, as elucidated by radioimmunoassay and competitive protein-binding techniques. A relationship has been established between the pituitary cell types and hormonal secretions (Table 9-1). Growth hormone secretion has been linked to somatotrophic cells predominantly located in the lateral wings of the pituitary. Lactotropic cells, which contain eosinophilic granules, have been identified by immunofluorescent staining with an antiserum against bovine prolactin. The relative number of lactotropic cells is increased in fetal pituitaries and during pregnancy. This proliferation is related to a high concentration of circulating estrogen associated with human pregnancy. Identification of human thyrotropic cells was accomplished, again by immunofluorescent staining techniques, which identified thyrotropic cells located predominantly in the central or mucoid wedge of the pituitary. The gonadotropic cells secreting human luteinizing hormone (LH) are characterized as granulated and are distributed sparsely throughout the entire pituitary. The FSH gonadotropic cell remains less well identified but is believed to be a member of the basophilic group of cells of the pituitary. Cells that secrete corticotropin are identified by immunoreaction in the medial mucoid wedge of the pituitary and less frequently in the lateral somatotropin ridge areas. Corticotropic cells have also been identified in the neurohypophysis in apposition to the adenohypophysis. Melanotropic cells, which secrete the melanocyte-stimulating hormone (MSH), appear to react similarly in terms of antiserums with corticotropic cells of the adenohypophysis and neurohypophysis. Thus it appears that MSH and ACTH are most likely secreted by the same cell; however, this assumption cannot be considered as firmly established. Analyzing the remainder of cell types, one finds that approximately one fourth of the pituitary cells appear to have no characteristic secretory granules. It is hypothesized that these cells, which are classified as chromophobe cells in the historic classifications, may also participate in pituitary function. Some of these cells may represent undifferentiated precursors to secretory cells, whereas others may have been temporarily depleted of stored secretions and represent reserve cells in a resting state. Another identified cell is characterized as the follicular or stellate cell. The function remains uncertain.

Physiologic role

Peptide hormones. On a biochemical and physiologic basis the pituitary produces six principal hormones of established functional significance. These peptide and protein hormones as well as related hormones produced by the placenta have been assigned to three distinct families on the basis of molecular structure as well as biochemical synthesis. The corticotropins, as related peptide hormones, represent the first general group of pituitary hormones. Corticotropin binds with specific receptors on the surface of the adrenocortical cell, which permits concentration of ACTH from plasma. Adenyl cyclase is activated when the ACTH is bound to the receptors in the presence of calcium, which in turn increases the concentration of cyclic AMP in the adrenal cell. The net result of

Table 9-1. Production, control, and effects of pituitary hormones

Pituitary gland (hypophysis cerebri)	Hormone	Source (cell type or location)	Control mechanism	Effect
Anterior pituitary gland (adenohypophysis)	Growth hormone (GH, somatotropin [STH])	Acidophils	GRH (growth hormone–releasing hormone) from hypothalamus	Promotes body growth, protein anabolism, and mobilization and catabolism of fats; decreases glucose catabolism; increases blood glucose levels
Pars anterior	Prolactin (lactogenic or luteotropic hormone [LTH])	Acidophils	Prolactin-inhibitory factor (PIF); prolactin-releasing factor (PRF) from hypothalamus and high blood levels of oxytocin	Stimulates milk secretion and development of secretory alveoli; helps maintain corpus luteum
	Thyrotropin (TH); thyroid-stimulating hormone (TSH)	Basophils	Thyrotropin-releasing hormone (TRH) from hypothalamus	Growth and maintenance of thyroid gland and stimulation of thyroid hormone secretion
	Adrenocorticotropin (ACTH)	Basophils	Corticotropin-releasing factor (CRF) from hypothalamus	Growth and maintenance of adrenal cortex and stimulation of cortisol and other glucocorticoid secretions
	Follicle-stimulating hormone (FSH)	Basophils	Follicle-stimulating hormone–releasing hormone (FSH-RH) from hypothalamus	In female—stimulates follicle growth and maturation and estrogen secretion In male—stimulates development of seminiferous tubules and maintains spermatogenesis
	Luteinizing hormone (LH in female, ICSH in male)	Basophils	Luteinizing hormone–releasing hormone (LH-RH) from hypothalamus	In female (LH)—induces ovulation and stimulates formation of corpus luteum and progesterone secretion In male (ICSH)—stimulates interstitial cell secretion of testosterone
Pars intermedia	Melanocyte-stimulating hormone (MSH); intermedin	Basophils	Unknown in humans	May cause darkening of skin by increasing melanin production
Posterior pituitary gland (neurohypophysis)	ADH (vasopressin)	Hypothalamus, mainly supraoptic nucleus	Osmoreceptors in hypothalamus stimulated by increase in blood osmotic pressure, decrease in extracellular fluid volume, and stress	Decreased urine output
	Oxytocin	Hypothalamus, paraventricular nucleus	Nervous stimulation of hypothalamus caused by stimulation of nipples (nursing)	Contraction of uterine smooth muscle and ejection of milk into lactiferous ducts

From Anthony, C. P., and Thibodeau, G. A.: Textbook of anatomy and physiology, ed. 10, St. Louis, 1979, The C. V. Mosby Co.

the increased intracellular cyclic AMP concentration is the phosphorylation of key enzymes and histones, which results in the biologic actions of the hormone. Stimulation of steroid production by the adrenal cortex then ensues. Outside the adrenal gland, corticotropin has a number of actions, including the promotion of microlysis in fat cells and the stimulation of amino acids and glucose uptake by muscle. Corticotropin also stimulates the pancreatic beta cell to create insulin and somatotropic cells of the pituitary to secrete growth hormone. Measurement of ACTH originally involved rather demanding bioassay with hypophysectomized rats. The development of radioimmunoassays and the evolution of the field of in vitro nuclear medicine has resulted in the development of satisfactory assays for ACTH. Those techniques described are based upon competitive binding labeled and unlabeled ACTH for the binding protein–receptor action in cell membranes isolated from normal and tumorous adrenal cells.[10] This radioimmunoassay correlates well with the biologically active species of ACTH. In addition to its specificity, this procedure demonstrates a significant advance in sensitivity. The principal problem area with this assay is the difficulty in the preparation of stable membranes capable of specific binding, and thus this assay has had a relatively limited application, mostly in an investigative role.

Regulation of the secretion of ACTH by the anterior pituitary is characterized by a dual control system. The first control is a "long-loop" feedback inhibition of ACTH secretion by the circulating level of cortisone. The second control mechanism is exerted by the hypothalamus through the secretion of corticotropin-releasing hormone (CRH). This mechanism exemplifies again the neuroendocrine-system influence stemming from a number of neurogenic stimuli such as response to pain, anxiety, and hypoglycemia. Melanocyte-stimulating hormones (MSH) are released by corticotropic cells in both the adenohypophysis and the neurohypophysis. Radioimmunoassays exist for separate measurements of alpha and beta MSH. Regulation of MSH secretion appears predominantly under hypothalamic control, which is exerted by an MSH-inhibiting factor. The existence of an MSH-releasing factor has been postulated but not definitively established. In humans, the MSH secretion shares a similar feedback inhibition by cortisol as discussed in connection with ACTH. The relationship between these two hormones, ACTH and MSH, is so close that the secretion is usually considered to be simultaneous.

Glycoprotein hormones. A second class of pituitary hormones are those characterized as glycoprotein hormones. They are derived by biochemical synthesis from a common molecule. This group includes thyrotropic hormone, follicle-stimulating and luteinizing gonadotropins as well as chorionic gonadotropic hormone (HCG) produced by the placenta.

The pituitary gland secretes two hormones whose primary action is on the gonads. The follicle-stimulating hormone (FSH) stimulates follicular development in the ovary and gametogenesis in the testes. Luteinizing hormone (LH) acts primarily on the ovary in promoting luteinization and in the testes, the Leydig cell function. Measurement of these hormones until recently has primarily utilized the bioassay technique. Again, the precision and relative simplicity of radioimmunoassay provides substantial advantages, despite the fact that biologic activity and immunologic activity do not always directly correlate. The radioimmunoassay of LH correlates satisfactorily, whereas the radioimmunoassay of FSH is less well correlated with biologic activity. Cross-reactivity of FSH with LH has been seen, requiring extensive purification for specificity in the FSH assay. The regulation of secretion of FSH and LH is controlled by a hypophysiotropic hormone or hormones and by feedback inhibition by sex steroids. There is some evidence that the LH-releasing hormone (LRH) also stimulates the release of FSH, but there remains the unproved possibility of an additional FSH-releasing hormone.

Thyrotropin results in significant effects upon thyroid function. It increases the thyroid mass and vascularity, and on a microscopic basis an increase in molecular epithelial height may be appreciated. Thyrotropin increases iodine uptake, thyroglobulin synthesis, iodotyrosine and iodothyronine formation, thyroglobulin proteolysis, and thyroxin and triiodothyronine release from the thyroid gland. Binding of thyrotropin on the thyroid epithelium cell by specific receptors with subsequent activation of adenyl cyclase is the basic mechanism of activity. Subsequently, there is an increase in intracellular cyclic AMP with this secondary messenger regulating many intracellular receptors through phosphorylation of key proteins. Measurement of plasma concentration is principally by radioimmunoassay. The regulation of secretion of TSH by the pituitary is determined concurrently by the level of thyrotropin-releasing hormone (TRH) and by the level of circulating thyroid hormone.

Somatotropic hormones. The somatotropin family of hormones consisting of growth hormone (GH) and prolactin (Pr), secreted by the pituitary, along with chorionic somatomammotropin (HCS), produced by the placenta, are characterized by similar chemical structures and overlapping biologic actions. Growth hormone influences a variety of metabolic processes. A number of aspects of protein metabolism have been studied after growth hormone administration, and there appears to be augmented protein synthesis as a result of the effects of growth hormone. Stimulation of synthetic processes in cartilage by growth hormone have been shown by use of sulfur-35 sulfate incorporation in chondroitin sulfate. Growth hormone also induces a number of important alterations in fat metabolism, which include mobilization of fat from peripheral adipose depots. The latter effect is associated with increased fat metabolism. It appears that some abnormalities in carbohydrate metabolism associated with hypopituitarism are the result of growth hormone deficiency, but there is an interrelationship with corticotropin deficiency in this area. For clinical purposes the measurement of growth hormone may be accomplished by one of a number of radioimmunologic methods. There is some disparity between the immunologic quantitative activity of growth hormone and that measured by biologic activity. Utilizing the radioimmunoassay approach, more precise assays of end-organ function have been developed, based upon the capability of measuring pituitary polypeptide hormones. Detection of incomplete or early pituitary insufficiency using even more recent end-organ function assays is often unsatisfactory for early diagnosis. The function of the end organ may become abnormal only when the pituitary reserve has been greatly reduced; such a reduction necessitates the use of standardized provocative tests for evaluation of pituitary function. Growth hormone release is known to be sensitive to a wide variety of stimuli including emotional and physical stress, exercise, and food intake. Five standardized stimulation tests, including insulin, arginine, vasopressin, and glucagon, have been utilized, and, more recently, levodopa has been added to this list. In a comparative study of these provocative test parameters, levodopa- and insulin-stimulation studies were the most consistent, with arginine, vasopressin, and glucagon being significantly less consistent.[28]

The regulation of human growth hormone exemplifies a classic example of the physiologic antagonism that exists between growth hormones and insulin. The secretion of growth hormone is an important defense mechanism against hypoglycemia. Oral or intravenous administration of amino acids stimulate hormone secretion, which serves as the basis for the arginine provocative test. There are also believed to be effects of other hormones on growth hormone. For instance, plasma growth hormone levels are higher in women after exercise, hypoglycemia, or arginine infusion than are ordinarily seen in men. This sex difference is attributed to estrogens. Corticosteroid excess impairs the plasma growth hormone response to hypoglycemia and also inhibits the cyclic peak of growth hormone related to sleep. A reduced response in growth hormone level to hypoglycemia is also observed in patients with hypothyroidism. The hypothalamic regulation of growth hormone secretion is altered by a number of pharmacologic agents that affect the catecholamine neurotransmitters. For example, blockade of the hypothalamic alpha-adrenergic receptors will decrease growth hormone secretion in response to provocative stimuli. Conversely, beta-adrenergic blocking agents facilitate the secretion of growth hormone. As mentioned earlier, the administration of levodopa serves as a provocative test by increasing the hypothalamic release of dopamine and possibly norepinephrine, resulting in rapid discharge of growth hormone.

Prolactin is similar to growth hormone in that it acts directly on tissues and does not regulate the function through a secondary endocrine tissue. The established function of prolactin in the human is that of initiation and maintenance of lactation. In and of itself, prolactin evokes little effect on the mammary gland because full lactation requires preparation by estrogens, progestins, corticosteroids, and insulin. Prolactin also demonstrates general metabolic actions similar in nature to those seen with growth hormone. These include nitrogen retention, impairment of carbohydrate tolerance, hypercalciuria, and even skeletal growth. Fat mobilization, however, has not been observed. No known role has been identified for this hormone in the male.

Pathophysiologic derangements

Pathophysiologic derangements relating to the neuroendocrine axis and specifically related to the hypothalamus and the pituitary gland serve as primary indications for application for nuclear medicine techniques. The hypothalamus may be affected by a number of etiologic agents such as tumors, granulomas, infectious processes, and vascular lesions. Hypothalamic disorders produce various endocrinopathies as a result of damage to hypothalamic neurosecretory centers. Diseases of the anterior pituitary are relatively common. Eosinophilic adenomas are commonly associated with excess production of growth hormone and result in the clinical entity known as "acromegaly." Adenomas involving the chromophilic cells are generally nonfunctioning but rarely may secrete excess growth hormone or ACTH, resulting in clinical expression as acromegaly or as Cushing's syndrome. Hypopituitarism may result from tumor compression of normal tissue, a finding more common in the chromophobe adenoma.

As a general statement with respect to pathophysiologic disorders resulting in endocrinopathy, the following outline is suggested as a useful way of considering possible endocrine pathophysiologic derangements:

Primary dysfunctions

1. Overproduction
   a. Abnormal gland function
   b. Abnormal tropic stimulus
   c. Change in response to negative-feedback signal; change in threshold response point
   d. Inappropriate time course of tropic stimuli
2. Increased target-organ sensitivity; an increased peripheral tissue response with normal production of hormones
3. Underproduction
   a. Abnormal gland function
      (1) Lack of hydroxylase enzyme in biosynthesis of steroids
      (2) Lack of conversion of prohormone to hormone in the instance of peptide hormones
      (3) Secretion of an inactive product that retains immunologic cross-reactivity without biologic activity
   b. Lack of normotrophic stimulus
      (1) Lack of appropriate time sequence of hormonal stimuli or neurostimuli
      (2) Decreased target-organ sensitivity; decrease in peripheral-tissue response accompanied by normal production of hormone
         (a) Lack of peripheral-tissue receptors
         (b) Decrease of peripheral-tissue responsiveness as result of altered intracellular feedback responses

Secondary dysfunctions

1. Overproduction as a result of sustained normal physiologic stimulus
2. Underproduction resulting from a lack of normal physiologic stimulus

Nuclear medicine applications—in vitro techniques

Corticotropin. Assay of ACTH utilizes the sensitive and exacting method of radioimmunoassay. Prior to assaying, one must obtain heparinized blood samples and use plasma for analysis. Since the enzymes released during clotting destroy corticotropin, degradation of ACTH may begin as soon as blood is drawn. This can be alleviated to some extent by acidification and freezing of the plasma sample. There is also strong evidence that glass adsorbs ACTH, adding to the preliminary problems of sample collecting and handling. The diurnal variation in blood ACTH levels makes it imperative that standardization of sampling times be accomplished. Corticotropin levels are highest prior to waking and decrease throughout the waking day. One usually accomplishes the technique by adding antiserums to the patient sample, incubating the solution, and adding radioactive ACTH. Double antibody assays are affected by complement, and so a substance such as EDTA (ethylenediaminetetraacetic acid) must be added to inactivate complement. Competitive-binding assays or tissue-receptor assays using adrenal receptors appear to be the most sensitive, specific, and precise method. ACTH assays are usually done in conjunction with other assays such as cortisol because of the interrelationships of hormones of the anterior pituitary.

ACTH levels rise in response to stress. This fact is used for a stimulation test by induction of stress with pyrogens, insulin, or vasopressin. Another stimulation test utilizes the negative-feedback mechanism between cortisol and ACTH when one administers metapyrone or dexamethasone, which inhibit cortisol formation, thus increasing ACTH levels in normal subjects.

Growth hormone. The assessment of growth hormone (GH) is complicated by the varying levels of GH in a normal adult. Daily activities such as exercise, sleep, and fasting produce fluctuations in GH levels, which make a single-sample assay unreliable. A more reliable means of assessing GH utilizes stimulation and suppression tests after establishment of a base-line value. The stimulation tests are especially useful for children because their normal GH levels are low and a deficiency may be indistinguishable from normal secretion. There is evidence that normal levels of GH increase through childhood, reaching a maximum during adolescence, only to decrease at older ages.

Assay methods use plasma or serum samples analyzed by standard radioimmunoassay (RIA), double-antibody RIA, or radioreceptors using lymphocytes.[49] Cerebral spinal fluid assay may also be used in the RIA assay with increased GH levels seen in those patients with acromegaly.[84]

Stimulation tests artificially elevate growth hormone secretion in normal individuals. Therefore, they may be used to confirm hyposecretion of GH. These tests are of particular interest in children with suspected dwarfism. Exercise is the simplest approach for a preliminary test, but lack of patient cooperation may necessitate use of insulin, levodopa, L-arginine hydrochloride, glucagon, or vasopressin stimulation. Use of insulin and vasopressin also yields augmented levels of ACTH and cortisol, which may be of added clinical value. Prestimulation basal blood values are drawn and blood is sampled after stimulation at 15- or 30-minute intervals for up to 180 minutes after stimulation. Levodopa, arginine, vasopressin, and insulin stimulation may induce maximum GH levels as early as 60 minutes after stimulation. However, GH may not reach a maximum with glucagon stimulation until 150 minutes after stimulation in adults. To ascertain whether hypoglycemia is indeed induced with insulin administration, one should assay blood samples for glucose as well as GH levels.

Doses for suppression and stimulation tests are found in Table 9-2. The use of diethylstilbestrol modification in conjunction with arginine in female GH as-

Table 9-2. Supplemental growth hormone tests

Drug	Stimulant (S) or depressant (D)	Adult dose	Children's dose
Insulin	S	0.05 to 0.15 units/kg IV[25,28,69]	0.1 units/kg IV[45,58]
Levodopa	S	0.5 g orally[17]	500 mg orally[45]
L-Arginine hydrochloride	S	0.5 g/kg IV infusion[28,69]	0.5 g/kg IV infusion[45,58]
Glucagon	S	1 g IM[55]	15 mg/kg IV[45] 0.5 mg IM
Vasopressin	S	10 units IM[28]	Not available
Glucose	D	1.3 g/kg[58]	Not applicable

sessment stems from the cyclic estrogen-progesterone release and subsequent fluctuations in GH, since estrogen is a stimulant for GH release whereas progesterone has inhibitory effects. Controversy exists over the use and effect of diethylstilbestrol in the arginine stimulation test. Aside from possible carcinogenic ramifications, the efficacy of diethylstilbestrol use in males to promote GH release is in doubt.[28]

Normal values are difficult to precisely define; however, poststimulation values in children with normal GH secretion should rise about 7 ng/ml.[45,58] A thorough discussion of GH secretion may be found in reference 25, covering both normal and disease states, along with further discussion of levodopa effects in reference 69.

Thyrotropin (TSH). Using purified human thyrotropin (thyroid-stimulating hormone, TSH), radioimmunoassays for quantitative measurement of human TSH applying the double-antibody technique have been developed.[60,87] Problems which may be encountered with this radioimmunoassay include protein labeling with iodine radionuclides which produce some degree of alteration in the immunoreactive characteristics of the hormone. Purification using column chromatography usually allows for a sufficiently undamaged TSH for a sensitive assay. Cross-reactivity with other glycoprotein hormones may be circumvented by inclusion of human chorionic gonadotropin (HCG) in the assay procedure. Such problems must be considered in evaluating commercially available kits.

Thyrotropin-releasing factor–stimulation test. The availability of thyrotropin-releasing factor or hormone (TRF or TRH) with radioimmunoassays for pituitary and thyroid hormones have provided a contemporary method for more precise evaluation of the hypothalamic-pituitary-thyroid interrelationships in healthy and diseased states. Synthetic TRH also appears to act on the pituitary, resulting in the release of prolactin, which parallels the TSH response.[16,44,76] When TRH is administered intravenously to normal individuals, the serum TSH rises to a peak in 15 to 30 minutes, followed by a gradual decline, returning to basal levels in 1 to 4 hours. The TRH stimulation, when coupled with evaluation of both pituitary- and thyroid-hormonal responses, serves as a one-step procedure in the evaluation of the hypothalamic-pituitary-thyroid axis.[75] Since TSH, T_3, and T_4 respond rapidly to TRH stimulation (TSH within 30 minutes, and T_3 and T_4 in 2 to 4 hours), the procedure can be conveniently accomplished within 1 day.

Gonadotropins (LH, FSH). Since hormones involved in reproduction circulate at low concentrations, measurement for purposes of clinical diagnosis and treatment currently depend on evolving nuclear-medicine in vitro techniques that utilize either competitive-binding or displacement-measurement systems, that is, a specific high-affinity binding molecule, either a hormone receptor or an antibody. Such studies have found primary use in investigation of normal reproductive physiology; however, they hold considerable promise for clinical diagnostic purposes in the future. Glycoprotein gonadotropic hormones, LH and FSH, may be determined by quantitative radioimmunoassays. Historically, components of sufficient purity and specificity were available only from the National Pituitary Agency of the National Institutes of Health, or from specific investigators pursuing this area of research. Presently purified hormones for labeling and preparation of standards along with antiserums are becoming commercially available. Chemical similarity between portions of the LH, FSH, TSH, and HCG structures results in some degree of cross-reactivity. The basic methodology used for labeling LH and FSH (with ^{125}I), the incubation of assay tubes, and the separation of bound and free hormone fractions is similar to the assay of other peptide hormones.[9] Radioreceptor assays, employing specific binding sites on rat-testis cell membranes, have also been developed for LH and FSH.[20] Current evidence suggests that a single hypothalamic gonadotropin-releasing hormone (GnRH) stimulates the pituitary secretion of both FSH and LH. Thus a variability in the relative secretion of the gonadotropins appears to be modulated through additional control mechanisms. The concept of a negative-feedback mechanism involves the hypothalamic-pituitary-gonadal axis.

THE THYROID GLAND

Anatomic relationships

The thyroid gland is anatomically located low in the anterior cervical region lying adjacent to the anterior and lateral aspects of the larynx and trachea (Fig. 9-4). The gland consists of two lateral lobes joined by a thin band of tissue, the isthmus. This latter structure lies across the trachea below the level of the cricoid cartilate with the lobes extending along each side of the larynx to reach the level of the thyroid cartilage. The appearance of a narrow strip of the thyroid tissue, the pyramidal lobe, may be seen as an anomalous variation. Its prevalence depends on the functional status of the thyroid gland. For example, it is commonly found in patients with diffuse hyperthyroidism. The pyramidal lobe extends upward from the isthmus along the thyroid cartilage. This remnant of the embryonic thyroglossal tract, and the main primordium of the thyroid gland, develops in the embryo from endodermal tissue in the region of the primordial myocardium and the first pharyngeal pouch. Thus thyroid tissue may be found from the base of the tongue to the level of the diaphragm. This exemplifies the importance of knowledge of embryologic evolution when one applies tracer techniques in the diagnosis of thyroid disease.

The thyroid gland is exceedingly well vascularized, receiving its arterial blood supply from the external carotids through the superior thyroid arteries and the subclavian arteries through the inferior thyroid arteries. The lymphatics of the thyroid consist of a rich plexus intimately related to the individual follicles. The structural and functional histologic element of the thyroid gland is the thyroid follicle. Spheric in shape with an average diameter of 300 μm, the wall consists of a single layer of cuboid epithelium. The cells of the thyroid follicles are the site of synthesis of thyroid hormones, with the lumen of the follicles functioning as storage depots. In addition to the follicular cells, a second type of cell is found. These are parafollicular or C cells. These secrete calcitonin, a calcium-lowering polypeptide hormone that acts primarily by suppression of resorption of calcium from bone and in conjunction with parathyroid hormone regulates calcium metabolism of the body.

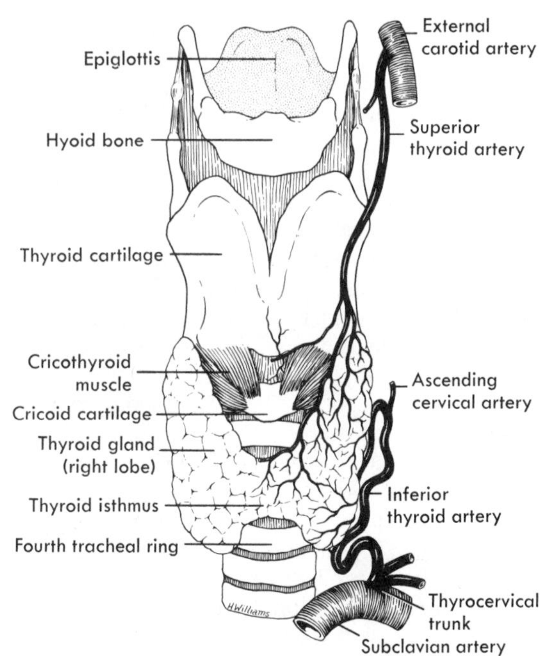

Fig. 9-4. Anterior view of thyroid gland and larynx. (From Francis, C. G.: Introduction to human anatomy, ed. 5, St. Louis, 1968, The C. V. Mosby Co.)

Physiologic role

Although portions of our understanding of thyroid physiology have been well established historically, during the last decade more contemporary findings have elucidated greater detail in the mechanisms of synthesis of thyroid hormone. Additionally, we have expanded our knowledge of control mechanisms as well as peripheral utilization of synthesized hormone. Intrathyroidal production of T_4 and T_3 are well established mechanisms, though detailed knowledge of some specific steps are lacking. The concentration of iodide by the thyroid follicular cells is followed by rapid oxidation, with subsequent iodination of tyrosyl residues catalyzed by thyroid peroxidase. Subsequently, a coupling reaction results in the formation of T_4 and T_3, depending on the constituents of the coupling reaction. Combined with globulin, a thyroglobulin thyroid hormone is stored for later use. Upon resorption into the thyroid cells it is hydrolyzed, and T_4 and T_3 are formed and released into the circulation. There is evidence that T_4 may be deiodinated to T_3 within the thyroid gland; however, the relationship to overall T_3 production is unknown.[37] Recent data on thyroid hormone production and metabolism resulting from development of methods to directly measure serum T_3 concentrations has altered some of our previous concepts in thyroid physiology. 3,5,3′-Triiodothyronine (T_3) is recognized as the more physiologically active of the two thyroid hormones despite its serum concentration, which is much lower than that of thyroxine (T_4). Until recently it was believed that the circulating T_3 level was derived solely from the thyroid. It is now apparent that the majority of T_3 results from the non-deiodination of T_4 in the peripheral tissues, that is, outside the thyroid gland.[18,62,81] This fact has led some workers in the field to speculate that T_4 itself might be biologically inactive and thus could be considered a prohormone requiring conversion to T_3 in order to exert its effect. The presence of intracellular T_4 and T_3 receptors as well as clinical situations in which T_4 correlates better than T_3 with the physiologic or pathophysiologic status suggests that both exert biologic activity.[61,79] Further development of radioimmunoassay technics, which have been a key contribution to this detailed understanding of thyroid hormone production and metabolism, has elucidated an alternate monodeiodination product of T_4. 3,3,5′-Triiodothyronine, or reverse T_3 (rT_3), has been found circulating in the vascular bed. It is also formed principally from extrathyroidal sites.[22]

The synthesis pathways of thyroid hormones (iodothyronines, T_3, T_4, and rT_3) must be influenced not only by thyroidal production and its regulation (that is, the hypothalamic-pituitary-thyroid interactions), but also by the extrathyroidal metabolism that supplies the majority of T_3.

The thyroid contains approximately 600 $\mu g/g$ of total iodine and about 200 $\mu g/g$ of T_4 and 25 $\mu g/g$ of T_3.[23] Extrathyroidal conversion of T_4 to T_3 indicate that around 35% of released T_4 is monodeiodinated to T_3 in peripheral tissues and this route accounts for about 80% of the production of T_3.

The iodothyronines circulate in both free and bound forms. In the bound form three plasma proteins are involved: thyroxine-binding globulin (TBG), thyroxine-binding prealbumin (TBPA), and albumin. TBG and TBPA are specific thyroid hormone–binding proteins, with T_4 exhibiting the greatest affinity for these proteins. T_3 binds to TBPA and TBG; however, its affinity is less than that of T_4. Under normal conditions the free T_4 concentration is approximately 0.02% of the total, whereas the free T_3 concentration is 0.2%. Thyroid hormones mediate a variety of responses in virtually every organ system in the body. At this time the principal mechanism of action appears to be in the nucleus and accelerates RNA synthesis, which is followed by increased protein synthesis. Application of tracer techniques through a variety of procedural categories in assessment of thyroid function and structure exemplify the diversity of clinical nuclear medicine. These techniques may be used for evaluation of a multitude of aspects of thyroid hormone synthesis, metabolism as well as the influence of pathophysiologic derangements.

Nuclear medicine applications in the assessment of thyroid function and structure represent one of the oldest and still frequent techniques in an active practice. With the concurrent evolution of radiation biologic knowledge in the effects of ionizing radiation and increasing application of tracer techniques in the field of Nuclear Medicine, we must be aware of an increasing concern of late effects of exposure to ionizing radiation. In addition, increasing attention is directed to the potential deleterious sequelae of exposure to low-dose radiation, a concern based upon extrapolation from effects noted at higher dose and dose-rate irradiation. For example, the media have drawn attention to the association between exposure to ionizing radiation and the development of the thyroid nodules and in some cases thyroid cancer. This association is based primarily on epidemiologic studies of patients receiving external beam-radiation therapy, however, guilt by association appears to be the popular lay conclusion. Despite a considerable body of scientific data that shows no association between the diagnostic use of radiopharmaceuticals in the thyroid and the occurrence of thyroid carcinoma, it appears advisable to reduce the radiation exposure to the thyroid gland provided that diagnostic information will not be sacrificed. The evolution of radiopharmaceutical development offers new alternatives to traditional approaches, and when it is coupled with the burgeoning area of in vitro nuclear medicine, we may advance simultaneously the beneficial goal of radiation-dose reduction while maintaining diagnostic accuracy and in some instances enhancing the usefulness of our techniques. The Task Force on Short-lived Radionuclides for Medical Applications published a report, *Evaluation of Diseases of the Thyroid Gland with In Vivo Use of Radionuclides*,[71] recommending the use of newer radionuclides and techniques to yield comparable if not better information while providing lower radiation doses than more traditional approaches. The continuing primary use of ^{131}I in studies of the thyroid gland represents comparatively one of the larger increments of radiation dose delivered by nuclear medicine applications. Availability of sodium ^{123}I-iodide and the ubiquitously distributed sodium ^{99m}Tc-pertechnetate represent alternatives to commonly employed sodium ^{131}I-iodide. The pertechnetate form of ^{99m}Tc has significantly replaced the use of ^{131}I in many areas and offers advantages in the cost area as well as radiation dose to the thyroid. Although the absorbed dose to the thyroid is reduced, the critical organ is not the thyroid, and attention must be redirected to the large bowel, bone marrow, whole body, and gonadal dose calculations. ^{123}I by comparison delivers less radiation dose to the latter tissues. The variation in metabolic sequence between pertechnetate (on transport or trapping) and iodine radiopharmaceuticals, which trace the full metabolic pathway, must be recognized.

The following recommendations of the aforementioned task force represent a useful preamble to considerations of techniques in the assessment of thyroid gland function and structure.[71] The use of these recommendations for modifying traditional application approaches are suggested for consideration. (The references to Saenger et al. are located after the recommendations.)

Recommendations for use of radioactive iodine in thyroid disease*

1. Radioactive iodine should not be used for the following thyroid diagnostic studies:
   a. In screening for thyroid disease in an apparently healthy population.
   b. As a primary diagnostic test for hyperthyroidism or hypothyroidism.
   c. During pregnancy and lactation, except under special circumstances.
   d. In children, except under special circumstances.
2. Radioiodine-uptake testing is important and useful in the diagnosis of thyroid disease, as follows:
   a. For confirmation of the diagnosis of hyperthyroidism, that is, for confirmation that the thyroid gland is the source of elevated blood thyroid-hormone levels in clinical hyperthyroidism before instituting treatment, especially:
      (1) When the manifestations of hyperthyroidism are not clear as based on clinical findings and other laboratory tests.
      (2) When ruling out thyrotoxicosis factitia.
      (3) When determining the existence of ectopic secretion of thyroid hormone.
   b. For assistance in the diagnosis of subacute and chronic thyroiditis and in the evaluation of various types of goiter.
   c. For use in thyroid suppression tests to evaluate autonomy of functioning thyroid tissue.
   d. For stimulation tests to assist in the differentiation of primary from secondary hypothyroidism, when determination of serum TSH is not available or appropriate.
   e. For estimation of therapeutic doses of iodine 131 in the treatment of hyperthyroidism or thyroid cancer, or for thyroid ablation.
3. Thyroid imaging with radioiodine can provide useful information in the following circumstances:
   a. Detection and evaluation of function of solitary or multiple thyroid nodules.
   b. Evaluation of aberrant thyroid tissue such as substernal masses, possible lingual thyroid, functioning metastases of thyroid cancer, and other tumors containing thyroid tissue.
   c. Assistance in the estimation of thyroid size for radioiodine dosimetry.
   d. Management of thyroid cancer.
4. Technetium 99m, as sodium pertechnetate, is a suitable substitute for radioiodine for thyroid imaging in the following circumstances:
   a. Detection and evaluation of function of solitary or multiple thyroid nodules.
   b. It may be necessary to reimage the thyroid with radioiodine when:
      (1) The pertechnetate images demonstrate no abnormality corresponding to a palpable nodule or nodules.
      (2) The pertechnetate images demonstrate a hyperfunctioning nodule or nodules (without suppression of extranodular thyroid tissue).
      (3) The thyroid pertechnetate concentration is low and image contrast is unsatisfactory.
      (4) Unexplained extrathyroidal uptake is suspected of being an artifact.
      (5) Pertechnetate is generally a less satisfactory substitute for radioiodine for thyroid imaging in the following circumstances:
         (a) Evaluation of aberrant thyroid tissue, except in the lateral portion of the neck.
         (b) Management of thyroid cancer.
         (c) Suppression and stimulation testing.

Recommendations to decrease administered doses of ^{123}I and ^{131}I as iodides, and ^{99m}Tc as pertechnetate

In this section we discuss some combinations of satisfactory imaging and measuring devices, together with some "routine" doses of the above radiopharmaceuticals for adults; they yield adequate information and simultaneously minimize radiation exposure of the patient (Table 9-3).

Table 9-3, showing typical absorbed doses, lists the radiopharmaceuticals that are used in thyroid studies in relation to the recommended administered activities. The table illustrates the magnitude not only of critical-organ doses but also of the gonadal and whole-body doses where the information is available. Since pertechnetate is also concentrated in the stomach and lower large intestine, available data on these critical organs have been included. For different assumed administered activities or assumed uptake percentages, a simple ratio calculation may be applied for the critical-organ dose.

It is to be emphasized that ^{99m}Tc, ^{123}I, and ^{131}I should not be used during pregnancy and their use should be limited in young children. Recommended oral doses for children are given in Tables 9-3 and 9-4.

These recommendations should be posted wherever tracer doses of radiopharmaceuticals used for studies of the thyroid are prepared. The physician should make certain that the prescribed tracer doses are of appropriate amounts in accordance with these recommendations except under special circumstances. For greater detail, reference may be made to the thyroid radionuclide uptake recommendations of the International Atomic Energy Agency[a] and the American National Standards Institute.[b]

1. Iodine 131 as sodium iodide.
   A principal concern in preparing these recommendations is the observation that doses of 100 to 500 μCi of ^{131}I for "routine" thyroid imaging are frequently used to decrease the time required for imaging a patient.
   a. For uptake measurement using a single crystal, recommended doses are predicated upon a crystal with an average diameter of about 2 inches (5 cm), with

*Modified slightly from Saenger, E. L., et al.: J. Nucl. Med. **19:** 107-111, 1978.

Table 9-3. Typical absorbed doses from thyroid diagnostic radiopharmaceutical procedures[c,d] based on activities recommended accompanying this report*

Age range and procedure	Recommended administered activity	Critical organ	Critical organ (mrad/μCi)	Critical organ (actual mrads)	For administered activities: Whole-body dose (mrad)	Gonadal[f] dose (mrad)
Procedure for adults						
Uptake						
^{123}I (iodide)	10-20 μCi	Thyroid	11	110-220	0.3-0.6	M: 0.1-0.2 F: 0.2-0.4
^{131}I (iodide)	6 μCi	Thyroid	1100	6600	2.6	M: 0.52[e] F: 0.84
Scan						
^{99m}Tc (pertechnetate)	5-10 mCi	Thyroid†	0.20	1000-2000		M: 60-120
		Lower large intestine	0.20	1000-2000	60-120	
		Stomach[g]	0.10-0.30	500-300		F: 90-180
^{123}I (iodide)	100-400 μCi	Thyroid	11	1100-4400		M: 1-4
		Lower large intestine		Negligible	3-12	
		Stomach[e]	0.22	22-88		F: 2-8
^{131}I (iodide)	30 μCi	Thyroid	1100	33,000	14	M: 2.6[e] F: 4.2
Procedure at age 15						
Uptake						
^{123}I (iodide)	10-20 μCi	Thyroid	16	160-320	0.36-0.73	M: 0.12-0.24 F: 0.24-0.48
^{131}I (iodide)	2 μCi	Thyroid	1600	3200	1	
Scan						
^{99m}Tc (pertechnetate)	4.2 mCi	Thyroid†	0.35	1500	63	M: 59
		Lower large intestine	0.20	840		F: 92
^{123}I (iodide)	170 μCi	Thyroid	16	2700	6	F: 4
^{131}I (iodide)	25 μCi	Thyroid	1600	40,000	13	
Procedure at age 10						
Uptake						
^{123}I (iodide)	10 μCi	Thyroid	22	220	0.5	M: 0.53 F: 0.37
^{131}I (iodide)	2 μCi	Thyroid	2200	4400	1.6	
Scan						
^{99m}Tc (pertechnetate)	3 mCi	Thyroid†	0.47	1400	65	M: 200
		Lower large intestine	0.30	900		F: 100
^{123}I (iodide)	120 μCi	Thyroid	22	2600	6.2	M: 6.6 F: 4.4
^{131}I (iodide)	18 μCi	Thyroid	2200	40,000	15	
Procedure at age 5						
Uptake						
^{123}I (iodide)	10 μCi	Thyroid	38	380	0.9	M: 0.9 F: 0.5
^{131}I (iodide)	2 μCi	Thyroid	3800	7600	2.6	
Scan						
^{99m}Tc (pertechnetate)	2.2 mCi	Thyroid†	0.78	1700	75	M: 160
		Lower large intestine	0.40	880		F: 99
^{123}I (iodide)	86 μCi	Thyroid	38	3300	6.8	M: 5.4 F: 4.4
^{131}I (iodide)	13 μCi	Thyroid	3800	49,000	17	

*Modified from Saenger, E. L., et al.: J. Nucl. Med. **19:**107, 1978. See also p. 246 for letter references.

†Assumed a 1.6% uptake of pertechnetate for all ages except the newborn, where a 3.5% uptake is assumed, following Webster et al.[c]

Table 9-3. Typical absorbed doses from thyroid diagnostic radiopharmaceutical procedures[c,d] based on activities recommended accompanying this report—cont'd

Age range and procedure	Recommended administered activity	Critical organ	Critical organ (mrad/μCi)	Critical organ (actual mrads)	For administered activities: Whole-body dose (mrad)	Gonadal[f] dose (mrad)
Procedure at age 1 year						
Uptake						
^{123}I (iodide)	10 μCi	Thyroid	81	800	1.3	M: 0.67 F: 0.83
^{131}I (iodide)	2 μCi	Thyroid	8100	16,000	4	
Scan						
^{99m}Tc (pertechnetate)	1.5 mCi	Thyroid† Lower large intestine	1.30 0.70	2000 1000	76	M: 120 F: 110
^{123}I (iodide)	60 μCi	Thyroid	81	4900	7.8	M: 4.0 F: 5.0
^{131}I (iodide)	9 μCi	Thyroid	8100	73,000	18	
Procedure for newborn						
Uptake						
^{123}I (iodide)	10 μCi	Thyroid	160	1600	3.7	M: 0.87 F: 2.4
^{131}I (iodide)	2 μCi	Thyroid	16,000	32,000	20	
Scan						
^{99m}Tc (pertechnetate)	0.7 mCi	Thyroid† Lower large intestine	3.40 2	2400 1400	100	M: 71 F: 150
^{123}I (iodide)	28 μCi	Thyroid	160	4500	9.8	M: 2.4
^{131}I (iodide)	4 μCi	Thyroid	16,000	64,000	42	F: 6.8

Table 9-4. Fraction of adult administered radioactivity recommended for children[c,d]*

Age	Newborn	1 year	5 years	10 years	15 years	Adult
Body weight (kg)	3.54	12.1	20.3	33.5	55.0	70.0
Fraction of adult activity (based on ⅔ power of body weight)†	0.14	0.30	0.43	0.60	0.85	1

*Modified from Saenger, E. L., et al.: J. Nucl. Med. **19:**107, 1978. See also p. 246 for letter references.

†The fraction of adult activity used for imaging procedures in children was chosen on the basis of proportionality to the ⅔ power of body weight following Webster et al.[c] For the purpose of this calculation, adult values of 5 mCi of ^{99m}Tc and 100 μCi of ^{123}I are assumed.

a thickness of at least 1 inch (2.5 cm) at a standard distance of 10 inches (25 cm), measured from the surface of the neck at the thyroid isthmus to the front face of the crystal.

b. Based upon the instrumentation, recommended maximum doses for uptake-percentage measurement are as follows: for adults 6 μCi; for children of varying ages see Tables 9-3 and 9-4. In uptake measurements for children, consideration may be given for a shortened distance between detector and neck.

c. Recommended doses for imaging are predicated upon a crystal in a rectilinear scanner with an average diameter of 3 to 5 inches (8 to 13 cm) and a thickness of at least 2 inches (5 cm).

d. Imaging with the rectilinear scanner or scintillation camera, or both, is based upon percentage of iodine uptake and estimated thyroid gland weight for a euthyroid subject. For imaging, a dose of 30 μCi is recommended for euthyroid patients whose glands are of normal size. A dose of 100 μCi would be considered to be an upper limit, especially suitable for hypothyroid patients.

e. When a second dose is to be given for the completion of a "TSH stimulation test" or a "thyroid suppression test," and when the second part of the test immediately follows the first, the thyroid gland should always be "counted" and a repeat dose calculated to deliver to the thyroid gland between one and two times the number of microcuries of ^{131}I remaining in the gland from the first dose. If little or none of the first dose remains, the second dose need not exceed the first one.

f. After the diagnosis of hyperthyroidism or thyroid cancer has been made and when ^{131}I therapy is to be used, thyroid imaging studies can be done with ^{131}I; here ^{123}I or ^{99m}Tc offers no advantage.

2. Iodine 123 as sodium iodide.
   a. For uptake measurements using a single crystal, the same system collimators can be used as for ^{131}I. For imaging with currently available ^{123}I, the same rectilinear scanners and collimators can be used as for ^{131}I. With the available scintillation cameras, a pinhole collimator having an aperture 3 to 6 mm in diameter is recommended.
   b. For uptake measurements with the above instruments, the following oral doses are recommended:
      (1) Measurement at 4 to 6 hours, 10 μCi
      (2) Measurement at 24 hours, 20 μCi
   c. For imaging either with the rectilinear scanner or scintillation camera as described above, an oral-dose range of 100 to 400 μCi is recommended.
3. Technetium 99m as pertechnetate.
   a. The measurement of thyroid uptake with pertechnetate is more difficult than with the radioiodines, since the uptake must be measured within 20 minutes of administration, at which time body background is high compared to the activity in the thyroid gland, enough to threaten the test's reliability. Although it is possible to develop appropriate ranges for this use, with the decreasing use of uptake measurements as a measure of thyroid function, either an in vitro test or uptake with one of the radioiodines is preferable.
   b. For imaging, the preferred method is the scintillation camera with a pinhole collimator having a 3 to 6 mm aperture.
   c. An imaging dose of 3 to 10 mCi, given intravenously, is generally adequate. Recently, doses of 15 to 20 mCi have been used to improve visualization. At these dose levels the physician should consider the radiation dose delivered to the stomach, colon, and whole body, as well as that to the thyroid gland (see Table 9-3).

REFERENCES WITHIN SAENGER ET AL.[71]

a. International Atomic Energy Agency Panel: Thyroid radionuclide uptake measurements, Special Report No. 7. Br. J. Radiol. **46:** 58-63, 1973.

b. American National Standards Institute: Thyroid radioiodine uptake measurements using a neck phantom, ANSI N44.3, 1973.

c. Webster, E. W., Alpert, N. M., and Brownell, G. L.: Radiation doses in pediatric nuclear medicine and diagnostic x-ray procedures, as revised in July 1976, from James, A. E., Wagner, H. N., and Cooke, R. E., editors: Pediatric nuclear medicine, Philadelphia, 1974, W. B. Saunders Co.

d. Kereiakes, J. G., Wellman, H. N., Simmons, G., et al.: Radiopharmaceutical dosimetry in pediatrics, Semin. Nucl. Med. **2:** 316-327, 1972.

e. MIRD: Dose estimate report no. 5, J. Nucl. Med. **16:**859, 1975.

f. Kereiakes, J. G., Feller, P. A., Ascoli, F. A., et al.: Pediatric radiopharmaceutical dosimetry, unpublished data, 1976.

g. Hine, G. H., and Sorenson, J. A.: A guide to the absorbed dose from internally administered radionuclides. In Hine, G. H., and Sorenson, J. A., editors: Instrumentation in nuclear medicine, vol. 2, pp. 588-589, New York, 1974, Academic Press, Inc.

Nuclear medicine application—in vivo technique

Thyroid uptake. The use of iodine by the thyroid has been traditionally investigated with radioactive iodine in the thyroid uptake test (RAIU). The most commonly used iodine isotopes are ^{131}I and ^{123}I, though others used in the past include ^{125}I, ^{124}I, ^{132}I, ^{130}I, and ^{128}I.

The use of ^{99m}Tc-pertechnetate for evaluation of thyroid trapping ability may incorporate an uptake assessment. The technetium uptake may be done with a dose separately from the iodine,[1,5] or it may be given simultaneously orally, or it may be administered intravenously.[41]

Table 9-5 summarizes the pertinent data on nuclides used for thyroid uptake. Administration of the uptake dose is usually oral. The desire to standardize as many variables as possible precludes instructing the patient not to eat solid food several hours prior to dose administration. By having the stomach empty the radionuclide is absorbed in preference to any food, which may impede the absorption. A 24-hour-percent uptake is calculated, though 2-, 4-, or 6-hour uptakes may be routine in addition to or instead of a 24-hour calculation. Prior to dose administration, the patient should be questioned as to prior thyroid history, medication, and x-ray procedures. Many medications contain iodine, and those radiographic procedures using contrast expand the inorganic iodide pool, with a resultant low uptake. Medications that block the use of iodine also interfere with the uptake assessment.[34]

Table 9-6 gives a partial listing of influences on the radioactive iodine–uptake study. To assess uptake, one counts the standard dose prior to administration at the appropriate energy settings in a neck phantom for a time interval sufficient for a collection of a statistically adequate number of counts. A room background is taken and subtracted from the standard to obtain net counts. Two, 4, 6, and 24 hours after dose administration, one counts the radioactivity of the patient's neck. Using the same geometry in counting both the patient and the phantom is essential. The probe for counting (detector) should be centered on the thyroid cartilage. Since all the area in the neck is not thyroid, a method to subtract the background must be employed. A simulated lead thyroid shield can be placed over the patient's neck and a count taken. An assumption that the thigh is similar to the neck in shape and blood supply makes use of this count as an alternative method of background correction. If this method is used, care

Table 9-5. Thyroid uptake

Nuclide	Dose administered* (μCi/kg)	Method of administration	Method of localization	Patient preparation	Absorbed dose to thyroid (mrad/μCi)	Principal energy (keV)	Half-life
^{123}I	0.7 to 1.4	Oral	Active transport	No solids	7.5†[54]	159	13 hours
^{125}I	0.7 to 1.4[31]	Oral	Active transport	No solids	450†	35	60 days
^{131}I	0.07 to 0.14	Oral	Active transport	No solids	800†[54]	364	8.1 days
^{99m}Tc	0.7[5,52,80]	Oral or IV	Active transport	No solids if oral	0.2[66]	140	6 hours
	10 to 70[65]	IV					

*Based on 15% thyroid uptake.
†Based on average adult weight of 70 kg.

Table 9-6. Factors influencing iodine uptake

Factors	Time for excretion
Iodine-containing compounds	
Inorganic compounds	
Lugol's iodine	Approximately 2 to 4 weeks
Tincture of iodine	Approximately 2 to 4 weeks
Potassium iodide or sodium iodide	Approximately 2 to 4 weeks
Syrup of hydroiodic acid	Approximately 2 to 4 weeks
Kelp (seaweed)	Approximately 2 to 4 weeks
Mineral supplements and foods with more than 0.5 mg of iodine per day	Approximately 2 to 4 weeks
Organic compounds	
Radiopaque agents	
Cholecystographic	4 weeks to several months
Urographic	2 to 4 weeks
Angiographic	2 to 4 weeks
Bronchographic	4 weeks to indefinite
Myelographic	4 weeks to indefinite
Drugs	
Vaginal suppositories (diiodohydroxyquin)	2 to 4 weeks
Many proprietory expectorants, cough mixtures, and antispasmodics	2 to 4 weeks
Nonthyroidal factors affecting iodine uptake	
Decreased uptake	
Excess iodine (dilutional effect)	
Goitrogenic foods	
Genus *Brassica* (turnip, cabbage)	
Milk from cattle eating choumoellier fodder	
Thioamide derivatives (wait 6 days before testing)	
Thiouracil	
Propylthiouracil and methylthiouracil	
Methimazole and carbimazole	
Aromatic antithyroid drugs (possibly acting by binding iodine within gland)	
Resorcinol	
Aminobenzenes	
Sulfonylureas (only carbutamide, not drugs in current use for treating diabetes)	
Para-aminobenzoic acid	
Para-aminosalicylic acid (PAS)	
Monovalent ions (compete for thyroid trapping)	
Thiocyanate	
Perchlorate	

Continued.

Table 9-6. Factors influencing iodine uptake—cont'd

Factors	Time for excretion
Miscellaneous	
Cobalt (blocks organification)	
Phenylbutazone (only early in treatment with doses greater than 800 mg)	
Amphenone (blocks organification)	
Aminoglutethimide (blocks organification)	
Antihistamines (particularly chlorpheniramine and dexbrompheniramine)	
Thyroid hormones (wait at least 2 weeks before testing)	
Corticosteroids	
Edema (increased iodine pool)	
Renal failure (raised plasma inorganic iodide)	
Increased uptake	
Iodine deficiency	
Rebound after discontinuing antithyroid therapy	
Recovery phase after subacute thyroiditis	
Pregnancy (normal 6 weeks post partum)—loss of iodide to fetus	
Hydatidiform mole, choriocarcinoma—chorionic TSH production	
Acute renal failure (from lack of renal clearance of iodide)	
Soya-bean diet in children (enhanced fecal excretion of thyroxine)	
Chronic liver disease (probably dietary iodide deficiency)	
Nephrosis, diarrheal states—(excess thyroxine and iodine loss)	

must be taken not to include counts from the bladder.

The following is the equation for the uptake:

$$\text{Uptake (\%)} = \frac{P - T}{(S \times F_d) - B} \times 100$$

where P is patient neck counts per minute; T is patient background counts per minute; S is counts per minute from the dose; F_d is decay factor obtained from the time that the dose is counted to the time that the radioactivity in the patient is counted (specific for nuclide); and B is room background counts per minute.

Thyroid imaging. Rectilinear scanners at one time were the mainstay of nuclear medicine departments. These have been replaced in many institutions by the scintillation cameras. However, many rectilinear scanners are in use and a discussion of thyroid techniques would be inadequate without the inclusion of rectilinear scanning (Fig. 9-5). The imaging dose administered with ^{131}I is calculated to deposit 10 μCi in the gland. Higher doses are possible with ^{123}I or ^{99m}Tc. With the majority of rectilinear systems presently in use, this level of activity will allow imaging at an adequate informational density in a reasonable time period. The patient is positioned supine for an anterior view with a pillow under the shoulders so that the neck is hyperextended with the chin level with the neck. To determine the scan speed, one determines the maximum count rate over the thyroid. The scan speed selected should yield an informational density between 800 to 1000 counts/cm^2. Right and left margins are set as needed to include the entire neck area. The chin, suprasternal notch, and thyroid cartilage, which should all be parallel to the collimator indexing motion, are marked on the film as well as the left and right sides of the patient. The area imaged should include the anterosuperior mediastinum as a routine part of the procedure. During the scan the patient should not swallow while the probe is over the thyroid. In a thorough search for extrathyroid tissue, scanning may continue down to the level of the diaphragm and possibly the ovaries of a female. Additional views may include oblique views at 45 degrees to obtain information in a second plane. The same landmarks are used as in the anterior scan. The physician may request identification of nodules or suspected thyroid masses by placing marks on the image film for anatomic regional correlation.

Currently visualization and localization of tracer in the thyroid gland for regional functional evaluation may make use of scintillation-camera systems with pinhole collimation. Particularly when one uses radiopharmaceuticals with increased photon yield, that is, ^{99m}Tc as pertechnetate or ^{123}I, significant advantages accrue. The small field size required, coupled with the close approximation of the pinhole collimator, allows magnification, which increases resolution. Oblique projections are more efficiently accomplished when compared with the rectilinear studies in which the large shielded detector encounters the patient's shoulder during its traverse and indexing. The photon yield and

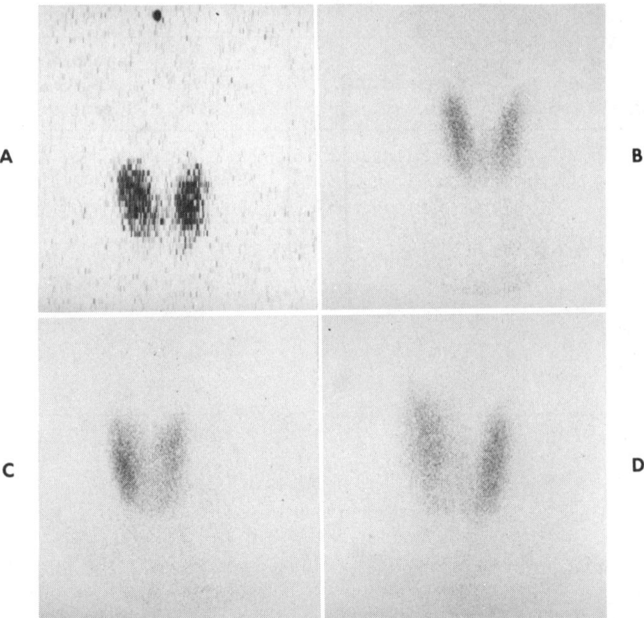

Fig. 9-5. Normal thyroid image. Contour and configuration of both lobes of thyroid gland as well as isthmus are visualized. Distribution of radionuclide varies proportionally with tissue volume being viewed by collimated detector system. Some neck background should be seen to establish that contrast enhancement or other means of image modification has not occurred. These general guidelines apply in imaging with rectilinear as well as scintillation camera. **A,** Rectilinear scan with iodine 131 (anterior projection). Scintillation-camera images with ^{99m}Tc-pertechnetate. **B,** Anterior. **C,** Left anterior oblique. **D,** Right anterior oblique.

energy of the two foregoing radionuclides offer advantages over the more traditional use of ^{131}I. The thin (0.5 inch thick) crystal of the Anger scintillation camera is more efficient with the lower energies afforded by ^{99m}Tc and ^{123}I.

^{75}Se as selenomethionine and ^{67}Ga as gallium citrate have been used to further identify solitary hypofunctional areas such as carcinomas with limited success.[46,77,83] Both nuclides are suited for scintillation camera scintigraphy or rectilinear scanning. See Table 9-7 for energies. Fluorescent scanning utilizing ^{241}Am bombardment of nonradioactive ^{127}I in the thyroid is used to assess size and iodine content, but it cannot be used to evaluate trapping. Table 9-7 outlines nuclides used for scanning.

When performing in vivo thyroid studies on pediatric patients, one must realize that the thyroid at birth is one tenth the weight of an adult's thyroid, even though body weight is approximately one twentieth. The critical organ in radioiodine studies is the thyroid; so radiation dose to a smaller thyroid must be considered when an administered dose is calculated. The nuclide of choice is ^{123}I (if one wishes to assess the iodine cycle) because of its pure gamma emissions and relatively short half-life of 13 hours. The euthyroid range for newborns and very young children is higher than that of adults; so radiation dose to the thyroid for the same adult administered dose will be increased because of this factor as well as the decreased thyroid weight.[47] ^{99m}Tc-pertechnetate offers another alternative; however, this radionuclide is trapped but not organified by the thyroid.[38,90]

T_3 suppression test. Using the pituitary-thyroid axis feedback mechanism, the T_3 suppression test allows the evaluation of the function of the thyroid gland in relationship to its dependence on TSH secretion. The principal clinical application relates to the evaluation of functional autonomy in the thyroid gland either generally, as in Graves' disease, or regionally, as in toxic nodular goiter (Plummer's disease), using the parameter of concentration or trapping as measured by the radioactive-iodine uptake. In addition, one may make regional assessment by visualization and localization of the tracer distribution within the thyroid (thyroid imaging). Parameters such as T_4 and T_3 measurement by in vitro techniques concurrently augment the diagnostic evaluation.

The most common method of performing the T_3 sup-

Table 9-7. Thyroid visualization

Nuclide	Dose administered* (μCi/kg)	Method of administration	Method of localization	Patient preparation	Absorbed dose to thyroid (mrad/μCi)	Principal energy (keV)	Half-life
^{123}I	0.7 to 1.4[4]	Oral	Active transport	None	7.5†[54]	159	13 hours
^{125}I	0.7 to 1.4[31]	Oral	Active transport	None	450†	35	60 days
^{131}I	1.4	Oral	Active transport	None	800†[54]	364	8.1 days
^{127}I	—	—	—	—	15[66]	28	Stable
^{99m}Tc	10 to 140	Oral or IV	Active transport	None	0.2[66]	140	6 hours
^{75}Se	3[77,83]	IV	Active transport	None	6[66]	136 265	120 days
^{67}Ga	35 to 50[46]	IV		None		93 184 296	77 hours

*Based on average adult weight of 70 kg.
†Based on 15% uptake.

pression tests utilizes the administration of 75 to 100 μg of T_3 for a period of approximately 1 week after establishment of base-line data.[91] Repeat thyroid uptake after the T_3 administration under normal conditions will reveal suppression of the original uptake. In patients with autonomous function, the values will not be suppressed. Regional functional evaluation by imaging is an exceedingly useful concurrent evaluation procedure. See Fig. 9-6 depicting an autonomous nodule.

TSH stimulation. Since the thyroid gland is under the regulatory control of TSH, evaluation of the end-organ (thyroid) functional capability may be assessed where there is concern with respect to hypofunction. The administration of TSH permits the evaluation of the capacity of the gland to respond. The usual parameter of measurement is the radioactive iodine in the thyroid uptake (RAIU), which under normal circumstances doubles or triples. Such a study may be used to evaluate borderline hypofunction with a normal RAIU. Failure to respond suggests a decrease in thyroid reserve. Although most cases of hypothyroidism are the result of primary disease in the thyroid gland, occasionally cases of pituitary hypothyroidism are encountered. In such cases the TSH stimulation test will establish the functional capability of the thyroid gland and incriminate the pituitary. The TSH stimulation test is also of value in the assessment of patients with autonomously functioning tissue after evaluation with the T_3 suppression test. Here the response of the suppressed thyroid tissue to TSH ensures its normality. See Fig. 9-7 demonstrating normal functional capability of suppressed tissue seen in Fig. 9-6 under the influence of TSH.

In practice, the procedure is usually accomplished by administration of 10 units of TSH intramuscularly on a daily basis for three successive days after establishment of base-line data. On the third day the patient begins the second uptake. Normally, patients will increase their RAIU by 100% or more.

Although still a valuable tool in specific cases, the procedure has been largely replaced by the RIA-TSH in evaluation of hypothyroidism. The use of TRH has also begun to replace the use of TSH in the identification of pituitary hypothyroidism.

Perchlorate-washout test. Perchlorate, a ''large'' anion, has been utilized to detect a synthesis defect at the stage of organification in the metabolism of iodine. Under normal circumstances there is a continuous progression from the concentration or trapping of iodide through organification, coupling, storage, and release. When an organification defect is present, the trapped iodide is not organified and builds up in the trapping stage of the metabolism of iodine. The TSH-stimulated trap maintains an abnormally high level of iodide. If the trapping mechanism is altered, that is, inactivated, the nonorganified iodide would be released from the thyroid into the circulating vasculature. Anions such as thiocyanate or perchlorate may be used to evaluate impaired iodination of tyrosine (organification) through its effect on the trapping mechanism. The administration of perchlorate after a tracer dose of radioiodine shows no appreciable decline in radioactivity in normal subjects as compared with the level before perchlorate. However, if there is a defect in organification, which, for example, may be present in Hashimoto's thyroiditis, a significant fall in tracer activity will be seen after the perchlorate administration.

The methodology of the perchlorate-washout test has varied widely with respect to the timing of radiometric analysis. In general a tracer dose of $Na^{131}I$ is administered to the fasting patient in a fashion analogous to

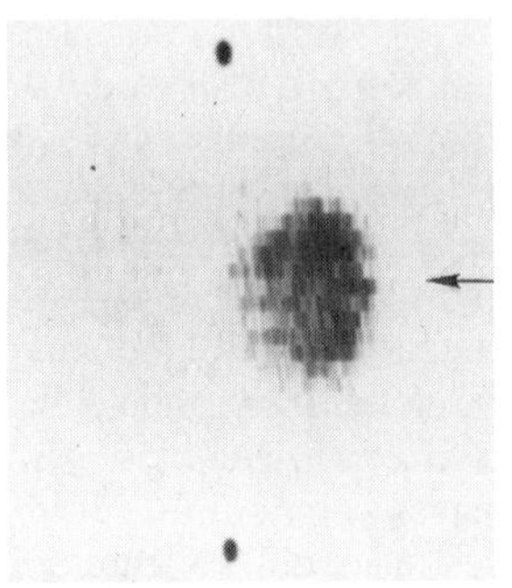

Fig. 9-6. Functional autonomy demonstrated by T_3 suppression. Normal thyroid tissue reflects suppression by biofeedback mechanism. The region that functions autonomously is clearly visualized by differential accumulation of tracer, *arrow*.

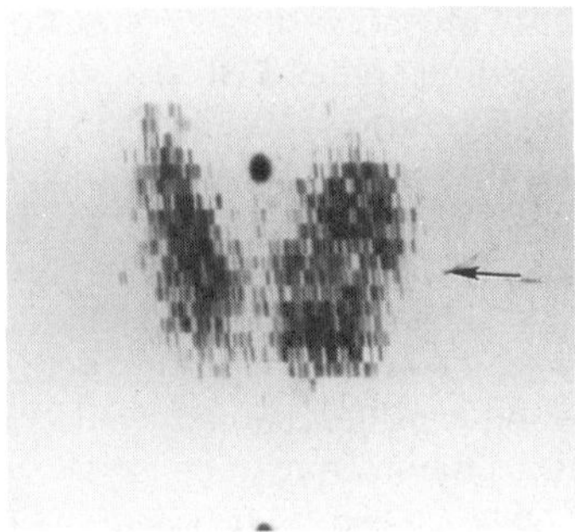

Fig. 9-7. Demonstration of normally functioning but suppressed tissue by TSH stimulation. After TSH stimulation of patient shown in Fig. 9-6 (T_3-suppression study), the suppressed tissue is shown to be capable of normal function by TSH stimulation, *arrow*.

the initiation of an RAIU test. The uptake is measured at 2 hours as a base-line value, and perchlorate in doses varying from 200 to 1000 mg is given orally. The thyroid activity is measured 1 hour later. An abnormal response is indicated by a fall in excess of 5% from the 2-hour value. Others have required a 50% decrease before diagnosing an organification defect. In addition to Hashimoto's thyroiditis, a similar defect may be seen in some patients with adenomatous colloid goiters, sporadic goitrous cretinism, nontoxic goiter, congenital deformation without goiter, Pendred's syndrome, untreated Graves' disease, as well as ^{131}I-treated hyperthyroidism.

Nuclear medicine applications—in vitro techniques

Hormones produced by the thyroid have been reviewed extensively, particularly since Yalow and Berson's initial method for radioimmunoassay and Murphy-Pattee's competitive protein-binding assay for T_4. T_4 and T_3 are bound to serum proteins, namely, thyroxine-binding globulin (TBG), and to some extent prealbumin (TBPA), and albumin in the case of T_4. T_3 is more loosely bound to serum proteins than is T_4. T_4 comprises the major compound (90%) released from the thyroglobulin molecule. Some T_4 and T_3 is "free" or not bound to serum protein, and this unbound portion is the major contributor to the hormonal activity and feedback mechanism. T_3 is felt to be three to five times more powerful in biologic activity.

Protein-bound iodine (PBI) and butanol-extractable iodine (BEI). For many years the standard assay for thyroidal activity was the amount of protein-bound iodine (PBI). Difficulties arose, however, since exogenous iodide is also measured, as well as any circulating iodoproteins or iodotyrosines (monoiodotyrosine [MIT], diiodotyrosine [DIT], thyroglobulin). Inorganic iodide may contribute significantly to elevated PBIs. A partial solution came with the development of the butanol-extractable iodine (BEI). Inorganic contamination is eliminated but organic iodide, for example, from radiographic contrast agents is still measured. The BEI and PBI can be used together to estimate increased amounts of circulating thyroglobulin, MIT, or DIT, which are included in a PBI measurement but not by BEI.

T_4 and T_3. In the 1960s BEI was replaced by the Murphy-Pattee T_4 analysis, in which ethanol denatured the serum protein to release T_4 and some T_3. By adding radiolabeled T_4 and establishing a competitive system between labeled and unlabeled T_4 in relation to TBG, one could determine the amount of total, free and bound, T_4. The first separation was by gel filtration, but that method has been replaced by anion-exchange resins.[59] Radioimmunoassay for T_4 has to some extent replaced the extraction methods in which the percent extraction of T_4 varied around 80% to 90%. The addition of agents that directly displace T_4 from serum protein allows analysis to proceed directly on the serum sample. Agents that displace T_4 include salicylates, thimerosal (sodium [(*o*-carboxyphenyl)thio]ethylmercury), phenytoin, tetrachlorthyronine, and ANS (8-anilino-1-naphthalene sulfonic acid). The assay proceeds with the addition of T_4 antibody and radioiodinated T_4 and separation of bound T_4 from the free form.

A variation on the competitive protein binding (CPB) assay has been developed. It involves the addition of a fraction of the patient's serum back into the sample extracted with ethanol. This assay is called a normalized serum thyroxine (T_4N) level, free thyroxine index (FTI), or effective thyroxine ratio (ETR), in which patients with protein-moiety alterations but without thyroid disorder remain in the normal range.[3,53]

A measure of unoccupied sites of thyroxine-binding globulin utilizing red blood uptake of TBG has erroneously been called a "T_3 uptake." It is not an analysis for T_3 but TBG. Radiolabeled T_3 fills the available TBG sites without displacing T_4 and thus is an indirect method of assessing TBG binding. The use of other separation vehicles in preference to red blood further confuses the interpretation as does the fact that total T_3 is now analyzed with a radioimmunoassay method.

Mathematical manipulation may be done on the results of various tests such as the "T_7," or free thyroxine index, which is a product of the T_3 uptake test and the T_4 serum analysis. The original data would seem to be the most reliable for diagnostic purposes, with the mathematical manipulations being an attempt to simplify the diagnosis of hormone-related disease states by normalization of variations resulting from protein-moiety alterations. Measurement of TSH levels in the blood is accomplished with great sensitivity by radioassays that usually make use of a double-antibody method. To ascertain whether the normal thyroid-pituitary-hypothalamic feedback is functional, one includes TSH levels with T_3 and T_4 assays. Exogenous T_3 may be administered to suppress TSH release and TRF to stimulate TSH release.

Long-acting thyroid stimulator (LATS) and associated antibodies. The assay of long-acting thyroid stimulator (LATS) may be used in the evaluation of autoimmune disorders of the thyroid, for example, Graves' disease and thyroiditis. Historically, LATS has been evaluated by bioassay. In the common pattern of technique evolution noted elsewhere in this chapter, radioimmunoassay may be applied in this area. Potentially useful assays for antithyroglobulin and antimicrosomal antibody should also be mentioned in this context. Both of the foregoing are present in patients with autoimmune thyroid diseases. They may be measured by radioimmunoassay techniques; however the approach is a "reverse" analysis in that the substance to be measured is the antibody rather than the antigen. Purified antigen must be obtained from human rather than animal sources.[13]

Calcitonin. Secreted by the parafollicular cells of the thyroid, the complete role of calcitonin in calcium and phosphate metabolism is still developing. It is known that calcitonin reduces calcium and phosphate levels in the blood by inhibiting bone resorption. The heterogeneous composition of calcitonin and nonspecificity of antiserum used for radioimmunoassay makes detection in normal adults difficult. However, bioassay is even less sensitive. Elevated levels evident in medullary thyroid carcinomas can be detected and confirmed by use of a calcium infusion test in which 15 mg of $CaCl_2$ per kilogram of body weight is infused over a 3-hour period. Blood samples are taken before infusion and 1 hour after. Increased calcitonin levels result during the infusion process in patients with medullary carcinoma.[82] Catheterization of thyroid venous drainage and comparison of blood values of the thyroid veins and selected adjacent veins, such as the internal jugular and superior vena cava, will more precisely define the increased calcitonin level in the thyroid vein samples in cases of medullary carcinoma.

Nuclear medicine therapy in thyroid disease

Therapeutic doses of radioiodine have been utilized in the treatment of hyperthyroidism,[42] metastatic foci of thyroid carcinoma,[67] and the ablation of thyroid tissue in patients with intractable angina pectoris, congestive heart failure,[15] or severe pulmonary insufficiency.[30]

Nuclear medicine therapy, as exemplified by application in the endocrine system, is based upon the therapeutic effectiveness of radioiodine administered by the metabolic route, with the resultant selective localization and retention in functioning thyroid tissue.[36] This tissue is subjected to intense irradiation according to the amount of radionuclide and its decay scheme and characteristics, as well as the influence of its residence time in the tissue (effective half-life). These components make up the time-dose factor, a keystone in the therapeutic effectiveness of this modality. The amount of tissue, its geometric configuration, and the distribution of radionuclide also exert an influence upon the therapeutic outcome. This is the volume distribution factor. Finally, biologic factors, conditions within the thyroid tissue, and disease processes, as well as disease in the patient as a whole, also affect the ultimate outcome of the treatment. In radiation biologic terms, the thyroid cell–renewal system is simple epithelium in the reverting postmitotic state. Although the thyroid epithelial cells are relatively radioresistant to the direct cytocidal effects of radiation, the thyroid is moderately radiosensitive in terms of delayed degeneration and loss of epithelium through the indirect mechanism of vascular damage.

Consideration of precautions in the management of patients who have received therapeutic amounts of radionuclides is paramount in proper care. In addition, radiologic health and safety aspects are necessary concomitant considerations with respect not only to attending personnel but also fellow patients, visitors, and other workers in the hospital environment, as well as the general public who might casually encounter potential exposure from such a source. The following four situations highlight the possible exposure to others from patients involved in nuclear medicine therapy:

(1) the patient receiving regular nursing care as an inpatient, (2) the patient referred for emergency operation after therapy, (3) the patient released from the hospital while still containing an appreciable quantity of radionuclide, and (4) the patient who dies while appreciably radioactive. The reader is referred to the chapter on radiation safety for basic information on this area of management. In addition, a primary resource for guidance is the *NCRP Report No. 37,* 1970 (available from NCRP Publications, P.O. Box 4867, Washington, D.C.). This document should be considered mandatory reading for every member of the ''nuclear medicine team'' involved in therapeutic application of radioactive material. It is important to recognize that in addition to the external radiation exposure potential from the relatively energetic gamma emissions, there exists the potential for contamination from the metabolized and excreted radiopharmaceutical. The latter raises the dual possibility of external exposure to both beta and gamma irradiation, as well as the opportunity for internal deposition of the radionuclide by ingestion or inhalation of this volatile element. Thus, health physics principles and practices relating to contamination control and decontamination must be an integral part of the body of knowledge and skills of nuclear medicine personnel. They must be able to communicate, by precept as well as by example, the facets of radiologic health and safety to other members of the health care team, the patient, and the public at large in order to maintain control of the radioactive material involved and assure the safety of those who might potentially receive exposure. Specific guidance for use of radioactive iodine is contained in the aforementioned *NCRP Report No. 37*. More recently publication of revised regulatory guides by the NRC (8.23 and 10.8) have pointed up contemporary standards for medical applications and radiation safety surveys in medical institutions. The regulatory guides, in addition to speaking to the traditional radiation safety concerns with therapeutic levels of radioactive iodine, also point up the issue of bioassay of personnel for evidence of internal deposition of iodine. The application of radioactive iodine (^{131}I) in therapeutic doses to the treatment of thyroid disease allows reinforcement of the need for a continuing awareness of the principles and practices of radiation safety.

Treatment of hyperthyroidism. The purpose of the therapeutic application of radioiodine to hyperthyroidism is to control the disease and return the patient to a euthyroid status. The accumulation and retention of radioiodine with the subsequent radiation effects upon the cellular renewal system of the thyroid and its supporting stroma serve as the basic principle.[36] The radiopharmaceutical of choice remains ^{131}I, though, historically, other radionuclides of iodine have been utilized and currently some centers are exploring the efficacy of ^{125}I. The patient selection remains related to the accurate diagnosis of the disease entity, with evaluation of the etiologic variations, primarily the problem of diffuse versus toxic nodular hyperthyroidism (Figs. 9-6 and 9-8). Age,[35,40] which has historically been a primary criterion for selection, currently causes consideration only from the medicolegal standpoint, reflecting some residual from the age of radiation hysteria. No noteworthy morbidity, other than hypothyroidism, has occurred as a result of radioiodine therapy in children with childhood thyrotoxicosis. Such treatment not only is simple to administer and efficacious, but also is comparable with surgery and antithyroid drug therapy with regard to safety. Editorially speaking, the *New England Journal of Medicine* in 1971[21] stated that radioiodine has practically replaced thyroidectomy in the treatment of Graves' disease in adults and, further, the apprehension concerning radiation-induced thyroid cancers and leukemia has been dispelled by careful long-term observations. Pregnancy and lactation remain contraindications to the therapeutic application.[70]

Preparation of the patient for radioiodine therapy requires primarily a correlation of the clinical findings with an assessment of the thyroidal status in terms of function and size. Because the therapeutic effect of ^{131}I is not immediate, three possible regimens of management have been employed: (1) Potassium iodide utilized in the postradioiodine period may achieve control; however, an appreciable number of severely hyperthyroid patients may not be controlled.[33] The expansion of the inorganic iodide pool by stable iodide interferes with effective reutilization of radioiodine, and the use of tracer diagnostic studies involving the

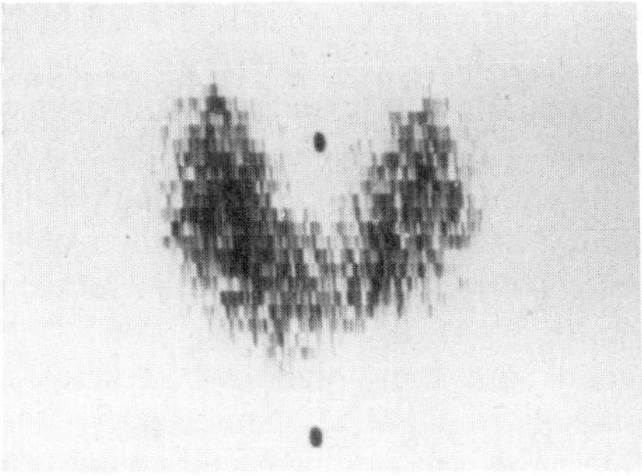

Fig. 9-8. Diffusely enlarged thyroid gland in Graves' disease depicts relatively uniform distribution of tracer varying proportionately with tissue volume being viewed by collimated detector. Contrast this study with that seen in Figs. 9-6 and 9-7 showing an autonomously hyperfunctioning adenoma. Planimetric measurement of image is used in calculating size of gland for therapy dose planning.

iodide cycle. (2) Antithyroid drugs such as methimazole and propylthiouracil may be introduced into the treatment plan as soon as the diagnosis is confirmed and then discontinued prior to the ^{131}I treatment.[24] Medications may then be reintroduced later than a week after treatment if clinical status warrants. Problems may be encountered in such utilization: antithyroid drugs may manifest varying lengths of block after discontinuance of the drug, or such agents may exert a radioprotective effect on tissues through the sulfhydryl (SH) groups. (3) Beta-adrenergic receptor blockade using propranolol[78] in doses of 40 mg every 6 hours offers the major advantage of peripheral action with thyroid functional parameters being left unaffected and utilization possible at any stage in the treatment regimen.

In our opinion, the availability of the thyroid tissue in its unadulterated pathophysiologic state is optimal for radioiodine therapy. Thyroid-blocking agents or expansion of the inorganic iodide pool, or both, significantly influence therapeutic effectiveness and, indeed, in the posttreatment period, effect the reutilization of the radioiodine, thus giving full use to the administered therapeutic dose.

Selection of the therapeutic dose invites the usual empirical versus calculated dose debate. The empirical dose, on the average, probably does as well; however, by its very nature it excludes patients with variations from the mean in terms of their pathophysiology and does not allow tailoring of the therapeutic plan to cope with unique situations. Thus we recommend consideration of the functional status of the thyroid gland, the size of the thyroid gland, and the inclusion of other biologic-variation considerations present in the individual case. The basis of our treatment plan, in diffuse disease, is the deposition of 80 μCi/g of thyroid tissue for the first 50 g, and 40 μCi/g thereafter. The weight is calculated by planimetry and adjusted by the functional level (24-hour RAIU) in order to derive the activity to be administered. In toxic nodular disease, the desired deposition activity is increased to 120 μCi/g.

The patient follow-up and spacing of treatments must allow sufficient time for evolution of the therapeutic effect prior to retreatment. A retreatment decision must be made after integration of total case information indicating significant residual disease, never on isolated abnormal parameters.

The literature is replete with suggestions of radiation thyroiditis,[7] thyroid crisis,[74] abnormalities of calcium metabolism,[29] leukemia,[72,85] thyroid cancer,[39] genetic effects,[14] and the widely variable percentages of hyperthyroidism.[19,27,57] Immediate problems are extremely uncommon and predictions of long-term hazards, that is, neoplastic disease, are becoming increasingly difficult to support with scientific data.

Although thorough consideration should be given to all these areas, the major problem, if indeed it is a problem, remains the occurrence of the hypothyroid state and its progressively increasing incidence with time.

Treatment of hyperthyroidism with radioiodine (^{131}I) has proved to be simple, effective, and inexpensive. Virtually every case of hyperthyroidism can be controlled with doses of ^{131}I that can be tolerated by the patient. The treatment delivers a sufficient amount of radiation resulting in damage to functioning thyroid cells and supporting stroma so that the hormonal production is permanently reduced. Myxedema, an undesirable result, may be controlled by replacement therapy.

Treatment of thyroid carcinoma. The treatment of thyroid carcinoma with radioiodine is directed toward the control of metastatic foci and palliation of patients with thyroid carcinoma. The principle of therapy is the same as that in hyperthyroidism but with delivery of larger amounts of radioactivity to achieve effects on the neoplastic cellular renewal system.

The selection of patients for radioiodine therapy necessitates a search for tumors that are likely to develop efficient radioiodine uptake. The biochemical function and the histologic character of thyroid carcinoma tissue correlate closely. Many adenocarcinomas of the gland develop uptake, 50% or more, provided that a diagnostic survey is made with ^{131}I after complete thyroid ablation (Fig. 9-9).

For known or inoperable differentiated tumors showing evidence of advancing, two major opinions with respect to therapy have evolved: (1) Thyroid adenocarcinoma is a relatively benign disorder with a long survival—successive recurrences can be removed surgically as they occur, with no other therapy than TSH-suppressive doses of thyroxine. (2) Any known or suspected functioning tumor tissue remaining after surgery requires treatment by therapeutic doses of radioiodine.

Preparation of the patient with histologically differentiated tumor, at biopsy or operation, includes a near total thyroidectomy as well as total removal of recognizable neoplastic tissue. Subsequently, a diagnostic dose of radioiodine should be administered sufficient to accomplish a total body survey for visualization and localization of residual functional tissue prior to any thyroid suppression. If any residual normal thyroid tissue remains in the neck, and it usually does, an ablative dose of radioiodine should be administered. In a patient with known inoperable and differentiated metastases, radioiodine therapy should be given if tumor tissue develops radioiodine uptake. In all cases, thyroxine would be administered in maximally acceptable dose during the intervals between radioiodine

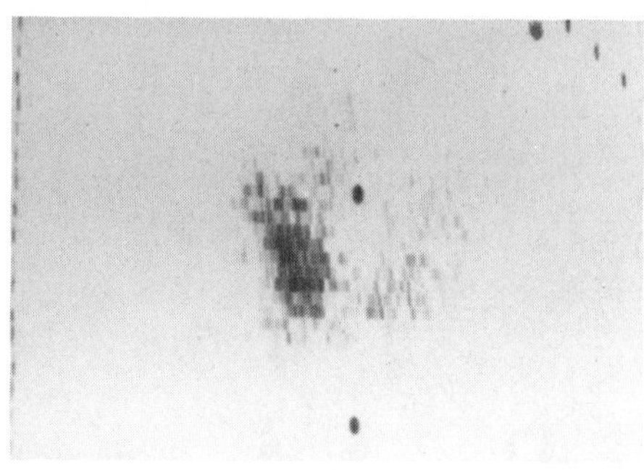

Fig. 9-9. Thyroid carcinoma presenting as hypofunctional region. Although thyroid carcinoma often presents as hypofunctional area of tissue illustrated by altered distribution of radioactive tracer, more than half of such tumors retain sufficient functional capability to allow identification by nuclear medicine imaging techniques. This necessitates removal or ablation of competing normal thyroid tissue.

administration for diagnostic survey or treatment, or both.

An attempt should be made to deliver a tumor dose of 10,000 rads in a series of ^{131}I administrations in the order of 100 mCi per administration.[63] A careful and extended follow-up is mandatory in all patients. Astute clinical evaluation with use of appropriate adjuncts, such as whole body scanning for functional foci and diagnostic radiographic surveys for metastatic sites, will dictate the management during this protracted follow-up.

Fifty percent of all patients who have active disseminated thyroid adenocarcinoma are benefited by therapy with radioiodine. A recent report indicates that in patients 40 years of age or older, the group treated with ^{131}I had a significantly lower death rate than the surgery-only group.[88]

Problems are primarily related to the delivery of significantly larger doses of ionizing radiation than are encountered elsewhere in nuclear medicine therapy. Radiation-induced hypoplasia of the bone marrow serves as a major limiting factor. A balance must be maintained between frequency of treatment to obtain a result as rapidly as possible and the effects of therapy in terms of whole body radiation. In the area of long-term effects, leukemia must be considered, and in one reported series, four of 250 patients treated developed leukemia, where statistically, only 0.1 case was predicted. With regard to other neoplasia, no evidence has been found to support increased mortality from other malignant neoplasms.[63]

Treatment of cardiorespiratory disease. The purpose of the administration of radioiodine in euthyroid patients with cardiorespiratory disease cases is the deliberate induction of a hypothyroid state in the face of progressive and irreversible disease processes associated with a high and often sudden mortality. The result is a reduced metabolic rate and a decreased oxygen requirement. Patients in whom the basic disease process is progressive and irreversible under conditions of optimal standard therapeutic regimen should be considered for this form of therapy.

As in the aforementioned disease entities, a functional assessment of the thyroid is prerequisite to effective delivery of an ablative dose of radioiodine. A retained dose in the order of 10 mCi of ^{131}I appears to be a useful point of departure in dose selection. Clinical improvement should not be expected for 6 to 8 weeks, and a decision to re-treat should not be made until at least 3 months after therapy.

This modality is effective in approximately 50% of patients. One must remember that this form of therapy is primarily symptomatic and does not reflect definitive attack on the primary etiology.

Problems encountered with this form of therapy are the occasional aggravation of clinical symptoms seen some 2 to 3 weeks after treatment. This is most likely attributable to the release of the thyroid hormone from disrupted follicles as a result of the effects of ionizing radiation. A variety of troublesome symptoms may accompany the resultant myxedema, which requies small replacement doses of thyroxine. One must exercise caution in order to prevent reactivation of the primary disease disability while reducing the complaints referable to the hypothyroid state.

THE PARATHYROID

Anatomic relationships

The parathyroid gland of man consists of four separate (two superior and two inferior) parathyroid glands situated close to the posterior surface of the thyroid gland (Fig. 9-10). However, the number of parathyroid glands may vary from less than four to 12. The size of the single parathyroid gland averages 6 × 4 × 2 mm, with an approximate weight of 30 mg. The parathyroid glands are derived from the third and fourth branchial pouches. In about 10% of the population the parathyroid glands are found in an aberrant location (near the mediastinum, inside the thyroid gland, and, rarely, behind the esophagus). Each gland is surrounded by an ill-defined fibrous capsule and has distinct stalks containing the blood vessels and the nerves, which enter each gland independently. The blood supply of the parathyroid glands is from superior and inferior thyroid arteries and in some cases from the small vessels surrounding the esophagus and trachea.

Histologically, the normal parathyroid gland consists of two types of epithelial cells: the chief cells (the light and the dark), and the oxyphil cells. The third type of epithelial cell, water-clear cells, present

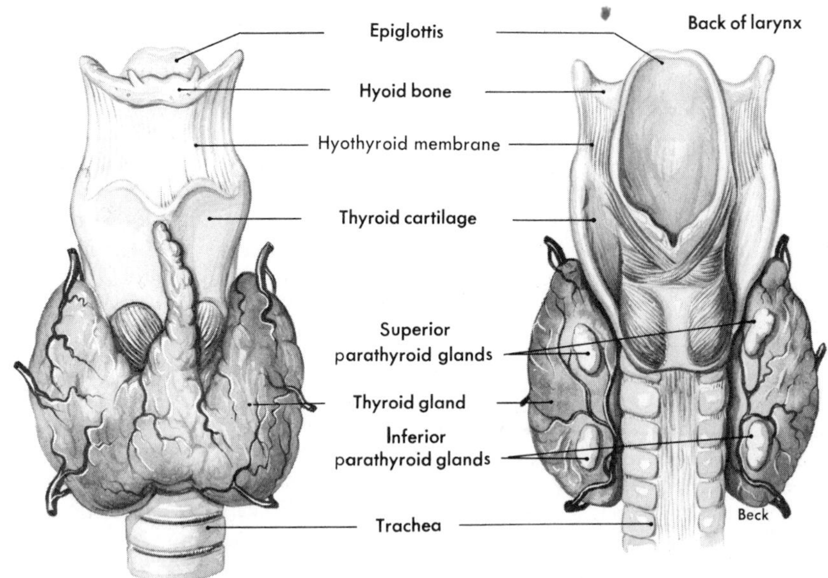

Fig. 9-10. Thyroid and parathyroid glands. Note their relations to each other and to larynx (voice box) and trachea. (From Anthony, C. P., and Thibodeau, G. A.: Textbook of anatomy and physiology, ed. 10, St. Louis, 1979, The C. V. Mosby Co.)

as large polygonal cells 10 to 15 μm in diameter and can be seen in hyperplasia.

Physiologic role

Parathyroid hormone (PTH) is the only known secretory product of the parathyroid glands. Dark chief cells are considered to be the main source of PTH. Oxyphil cells and water-clear cells have not been identified with any special function. The principal function of PTH is the regulation of calcium-ion concentration in the body fluids to provide optimal functioning of the different cells (the beta cells of the Langerhans' islands in the pancreas, and nerve and muscle cells throughout the body). PTH also functions as a tropic hormone, regulating the kidney oxidation of 25-hydroxy-vitamin D_3 to 1,25-hydroxyvitamin D_3. The latter form is the most active form of vitamin D_3.

Parathyroid hormone is a polypeptide with a molecular weight of 9500 and a single polypeptide chain that consists of 84 amino acid residuals. Human PTH consists of small amounts of intact hormone molecule as well as different fragments in the blood, that is, biologically inactive C (carbon) and biologically active N (nitrogen) fragments, and the N-terminal portion and has been shown to differ from both the bovine and porcine hormones. It was recently shown that those fragments can be separately estimated by different radioimmunoassay techniques and carry the different diagnostic information.

Physiologically, PTH acts primarily on kidney and bone. It also acts upon the small intestine, but its effect is considered to be indirect. In bone, PTH (1) inhibits collagen synthesis, (2) enhances osteolysis, both osteolytic and osteoclastic, (3) increases the rate of maturation of both osteoclasts and osteoblasts, (4) causes a release of Ca^{++} and acidic mucopolysaccharide from the bone matrix, (5) increases the accumulation of lactic acid and isocitric acids, and (6) increases a collagen breakdown. In kidneys, PTH increases tubular absorption of Ca^{++} and Mg^{++} and decreases the reabsorption of inorganic phosphate (P_i). The effect of this action is to increase serum Ca^{++} and to cause phosphaturia. In the gut, PTH promotes the absorption of Ca^{++} and P_i, but only in the presence of vitamin D. PTH activates adenyl cyclase in the cells of its target tissues and causes an initial increase in calcium entry into cells of target tissue. PTH is also responsible for altering the acid-base balance of the body.

Conditions that cause the calcium-ion concentration level in the body fluids to fall too low result in proliferation of and increased secretion of PTH by the parathyroid cells. Among the conditions that increase the output of parathyroid hormones are (1) low calcium-ion concentration in rickets, (2) low calcium-ion concentration in osteomalacia (adult rickets), (3) lactation, in which a large amount of calcium ion is secreted in the milk, and (4) low-calcium diet. Thus one can show that secretion of PTH is closely regulated by serum Ca^{++}, increasing as its falls and decreasing as it rises. The size and activity of the glands are inversely related to the dietary intake of the calcium.

Pathophysiologic derangements

Pathophysiologic derangements of the parathyroids may be generally characterized by states of hypofunction and hyperfunction. In brief, in hypoparathyroidism (low PTH level in plasma), serum Ca^{++} falls and inorganic phosphate rises. Hypoparathyroidism is seen either as an idiopathic disease or, much more commonly, as a complication of operation of the thyroid gland. It is manifested early by paresthesia, signs of increased neuromolecular excitability, and frank tetany. In hyperparathyroidism (excessive PTH secretion), serum Ca^{++} is increased and inorganic phosphate is decreased, leading in severe cases to pathologic development of osteitis fibrosa cystica, peptic ulcers, and metabolic acidosis. The renal excretion of Ca^{++} is greatly increased, leading often to the formation of urinary calculi. Primary hyperparathyroidism results from hyperplasia of the parathyroid glands (about 11%) and from functioning tumors (about 89%). Primary hyperparathyroidism is usually caused by a single benign adenoma of one parathyroid gland (over 80%) and, rarer, by the carcinoma (less than 2%). Multiple adenomas and hyperplasia (especially chief cells) of the parathyroid glands are often associated with a multiglandular endocrinopathy, classified as multiple endocrine adenomatosis type I (acidophilic or chromophobic adenomas of the pituitary, functioning islet tumors of the pancreas, adenomas of the parathyroid and adrenal cortex) or type IIa (medullary carcinoma of the thyroid, pheochromocytoma, and parathyroid hyperplasia). Hyperparathyroidism may arise secondary to chronic renal insufficiency. Retention of inorganic phosphate depresses serum Ca^{++} and this, in turn, stimulates PTH production. Among the other conditions leading to the secondary hyperparathyroidism as a compensatory mechanism in any abnormal state tending to produce true hypocalcemia are (1) hypovitaminosis D, (2) vitamin D–dependent rickets, (3) malabsorption of Ca^{++}, (4) hyperphosphatemia, and (5) renal tubular acidosis.

A very sensitive carboxyl-terminal assay (C-fragment assay) is used to measure serum PTH in routine clinical analysis. Assessment of serum PTH level in children and adolescents with low calcium concentration in the blood and the aforementioned clinical manifestations of hypoparathyroidism allows differentiation of idiopathic hyperparathyroidism from pseudohypoparathyroidism. The latter is genetic disease transmitted as a sex-linked dominant trait. The clinical characteristics and chemical findings (hypocalcemia, hyperphosphatemia, and low urinary calcium) are similar to those of idiopathic or postoperative hyperparathyroidism. However, this disease (pseudohypoparathyroidism) is characterized by a normal secretion and a serum concentration of PTH but a lack of response of the receptor tissue. A normal to high PTH plasma level, together with the minimal effect of exogenously administrated parathyroid hormone (in terms of urinary excretion of 3′,5′-AMP) allows differentiation between the two groups.

The signs of primary and secondary hyperparathyroidism and the serum PTH level are very important in the differential diagnosis of other causes of hypercalcemia, which are (1) malignant diseases (metastasis to bone, multiple myeloma, ectopic PTH secretion), (2) thyrotoxicosis, (3) immobilization of patients with Paget's disease, (4) vitamin D intoxication, (5) vitamin A intoxication, (6) milk-alkali syndrome, (7) sarcoidosis, (8) adrenocortical insufficiency, and (9) thiazide diuretics. It is valuable in the clinical setting to evaluate the serum PTH level together with the serum calcium and phosphate.

Nuclear medicine applications—in vivo techniques

Visualization and localization studies of the parathyroid glands may be attempted with a labeled amino acid that concentrates in hyperfunctioning parathyroid tissue. Selenomethionine (with ^{75}Se) is rapidly removed from the vascular bed by tissue involved in protein synthesis after intravenous administration. Subsequently, there is a reappearance of tracer in the form of labeled plasma proteins.[6] The application of this technique appears to be of primary value in the preoperative assessment of hyperactive parathyroid tissue. The mechanism of the successful study relates to the differential accumulation of the gamma-emitting amino acid analog relative to the concentration of tracer in neighboring tissues. The relative affinity of each of the adjacent tissues becomes exceedingly important and depends primarily on the cellular nature of the tissue and its rate of metabolic activities. Additionally, with the ability to localize and visualize functioning parathyroid tissue one must consider the variable blood background of tracer. As in all imaging studies the crux of the success or failure in diagnostic interpretation depends on the target to nontarget ratio of information being reviewed. Using the kinetic relationship of the levels of tracer (^{75}Se-selenomethionine) in the blood-tissue background and the parathyroid differential accumulation, the clinical application in imaging may prove useful in a given case. A patient with suspected hyperparathyroidism is placed on a TSH suppressive dose of triiodothyronine (T_3) so that the background level of tracer in the thyroid gland (usually 100 μg of T_3 per day for a week) may be suppressed.

After this pretreatment, 250 μCi of ^{75}Se-selenomethionine is administered intravenously and imaging begun 5 to 10 minutes after radiopharmaceutical administration. Rectilinear imaging is usually utilized for the optimal sensitivity resolution. Proper attention to energy in collimation selection would allow camera imaging, though the photon flux available from the tracer dose would require a considerable time to achieve adequate informational density. One images the anterior cervical region from the upper aspect of the thyroid to the sternum, using sequential repetitive studies with one study including the anterior mediastinum. The total elapsed time in the sequence is ordinarily 2 to 2½ hours spanning the optimal tracer kinetic relationships.

The images may then be evaluated individually and by superimposition of a composite of all studies. The criterion of diagnosis requires a persistent differential accumulation of tracer over that of the background. In one series of 40 selected patients undergoing parathyroid operation for suspected hyperparathyroidism, 20 of 36 with identified abnormality were correctly identified by the tracer study.[64] Parathyroid adenoma was the most common pathologic finding in these cases. One must recognize that this series was selected in terms of patient population and that it included five instances of false-positive studies. These represented in four of the five patients autonomous (nonsuppressed) thyroid adenomas. Addition of concurrent evaluation of the thyroid by tracer techniques would allow correct identification of this pitfall. False negatives remain the major constraint in application of this study.

Nuclear medicine applications—in vitro techniques

The most sensitive method of analysis for parathyroid hormone is the application of radioimmunoassay techniques. Since purified human PTH is not available as an antigen, antibodies are prepared primarily by use of bovine or porcine PTH. Antiserums from the bovine source vary in specificity from animal to animal, such that restandardization of the assay is required with each new batch of antiserums. The greatest success has been achieved with antiporcine antibody. Most workers establish their own pooled serums from normal subjects for a PTH standard. The best correlation between other parameters of disease and the level of circulating PTH is seen when the amount of 7000 molecular-weight PTH is assayed with antiporcine antibody. Studies applying the double-antibody radioimmunoassay methodology have shown a significant problem relating to the labeled PTH, which may be bound to serum protein rather than to the antiserum. Studies have shown that the amount of radiolabeled PTH that combines with serum protein is dependent on the amount of protein present. Thus the amount of unknown patient sample influences the binding requiring correction.[2] Studies using both antiporcine and antibovine hormone have demonstrated at least two species of circulating PTH. This heterogenicity reflects the principal problem in routine clinical application, the lack of standardization of techniques.

THE ADRENAL GLANDS

Anatomic relationships

The adrenal (suprarenal) glands are paired small bodies of a yellowish tissue, topographically located in the retroperitoneal median plane, immediately anterosuperior to the upper pole of each kidney (Fig. 9-11). They are somewhat pyramidal in shape and normally weigh about 10 to 12 g (5 to 6 g for each gland). The adrenal glands are divided into two major components: a mesodermally derived cortex (during 4 to 6 weeks of fetal life) and a neuroectodermally derived medulla (during the seventh week of embryonic development). A thick connective tissue capsule covers the glands, which are then enclosed together with kidneys in the renal fascia. One may also encounter small amounts of tissue identical with the adrenal cortex (accessory suprarenal glands) near the normal adrenals or in other locations, such as in the spermatic cord, epididymis, or broad ligament of the uterus. Certain anatomic features of each of the adrenal glands that appear on the images of the adrenal cortex are exceedingly important in the interpretation of nuclear medicine studies. The right adrenal is round in contour and is situated posterior to the inferior vena cava and the right lobe of the liver, and anterior to the diaphragm and superior pole of the right kidney. The left adrenal gland is oval in contour and is located in a more anterior position than is the right gland. The right gland lies in a more cephalad position than does the left. The overall dimensions are similar for both adrenals (50 mm vertically, 30 mm transversely, and 10 mm in the anteroposterior plane).

The arterial blood supply of the adrenal glands is derived from the aorta, the phrenic arteries, the renal arteries, and occasionally the ovarian, spermatic, or intercostal arteries as well. Venous drainage is through the central vein on the left, which empties into the renal vein, and on the right, which empties into the inferior vena cava. Histologically, the adrenal cortex consists of a narrow outer zona glomerulosa, which produces mineralocorticoids, a wider zona fasciculata, which produces glucocorticoids and sex hormones, and the zona reticulosa, which produces androgens. The inner portion of the adrenal gland, the medulla, is soft and reddish brown. Its polyhedral basophilic cells produce epinephrine and norepinephrine.

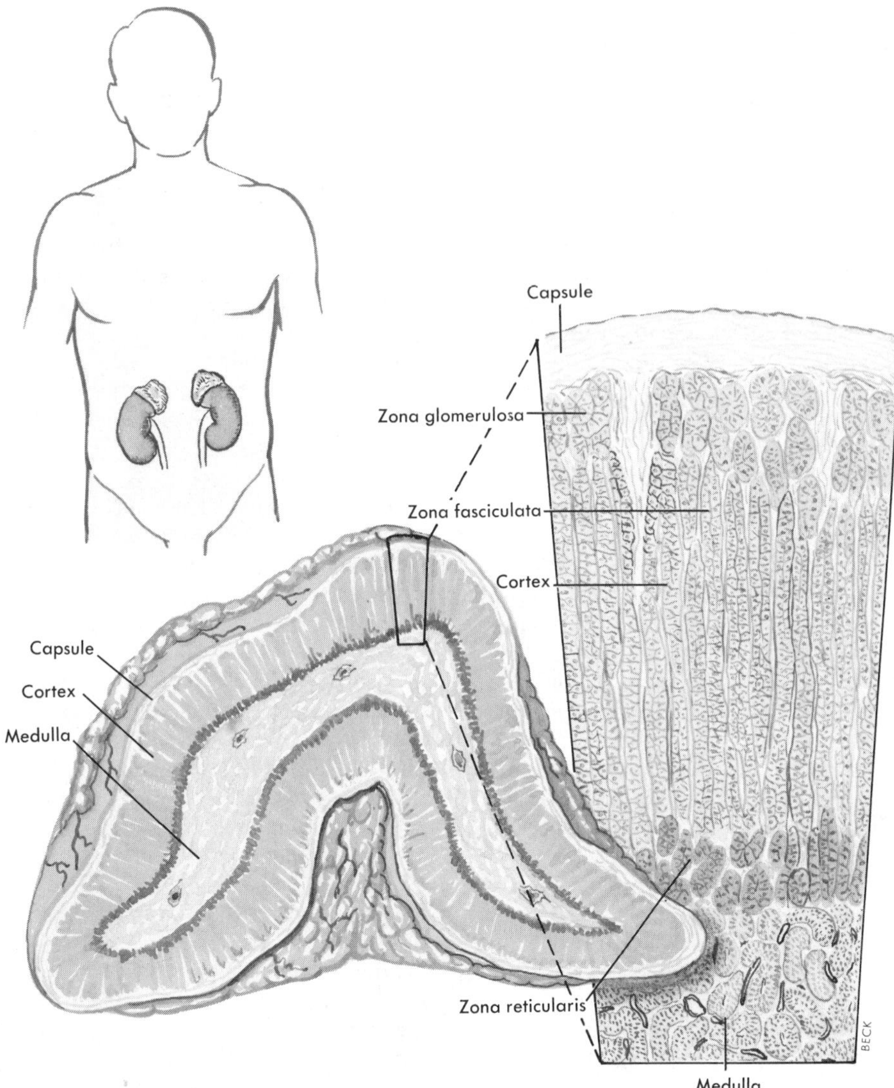

Fig. 9-11. Structure of adrenal gland showing cell layers (zona) of cortex. Zona glomerulosa secretes aldosterone. Zona fasciculata secretes abundant amounts of glucocorticoids, chiefly cortisol. Zona reticularis secretes minute amounts of sex hormones and glucocorticoids. (From Anthony, C. P., and Thibodeau, G. A.: Textbook of anatomy and physiology, ed. 10, St. Louis, 1979, The C. V. Mosby Co.)

Physiologic role

All hormones of the adrenal cortex (steroid hormones) are derivates of cholesterol. The side chain of cholesterol is shortened to yield the 21-carbon derivative pregnenolone. The zona glomerulosa converts pregnenolone to aldosterone (principal mineralocorticoid) through a series of enzymatically regulated steps. 11-Deoxycorticosterone (DOC) is secreted at approximately the same rate as aldosterone (0.1 mg per day), but since it has only one thirtieth the mineralocorticoid potency of aldosterone, it is usually of little physiologic importance. DOC normally occurs in the biosynthetic pathway as a precursor of aldosterone, but in certain forms of congenital adrenal hyperplasia it may be secreted in increased quantity, causing hypertension. Aldosterone is secreted by the zona glomerulosa in response to angiotensin, potassium, sodium, and ACTH. A very small mineralocorticoid effect is noted for cortisol, the principal glucocorticoid secreted by zona fasciculata. The biologic effect of mineralocorticoids stems from their property of stimulating transport of electrolytes. In response to mineralocorticoids, all these tissues tend to conserve sodium and lose potassium, magnesium, and hydrogen ions. Mineralocorticoids are also important in the maintenance of blood pressure and blood volume. In clinical practice serum concentration and urinary excretion of aldosterone are measured by radioimmunoassay, with specific antialdosterone serum and tritiated aldosterone as the marker. The normal value for serum aldosterone is 1 to 21 μg/dl (morning peripheral vein specimen) and for urine excretion is 2 to 16 μg per 24 hours. Usually the clinical study of aldosterone metabolism is combined with evaluation of the renin-angiotensin system.

Among naturally occurring steroids, only cortisol, cortisone, corticosterone, and 11-dehydrocorticosterone (compound A) have appreciable glucocorticoid activity. Of these, cortisol is the most potent. The biosynthetic steps of cortisol are as follows: cholesterol → pregnenolone → progesterone → hydroxyprogesterone → 11-deoxycortisol → cortisol. The normal adrenal gland secretes significant quantities of cortisol only in response to ACTH, which acts through the mediation of cyclic AMP. The ACTH regulates cortisol secretion by classic negative feedback, or servomechanism, which is so important in maintaining homeostasis. It is very improtant to note that, of the hormones synthesized by the human adrenal cortex, only cortisol itself has much ACTH-suppressing activity, though a number of synthetic corticosteroids may produce this effect. Biologic effects of glucocorticoids include (1) promotion of breakdown and possible inhibition of protein synthesis (protein-wasting activity); (2) promotion of glycogen deposition, gluconeogenesis hyperglycemia, and glucosuria; (3) anti-inflammatory and antiallergic effects; (4) inhibition of the lymphatic system and fibroblast proliferation; (5) stimulation of erythropoiesis and production of platelets; (6) stimulation of gastric acid production; and (7) inhibition of bone growth, matrix formation, and calcification. Although an estimate of the plasma cortisol could be obtained from the level of corticosteroids "17-OH CS" (together with cortisone, 11-deoxycortisol, and their derivatives) during the last two decades, the radioimmunoassay technique for plasma and urine determination of cortisol appears to be the preferred method in clinical practice. The most useful technique at the present time is determination of free (unconjugated) cortisol in urine, by competitive protein-binding assay. The normal value of this test is 27 to 108 μg per 24 hours. This level may be increased in patients taking estrogens or oral contraceptives. Plasma cortisol determination together with plasma ACTH plays an important role in differential diagnosis of Cushing's syndrome (adrenal tumor, Cushing's disease, and ectopic ACTH syndrome) when used in conjunction with functional modified procedures involving metyrapone, dexamethasone, and ACTH.

Androgens and estrogens are also by-products of the adrenal gland cortex. The most important of these is dehydroepiandrosterone. It is secreted mostly without any biotransformation, but a very small amount is converted to classic androgens (androsterone and testosterone). Although there is no doubt about adrenal synthesis and secretion of small amounts of estrogen, the exact structure has been difficult to prove. It is assumed that they are produced by enzymatic conversion of androsterone.[51]

Pathophysiologic derangement

Primary aldosteronism is usually associated with a solitary suprarenal adenoma (Conn's syndrome). Occasionally it may be associated with multiple adenomas or adrenocortical hyperplasia, and in extremely rare cases the source of aldosteronism is adrenocortical carcinoma. Differential diagnosis of hyperaldosteronism demonstrates a unique interplay of in vivo and in vitro techniques of nuclear medicine. By applying parameters of renin activity, along with adrenal imaging modified by dexamethasone suppression, one may differentiate the characteristics of solitary adenoma (Conn's syndrome) from idiopathic cortical hyperplasia. For example, the solitary adenoma demonstrates a unilateral differential accumulation that is not suppressed by dexamethasone associated with low plasma renin activity. Idiopathic cortical hyperplasia, on the other hand, exhibits a bilateral uptake of radiopharmaceutical that can be suppressed by dexamethasone. Low renin levels are noted in the latter, whereas high levels are seen in hyperplasia with secondary hyperaldosteronism, which may also be seen in chronic renal disease.

The value of adrenal imaging has been demonstrated in the diagnosis of patients with Cushing's syndrome. Three distinct imaging patterns are observed. Patients with bilateral hyperplasia have prominent bilateral activity contrasting with the normal pattern, which usually shows less striking activity bilaterally, and bilateral hyperplasia is often asymmetric. Patients with adenoma of the adrenal glands show intense activity in one adrenal gland and decreased or absent activity in the contralateral gland. Focal unilateral uptake is seen in patients with adrenal remnants and recurrent Cushing's syndrome. Dexamethasone suppression helps in differentiation of adenoma from asymmetric bilateral hyperplasia.

Preoperative demonstration of a tumor is useful in a differential diagnosis between primary hyperaldosteronism caused by adenoma, and so-called idiopathic hyperaldosteronism (bilateral adrenocortical hyperplasia). Nonfunctional adrenal adenoma may be visualized on scan, probably because of uptake of iodocholesterol in nonsteroid lipid fraction.[68]

NM-145 and NP-59 (see below) do not concentrate in adrenal medulla tissue but may show the distortion or destruction of the adrenal cortex by the pheochromocytoma. Adrenal imaging appears to offer a valuable initial study if one attempts to preoperatively localize the pheochromocytoma. If positive, it may spare the patient more complicated procedures. Bilateral nonvisualization of adrenal glands is characteristic of carcinoma.

Nuclear medicine applications—in vivo techniques

Adrenal gland imaging. Visualization and localization of radioactive nuclides in the adrenal gland was introduced into our clinical armamentarium in 1971 with the demonstration of differential accumulation of ^{131}I-labeled 19-iodocholesterol.[8] In this study aldosterone-producing adenomas were shown to concentrate the foregoing radiopharmaceutical based upon the synthesis of adrenocorticosteroids from cholesterol. This biochemical basis has led to the evolution of radiopharmaceuticals for adrenal imaging by use of labeled cholesterol compounds.[26] ^{131}I-19-iodocholesterol (NM-145) was the initial tracer.[56] Subsequently, ^{131}I-6β-iodomethyl-19-norcholesterol (NP-59) was introduced with significant advantages over its predecessor.[48,73]

Procedures utilizing iodine (^{131}I)–containing radiopharmaceuticals for adrenal gland imaging require proper patient preparation to preclude any unnecessary radiation dose to the thyroid from free or metabolized ^{131}I. Thyroid "block" with either Lugol's solution or SSKI is recommended, beginning prior to the administration of the radiopharmaceutical and continuing for approximately 2 weeks. The tracer is administered slowly intravenously, and in the case of ^{131}I-19-iodocholesterol, serial images using a scintillation camera with suitable collimation for ^{131}I is accomplished in approximately 1 week after injection. Some protocols suggest images at 7, 10, and 13 days to maximize the probability of successful imaging, with recognition of individual metabolic variation from patient to patient. Particular attention should be directed toward the acquisition of adequate informational density to facilitate interpretation. For anatomic reference localization, it is useful to accomplish renal imaging with ^{99m}Tc-labeled pentetic acid (diethylenetriaminepentaacetic acid, DTPA), ferrous ascorbate, or DMSA (2,3-dimercaptosuccinic acid) after completion of the adrenal imaging procedure. This maneuver allows one to confirm tracer localization in adrenocortical tissue using the renal structures as the primary landmark. The evolution of radiopharmaceuticals such as ^{131}I- or ^{123}I-labeled 6β-iodomethyl-19-norcholesterol may allow diagnostic studies within 24 hours of tracer administration. Evaluation of this radiopharmaceutical in human subjects employing ^{123}I-NP-59 has demonstrated an improved image quality and a radiation dose reduction, properties implying that adrenal gland imaging may progress from its present investigational status to a useful member of our armamentarium of routine nuclear medicine consultative procedures.[89]

Modification of the base-line studies with dexamethasone, which suppresses uptake, offers useful differential diagnostic information with reference to adrenal pathology. Application of automated data-processing techniques (scintillation camera–coupled computer) may be useful in image processing and definition of more quantitative data for interpretation.

Nuclear medicine applications—in vitro techniques

Cortisol. Adrenocorticotropin hormone acts upon the adrenal cortex to produce cortisol (compound F) in the zona fasciculata and zona reticularis. A negative-feedback mechanism regulates the secretion of cortisol. However, diurnal rhythm and stress are two factors that increase both corticotropin and cortisol daily. Cortisol is one of a series of steroids important in adrenal physiology, and analysis of cortisol without cross-reactivity with some of the other steroids is not possible. Analysis can be carried out by a number of methods using either plasma or urine samples. Competitive protein binding is preferred over Porter-Silber, fluorometric, or chemical determination of 17-hydroxysteroids.

The analysis by competitive protein binding requires that the protein normally present in plasma first be removed. The binding protein, in this case cortisol-binding globulin, is added and subsequently a tracer that is cortisol labeled with either ^{3}H or ^{75}Se. The ^{75}Se label allows the samples to be counted in gamma equipment more readily available in nuclear medicine laboratories. Corticosterone, cortisone, 11-deoxycortisol, and cortisol are detected with CPA.

One may measure the cortisol secretion rate by injecting a known amount of labeled compound F and collecting urine. The specific radioactivity of cortisol in the urine is related back to the amount injected.

Inducing stress by administering pyrogens, insulin, or vasopressin is a test to assess the integrity of the ACTH-cortisol mechanism, since stress should increase both ACTH and cortisol. Also exogenous ACTH can be used as a stimulation test. Suppression of cortisol can be induced with dexamethasone and metyrapone injection.

Although urinary samples are still analyzed, radioassays utilizing plasma samples are the easiest to manipulate.

THE PANCREAS

Anatomic relationships

The pancreas is unique in our consideration of the endocrine system in that it offers an example of an anatomic structure that carries out dual roles in the digestion and assimilation of food (Fig. 9-12). One of these roles is exocrine in nature; the other, of our primary interest in this chapter, is endocrine in nature. The islet cells of the pancreas influence metabolism throughout the body, principally through the actions of insulin and glucagon. For better understanding of the pancreatic secretory mechanisms relating to the endocrine function, a few anatomic features should be highlighted. The endocrine portion of the pancreas, that is, the islets of Langerhans, make up only about 1% of the weight of the organ. This 1%, however, is comprised of 2 million islets from 20 to 300 μm in diameter. In the human the islets are composed of at least three cell types, designated A, B, and D cells. The A cells secrete glucagon, and the B cells produce and secrete insulin. The D cells have been identified as containing secretory granules, but their product at this point in time has not been identified. The hormone gastrin has been identified with islet cell function, but whether this is related to the D cell or a postulated fourth cell, the F cell, is yet to be established. The islets are surrounded by a basement membrane, which encloses the foregoing three types of cells. The capillaries permeating the islets likewise have a basement membrane, therefore, the hormones must cross two

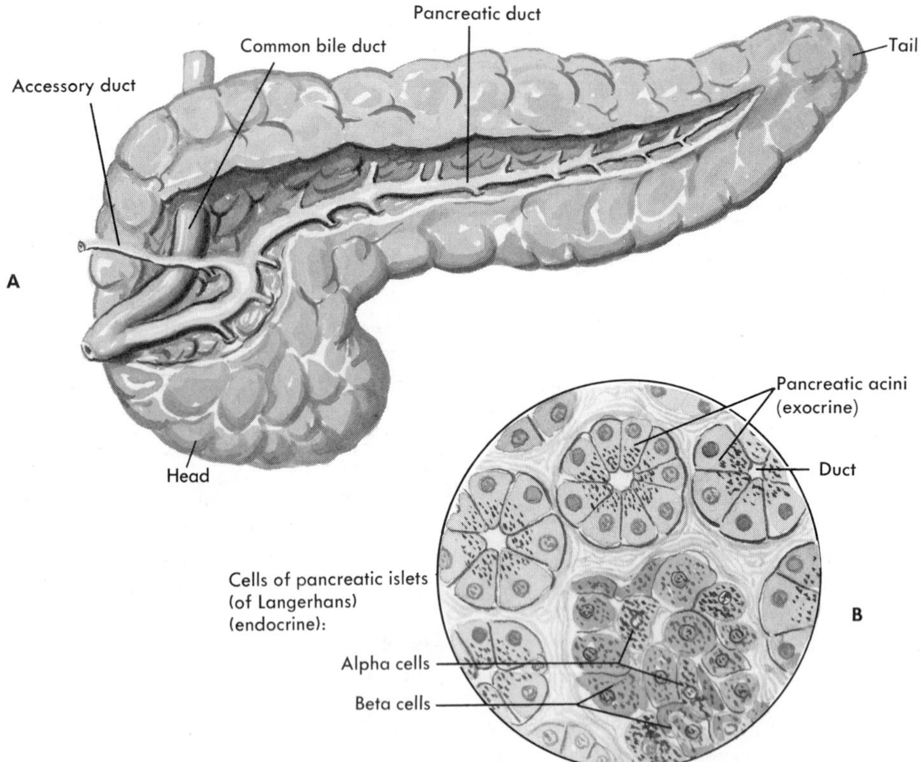

Fig. 9-12. A, Pancreas dissected to show main and accessory ducts. Main duct may join common bile duct, as shown here, to enter duodenum by a single opening at major duodenal papilla, or the two ducts may have separate openings. Accessory pancreatic duct is usually present and has separate opening into duodenum. **B,** Exocrine glandular cells (around small pancreatic ducts) and endocrine glandular cells of islands of Langerhans (adjacent to blood capillaries). Exocrine pancreatic cells secrete pancreatic juice, alpha endocrine cells secrete glucagon, and beta cells secrete insulin. (From Anthony, C. P., and Thibodeau, G. A.: Textbook of anatomy and physiology, ed. 10, St. Louis, 1979, The C. V. Mosby Co.)

basement membranes in order to enter the bloodstream. Electron microscopic studies have elucidated some of the intimate details of the rapid passage of hormonal elements, for example, insulin, between the islets and the vascular bed after islet-cell stimulation. Insulin is made up of a single polypeptide, which initially is identified as proinsulin. The conversion of proinsulin to insulin occurs by proteolytic cleavage with a reduction in molecular weight of the protein and two identifiable products, one being insulin and the other identified as C-peptide. Insulin is subsequently complexed with zinc and stored. The proinsulin synthesis and cleavage with subsequent insulin storage are not directly coupled with the release mechanism. These processes, rather, appear to be regulated separately. The insulin synthesis is sensitive to glucose level. Insulin release from the beta cells of the islets is related to the degree of glucose stimulation and is also correlated with the rate of calcium uptake by the islet. The products of the islet cells, namely, insulin, proinsulin, and C-peptide, circulate freely in the plasma. The principal mode of measurement in contemporary medical practice, either investigative or clinical, is by radioimmunoassay. Both proinsulin and insulin interact with the same antibodies and thus are measured unless the plasma is specifically pretreated in a way to differentiate between these hormones. The insulin secretion rate has been identified by radioimmunoassay techniques to consist of a biphasic pattern resulting from glucose stimulation. There is an immediate islet-cell response (within 30 seconds to 1 minute) when the glucose level is increased and held above 100 mg/dl. This response peaks within a few minutes and gradually falls. This fall is followed by a gradual rise, which reaches another steady-state level. The second phase appears primarily influenced by the metabolism of glucose. When the circulating level of glucose falls to normal levels, the insulin secretion rapidly returns to basal level.

Physiologic role

Glucagon synthesis and storage has been related to the A cells of the pancreatic islets; however, the intimate detail of knowledge about this hormone does not parallel that of insulin. The details of synthesis of glucagon are yet to be defined. The measurement of glucagon in plasma is more difficult than that of insulin because of interference by a number of larger molecular weight products arising from the gastroenteric tract that are similar in immunologic reactivity to glucagon. There are, however, several antibodies that have been identified as specific for this hormone. One concept that has been advanced suggests that glucagon and insulin participate together in regulation at the peripheral-tissue level. This coupling of the two hormones in a regulatory effect results in tissue effects that depend on the relative concentration of two hormones.[86] This hypothesis would give an exceedingly important role to glucagon as a regulator of metabolism in conjunction with insulin.

Pathophysiologic derangement

In terms of pathophysiologic effects, too much insulin results in hypoglycemia, whereas too little produces diabetes mellitus. An excess of glucagon results in diabetes, whereas too little permits hypoglycemia.

Nuclear medicine applications—in vitro techniques

Insulin. The initial work of Yalow and Berson on insulin led the way for the large number of radioimmunoassay techniques available today.[93] Insulin levels may be measured with great sensitivity by radioimmunoassay techniques, which utilize varying methods of separation of free from bound. The recent injection of insulin gives false results, since insulin antibodies are produced in the blood. These antibodies thus interfere with the assay. Stimulation of insulin secretion by glucose provides a means of artificially inducing insulin secretion with the glucose tolerance test. Other stimulation test alternatives include growth hormone, glucagon, arginine, and pancreozymin, but the inhibitors include epinephrine and thiazide diuretics.[50] The potential influence of such factors must be considered when one assesses a patient's insulin values. Stimulation tests utilizing tolbutamide, glucagon, or leucine may assist in the diagnosis of islet-cell tumors.[32]

Glucagon. Glucagon assays have not gained widespread use because of their lack of sensitivity. Adding a protease inhibitor to the serum samples and handling them at low temperatures are necessary to prevent the destruction of glucagon. Radioimmunoassay of glucagon may be useful in the diagnosis of deficiencies such as idiopathic hypoglycemia or hypopituitarism. Glucagon's main use is as a stimulant for the secretion of other hormones (see growth hormone, calcitonin, and insulin discussions). As our knowledge of glucagon's physiologic role increases, glucagon assays will expand beyond clinical investigation.

Gastrin. Gastrin, secreted by the mucosal lining of the stomach, and under pathologic conditions from gastrinomas, can be assayed by radioimmunoassay. The heterogeneous nature of gastrin is not completely understood. Antibodies that will incorporate all the various forms of gastrin must be prepared until more is known about their individual specificity in physiologic reactions.

Since proteins stimulate gastrin secretion, serum is obtained from patients who are fasting. Screening for

Zollinger-Ellison syndrome is most commonly accomplished by gastrin analysis.

THE GONADS

Anatomic relationships and physiologic role

The dual role of the gonadal tissue demonstrates another crossover in the organ system approach, which is partially covered under the category of genitourinary system and partially under the category of endocrine system. The testicular tissue in the male and the ovarian tissue in the female provide, on the one hand, hormonal secretions while simultaneously providing the cellular constituents for reproductive function. The testicular tissues involved in hormonal synthesis and the secretion of testosterone are the interstitial cells of Leydig. These cells are found interspersed in groups between the seminiferous tubules. The close interrelationship between the pituitary tissues and the gonadal tissues is demonstrated in the finding that both spermatogenesis and testosterone secretion are under the control of the gonadotropic hormones secreted from the anterior pituitary. FSH acts on the germinal epithelium to promote full spermatogenesis, whereas the interstitial cell–stimulating hormone (ICSH), or luteinizing hormone (LH), causes the Leydig cell to secrete androgens and estrogens. In the endocrine system, regulation by feedback appears the rule. Control of testicular function appears consistent with this concept. In the testes the interrelationship between LH and testosterone appears reciprocal; that is, when the Leydig cells are damaged so that the testosterone levels decrease, the LH levels increase. Conversely, when the testosterone levels increase, the LH levels decrease. The regulation mechanism for FSH secretion is less certain. Two postulates have been advanced: one is based upon a negative-feedback mechanism and the other upon utilization. Utilization, possibly by the germinal epithelium, lowers the level of FSH; thus the FSH levels are controlled. The understanding of this concept is further complicated by the role of releasing hormones identified from the hypothalamus. This area has been discussed previously in relation to neuroendocrine influences and the pituitary gland.

In the female the reproductive process is even more complex. Interactions of the hypothalamus, pituitary, ovaries, and genital tract are a continuing cyclic function in the mature adult with variations in the premenarchal and menopausal subjects. The ovaries serve to coordinate interactions of the foregoing interactive constituents. Normal ovarian function results in two major classes of products, sex steroid hormones and ova. As we noted for the male, the dual functions are products of the ovarian tissue and, in the female particularly, are products of the follicular apparatus under the stimulus of hormones produced by the anterior pituitary, which in turn is influenced by the releasing hormones. During the process of reproduction the estrogens act at the local tissue level to mediate some of the effects of gonadotropins resulting in follicular maturation. They also act peripherally, mediated by the hypothalamus, to moderate anterior pituitary gonadotropin secretion. An additional role played by the sex steroid hormones is in relationship to gamete transportation and also in fertilization, as well as conditioning the uterus for implantation of the ovum.

As we have seen throughout other areas of the endocrine system, the development of specific, sensitive radioimmunoassay and competitive protein-binding methodology has allowed the measurement, in this instance, of gonadotropin and sex steroid levels present in the serum. This has added tremendously to our body of knowledge in understanding both testicular and ovarian control mechanisms, as well as function and structure correlation. Specific detail with respect to techniques is provided in the chapter on radioimmunoassay and is not dealt with in detail here. Suffice it to say that the majority of applications with respect to the gonads have been investigative in nature to elucidate further not only physiologic interrelationships in the endocrine system but also pathophysiologic phenomena associated with disease states. This knowledge of pathophysiologic derangements is making a gradual transition into routine clinical application. One may anticipate that nuclear medicine will play an ever increasingly important role in the assessment of disease states involving aspects of the endocrine system other than our more traditional emphasis upon the thyroid gland.

Nuclear medicine applications—in vitro techniques

Sex steroids. The initial radionuclide assays for androgens, estrogens, and progesterone involved laborious double-isotope derivative techniques that limited a more general clinical application. Subsequent methodology has involved use of binding proteins in serum, intracellular receptor proteins, and antibodies produced against steroid protein complexes as specific binding reagents for so-called radioligand assays.[59] Steroid hormones circulate in three forms: conjugates, those bound to specific binding proteins in serum, and those that are free. The most useful assays utilized clinically for reproductive steroids appear to be those involving the unconjugated serum concentration of a given hormone. To accomplish the assay, one must separate the hormone from its conjugates or the conjugates must be inactivated within the assay system.

The usual methodology involves the extraction of the serum sample with an organic solvent, commonly diethyl ether. By this means the bound steroid is removed from its binding protein and, together with the free fraction, is distributed in the ether layer so that the conjugates are left nearly completely in the aqueous phase. Subsequent purification of the extraction depends on the specificity of the binding reagent as well as the presence or absence of interfering substances. For the more important reproductive steroids, sufficiently specific antiserums are available so that the requirement for involved purification steps such as chromatography is precluded. Although steroids are not antigenic, they can be made antigenic by combination of the steroid with a large molecule, such as bovine serum albumin, or thyroglobulin. To obtain maximum specificity, one must cause the steroid to link with the protein in a manner that preserves all its reactive groups.

Use of such assays remains contingent upon the user's validation of the antiserum to ensure the integrity of the technique. Many commercially available forms involve tritiated steroids as well as radioiodinated steroid tyrosine esters for use as radioligands. The bound and free hormones are separated in the assay procedures by use of activated charcoal or nonspecific absorbents, by second-antibody techniques or precipitation of the complex with ammonium sulfate, or by column chromatography.

Although such techniques appear straightforward or even simple in procedural-flow diagrams, it is well to remember that useful application is dependent on the quality assurance, which dictates meticulous attention to detail. For example, the extraction step requires attention to the fact that organic solvents deteriorate with storage. Strict cleanliness of glassware is required. Antiserums may adsorb to the surfaces of storage containers or become inactivated by contaminating substances. Separation of the bound-free fractions may be incomplete, so that the assay's sensitivity is reduced. In general, implementation of assay procedures for the steroid sex hormones should result from a sufficiently sustained requirement to ensure a continuing familiarity with the procedure and a sufficient turnover of reagents to preclude pitfalls in the technical aspects of the study. In terms of routinely available clinically useful information, the need for such assays appears limited at the current "state of the art."

THE PROSTAGLANDINS

Physiologic role

A final area of brief consideration in the endocrine system is the unique group of cyclic fatty acids known as "prostaglandins" (PGs). These somewhat ubiquitously distributed hormonal elements exhibit potent biologic effects in virtually every organ system of the body. Since the discovery of their action in the early 1930s and the isolation and identification of the initial two classes of prostaglandin (PGE and PGF) in 1960, a voluminous literature has evolved because of the diversity of action and potent biochemical and physiologic effects that these compounds exert. A variety of physiologic stimuli may evoke release of prostaglandins. It appears that prostaglandins are released into the venous circulation as a result of increased prostaglandin synthesis within a particular tissue or organ and that release subsequently leads to a functional change in that system followed by a secondary "overflow" into the circulatory bed with possible other effects within the organism. As an illustration of some of the diverse influences of these compounds, the cardiovascular-renal system is influenced by an antihypertensive renal functional effect as well as a blood pressure–lowering effect in normotensive animals. An antihypertensive effect is seen in hypertensive human subjects. Influences, which include effects on the estrus cycle, abortion, and induction of labor, are seen in the reproductive system. In the hematopoietic system, platelet inhibition and stimulation activities are ascribed to various prostaglandins in the aggregation of platelets. Erythrocytes are influenced in the microcirculation by the ability of the prostaglandins to alter deformability. Local and systemic influences on inflammatory processes have been reported, along with a broad influence upon immune response. The recitation goes on with respect to other organ systems, but in our frame of reference the endocrine system is of primary interest. The prostaglandins appear to influence the metabolic process by increasing the cyclic AMP with target-cell function augmented. In other cell systems function may be reduced, with a concomitant decrease in cyclic AMP. Interaction between tropic hormones and a receptor site in all membranes may require activation by prostaglandins as a specific intermediary. Investigation of prostaglandin action offers an opportunity to further define cellular events. There exists some evidence of therapeutic potential with prostaglandins.

REFERENCES

1. Arkles, L. B.: Quantitative thyroid scanning: a reliable thyroid function test, Am. J. Roentgenol. Radium Ther. Nucl. Med. **121:**705-713, Aug. 1974.
2. Arnaud, C. D., Tsao, H. S., and Liddledike, T.: Radioimmunoassay of human parathyroid hormone in serum, J. Clin. Invest. **50:**21, 1971.
3. Ashkar, F. S., and Bezjian, A. A.: Use of normalized serum thyroxine (T_4N). A new approach to thyroid hormone measurement, J.A.M.A. **221:**1483-1485, Sept. 25, 1972.
4. Atkins, H. L., Klopper, J. F., Lambrecht, R. M., and Wolf, A. P.: A comparison of technetium 99m and iodine 123 for thyroid imaging, Am. J. Roentgenol. Radium Ther. Nucl. Med. **117:**195-201, Jan. 1973.
5. Atkins, H. L., and Richards, P.: Assessment of thyroid function and anatomy with technetium-99m as pertechnetate, J. Nucl. Med. **9:**7-15, Jan. 1968.

6. Awwad, H. K., Adelstein, S. J., Potchen, E. J., and Dealy, J. B., Jr.: The interconversion and reutilization of injected ^{75}Se-selenomethionine in the rat, J. Biol. Chem. **242**:492-500, 1967.
7. Becker, D. V., and Hurley, J. R.: Complications of radioiodine treatment of hyperthyroidism, Semin. Nucl. Med. **1**:442, 1971.
8. Beierwaltes, W. H., Liekerman, L. M., et al.: Visualization of human adrenal glands in vivo by scintillation scanning, J.A.M.A. **216**:275-277, 1977.
9. Berson, S. A., and Yalow, R. S.: Measurement of hormones—radioimmunoassay. In Berson, S. A. and Yalow, R. S., editors: Methods in investigative and diagnostic endocrinology, New York, 1973, American Elsevier Publishing Co., Inc., p. 94.
10. Berson, S. A., and Yalow, R. S.: Radioimmunoassay of ACTH and plasma, J. Clin. Invest. **47**:2725, 1968.
11. Berson, S. A., and Yalow, R. S.: Recent studies on insulin binding antibodies, Ann. N.Y. Acad. Sci. **82**:338-344, 1959.
12. Berson, S. A., Yalow, R. S., Bauman, A., Rothschild, M. A., and Newerly, K.: Insulin–I-131 metabolism in human subjects: demonstration of insulin binding globulin in the circulation of insulin treated subjects, J. Clin. Invest. **35**:170-190, 1956.
13. Blahd, W.: Nuclear medicine, New York, 1971, McGraw-Hill Book Co.
14. Blomfield, G. W., et al.: Treatment of thyrotoxicosis with 131-I: a review of 500 cases, Br. Med. J. **1**:63, 1959.
15. Blumgart, H. L., Freedberg, A. S., and Kurland, G. S.: Treatment of incapacitated euthyroid cardiac patients with radioiodine: summary of results in treatment of 1,070 patients with angina pectoris or congestive heart failure, J.A.M.A. **157**:1, 1955.
16. Bowers, C. Y., Friesen, H. G., Hwant, P., et al.: Prolactin and thyrotropin release in man by synthetic pyroglutamyl-histidyl-prolinamide, Biochem. Biophys. Res. Commun. **45**:1033, 1971.
17. Boyd, A. E., III, Lebovitz, H. E., and Pfeiffer, J. B.: Stimulation of human-growth-hormone secretion by L-dopa, N. Engl. J. Med. **283**:1425-1429, 1970.
18. Braverman, L. E., Ingbar, S. H., and Sterling, K.: Conversion of thyroxine (T_4) to triiodothyronine (T_3) in athyreotic human subjects, J. Clin. Invest. **49**:855-864, 1970.
19. Burke, G., and Silverstern, G. E.: Hypothyroidism after treatment with sodium iodide I-131. Incidence and relationship to antithyroid antibodies, long-acting thyroid stimulator (LATS), and infiltrative ophthalmopathy, J.A.M.A. **210**:1051, 1969.
20. Catt, K. J., Dufau, M. L., Tsuruhara, T.: Radioligand-receptor assay of luteinizing hormone and chorionic gonadotropin, J. Clin. Endocrinol. Metab. **34**:123-132, Jan. 1972.
21. Chapman, E.: Which radioiodine? (editorial) N. Engl. J. Med. **285**:1142-1143, 1971.
22. Chopra, I. J.: An assessment of daily production and significance of thyroidal secretion of 3,3′,5′-triiodothyronine (reverse T_3) in man, J. Clin. Invest. **58**:32-40, July 1976.
23. Chopra, I. J., Fisher, D. A., Solomon, D. H., et al.: Thyroxine and triiodothyronine in the human thyroid, J. Clin. Endocrinol. Metab. **36**:311-316, Feb. 1973.
24. Crooks, J., Buchannan, W. W., Wayne, E. J., and McDonald, E.: Effect of pretreatment with methylthiouracil on results of 131-I therapy, Br. Med. J. **5167**:151-154, Jan. 16, 1960.
25. Daughaday, W.: Normal and abnormal secretion of growth hormone in man. In Hayes, R. L., Goswitz, F. A., and Murphy, B. E. P., editors: Radioisotopes in medicine: in vitro studies, Oak Ridge, Tenn., 1968, U.S. Atomic Energy Commission.
26. Dexter, R. N., Fishman, L. M., et al.: Stimulation of adrenal cholesterol uptake from plasma by adrenocorticotropin, Endocrinology **87**:836, 1970.
27. Dunn, J. T., and Chapman, E. M.: Rising incidence of hypothyroidism after radioactive iodine therapy in thyrotoxicosis, N. Engl. J. Med. **271**:1037, 1964.
28. Eddy, R. L., Gilliland, P. F., Ibarra, J. D., Jr., et al.: Human growth hormone release—comparison of provocative test procedures, Am. J. Med. **56**:179-185, Feb. 1974.
29. Eipe, J., Johnson, S. A., Kiamko, R. T., et al.: Hypoparathyroidism following 131-I therapy for hyperthyroidism, Arch. Intern. Med. (Chicago) **121**:270-272, March 1968.
30. Ellison, L. T., Gallaher, B. S., LaMotte, I. F., Hamilton, W. F., Jr., and Ellison, R. G.: Clinical and physiologic results following radioactive iodine in the treatment of chronic pulmonary insufficiency, Am. Rev. Respir. Dis. **80**:181, 1959.
31. Endlich, H., Harper, P., Beck, R., Siemens, W., and Lathrop, K.: The use of I-125 to increase isotope scanning resolution, Am. J. Roentgenol. **87**:148-155, Jan. 1962.
32. Fajans, S. S.: Diagnostic tests for functioning pancreatic islet cell tumors: diabetes. Proceedings of 6th Congress of the International Diabetes Federation, pp. 894-897, Amsterdam, 1969, Excerpta Medica Foundation.
33. Goldsmith, R. E., and Eisele, M. L.: The effect of iodide on the release of thyroid hormone in hyperthyroidism, J. Clin. Endocrinol. Metab. **16**:130, 1956.
34. Grayson, R. R.: Factors which influence the radioactive iodine thyroidal uptake test, Am. J. Med. **28**:397-415, March 1960.
35. Greene, W., and Wessler, S.: Management of juvenile hyperthyroidism, J.A.M.A. **213**:1652-1655, Sept. 7, 1970.
36. Greig, W. R., Boyle, J. A., Buchanan, W. W., and Fulton, S.: Radiation, thyroid cells and 131-I therapy—a hypothesis, J. Clin. Endocrinol. Metab. **25**:1411, 1965.
37. Haibach, H.: Evidence for a thyroxine deiodinating mechanism in the rat thyroid different from iodotyrosine deiodinase, Endocrinology **88**:918-923, April 1971.
38. Handmaker, H., and Lowenstein, J. M., editors: Nuclear medicine in clinical pediatrics, New York, 1975, The Society of Nuclear Medicine, Inc.
39. Hanford, J. M., Quimby, E. H., and Frantz, V. K.: Cancer arising many years after radiation therapy. Incidence after irradiation of benign lesions in the neck, J.A.M.A. **181**:404-410, Aug. 4, 1962.
40. Hayek, A., Chapman, E. M., and Crawford, J. D.: Long term results of treatment of thyrotoxicosis in children and adolescents with radioactive iodine, N. Engl. J. Med. **283**:949, 1970.
41. Hayes, M. T., and Wesselossky, B.: Simultaneous measurement of thyroidal trapping ($^{99m}TcO_4^-$) and binding (^{131}I): clinical and experimental studies in man, J. Nucl. Med. **14**:785-791, 1973.
42. Hertz, S., and Roberts, A.: Application of radioactive iodine in therapy of Graves' disease, J. Clin. Invest. **21**:624, 1942.
43. Hine, G. J., and Williams, J. M.: Thyroid radioiodine uptake measurements. In Hine, G. I., editor: Instrumentation in nuclear medicine, New York, 1967, Academic Press, Inc.
44. Jacobs, L. S., Snyder, P. J., Wilber, J. F., et al.: Increased serum prolactin after administration of synthetic thyrotropin-releasing hormone (TRH) in man, J. Clin. Endocrinol. Metab. **33**:996, 1971.
45. Kaplan, S. L.: In vitro studies: endocrinological. In Handmaker, H., and Lowenstein, J. M., editors: Nuclear medicine in clinical pediatrics, New York, 1975, The Society of Nuclear Medicine, Inc.
46. Kaplan, W. D., et al.: ^{67}Ga-citrate and the nonfunctioning thyroid nodule, J. Nucl. Med. **15**:424-425, 1974.
47. Kereiakes, J. G., Seltzer, R. A., Blackburn, B., and Saenger, E. L.: Radionuclide doses to infants and children: a plea for a standard child, Health Phys. **11**:999, 1965.
48. Kojima, M., Maeda, M., Ogawa, H., et al.: New adrenal scanning agent, J. Nucl. Med. **16**:666-668, 1975.
49. Lesniak, M. A., Roth, J., Gorden, P., et al.: Human growth hormone radioreceptor assay using cultured human lymphocytes, Nature (New Biology) **241**:20-22, Jan. 3, 1973.
50. Levine, R.: Mechanisms of insulin secretion, N. Engl. J. Med. **283**:522-526, Sept. 3, 1970.

51. Liddle, G., and Melmon, K. L.: The adrenal cortex. In Williams, R. H., editor: Textbook of endocrinology, Philadelphia, 1974, W. B. Saunders Co.
52. Marion, M. A., Ronai, P. M., Pain, R. W., and Wise, P. H.: Simultaneous assessment of thyroid structure and function with the gamma camera using pertechnetate, Aust. N. Z. J. Med. **4:**379-384, Aug. 1974.
53. Mincey, E. K., Thorson, S. C., Brown, J. L., et al.: A new parameter of thyroid function—the effective thyroxine ratio, J. Nucl. Med. **13:**165-168, Feb. 1972.
54. MIRD: Dose estimate report No. 5, J. Nucl. Med. **16:**857, 1975.
55. Mitchell, M. L., Byrne, M. J., Sanchez, Y., and Sawin, C. T.: Detection of growth-hormone deficiency, N. Engl. J. Med. **282:**539-541, 1970.
56. Morita, R., Liebermen, L. M., Beierwaltes, W. H., et al.: Percent uptake of 131-I radioactivity in the adrenal from radioiodinated cholesterol, J. Clin. Endocrinol. Metab. **34:**36-43, 1972.
57. Nofal, M. M., Beierwaltes, W. H., and Patno, M. E.: Treatment of hyperthyroidism with sodium iodide I-131, J.A.M.A. **197:** 605, 1966.
58. Odell, W. D.: Growth hormone (GH). In Nichols, A. L., and Fisher, D. A., editors: Radioimmunoassay manual, ed. 3, San Pedro, Calif., 1977, Nichols Institute.
59. Odell, W. D., and Daughaday, W., editors: Principles of competitive protein-binding assays, Philadelphia, 1971, J. B. Lippincott Co.
60. Odell, W. D., Wilber, J. F., and Paul, W. E.: Radioimmunoassay of human thyrotropin in serum, J. Clin. Endocrinol. Metab. **14:**465-467, 1965.
61. Oppenheimer, J. H.: Initiation of thyroid-hormone action, N. Engl. J. Med. **292:**1068-1073, 1975.
62. Pittman, C. S., Chambers, J. B., Jr., and Read, V. H.: The extrathyroidal conversion rate of thyroxine to triiodothyronine in normal man, J. Clin. Invest. **50:**1186-1196, June 1971.
63. Pochin, E. E.: Radioiodine therapy of thyroid cancer, Semin. Nucl. Med. **2:**503, 1971.
64. Potchen, E. J., Watts, H. G., and Awwad, H. K.: Parathyroid scintiscanning, Radiol. Clin. N. Am. **5:**267-275, 1967.
65. Quaife, M. A., and Kotlyarov, E. V.: Unpublished work performed at University of Nebraska Medical Center, Omaha, 1978.
66. Quinn, J. L., III, and Henkin, R. E.: Scanning techniques to assess thyroid nodules, Annu. Rev. Med. **26:**193-201, 1975.
67. Rawson, R. W., Marinelli, L. D., Skanse, B. N., Trunnell, J., and Fluharty, R. G.: The effect of total thyroidectomy on the function of thyroid cancer, J. Clin. Endocrinol. Metab. **8:**826, 1948.
68. Rizza, R., Wahner, H., Spelsbert, T., Northcutt, R., and Moses, H.: Visualization of nonfunctioning adrenal adenomas with iodocholesterol: possible relationship to subcellular distribution of tracer, J. Nucl. Med. **18:**600, 1977.
69. Rothfeld, B., editor: Nuclear medicine in vitro, Philadelphia, 1974, J. B. Lippincott Co.
70. Russel, K. P., Rose, H., and Starr, P.: The effects of radioactive iodine on maternal and fetal thyroid function during pregnancy, Surg. Gynecol. Obstet. **104:**560, 1957.
71. Saenger, E. L., et al.: Evaluation of diseases of the thyroid gland with the in vivo use of radionuclides, J. Nucl. Med. **19:**107-112, 1978.
72. Saenger, E. L., Thoma, G. E., and Tompkins, E. A.: Incidence of leukemia following treatment of hyperthyroidism: preliminary report of the cooperative thyrotoxicosis therapy follow-up study, J.A.M.A. **205:**855-862, Sept. 16, 1968.
73. Sarkar, S. D., Beierwaltes, W. H., Ice, R. D., et al.: A new and superior adrenal scanning agent, NP-59, J. Nucl. Med. **16:**1038-1042, 1975.
74. Shafer, R. B., and Nuttal, F. Q.: Thyroid crisis induced by radioactive iodine, J. Nucl. Med. **12:**262-264, May 1971.
75. Shenkman, L., Mitsuma, T., Suphavai, A., et al.: Triiodothyronine and thyroid-stimulating hormone response to thyrotropin-releasing hormone. A new test of thyroidal and pituitary reserve, Lancet **1:**111-112, Jan. 15, 1972.
76. Snyder, P. J., and Utiger, R. D.: Response to thyrotropin-releasing hormone (TSH) in normal man, J. Clin. Endocrinol. Metab. **34:**380-385, Feb. 1972.
77. Spencer, R., and Holroyd, A. M.: The value of ^{75}Se-selenomethionine scanning in solitary nodules of the thyroid gland, Br. J. Radiol. **47:**457-463, Aug. 1974.
78. Sterling, K., and Hoffenberg, R.: Beta blocking agents and antithyroid drugs as adjuncts to radioiodine therapy, Semin. Nucl. Med. **1:**422, 1971.
79. Sterling, K., and Milch, P. O.: Thyroid hormone binding by a component of mitochondrial membrane, Proc. Natl. Acad. Sci. U.S.A. **72:**3225-3229, 1975.
80. Strauss, H. W., Hurley, P. J., and Wagner, H. N., Jr.: Advantages of ^{99m}Tc pertechnetate for thyroid scanning in patients with decreased radioiodine uptake, Radiology **97:**307-310, Nov. 1970.
81. Surks, M. I., Schadlow, A. R., Stock, J. M., et al.: Determination of iodothyronine absorption and conversion of L-thyroxine (T_4) to L-triiodothyronine (T_3) using turnover rate techniques, J. Clin. Invest. **52:**805-811, April 1973.
82. Tashjian, A. H., Howland, B. G., et al.: Immunoassay of human calcitonin, N. Engl. J. Med. **283:**890, 1970.
83. Thomas, C. G., Pepper, F. D., and Owen, J.: Differentiation of malignant from benign lesions of the thyroid gland using complementary scanning with ^{75}selenomethione and radioiodide, Ann. Surg. **170:**396-408, Sept. 1969.
84. Thomas, F. J., Lloyd, H. M., and Thomas, M. J.: Radioimmunoassay of human growth hormone: technique and application to plasma, cerebrospinal fluid, and pituitary extracts, J. Clin. Pathol. **25:**774-782, 1972.
85. Tompkins, E. A.: Late effects of radioiodide therapy. In Cloutier, R. J., Edwards, C. L., and Snyder, P. J.: Medical radionuclides: radiation dose and effects, AEC Symposium Ser. **20:**431-440, 1970.
86. Unger, R. H.: Circulating pancreatic glucagon and extra-pancreatic glucagon-like materials. In Steiner, D. F., and Freinkel, N.: Handbook of physiology. I. Endocrinology, Washington, D.C., 1972, American Physiologic Society.
87. Utiger, R. D.: Radioimmunoassay of human plasma thyrotropin, J. Clin. Invest. **44:**1277-1286, Aug. 1965.
88. Varma, V. M., Beierwaltes, W. H., Nofal, M. M., Nishiyama, H., and Copp, J. E.: Treatment of thyroid cancer—death rates after surgery followed by sodium iodide I-131, J.A.M.A. **214:** 1439, 1970.
89. von Schuching, S., and Wellman, H. N.: Development and initial evaluation of 123-iodine labeled 6β-iodomethyl-19-norcholester-5(10)-3β-ol (NP-59) for adrenal scintiimaging, J. Nucl. Med. **18:**600, 1977.
90. Wellman, H. N., and Anger, R. T., Jr.: Properties, production, and clinical uses of radioisotopes of iodine, CRC Crit. Rev. Clin. Radiol. Nucl. Med. **6**(1):81-111, Feb. 1975.
91. Werner, S. C., and Spooner, M.: A new and simple test for hyperthyroidism employing L-triiodothyronine and the twenty-four hour ^{131}I uptake method, Bull. N.Y. Acad. Med. **31:**137-145, 1945.
92. Yalow, R. S., and Berson, S. A.: Assay of plasma insulin in human subjects by immunological methods, Nature **184**(suppl. 21):1648-1649, 1959.
93. Yalow, R. S., and Berson, S. A.: Introduction and general considerations. In Odell, W. D., and Daughaday, W. D., editors, Principles of competitive protein-binding assays, Philadelphia, 1971, J. B. Lippincott Co.

Chapter 10

THE RESPIRATORY SYSTEM

David J. Phegley and Roger H. Secker-Walker

Regional ventilation was first studied by Knipping and his colleagues, using radioactive xenon, more than 20 years ago.[21] Much of our present understanding of regional lung function, both in health and in disease, is based on the use of this gas and other radionuclides by respiratory physiologists working in London, and Montreal.[5,39] During this time considerable advances were also made in understanding the detailed anatomy of the lung[41] and in appreciating the mechanical interrelationships of airways, alveoli, and the thoracic cage.[23] Nonrespiratory functions have also been studied, particularly those dealing with lung defense mechanisms[15] and the metabolic activity of the lung.[12]

The development of macroaggregated albumin, at first labeled with iodine 131[35] and later with technetium 99m, led to the widespread use of perfusion scanning for the diagnosis of pulmonary embolism. The use of radioactive xenon to study regional ventilation has spread from the research laboratory to routine use in the last 5 years. This combined insight into regional ventilation and regional blood flow allows more accurate assessment of the disturbed physiology and, at the same time, increases both the diagnostic sensitivity and specificity of the procedure.[1,24]

NORMAL ANATOMY AND PHYSIOLOGY

The lungs lie within the thorax, protected by the rib cage. The ribs offer support to the intercostal muscles and the diaphragm. It is the action of these muscles that enlarges the chest during normal breathing (Fig. 10-1).

Air enters the lungs, first passing through the nose or mouth and then the pharynx, the larynx, and the trachea (Fig. 10-2). It is warmed, moistened, and filtered during this time. The trachea divides into right and left main-stem bronchi and these in turn divide into lobar bronchi (upper, middle, and lower on the right, and upper and lower on the left). The airways continue to divide in a somewhat irregular fashion, about 16 times from the trachea to the terminal bronchioles and a further four to seven times, as respiratory bronchioles, alveolar ducts, and alveolar sacs (Fig. 10-3). Bronchi have cartilage in their walls, which distinguishes them from bronchioles. Smooth muscle, collagen, and elastic fibers encircle the airways from the trachea to the alveolar ducts. The collagen and elastic fibers continue to the periphery of the lung as a three-dimensional lattice work in the walls of the alveoli. Alveoli first appear in the respiratory bronchioles but are most numerous around the alveolar sacs.

The alveoli are packed together like the cells of a honeycomb (Fig. 10-4). Each alveolus offers some support to its neighbors, and through the collagen and elastic fibers to the airways as well. This structural arrangement and the surfactant, which lines the surface of the alveoli, are responsible for the elastic properties of the lungs and provide the main force for expiration during normal breathing.

The bronchial epithelium is lined by ciliated cells interspersed with a few goblet cells and the openings of bronchial glands.[6] The alveoli, where oxygen and carbon dioxide are exchanged, are lined by alveolar type I cells. These are very thin and spread over the surface of the alveoli. Pulmonary capillaries lie in contact with these cells (Fig. 10-4). Two other important cells are found in the alveoli—alveolar type II cells, which are believed to make surfactant, and alveolar macrophages, which remove particulate matter that reaches the alveoli.

The pulmonary artery divides to form the right and left pulmonary arteries. These vessels follow the bronchi and bronchioles, dividing with them till they reach the alveoli (Fig. 10-2). Each alveolus, and there are about 250 to 300 million in an adult, is supplied by a terminal pulmonary arteriole, which has a diameter of about 35 μm and which gives rise to about 1000 capillaries per alveolus. The capillaries are 7 to 10 μm in diameter. The distance between the alveolar surface and the capillaries is only about 0.05 to 0.1 μm. The pulmonary capillaries drain into the pulmonary veins and thence into the left atrium.[41]

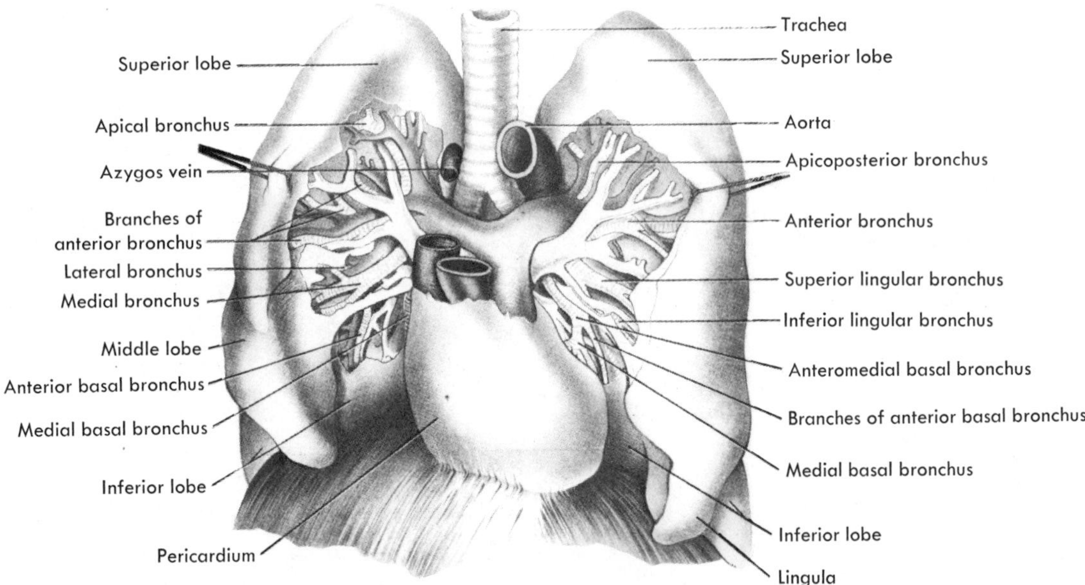

Fig. 10-1. Anatomic diagram showing relationships of heart, pulmonary vessels, airways, and lungs. (From Wyburn, G. M.: The respiratory system. In Romanes, G. J., editor: Cunningham's textbook of anatomy, London, 1972, Oxford University Press, p. 495.)

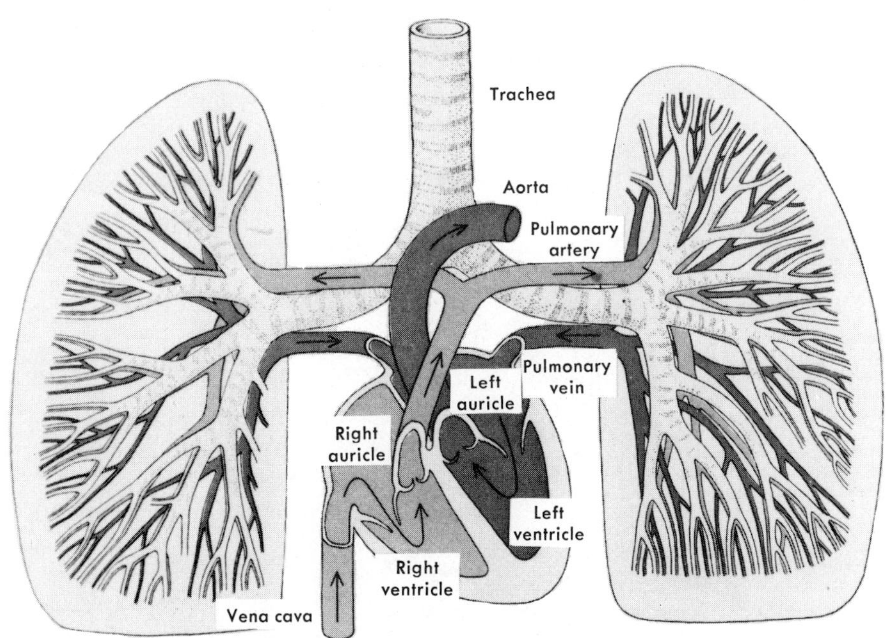

Fig. 10-2. Schematic diagram of pulmonary circulation and airways. (From Hammond, E. C.: The effects of smoking, Sci. Am. **39:**207, 1962. Copyright © 1962 by Scientific American, Inc. All rights reserved.)

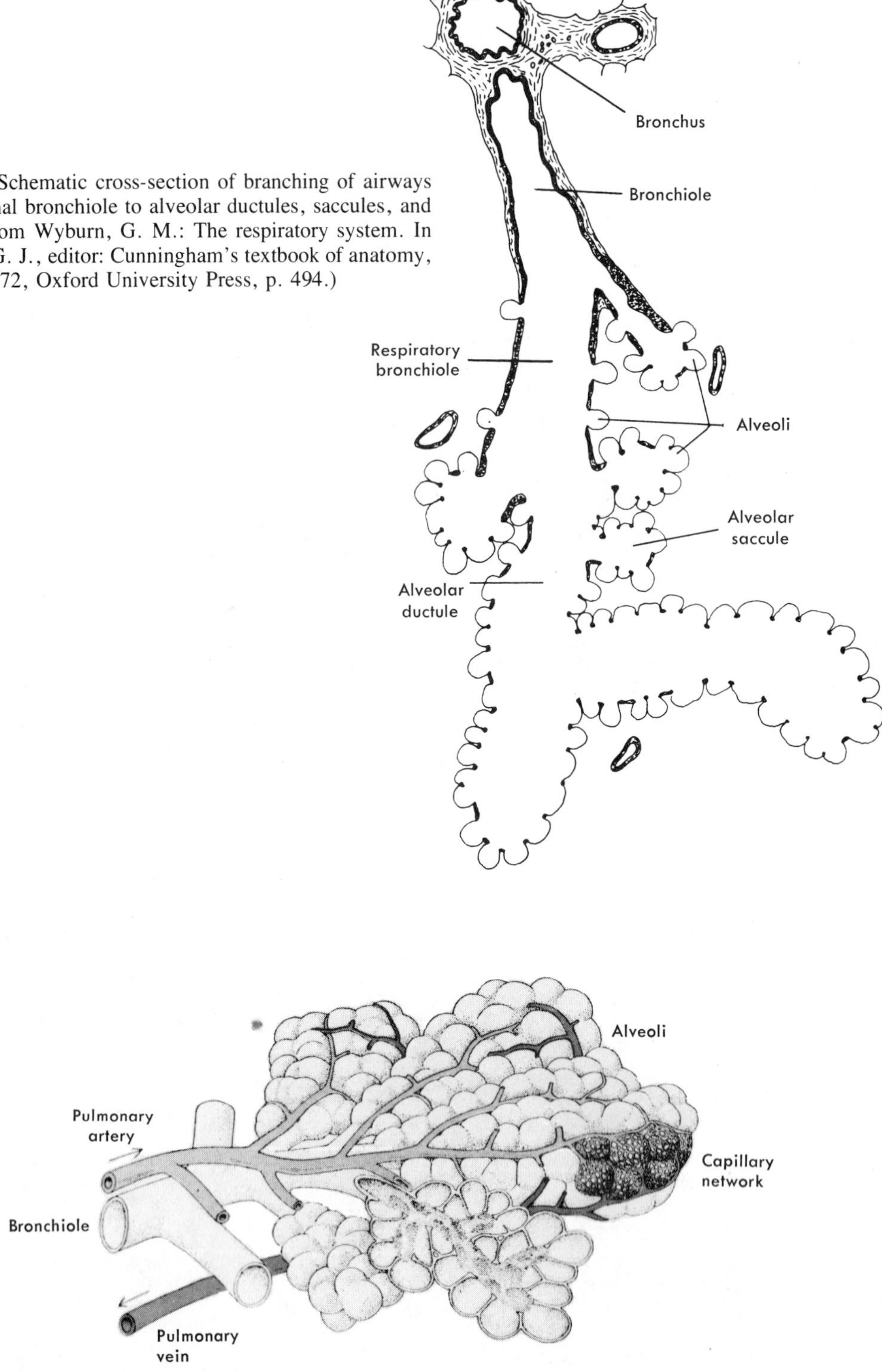

Fig. 10-3. Schematic cross-section of branching of airways from terminal bronchiole to alveolar ductules, saccules, and alveoli. (From Wyburn, G. M.: The respiratory system. In Romanes, G. J., editor: Cunningham's textbook of anatomy, London, 1972, Oxford University Press, p. 494.)

Fig. 10-4. Schematic drawing of peripheral airways and alveoli and their accompanying blood vessels. Bronchial circulation is not shown. (From Hammond, E. C.: The effects of smoking, Sci. Am. **39:**207, 1962. Copyright © 1962 by Scientific American, Inc. All rights reserved.)

The lungs also receive blood from the aorta, through the bronchial arteries. These are small, but also follow the bronchial tree as far as the respiratory bronchioles. They supply nourishment to the bronchi, surrounding blood vessels, nerves, and lymphatics. Anastomoses are formed between the bronchial and pulmonary circulations at the capillary level around the respiratory bronchioles. Most of the blood from the bronchial circulation drains into the left atrium through the pulmonary veins.[10]

The lungs are richly supplied with lymphatics. Some course over the pleura and pass into the lungs, whereas others arise in the interstitial spaces of the lungs. Lymphatic vessels travel toward the hilum of the lung, with airways and the blood vessels, reaching lymph nodes there and then continuing into the mediastinum.

The volume of air breathed out in a normal breath is called the "tidal volume," and the volume of air in the lungs at the end of a normal breath is called "functional residual capacity." "Total lung capacity" is the volume of air in the lungs when as much air has been inhaled as possible, whereas "residual volume" is the volume of air left in the lungs after a complete exhalation (Fig. 10-5). These volumes are measured by standard pulmonary function tests.[40]

During tidal breathing only a small porportion (about 10% to 15%) of the air within the lungs is exchanged with each breath. More will be exchanged with deeper breaths or a faster rate of breathing. About one third

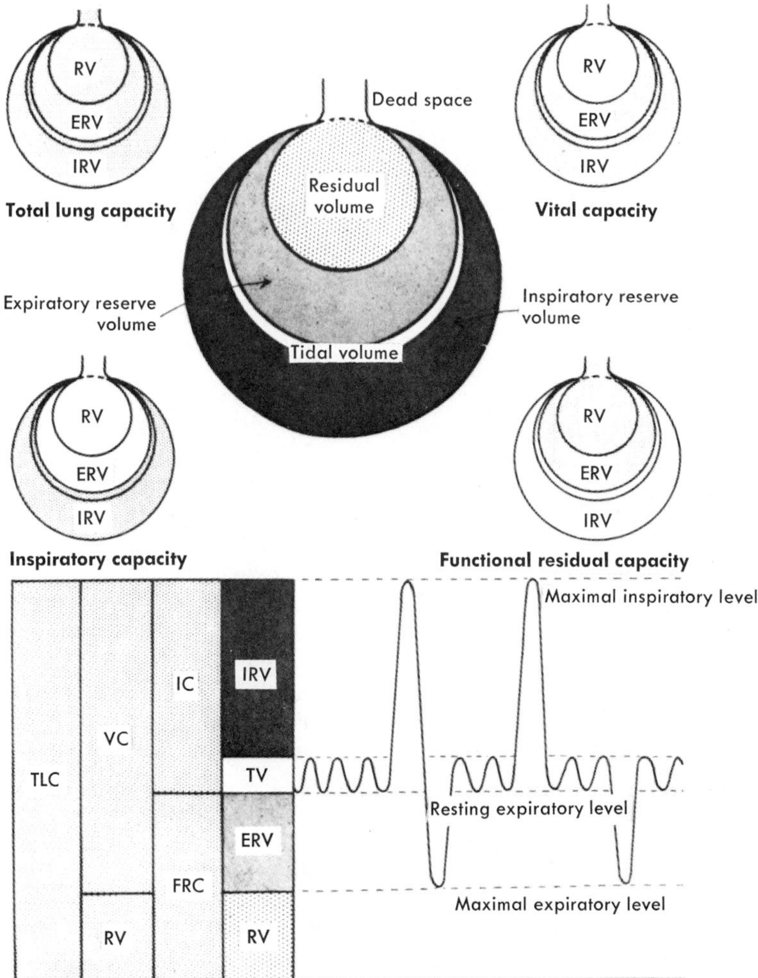

Fig. 10-5. Static lung volumes. Graphic tracing shows the volumes that can be measured by spirometry. (From Comroe, J. H., Jr., et al.: Lung volumes. In Comroe, J. H., et al., editors: The lung, Chicago, 1962, Year Book Medical Publishers, Inc., p. 8.)

of each breath is wasted because the air in the bronchial tubes, at the end of the breath, does not reach the alveoli. This is called ''anatomic dead space,'' because it takes no part in gas exchange.

The structure of the lung is well suited to its chief function of gas exchange, that is, delivering oxygen to the bloodstream and removing carbon dioxide, so that the body's cellular metabolism may continue.

Despite the numerous divisions of the bronchial tree, the resistance to air flow is low. Most of this resistance (80% to 90%) is found in the larger bronchial tubes where air flow is turbulent. It requires only small pressure changes within the chest for normal breathing. The change in volume for a change in pressure is called ''compliance,'' which is thus a measurement of the ease with which air enters or leaves the lungs.

The pressure in the pulmonary artery is considerably lower than that in the systemic circulation and there is very little resistance to blood flow. The entire cardiac output passes through the pulmonary capillaries, in an almost continuous sheet, in the alveolar walls.

These thin walls, which have a surface area of 70 to 80 square meters, offer an almost negligible barrier to the diffusion of gases from alveoli to blood or vice versa.

As the lung ages, its elastic properties diminish and the smaller bronchial tubes tend to collapse during a full expiration. The volume of air in the lungs when closure begins is called ''closing capacity.'' Both radioactive xenon and nonradioactive tracer gases, for example, nitrogen, helium, or argon, have been used to measure this volume. Early damage to the small airways from any cause increases this volume, an increase that is therefore a sensitive, but nonspecific, indication of small-airways disease.[2,7]

In the 1960s it was shown that both ventilation and blood flow are not evenly distributed within the lungs. Posture and the direction of gravity or of acceleration play an important part in healthy lungs.

In the upright position ventilation of the upper parts of the lung increases about 1.5 to 2 times over that of the lower parts.[5,20,39] In the supine position the distribution is more uniform from top to bottom, but there is then a gradient from front to back! If a person lies on one side, more air is exchanged in the lower part of the lung compared to the upper part. The distribution is modified by exercise, the rate of breathing, and diseases affecting the bronchial tubes or the lung parenchyma. These are discussed later.

In the upright position blood flow increases threefold to fivefold from the upper parts of the lung to the base. In fact the upper one fourth of the lungs gets very little blood flow at rest during upright sitting.[3,39] In the supine position blood flow is more uniform from apex to base, but then a gradient exists from front to back. Lying on one side will cause more blood to flow to the lowermost part of the lung. Apart from the disease states that usually alter blood flow within the lung, exercise will cause a more even distribution. Lowering the oxygen tension in the bronchial tubes also alters blood flow by causing local constriction of the pulmonary arterioles and diverting blood flow away from this region.

The distribution of blood flow within the upright lung shows the largest gradient from top to bottom when the measurements are made at total lung capacity. At functional residual capacity, blood flow increases from the apex to about the level of the fourth or fifth rib and then decreases a little toward the base. If the distribution of blood flow is measured at residual volume, it is almost even throughout the lungs.[19]

The ratio in which ventilation and blood flow are mixed is not uniform from top to bottom in the upright position. Ventilation exceeds blood flow by about 2:1 to 3:1 in the upper zones. In the midzones they are more closely matched, whereas in the lower parts of the lung blood flow exceeds ventilation. The closer the matching of ventilation and blood flow, the better is the oxygenation of the blood. Whenever ventilation is reduced in comparison to blood flow, the oxygenation of the blood is also reduced. If ventilation exceeds blood flow, the red cells will quickly take up their maximum load of oxygen (4 molecules per hemoglobin molecule, or 1.34 ml of O_2 per gram of hemoglobin) and the excess ventilation is then wasted.[40]

PATHOPHYSIOLOGY

The distribution of blood flow within the lungs is altered by many disease processes affecting either the lungs, the heart, the chest wall, or the diaphragm. The mechanisms underlying these disturbances are outlined schematically in Fig. 10-6. Fig. 10-6, *A* to *C* represent disease processes affecting the pulmonary vasculature. The most obvious cause, represented by *A*, is pulmonary embolism, in which the embolus (usually a small blood clot) blocks one of the branches of the pulmonary artery so that no blood can flow past this obstruction. The defect produced on the perfusion scan corresponds to the anatomic segment or lobe of the lung involved.

Other causes of defects in blood flow from disease processes affecting the pulmonary vessels are shown in Fig. 10-6, *B* and *C*. *B* represents enlarged lymph nodes at the hilum of the lung, as might be seen in advanced lung cancer, causing compression of the pulmonary vessels and hence alterations in blood flow. *C* represents disease processes involving the smaller pulmonary arterioles, for example, a vasculitis or multiple small pulmonary emboli.

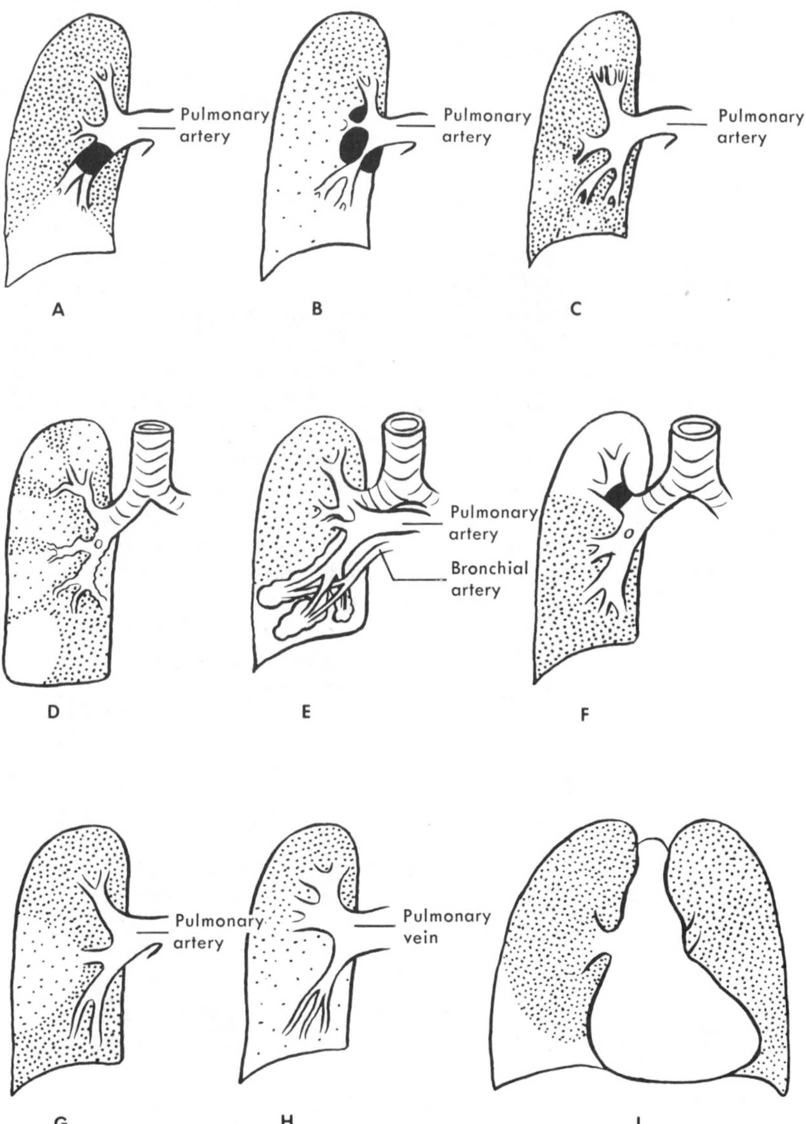

Fig. 10-6. Schematic representation of major mechanisms of abnormal perfusion scans. See text. *Spotted areas,* Blood flow; *clear areas,* regions with absent blood flow.

D to *F* in Fig. 10-6 represent diseases in which the initial problem is in the airways (or bronchial tubes) and blood flow is reduced as a result of the diminution in ventilation. *D* is a composite diagram to represent the changes seen in chronic bronchitis, emphysema, and asthma. *E* represents bronchiectasis in which there is dilatation of the peripheral bronchi and surrounding inflammation. The bronchial arteries to the affected region are often much enlarged. There is virtually no blood flow through the pulmonary artery and very little exchange of air in the bronchiectatic segment. *F* represents obstruction of a bronchus by tumor or foreign body. Blood flow is reduced in part by the local hypoxia.

G to *I* in Fig. 10-6 represent miscellaneous conditions. In *G*, the lung parenchyma is filled with inflammatory exudate as is seen in pneumonia, or blood as is seen in a pulmonary infarct. Blood flow is much reduced and there is no ventilation of the affected region. *H* represents the interesting phenomenon of a reversal of the normal gradient of blood flow. This is seen when there is elevation of the pressure in the left atrium, for example, in mitral stenosis or left ventricular failure. *I* represents the situation when there is a pleural effusion or a large heart compressing lung tissue and hence reducing blood flow in that region.

The mechanisms responsible for the disturbances in ventilation are shown in Fig. 10-7. Fig. 10-7, *A*, represents diseases that cause obstruction to air flow by narrowing or distortion of the airways. In chronic bronchitis there is excess mucus production and some inflammatory swelling of the bronchial walls. Both processes narrow the lumen of the airways, usually in an irregular fashion, producing variable patterns of airways obstruction.

In emphysema the main damage is in the alveoli, which are steadily destroyed, losing surface area and capillaries. The small airways are not properly supported, become kinked and distorted, and collapse readily on expiration. All this leads to inefficient exchange of air. Chronic bronchitis and emphysema are usually found together because both diseases are caused, for the most part, by cigarette smoking.

In bronchial asthma there is spasm of the bronchial smooth muscle, which causes narrowing of the airways and increased mucus production and edema of the bronchila mucosa. Severe abnormalities of ventilation and blood flow may be seen.

Fig. 10-7, *B*, represents bronchiectasis. Little or no air exchange takes place in the dilated bronchi, which are often the seat of chronic infection.

Fig. 10-7, *C*, represents narrowing or complete obstruction of a bronchus because of a tumor or foreign body. The worse the obstruction, the more obvious is the abnormality in ventilation. If the obstruction is in a lobar bronchus, the affected lobe of the lung will collapse as its lumen closes off. If the obstruction is in a segmental, or smaller bronchus, collateral ventilation through the pores of Kohn can prevent complete collapse by allowing air to enter the segment from a neighboring segment.

Fig. 10-7, *D*, represents the situation in pneumonia or pulmonary infarction, when the alveoli are filled with exudate or blood and hence will not exchange any air.

Fig. 10-7, *E*, represents pleural fluid or a large heart, both of which occupy lung volume and hence reduce ventilation.

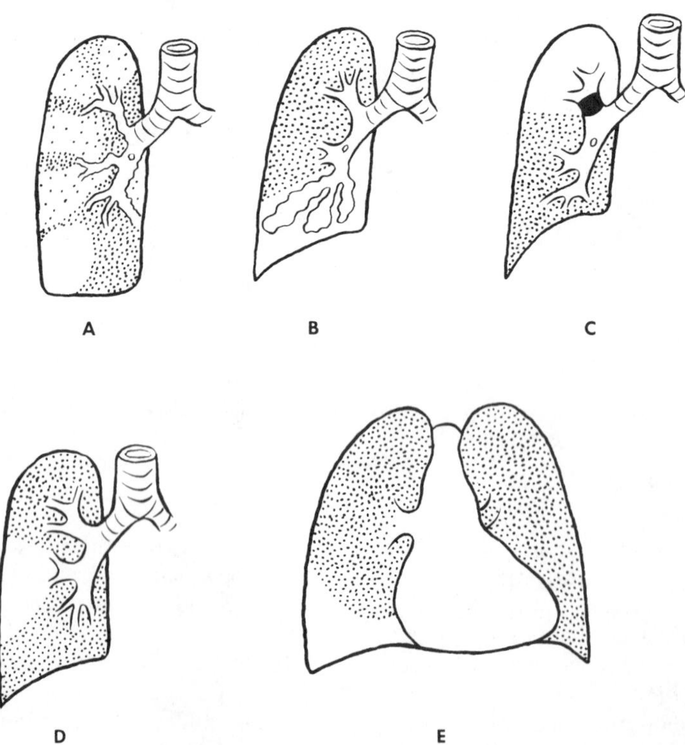

Fig. 10-7. Schematic representation of major mechanisms of abnormal ventilation studies. See text. *Spotted areas,* Ventilation; *clear areas,* regions of abnormal ventilation.

PERFUSION SCANS

The distribution of pulmonary arterial blood flow is usually demonstrated by the intravenous injection of radioactive particles. The method was shown to be effective by Haynie and his colleagues, who injected labeled ceramic microspheres into dogs.[17] The development of macroaggregated albumin (MAA), labeled with ^{131}I, by Taplin et al.[35] and Wagner et al.[38] in 1964 led to the first successful lung scans in human beings. Table 10-1 lists some of the radiopharmaceuticals that have been used for perfusion scans, along with their physical and biologic properties.

After intravenous injection the particles, which measure 30 to 40 μm in diameter, pass through the right atrium and right ventricle, where they are well mixed with blood, and then into the pulmonary artery. They pass out into the blood vessels of the lung until they become impacted in the terminal arterioles and capillaries because they are too large to pass through them. The usual diameter of human albumin microspheres corresponds to the size of the smallest pulmonary arterioles. The distribution of particles has been shown experimentally to be closely related to the distribution of pulmonary arterial blood flow,[27] by comparison of their relative distribution to the uptake of oxygen by each lung and also by comparison of the distribution of particles to that of labeled red blood cells.[37] A normal perfusion scan is shown in Fig. 10-9.

It is to be understood that the distribution is that which exists at the time of injection.

Macroaggregated albumin, human albumin microspheres, and other particles break up and pass through the pulmonary capillaries and are removed from the circulation in the liver and spleen. These particles have variable biologic half-lives in the lung, as shown in Table 10-1, which depend not only on the nature of the particles but also, to some extent, on the underlying disease processes. Clearance is delayed in chronic lung disease and heart failure.

With the usual dose of particulate material of the appropriate size, fewer than 1 in 1000 pulmonary arterioles are blocked.[16,35] No abnormalities of pulmonary function can be demonstrated after such an injection.[13,28]

Perfusion scanning has a reputation for great safety, but special care should be taken in patients known to have severe pulmonary hypertension because their available vascular bed is reduced in diameter.[9] Special care should also be taken in patients with right-to-left shunts,[26] because the particles will pass through to the systemic circulation and embolize to the brain, kidneys, heart, and other organs. Half the usual dose should be given to patients who have had a pneumonectomy.

Radioactive xenon dissolved in saline solution is occasionally used to demonstrate the distribution of blood flow. It is given intravenously, and because the gas is relatively insoluble, it comes out of solution as it reaches the air contained in the alveoli. Its distribution can be measured during breath holding and corresponds to pulmonary capillary blood flow. Regions of the lung that are collapsed or consolidated, as in pneumonia, will appear to have no blood flow because the alveoli contain no air. Krypton 81m may also be infused intravenously, and images of capillary blood flow can be made in any projection during natural breathing. Krypton 81m has the advantage that rapid changes can be followed.[11]

VENTILATION STUDIES

Table 10-2 shows some of the radioactive gases that are used to study regional ventilation. Xenon 133 has been used for quasi-static measurements of regional ventilation and blood flow, for dynamic measurements of regional ventilation, for measurements of regional lung volumes, for closing volume, and for studying factors that influence the distribution of a single breath.

Clinical studies of regional ventilation are usually done with xenon 133 although xenon 127 is becoming more readily available and has the advantage of a more energetic gamma emission.[4] Techniques for ventilation

Table 10-1. Radiopharmaceuticals used for perfusion lung imaging

	Agent	
	Technetium-99m macroaggregated albumin	**Technetium-99m albumin microspheres**
Dosage	2 to 4 mCi	2 to 4 mCi
Physical half-life	6 hours	6 hours
Biologic half-life	2 to 9 hours	7 hours
Principal gamma energy	140 keV	140 keV
Particle size	5 to 100 μm	20 to 40 μm
Radiation absorbed dose per millicurie in lungs	260 mrad	290 mrad

Table 10-2. Radiopharmaceuticals used for ventilation lung imaging

	Agent		
	Xenon 133	**Xenon 127**	**Krypton 81m**
Physical half-life	5.3 days	36.4 days	13 seconds
Biologic half-life	30 seconds	30 seconds	30 seconds
Principal gamma energy	80 keV	203 keV	190 keV
Particle size	Gaseous	Gaseous	Gaseous
Radiation absorbed dose per millicurie in lungs	12 mrad*	17 mrad*	7.5 mrad*

*The radiation absorbed dose has been estimated with a rebreathing time of 3 minutes being assumed.

studies are not yet standardized, but three aspects of ventilation are often examined: (1) the distribution of a single breath, (2) the distribution of lung volume, and (3) the distribution of the efficiency of ventilation from the clearance of radioactive xenon. Single-breath studies show the distribution of a bolus of radioactive xenon inhaled, with air, to total lung capacity—a somewhat unphysiologic situation. If the tracer gas is rebreathed to equilibrium, that is, until the concentration of xenon in the lungs and in the rebreathing system is constant, the distribution of xenon within the lungs corresponds to lung volume.

Measurements made during a washin of xenon to equilibrium reflect the efficiency of ventilation—the faster a region reaches equilibrium, the better its ventilation and vice versa. When air is breathed after a washin, the subsequent washout provides excellent evidence of the regional variations in ventilation. The best ventilated regions clear fastest, and the poorly ventilated ones stand out by contrast, as regions where the clearance of radioactivity is delayed.

Single-breath studies require considerable patient cooperation, whereas washin and washout studies can be done in virtually any circumstance from infancy to old age. Simple washin-washout studies have been found perfectly satisfactory in clinical practice[31] (Figs. 10-8 to 10-10).

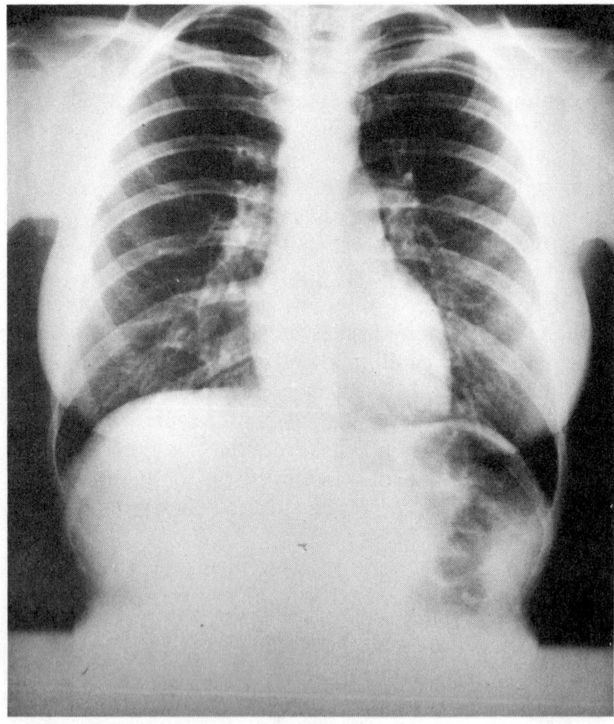

Fig. 10-8. Normal chest radiograph of healthy woman aged 23.

Krypton 81m is being used in a few centers. This gas has such a short half-life that when inhaled continuously during normal tidal breathing, an equilibrium count rate that is proportional to ventilation is reached. This means that images can be made in the same projections used for perfusion scanning and are directly comparable. Images made in this way show the distribution of regional ventilation, whereas images made with ^{99m}Tc–human albumin microspheres shows the distribution of regional blood flow. Visual comparisons of the matching of ventilation and blood flow are thus considerably easier with krypton 81m than with radioactive xenon[11,14] (Figs. 10-11 and 10-12).

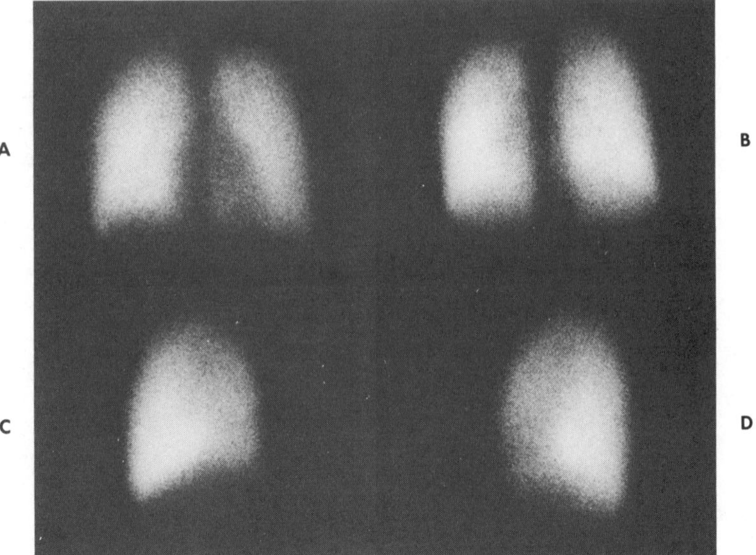

Fig. 10-9. Normal four-view perfusion scan of woman in Fig. 10-8. Injection was given with her seated upright. Images here and in all subsequent perfusion scans are arranged as follows: *top left,* anterior; *top right,* posterior; *bottom left,* right lateral; *bottom right,* left lateral.

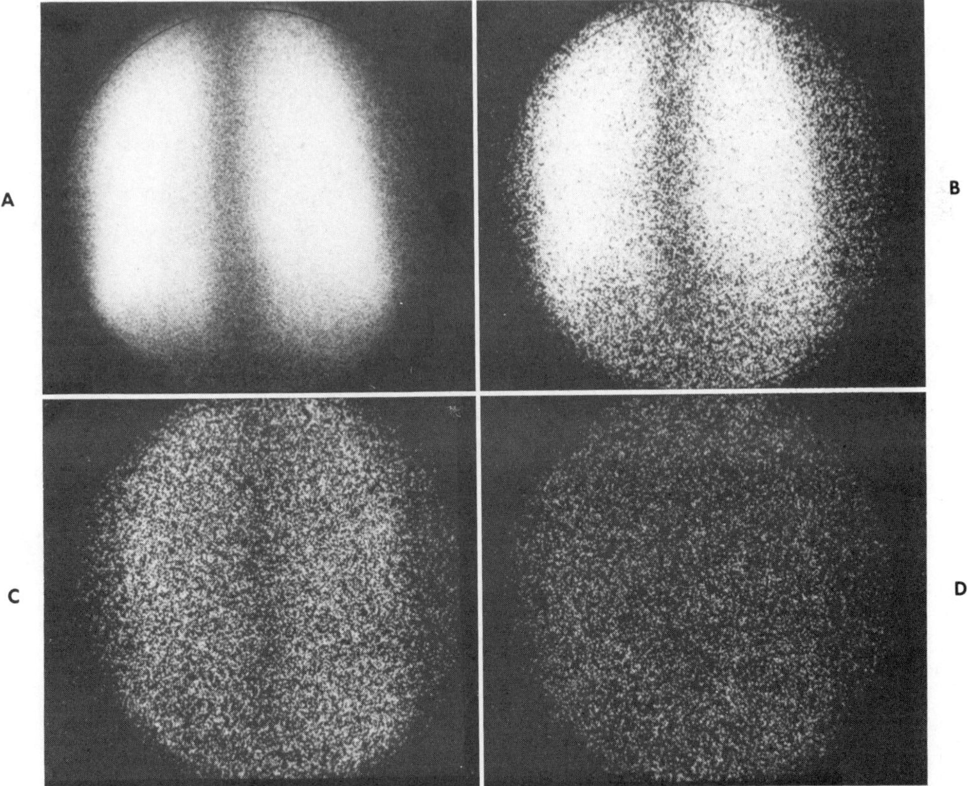

Fig. 10-10. Normal ventilation study of woman in Fig. 10-8. Images are arranged as follows: *top left,* washin; *top right,* washout at 0.5 minute; *bottom left,* washout at 1 minute; *bottom right,* washout at 3 minutes. All subsequent radioactive xenon images are arranged in this fashion. Different washout times are indicated. Note rapid clearance, with bases clearing slightly faster than regions elsewhere.

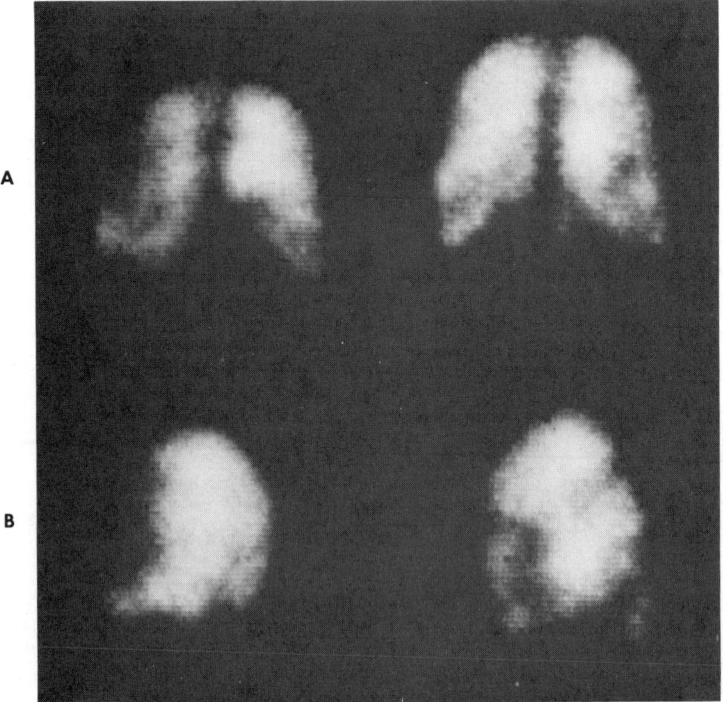

Fig. 10-11. Four-view krypton-81m ventilation study of a coal worker, aged 54. *Top left,* Anterior; *top right,* posterior; *bottom left,* right lateral; *bottom right,* left lateral. Numerous abnormalities in pattern of ventilation are visible in each view.

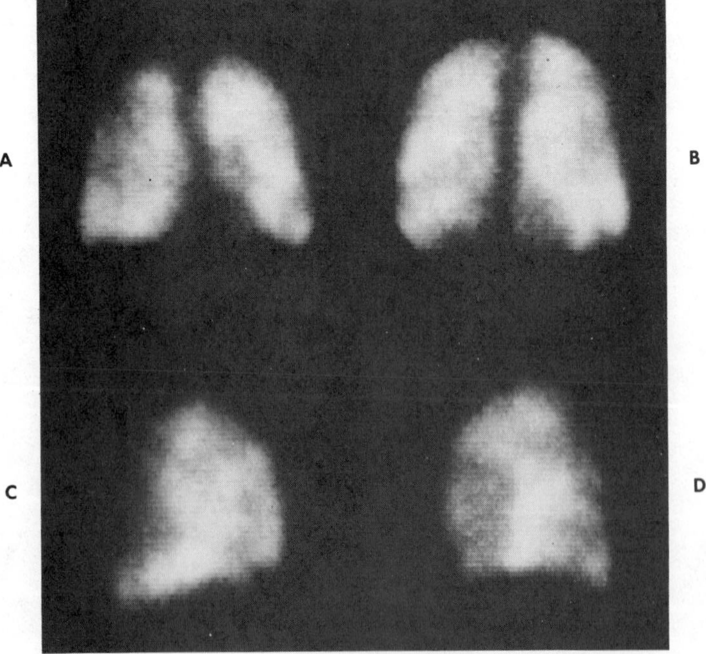

Fig. 10-12. Four-view ^{99m}Tc-HAM perfusion scan of coal worker in Fig. 10-11. Views are arranged in same way. Direct visual comparison of corresponding images shows that in several areas ventilation is worse than blood flow. These findings are consistent with chronic obstructive airway disease.

VENTILATION-PERFUSION STUDIES

By combining studies of ventilation and perfusion one can determine whether defects in blood flow are associated with defects in ventilation. The pulmonary diseases commonly met with in clinical nuclear medicine tend to fall into two categories: (1) Those with abnormal regional pulmonary blood flow, but normal (or almost normal) regional ventilation. Pulmonary embolism is by far the most important one of these, but early heart failure, interstitial lung diseases, some lung cancers and other abnormalities of the pulmonary vasculature may show this pattern. (2) Those with abnormal ventilation and abnormal blood flow. Here, the most common conditions are chronic bronchitis, emphysema, and asthma, with cystic fibrosis and bronchiectasis causing similar patterns. Cancers of the bronchus, other bronchial tumors, or foreign bodies obstructing a bronchus can all produce localized abnormalities of ventilation and blood flow. In general the disturbance of ventilation is more pronounced than that of blood flow and is detected as a regional delay in the clearance of xenon. When this delay is great, a corresponding defect is usually visible on the washin image as an area of diminished activity, where this part of the lung has not reached equilibrium with the tracer gas.

Pneumonias, pulmonary infarcts, and severe pulmonary edema are all associated with defects in the equilibrium images, which correspond to the infiltrates seen on the chest x-ray film. No retention of radioactive xenon is seen during the washout because no radioactive xenon can enter the fluid-filled alveoli.

Normal perfusion scans show an even gradation of activity, with more activity visible in the lower lobes than in that in the upper lobes, if the injection is given with the patient in the upright posture. The outline of the lungs and mediastinum corresponds closely to that seen on the chest x-ray film.

A normal washin image shows an even distribution of activity throughout the lungs, and a normal washout is usually complete within 3 to 4 minutes of breathing air. Occasionally the bases can be seen to clear a little faster than the upper zones do (Figs. 10-8 to 10-10).

Pulmonary embolism

In pulmonary embolism the defects in blood flow correspond to anatomic subdivisions of the lung, such as segments or lobes, in 75% of patients. The remaining 25% have ill-defined nonsegmental defects. If the patient had previously healthy lungs, ventilation is usually well maintained to the affected parts of the lung because their bronchial tubes are patent (Figs. 10-13 to 10-15). Only a small proportion (10% to

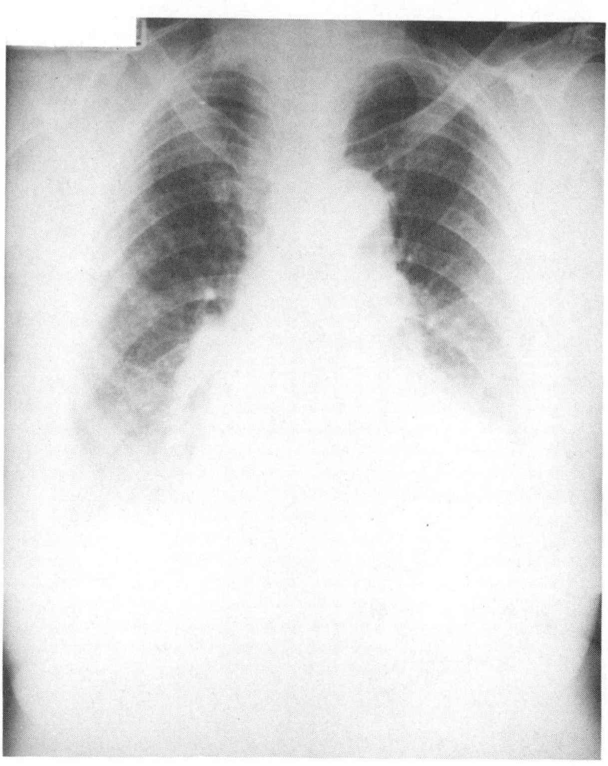

Fig. 10-13. Chest radiograph of 77-year-old lady with heart failure and pulmonary embolism. Heart is enlarged, and lung fields are congested.

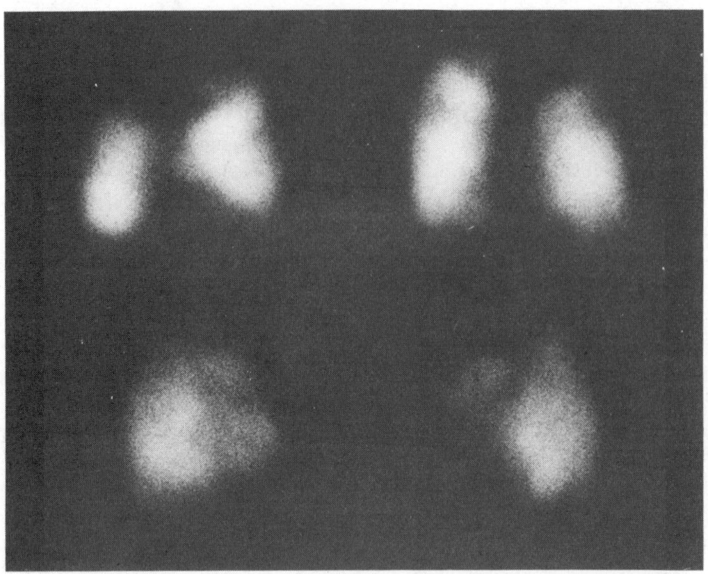

Fig. 10-14. Four-view perfusion scan showing segmental and subsegmental defects in blood flow in both lungs. Right upper lobe is most severely affected.

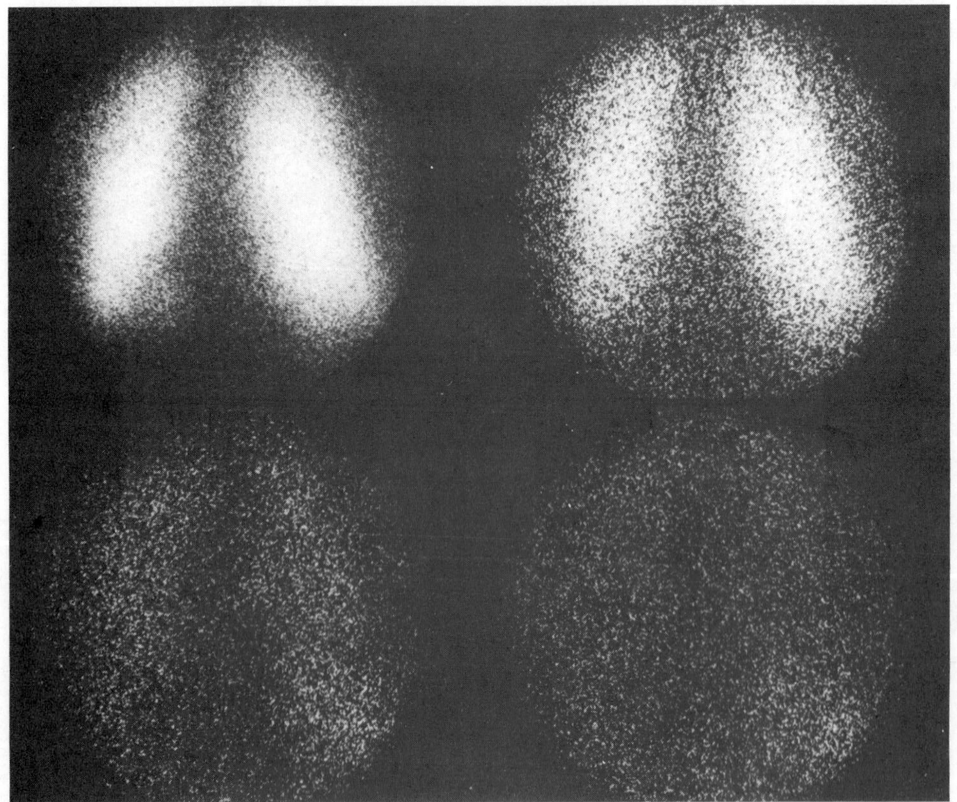

Fig. 10-15. Ventilation study. Washin; washout at 1, 2, and 4 minutes. Lungs fill evenly during washin, except for left base, where a defect caused by large heart is seen. Clearance is only minimally delayed from both lungs, except at right base. Combination of segmental and subsegmental defects in blood, with ventilation well preserved, is strong evidence for pulmonary embolism.

15%) of patients with emboli develop pulmonary infarction with its associated infiltrates seen in the chest x-ray film. Both the true-positive rate, or sensitivity, and the true-negative rate, or specificity, of ventilation-perfusion scanning are more than 90%.[1,24]

Interpretation is more difficult, and a little less reliable, when the patients already have chronic obstructive airway disease such as chronic bronchitis, emphysema, or asthma.

Most, but not all, pulmonary emboli are eventually lysed by the body's own fibrinolytic systems, so that defects in blood flow tend to disappear with time. Most improvement is seen in the first few days. Further improvement occurs rather more slowly over the following 3 to 4 weeks and may continue for several months.[34] Anticoagulant treatment is important and prevents the formation of new blood clots and the extension of those already present in the lungs.

Chronic obstructive airway disease

Radioactive xenon ventilation studies provide one of the most sensitive ways of detecting damage to the small airways.[36] Patients with chronic bronchitis and emphysema show an endless variety of defects in blood flow and ventilation. Eighty percent of the time the defects in blood flow cannot be strictly related to anatomic subdivisions of the lung. In general both lungs tend to be affected to a similar, though rarely identical, degree. In some patients most of the damage is in the lower zones, in others in the upper zones, and in yet others scattered throughout both lungs. It is by no means rare for one lung to be distinctly more severely affected than the other. See Figs. 10-16 to 10-21.

In chronic bronchitis, ventilation tends to be more severely affected than blood flow, and some changes in the pattern of ventilation and blood flow may be seen with exacerbations of this disease. In emphysema the defects in ventilation and blood flow correspond more closely and tend to be more stable from year to year.

Patients with bronchial asthma also show considerable changes in both ventilation and blood flow, with ventilation being more severely affected. Often the defects are recognizably segmental, or

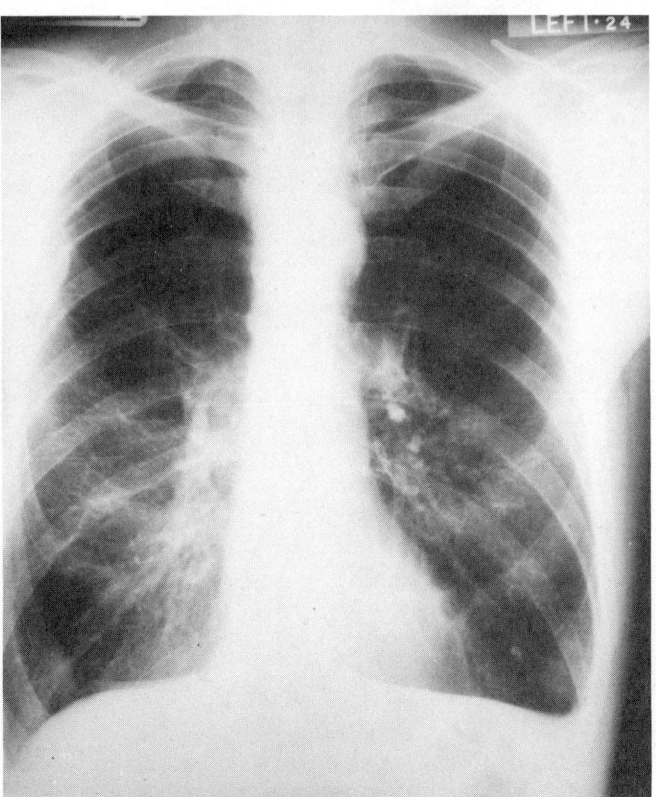

Fig. 10-16. Chest radiograph of 52-year-old man with severe emphysema. He has been a heavy cigarette smoker. He has large lungs and bullous areas in upper lobes.

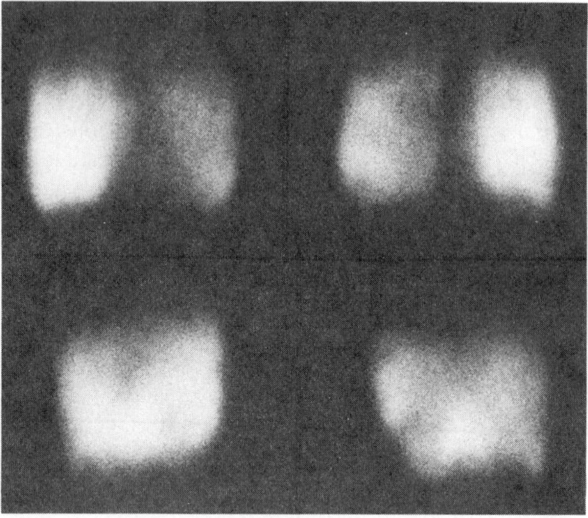

Fig. 10-17. Four-view perfusion scan showing absent perfusion in upper one third of each lung, with rather more blood flow to right lung. Irregular defects are visible in both lower lung fields.

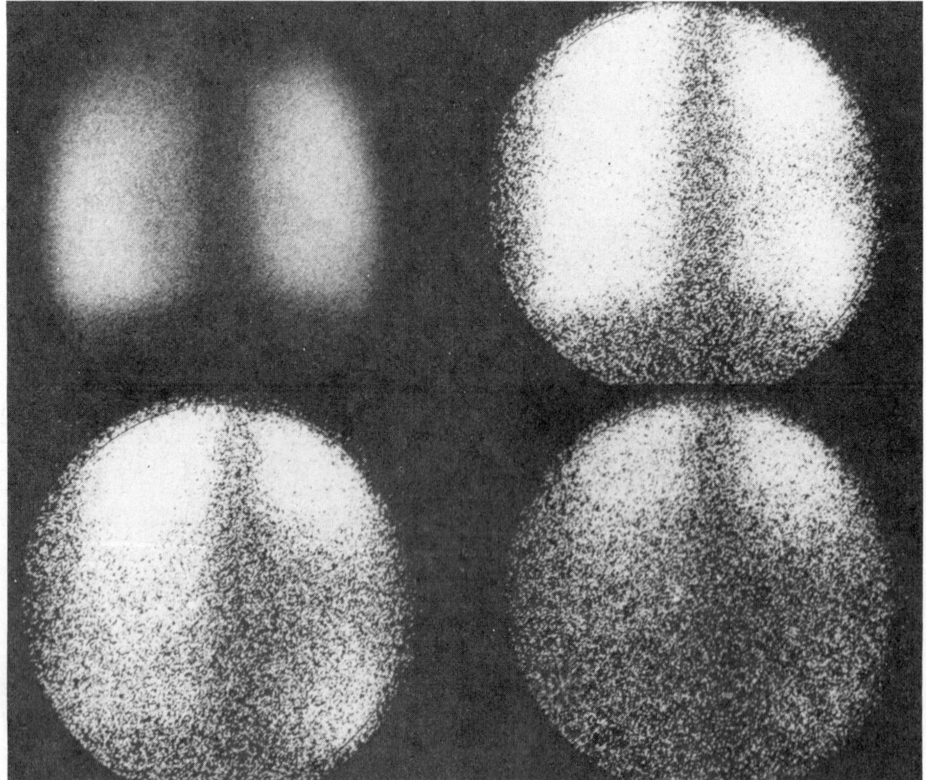

Fig. 10-18. Ventilation study. Washin; washout at 1, 5, and 10 minutes. There is diminished filling of both upper zones at end of washin and delayed clearance from both lungs during washout. Left lung is rather worse than right. These findings are fully consistent with severe bullous emphysema.

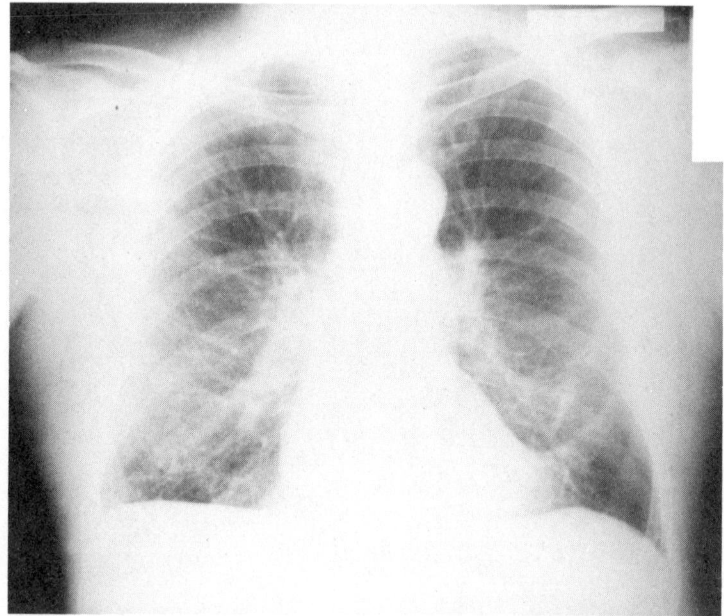

Fig. 10-19. Chest radiograph of 65-year-old man with symptoms of chronic bronchitis. Lung markings are less prominent in left lung.

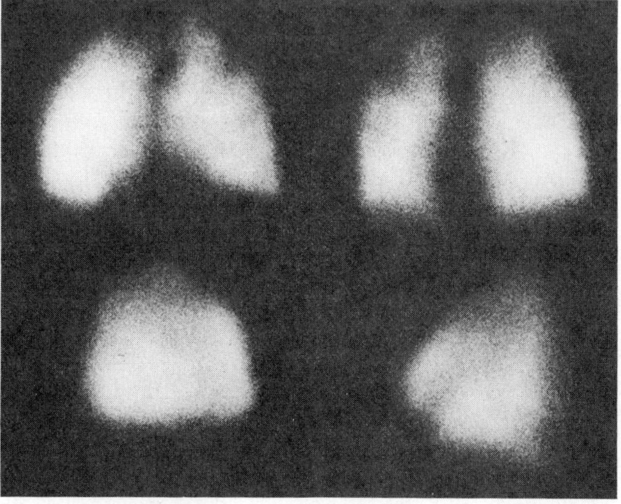

Fig. 10-20. Four-view perfusion scan. Less blood flow to left lung and defects in blood flow are visible in left upper zone, lingula, and left base. Blood flow is also diminished to right apex.

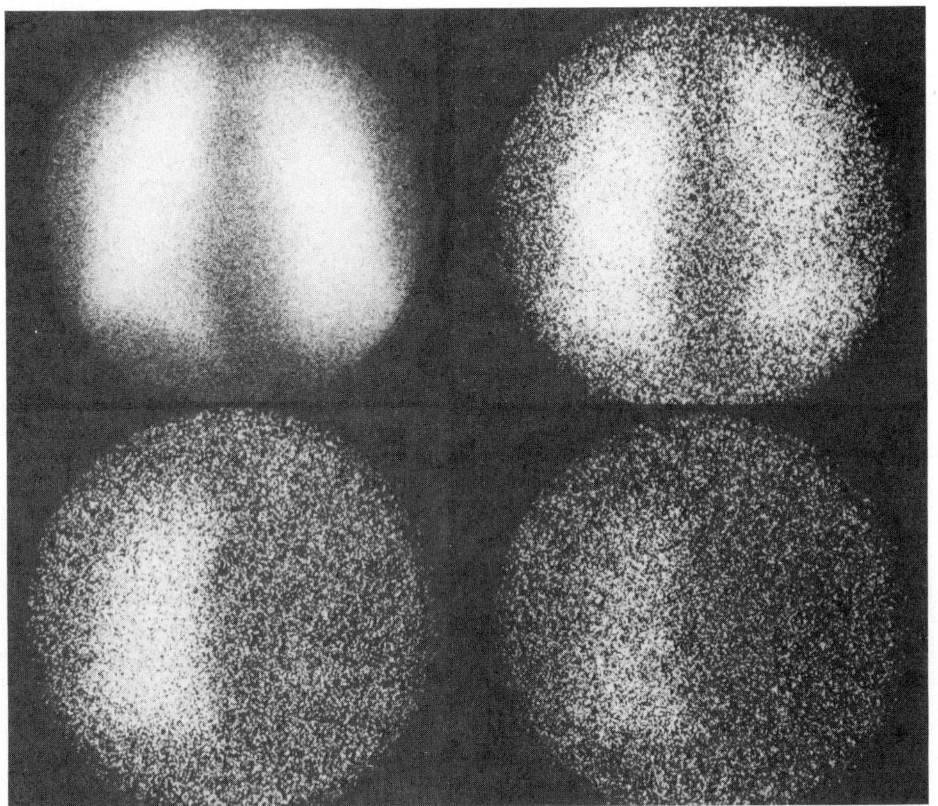

Fig. 10-21. Ventilation study. Washin; washout at 1, 5, and 10 minutes. There is even filling of both lungs during washin except for left base. Clearance is greatly delayed from left lung during washout, and slightly from right lung. These findings indicate predominantly left-sided obstructive airway disease.

even lobar, in nature, leading to a false diagnosis of pulmonary embolism, if only a perfusion scan is done.

In cystic fibrosis the upper lobes are usually the more severely affected and fissure signs are often seen on the lateral views. The sign is attributable to a defect in blood flow along the greater fissure. It is also seen in other obstructive airways diseases, as well as in pulmonary edema with pleural fluid and occasionally in pulmonary embolism. The segments or lobes of lung involved with bronchiectasis are clearly outlined by lack of ventilation and absent pulmonary arterial blood flow (Figs. 10-22 to 10-24).

Lung cancer

In cancer of the bronchus ventilation-perfusion studies may be used to determine individual lung function when a pneumonectomy is planned. The relative distribution of blood flow calculated from an upright perfusion scan enables postoperative lung function to be predicted with considerable accuracy (Figs. 10-25 to 10-27). A successful resection of the tumor tissue is unlikely if the affected lung receives less than about 25% to 30% of the total pulmonary blood flow. Occasionally the site of a tumor may be identified by ventilation-perfusion scanning when it cannot be found by conventional means. After radiation treatment for lung cancer, ventilation will usually improve, but blood flow is restored in a much smaller proportion of such patients.

The most important indication for ventilation-perfusion scanning is in the differential diagnosis of pulmonary embolism. Lesser indications are for the follow-up of this condition and for the assessment of regional and individual lung function in the preoperative assessment of patients with lung cancer or other conditions in which lung tissue may be resected. Ventilation-perfusion scans may sometimes be helpful in the management of patients with obstructive disease of the airways. They may also play some part in the follow-up of patients who have had surgical correction of certain congenital heart defects.

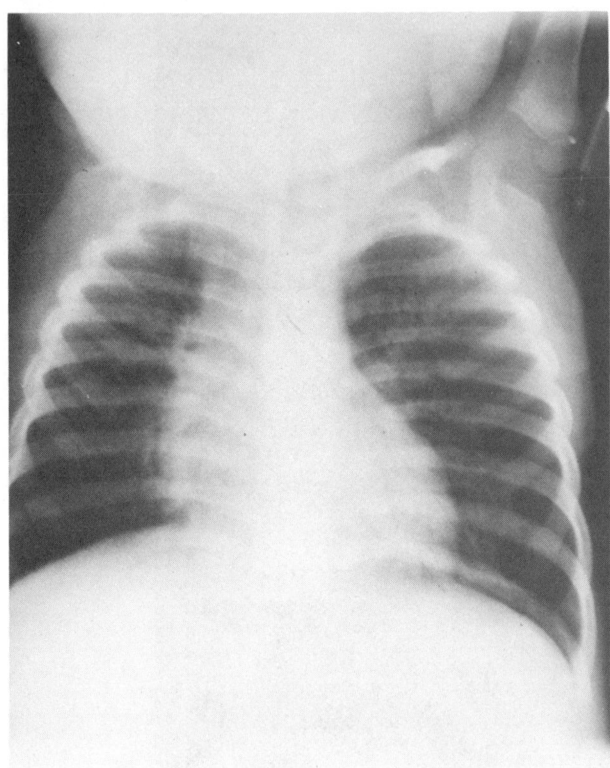

Fig. 10-22. Chest radiograph of 1-year-old infant. No localizing signs are seen. He suffered from chronic cough and wheezing. Bronchograms showed bronchiectasis in several segments of the right lung, particularly in right upper and middle lobes.

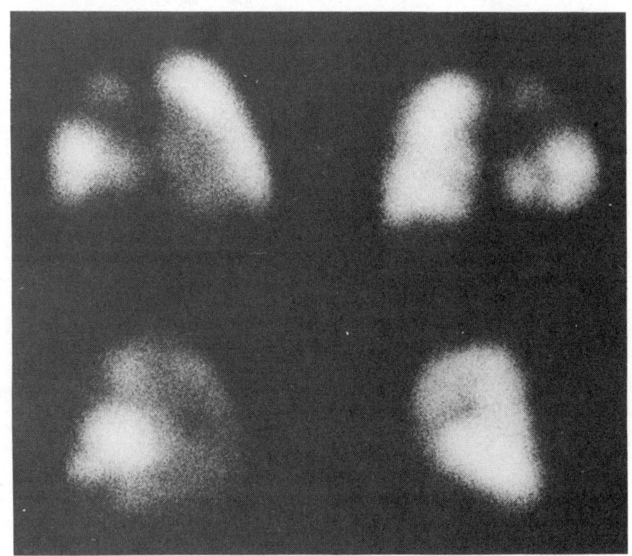

Fig. 10-23. Four-view perfusion scan of infant in Fig. 10-22 showing severe abnormalities of blood flow in right lung and several smaller defects in left lung.

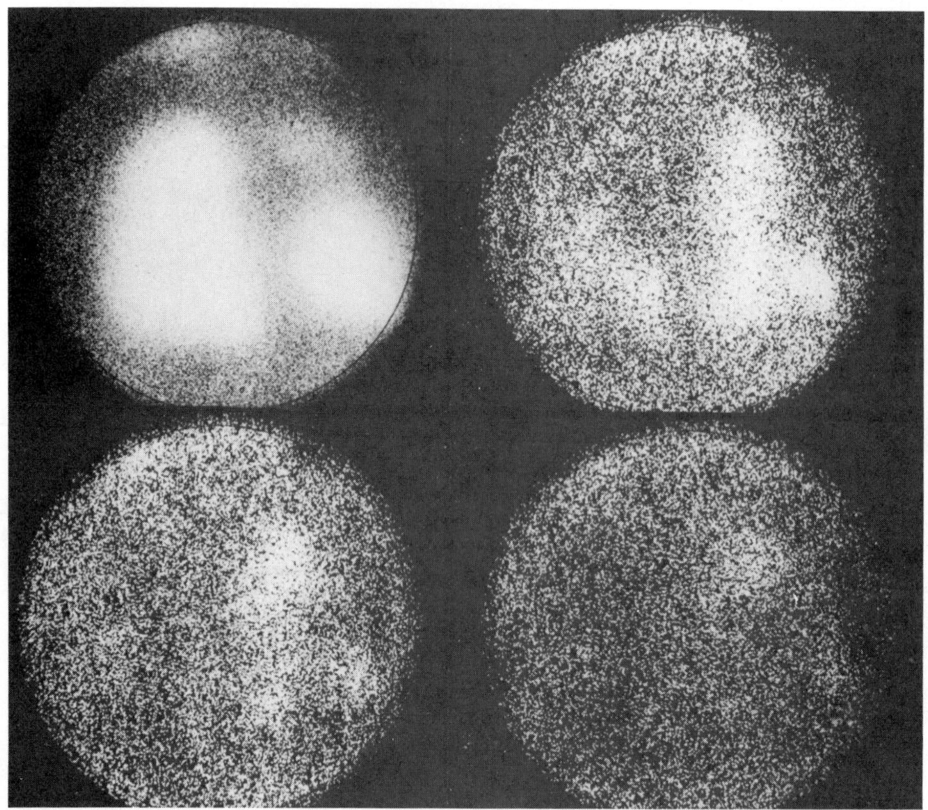

Fig. 10-24. Ventilation study of infant in Fig. 10-22. Washin; washout at 1, 5, and 10 minutes. During washin, right upper zone fails to fill properly. During washout, clearance is greatly delayed from right upper and lower zones. Slight delay is seen on left side. These findings are compatible with findings of bronchiectasis.

Computer processing of ventilation-perfusion images

Increasingly ready access to digital computer processing of image data has led to several different ways of processing the information from ventilation-perfusion imaging. The partitioning of ventilation, lung volume, and blood flow between the lungs can be obtained with considerable ease. However measurements of regional ventilation and regional ventilation-perfusion ratios are less readily obtained. In most instances, the numerical values obtained do not correspond to how much air is exchanged nor to the physiologic ventilation-perfusion ratios. Furthermore there is no convincing evidence that these numerical values actually help in clinical decision making, so that their benefit to the patient is dubious.[33]

Aerosols

Aerosols are deposited in the bronchial tree in relation to particle size, air-flow rates, and turbulence. The hose effectively filters out larger particles, 10 to 15 μm in diameter. Smaller ones are deposited in the larger airways during both inspiration and expiration. Particles less than 2 μm may reach the alveoli and be deposited there, whereas even smaller particles, less than 0.1 μm, will probably escape in the expired air.

Radioactive aerosols have been used for more than a decade to study the patency of the airways. It is important that aerosol particle size be well controlled for reproducible studies. Many radionuclides have been used, but currently $^{99m}TcO_4^-$, ^{99m}Tc-sulfur colloid, ^{99m}Tc-HSA, and $^{113m}InCl_2$ are most popular.

The aerosol is generated from an ultrasonic nebulizer or a positive-pressure nebulizer. It is inhaled through a face mask. Exhaled material must be collected, and the procedure is best done near a fume hood with an extraction fan. Eight to 10 ml of fluid containing up to 10 mCi of the radiopharmaceutical are inhaled. Only

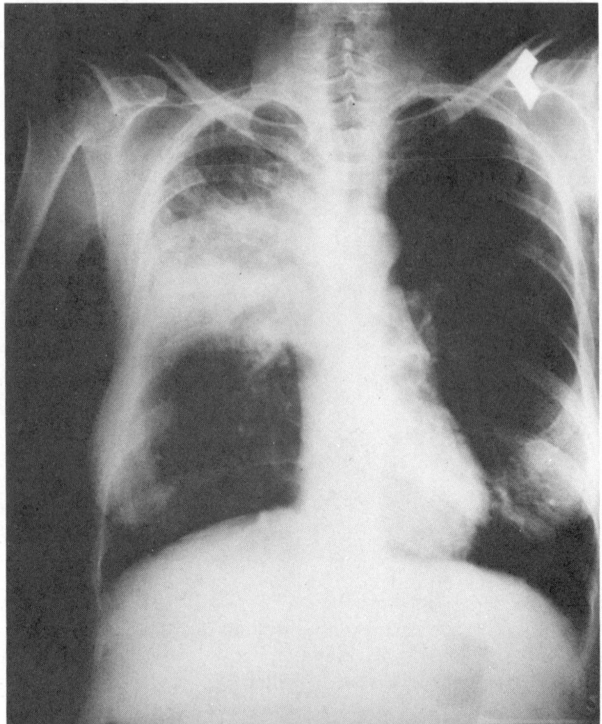

Fig. 10-25. Chest radiograph of 51-year-old woman with cancer of right upper lobe. Dense infiltrate can be seen in this region. She was a heavy cigarette smoker and also had symptoms of chronic bronchitis.

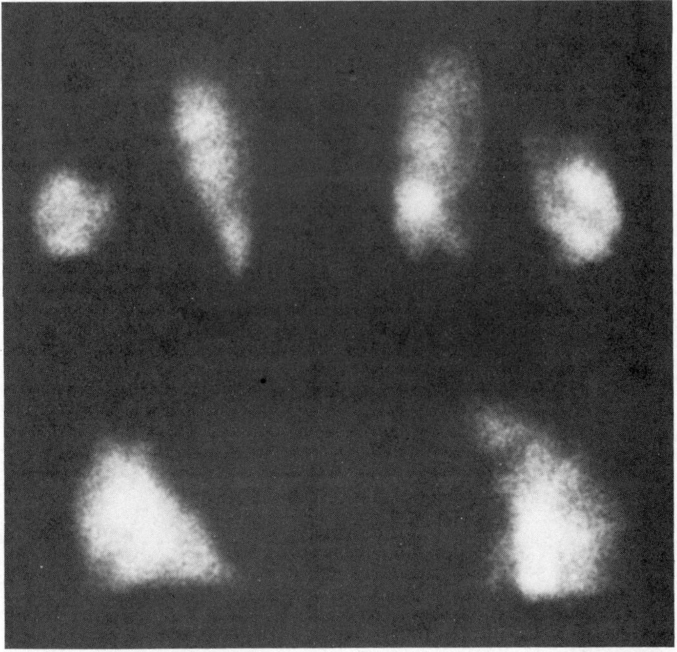

Fig. 10-26. Four-view perfusion scan shows absent perfusion of right upper lobe and some irregularities in perfusion of right lower lobe. Perfusion is also abnormal throughout left lung.

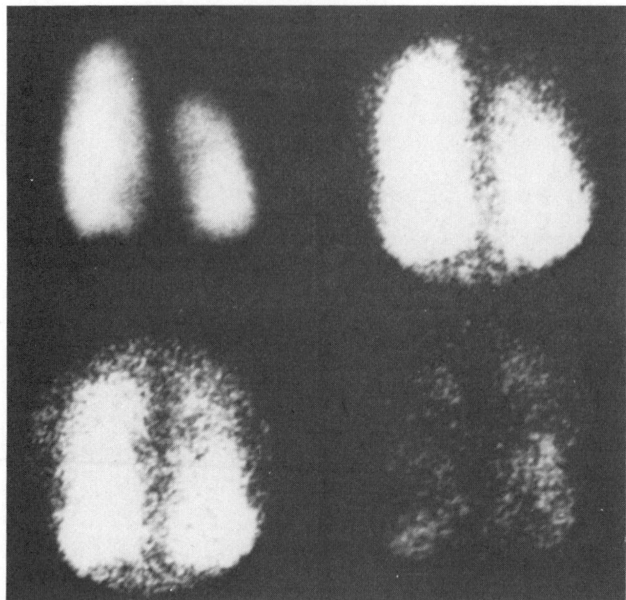

Fig. 10-27. Ventilation study. Washin; washout at 1, 5, and 10 minutes. There is no filling of right upper lobe during washin. Clearance is delayed in irregular fashion from both lungs but especially the right. Some radioactive xenon reaches right upper lobe through bronchial circulation but clears very slowly. These findings are consistent with a lung cancer obstructing right upper lobe bronchus.

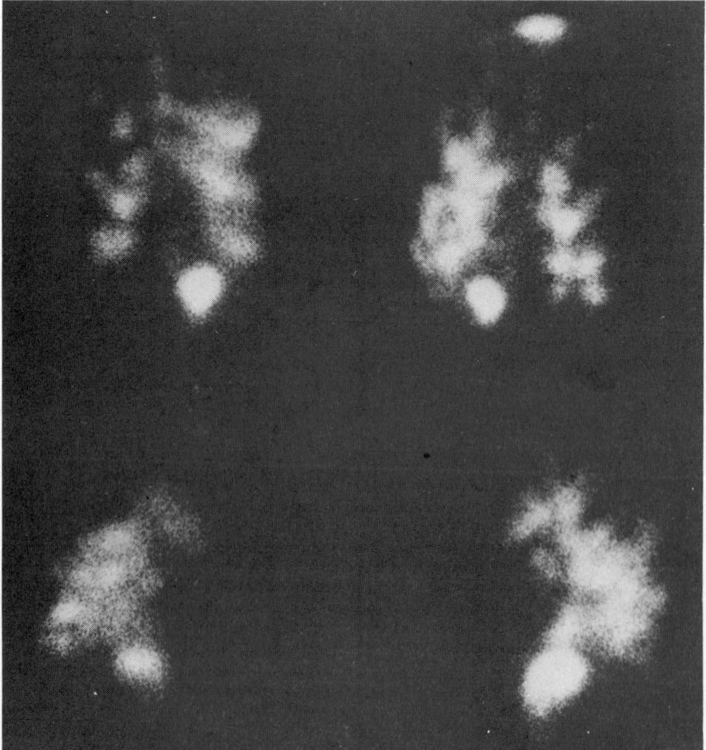

Fig. 10-28. Four-view ^{99m}Tc-sulfur colloid aerosol inhalation scan. The images are arranged as for a perfusion scan. Patient had cystic fibrosis. Images show much central irregular deposition, with very poor peripheral filling, as is seen with severe bronchial obstruction. In addition, activity can be seen in pharynx, esophagus, and stomach.

10% to 15% actually reaches the lungs. Images can then be made in the four standard views.

Normal aerosol scans look much like perfusion scans, except that the trachea and main-stem bronchi can usually be seen, as well as the esophagus and stomach from swallowed material.

In the presence of obstructive disease of the airways there may be much central deposition in the larger bronchial tubes with little or no peripheral filling—a pattern seen in severe bronchial asthma and emphysema. Less central, but definitely patchy peripheral filling tends to be seen in chronic bronchitis, cystic fibrosis, and mild bronchial asthma (Fig. 10-28). Delayed views, 4 to 6 hours after the initial images, may help resolve some central deposition. This will be cleared by mucociliary transport in otherwise normal subjects, leaving normal delayed images. Aerosol scans are almost as sensitive as xenon studies in detecting early disease of small airways. Sequential images for several hours after aerosol inhalation have been used to measure mucociliary clearance rates in smokers, nonsmokers, and children with cystic fibrosis.[29]

TECHNICAL CONSIDERATIONS

Patient preparation

No special patient preparation is required for either ventilation or perfusion lung imaging. There are, however, a few things that should be done in advance of the examination. A recent chest x-ray film (within 24 hours) should accompany the patient to the nuclear medicine facility. The chest x-ray film will allow the physician to be more specific when interpreting the images. Many physicians also require that a blood-gases report accompany the patient. Again this additional information may provide another clue to the correct diagnosis of the patient. It will not be the technologist's responsibility to set laboratory policy with regard to this type of advance information. It will, however, generally be his responsibility to enforce it.

Dosage

In addition to the amount of radioactivity given, the number of particles and the amount of albumin injected are of special importance. Since, as previously discussed, a small percentage of the capillary bed is being obstructed so that the perfusion image may be performed, care must be taken to ensure that the patient's respiratory ability is not further impaired by a test intended to help him.[16] A satisfactory perfusion image can be obtained with anywhere between 60,000 and 150,000 particles in the "normal" patient.[18] An appropriate reduction in the number of particles should be applied for pediatric patients, those with pulmonary hypertension and those who have had a pneumonectomy. To help control the number of particles used in perfusion imaging, one should prepare aggregated albumin kits to the same volume every day and schedule patients as close as possible to the preparation time. Every technologist in the laboratory should know the total number of particles in whichever kit the laboratory uses.

If too few particles are given, the scans have an obvious blotchy appearance. An even more blotchy appearance is seen if small blood clots or incompletely separated particles are inadvertently injected.

Albumin appears to have an affinity for the plastic tubing of intravenous sets, catheters, and syringes. If these avenues of administration are used, a variable proportion of the dose never reaches the patient. We recommend a saline-syringe, three-way stopcock, and dose syringe set up (Fig. 10-29) for aggregated albumin injections. This arrangement also eliminates drawing blood back into the dose and prevents the possible formation of small thrombi as a result of the mixing of whole blood and macroaggregated human serum albumin (MAA).

Always inject labeled particles slowly over 30 seconds or more. Some physicians recommend having the patient take a few deep breaths during the injection in order to assist the homogeneous distribution of the particles.

Method of injection

There is a difference in the patterns of perfusion depending on whether the particles are injected with the patient in the upright or supine position. As indicated earlier, gravity plays an important role in the pressure relationships within the lungs. Patients injected upright will tend to have a larger proportion of the particles distributed toward the bases. Patients injected supine demonstrate a more homogeneous distribution of particles from the bases to the apices. There are arguments and situations favoring each position for injection. As long as both technologist and physician are aware of the difference, either method is satisfactory. The method of injection should be noted somewhere on the film or film jacket.

Positioning

Standard perfusion imaging includes the four basic views: posterior, anterior, right and left laterals, and right and left posterior obliques.[30] We recommend doing the posterior view first, for 500,000 counts, and then each of the other views for the same time that it takes to do the posterior view. The lateral views can then be compared more easily. About one third of the counts from the contralateral lung are included during lateral imaging.

Unlike many radiographic procedures the radionuclide images provide the physician with very few land-

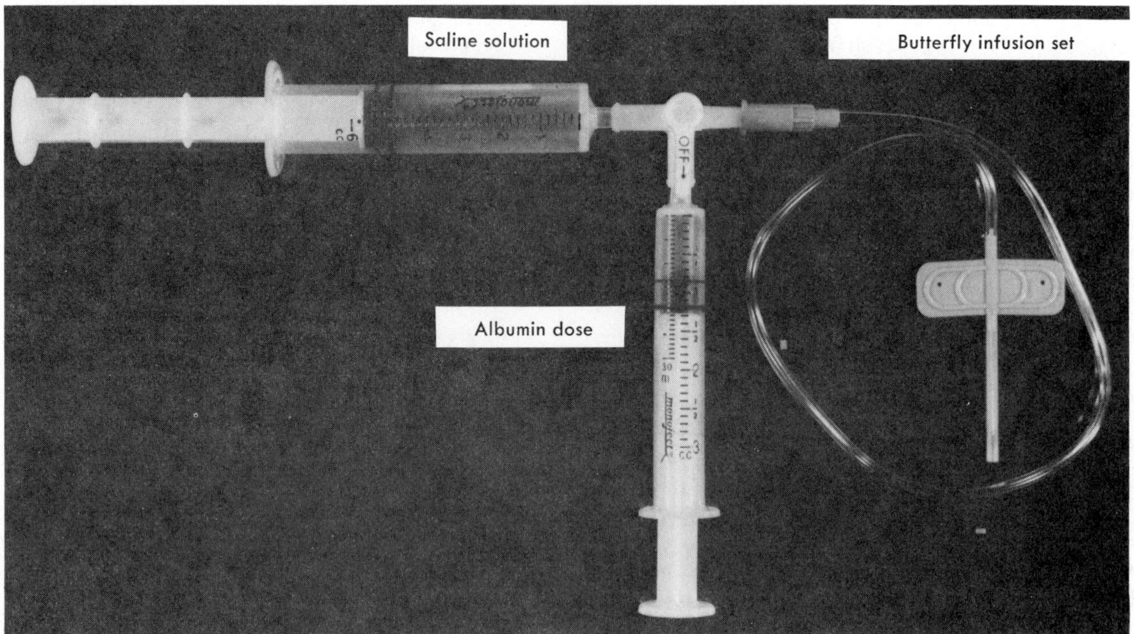

Fig. 10-29. This shows arrangement of recommended injection set for albumin particles. Its operation is described in text.

marks that indicate rotation or distance from the collimator face. The responsibility for good positioning in the nuclear medicine area is basically in the hands of the technologist.

Xenon 133

At present the most readily available nuclide for performing ventilation studies is xenon 133. Although it is not an ideal nuclide for this study because of its low energy, beta emission, and solubility in fat and blood, its price and ready availability have forced it into prominence. The energy 80 keV is not optimal for the Anger camera because so much scattered activity is included in the window. Ideally the perfusion study should be done first so that if a ventilation study is necessary the patient can be positioned for it on the basis of the perfusion scan. Several institutions do the perfusion image first, using only 1 mCi of ^{99m}Tc-labeled particles, and then procede with a ventilation study using 20 to 30 mCi of xenon 133 or more. However because the energy of xenon 133 is lower than that of technetium 99m and because of the importance of the washout phase, we find that it is technically more satisfactory to perform the ventilation study before the perfusion exam.

A number of commercially available gas delivery and rebreathing units are available for ventilation studies, but with a little imagination and some engineering skill you can build your own[32] (Fig. 10-30). An additional problem with xenon ventilation studies is disposal of the xenon when the study is finished. Many laboratories, if suitably located, simply vent the diluted xenon (half-life 5.27 days) into the atmosphere. The Nuclear Regulatory Commission requires that the average yearly concentration must be less than 3×10^{-7} μCi/ml. There are some arguments against this practice, but from a pragmatic standpoint this is the simplest solution. An alternative is to trap the xenon. Several commercial units are available for this purpose, most of which use activated charcoal.[22]

There are several methods for doing a ventilation study. Some laboratories use the single-breath technique, having the patient inhale a bolus of 10 to 20 mCi of xenon 133 and hold his breath for 10 to 20 seconds while a static image is taken. Serial washout images are then made at 30- to 60-second intervals as the xenon clears from the lungs. This method works well but requires a good deal of patient cooperation in taking a deep breath and then holding it for 10 to 20 seconds.

We favor the more straightforward washin-washout method, which can be used even on comatose patients. In this method 10 to 20 mCi of xenon 133 diluted in 2 liters of oxygen are rebreathed from a simple re-

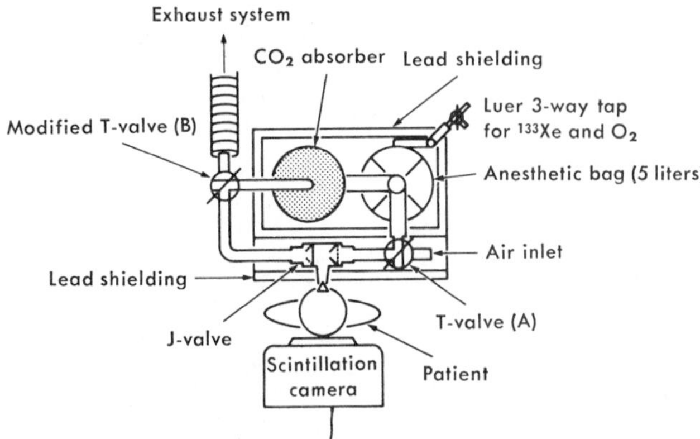

Fig. 10-30. Diagram of simple rebreathing apparatus that can be constructed from commercially available parts. (From Secker-Walker, R. H., Barbier, J., Weiner, S. N., and Alderson, P. O.: J. Nucl. Med. **14:**288, 1974.)

breathing apparatus for approximately 3 minutes while a static washin image is taken. Air is then breathed and serial images are taken at 1/2- to 1-minute intervals as the xenon clears from the lungs. With the variety of mouthpieces, respiratory masks, and harnesses available it is possible for a technologist to perform a ventilation study without assistance from the patient. We have successfully completed this type of examination on many patients and feel confident in saying that if the patient is breathing, a ventilation study can be done. Such studies can also be done on patients on mechanical ventilation.

The ventilation study may be done in any position. Routinely we use the posterior view in the upright position because this provides the best view of the greatest area of lung. The patient should be seated comfortably with his back to the scintillation camera. Every encouragement should be given to keep as still as possible during the study. The first few breaths of xenon, seen on the monitor, can be used to adjust the position of the camera, before the washin images are started.

The pediatric patient

A special note should be made here concerning the pediatric patient. If a rebreathing system is used, the tubing between the infant and the apparatus must be kept as short as possible to reduce dead space. In infants and children the washin and washout timing will often require modification. The washout phase in infants and small children is very rapid and usually requires serial images at 15-second intervals. As is the case with the full spectrum of nuclear medicine studies, pediatric studies require maximum skill, imagination, and flexibility on the part of the technologist.

Krypton 81m

Krypton 81m is a more promising nuclide for the performance of ventilation studies. This gas is obtained by elution of a rubidium-81 generator with a stream of air. Krypton 81m has a 13-second half-life and an energy of 190 keV so that the examinations can be performed in the preferred order. Its 13-second half-life also eliminates any problems of trapping, venting, or contamination. Since krypton 81m decays almost immediately, 4- or 6-view ventilation studies to match the perfusion images can be done routinely.[11,14]

Information density

Calculations of information density fell into the background after the rectilinear scanner was replaced by the Anger camera. Instead the interpreting physician generally accepts that combination of intensity and total counts (usually about 500,000) that give him a "good picture." Although this method leaves itself open to criticism, the physician's specialized training at handling visual information and the image processing of the mind and eye enable satisfactory clinical decisions to be made from such images. It is doubtful if any special calculations of information density are required today.

Collimation

Imaging either ventilation or perfusion generally requires a diverging collimator so that one may view both adult lungs on a standard-field-of-view camera. A parallel-hole collimator may be used for lung imaging on a large-field-of-view camera.[8] The gamma rays from xenon 133 and technetium 99m are easily resolved by the low-energy collimator; however the more energetic photons of krypton 81m may be better resolved with a medium-energy collimator.

REFERENCES

1. Alderson, P. O., Rujanavech, N., Secker-Walker, R. H., and McKnight, R. C.: The role of ^{133}Xe ventilation studies in the scintigraphic detection of pulmonary embolism, Radiology **120:** 633, 1976.
2. Anthonisen, N. R., Danson, J., Robertson, P. C., and Ross, W. R. D.: Airway closure as a function of age, Respir. Physiol. **8:**58, 1969.
3. Anthonisen, N. R., and Milic-Emili, J.: Distribution of pulmonary perfusion in erect man, J. Appl. Physiol. **21:**760, 1966.
4. Atkins, H. L., Susskind, H., Klopper, J. F., Ansari, A. N., Richards, P., and Fairchild, R. G.: A clinical comparison of Xe-127 and Xe-133 for ventilation studies, J. Nucl. Med. **18:**653, 1977.
5. Ball, W. C., Jr., Stewart, P. B., Newsham, L. G. S., and Bates, D. V.: Regional pulmonary studies with xenon 133, J. Clin. Invest. **41:**519, 1962.
6. Breeze, R. G., and Wheeldon, E. B.: The cells of the pulmonary airways, Am. Rev. Respir. Dis. **116:**705, 1977.
7. Buist, A. S., Van Fleet, D. L., and Ross, B. B.: A comparison of conventional spirometric tests and the test of closing volume in an emphysema screening center, Am. Rev. Respir. Dis. **107:**735, 1973.
8. Burdine, J. A., and Murphy, P. H.: Clinical efficacy of a large-field-of-view scintillation camera, J. Nucl. Med. **16:**1158, 1975.
9. Child, J. S., Wolfe, J. D., Tashkin, D., and Nakano, F.: Fatal lung scan in a case of pulmonary hypertension due to obliterative pulmonary vascular disease, Chest **67:**308, 1975.
10. Daly, I. de B., and Hebb, C.: Pulmonary and bronchial vascular systems, Baltimore, 1966, The Williams & Wilkins Co.
11. Fazio, F., and Jones, T.: Assessment of regional ventilation by continuous inhalation of radioactive krypton-81m, Br. Med. J. **3:**673, 1975.
12. Fishman, A. P., and Pietra, G.: Handling of bioactive materials by the lung, N. Engl. J. Med. **281:**884 and 953, 1974.
13. Gold, W. M., and McCormack, K. R.: Pulmonary function response to radioisotope scanning of the lungs, J.A.M.A. **197:** 146, 1966.
14. Goris, M. L., Daspit, S. G., Walter, J. P., McRae, J., and Lamb, J.: Applications of ventilation lung imaging with ^{81m}krypton, Radiology **122:**399, 1977.
15. Green, G. M.: The Amberson Lecture: In defense of the lung, Am. Rev. Respir. Dis. **102:**691, 1970.
16. Harding, L. K., Horsfield, K., Singhal, S. S., and Cumming, G.: The proportion of lung vessels blocked by albumin microspheres, J. Nucl. Med. **14:**579, 1973.
17. Haynie, T. P., Calhoon, J. H., Nasjleti, C. E., Nofal, M. M., and Beierwaltes, W. H.: Visualization of pulmonary artery occlusion by photoscanning, J.A.M.A. **185:**306, 1963.
18. Heck, L. L., and Duley, J. W.: Statistical considerations in lung imaging with Tc-99m albumin particles, Radiology **113:** 657, 1974.
19. Hughes, J. M. B., Glazier, J. B., Maloney, J. E., and West, J. B.: Effect of lung volume on the distribution of pulmonary blood flow in man, Respir. Physiol. **4:**78, 1968.
20. Kaneko, K., Milic-Emili, J., Dolovich, M. B., Dawson, A., Bates, D. V.: Regional distribution of ventilation and perfusion as a function of body position, J. Appl. Physiol. **21:**767, 1966.
21. Knipping, H. W., Bolt, W., Vanrath, H., Ludes, H., and Endler, P.: Eine neue Methode zur Prüfung der Herz- und Lungenfunktion, Dtsch. Med. Wochenschr. **80:**1146, 1955.
22. Luizzi, A., Keaney, J., and Freedman, G.: Use of activated charcoal for the collection and containment of Xe-133 exhaled during pulmonary studies, J. Nucl. Med. **13:**673, 1972.
23. Mead, J., Takishima, T., and Leith, D.: Stress distribution in lungs: a model of pulmonary elasticity, J. Appl. Physiol. **28:** 596, 1970.
24. McNeil, B. J.: A diagnostic strategy using ventilation-perfusion studies in patients suspect for pulmonary embolism, J. Nucl. Med. **17:**613, 1976.
25. Nielsen, P. E., Kirchner, P. T., and Gerber, F. H.: Oblique views in lung perfusion scanning: clinical utility and limitations, J. Nucl. Med. **18:**967, 1977.
26. Rhodes, B. A., Stem, H. S., Buchanan, J. A., Zolle, I., and Wagner, H. N.: Lung scanning with Tc-99m microspheres, Radiology **99:**613, 1971.
27. Rogers, R. M., Kuhl, D. E., Hyde, R. W., and Maycock, R. L.: Measurement of the vital capacity and perfusion of each lung by fluoroscopy and macroaggregated albumin lung scanning, Ann. Intern. Med. **67:**947, 1967.
28. Rootwelt, K., and Vale, J. R.: Pulmonary gas exchange after intravenous injection of ^{99m}Tc-sulphur-colloid albumin macroaggregates for lung perfusion scintigraphy, Scand. J. Clin. Lab. Invest. **30:**17, 1972.
29. Sanchis, J., Dolovich, M., Rossman, C., Wilson, W., and Newhouse, M. T.: Pulmonary mucociliary clearance in cystic fibrosis, N. Engl. J. Med. **288:**651, 1973.
30. Sasahara, A. A., Belko, J. S., and Simpson, R. C.: Multiple view lung scanning, J. Nucl. Med. **9:**187, 1968.
31. Secker-Walker, R. H.: Nuclear medicine in lung disease. In Sagel, S. S., editor: Special procedures in chest radiology, Philadelphia, 1976, W. B. Saunders Co., pp. 147-202.
32. Secker-Walker, R. H., Barbier, J., Weiner, S. N., and Alderson, P. O.: A simple ^{133}Xe delivery system for studies of regional ventilation, J. Nucl. Med. **15:**288, 1974.
33. Secker-Walker, R. H., and Evens, R. G.: The clinical application of computers in ventilation perfusion studies, Progr. Nucl. Med. **3:**166, 1973.
34. Secker-Walker, R. H., Jackson, J. A., and Goodwin, J.: Resolution of pulmonary embolism, Br. Med. J. **4:**135, 1970.
35. Taplin, G. V., Johnson, D. E., Dore, E. K., and Kaplan, H. S.: Lung photoscans with macroaggregates of human serum radioalbumin: experimental basis and initial clinical trials, Health Phys. **10:**1219, 1964.
36. Taplin, G. V., Tashkin, D. P., Chopra, S. K., et al.: Early detection of chronic obstructive pulmonary disease using radionuclide lung imaging procedures, Chest **71:**567, 1977.
37. Tow, D. E., Wagner, H. N., Lopez-Majano, V., Smith, E. M., and Migita, T.: Validity of measuring regional pulmonary arterial blood flow with macroaggregates of human serum albumin, Am. J. Roentgenol. Radium Ther. Nucl. Med. **96:**664, 1966.
38. Wagner, H. M., Sabiston, D. C., McAfee, J. G., Tow, D., and Stern, H. S.: Diagnosis of massive pulmonary embolism in man by radioisotope scanning, N. Engl. J. Med. **271:**377, 1964.
39. West, J. B.: Pulmonary function studies with radioactive gases, Annu. Rev. Med. **18:**459, 1967.
40. West, J. B.: Respiratory physiology—the essentials, Baltimore, 1975, The Williams & Wilkins Co.
41. Weibel, E. R.: Morphometry of the human lungs, New York, 1963, Academic Press, Inc.

Chapter 11

THE CARDIOVASCULAR SYSTEM

Adel G. Mattar and Francine K. Schaffner

The cardiovascular system consists of the heart and blood vessels, which contain the circulating blood. The basic function of the heart is to act as a circulatory pump. This allows the blood to transport oxygen and nutrients to the cells of the body, to remove metabolic waste products, and to carry substances such as hormones from one part of the body to another.

The heart is subject to a wide variety of congenital and acquired diseases, which may involve the myocardium, valves, coronary vessels, or pericardium. Some diseases, such as coronary atherosclerosis, may be insiduous in onset and progress slowly, becoming evident only when the disease is far advanced. Others, such as myocardial infarction, which is the most serious complication of atherosclerosis, usually develop acutely and may run a catastrophic course.

At the present time, radionuclide techniques play an important role in the diagnosis of cardiovascular disorders and for the evaluation of cardiac function.

ANATOMIC CONSIDERATIONS

The heart (Fig. 11-1) is a hollow muscular organ, about the size of the fist of the same individual. It is located in the middle mediastinum enveloped by the pericardium with its inferior surface resting on the diaphragm. The heart is shaped like a blunt cone—the base is tilted backwards, upwards, and to the right, and the apex points downward, forward, and to the left. The apex of the heart is part of the left ventricle, and its beat normally can be palpated in the left fifth intercostal space just medial to the midclavicular line.

The heart is completely divided into right and left sides. Each side consists of a receiving chamber, or atrium, into which large veins open, and a delivering chamber, or ventricle, which propels the blood into the arteries. The atria are separated by the interatrial septum, and the ventricles by the interventricular septum. The right atrium and ventricle are separated by the tricuspid valve, and the left atrium and ventricle by the mitral valve. The right ventricle is separated from the main pulmonary artery by the pulmonary valve, and the left ventricle from the aorta by the aortic valve.

The right side of the heart is concerned with receiving the systemic (body) venous return and pumping this blood into the pulmonary circulation for oxygenation. The left side of the heart receives the oxygenated blood from the lungs and supplies this blood to the systemic arterial circulation for the body to carry out its various metabolic functions.

The heart muscle is supplied by two main coronary arteries, which arise from the ascending aorta. These are the left and right coronary arteries. The left coronary artery divides into two major branches, the left anterior descending and the left circumflex arteries (Fig. 11-2). The right coronary artery supplies the right atrium, right ventricle, and inferior wall of the left ventricle. The anterior descending branch of the left coronary artery supplies the interventricular septum and the anterolateral wall of the left ventricle. The left circumflex branch of the left coronary artery supplies the left atrium as well as the lateral and posterior wall of the left ventricle.

The heart wall is composed of 3 layers: (1) epicardium, or surface layer consisting of a thin serous membrane covering the heart and is reflected at the roots of the great vessels to line the inside of the pericardium, (2) myocardium, which is the heart muscle, and (3) endocardium, which is a thin endothelial layer lining the heart cavities and is continuous with the endothelial lining of the great blood vessels.

PHYSIOLOGIC CONSIDERATIONS

Blood circulation. The right atrium receives the systemic venous blood from the body through the major veins, the superior and inferior venae cavae. Blood then flows to the right ventricle through the tricuspid valve. The right ventricle pumps its blood into the main pulmonary artery through the pulmonary valve. Blood flows into the pulmonary arterial circulation, and after oxygenation in the lungs it drains into the left atrium

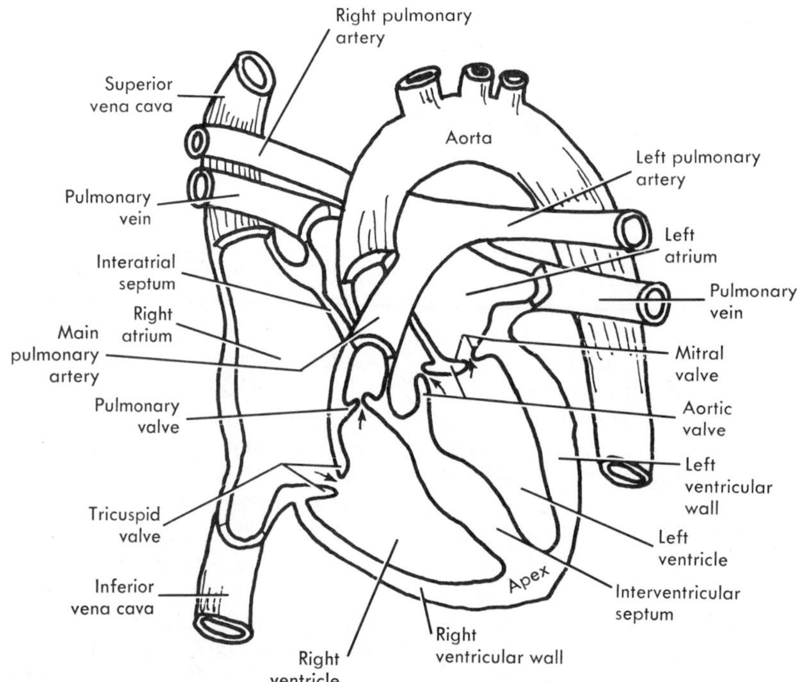

Fig. 11-1. Gross anatomy of heart.

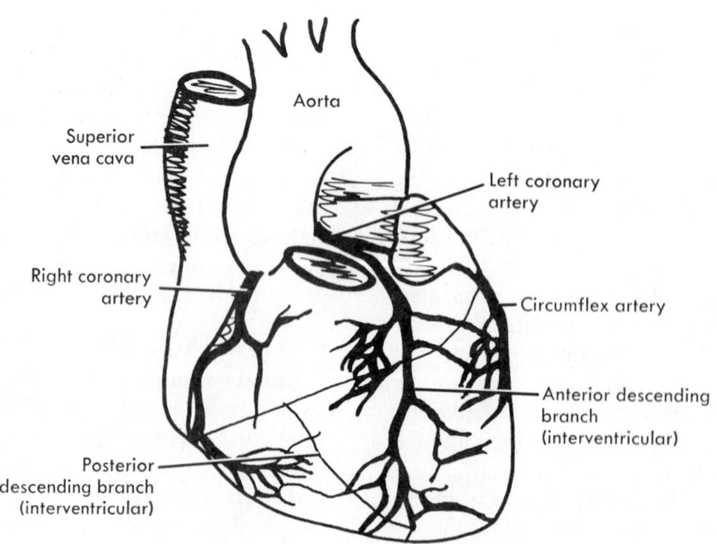

Fig. 11-2. Coronary arteries.

through the pulmonary veins. It then flows into the left ventricle through the mitral valve. The left ventricle ejects its blood into the aorta through the aortic valve. The aorta is the largest artery in the body and supplies the body's systemic circulation with arterialized (oxygenated) blood. Systemic venous blood finally collects and returns to the right atrium through the superior and inferior venae cavae.

The heart as a pump. Functionally, the heart consists of two major pumps, the ventricles, and two minor pumps, the atria. The heart valves maintain competency of the pumping action. Normally the valves open and close at specific intervals during the cardiac cycle and allow the blood to flow in a unidirectional manner.

During each cardiac cycle, the ventricles contract and relax in unison. The contraction phase is called "systole" and the relaxation phase, "diastole." During ventricular diastole, each ventricle fills with blood from the corresponding atrium. During ventricular systole, blood is ejected forward.

The strength of ventricular contraction is influenced by many factors, among which are the preload and afterload. The preload is determined by the volume and pressure within the ventricle prior to the beginning of contraction, that is, at end diastole. The afterload represents the arterial resistance against which the ventricle contracts. The strength of ventricular contraction increases as the preload or afterload increases.

Electrical activity of heart. The heart muscle contracts as a result of stimulation by an electrical impulse, and its relaxation occurs during recovery from this stimulation. The electrical impulse is generated by a specialized structure, the sinoatrial (SA) node, which is located at the junction of the superior vena cava and right atrium. The normal rhythmic contractions of the heart are the result of the rhythmic stimulation by the sinoatrial node, which is considered the physiologic cardiac pacemaker.

The small electrical activity of the heart is transmitted to the body surface, where it can be amplified and recorded externally by the electrocardiogram (ECG). A normal ECG tracing of a single cardiac cycle is illustrated in Fig. 11-3.

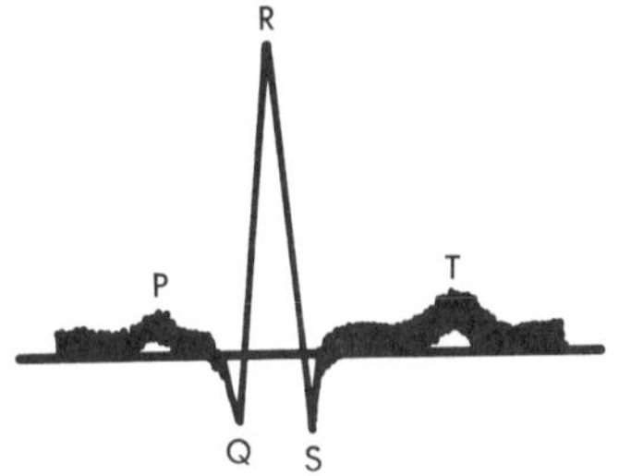

Fig. 11-3. Normal electrocardiograph deflection.

Stroke volume (SV). The stroke volume is the volume of blood ejected forward by either ventricle during a single ventricular systole. Normally the stroke volume of both ventricles is equal.

Cardiac output (CO). The cardiac output is the volume of blood pumped out by either ventricle over a period of 1 minute, that is, CO = SV × Heart rate/minute.

End-diastolic volume (EDV). The end-diastolic volume represents the capacity of the ventricle after completion of its filling with blood, that is, at the end of the diastolic (relaxation) phase. The end-diastolic volume is the largest volume reached by the ventricle during the cardiac cycle.

End-systolic volume (ESV). When the ventricle contracts, it does not completely empty all its blood content. The end-systolic volume represents the residual capacity of the ventricle at the end of the systolic (contraction) phase and is the smallest volume reached by the ventricle during the cardiac cycle.

Ejection fraction (EF). Since the ventricle does not fully empty its blood during contraction, the ejected stroke volume represents only a fraction of the total filling volume reached at end diastole.

Basic equations. From the above, the different parameters can be expressed mathematically as follows:

$$\mathrm{ESV} = \mathrm{EDV} - \mathrm{SV}$$
$$\mathrm{EDV} = \mathrm{SV} + \mathrm{ESV}$$
$$\mathrm{SV} = \mathrm{EDV} - \mathrm{ESV}$$
$$\mathrm{EF} = \frac{\mathrm{SV}}{\mathrm{EDV}}$$
$$\mathrm{EF} = \frac{\mathrm{EDV} - \mathrm{ESV}}{\mathrm{EDV}}$$
$$\mathrm{EF} = 1 - \frac{\mathrm{ESV}}{\mathrm{EDV}}$$

NUCLEAR CARDIOLOGY

Various radionuclide techniques are presently utilized for the diagnosis of cardiovascular diseases and the assessment of cardiac function. Some of the procedures are aimed at the evaluation of the hemodynamics of the cardiovascular system, and others are used for static imaging. The following is an outline of some of the procedures that are discussed in this chapter:

1. Quantitative radionuclide angiocardiography and cardiography
2. Evaluation of left ventricular function
3. Cardiac-shunt evaluation by use of radionuclide angiocardiography and cardiography
4. Myocardial perfusion imaging
5. Scanning of acute myocardial infarction
6. Diagnosis of pericardial effusion
7. Diagnosis of venous thrombosis

RADIONUCLIDE ANGIOCARDIOGRAPHY AND CARDIOGRAPHY

The technique of recording the passage of a radionuclide bolus through the cardiopulmonary circulation is called "radionuclide angiocardiography." The radionuclide cardiogram refers to the record of the bolus through the heart chambers. Both qualitative and quantitative information may be derived from the recording.

Serial imaging of the radionuclide flow is obtained by the scintillation camera. A scintillation probe system can also be used for such studies, but it lacks the benefit of imaging.

A computer is necessary for very rapid serial data acquisition and for sophisticated data analysis such as is required for the determination of the left ventricular ejection fraction.

Quality of injected bolus

For quantitative analysis of angiocardiographic data, the quality of the bolus is extremely important. The bolus spread in the area of interest must be of a short duration (compact) and not fragmented (intact). Bolus prolongation and fragmentation make quantitative analysis inaccurate.

The radionuclide should have a high specific activity so that the injected volume remains small (preferably less than 1 ml for adults, and less than 0.5 ml for infants). The saline flush technique satisfies the requirements for injection of a good bolus.

Saline flush technique of bolus administration[26]

A special injection set is used for this technique (Fig. 11-4). The set consists of an intravenous catheter (1¼ inches, 20G), a three-way stopcock, a 10-inch flexible connecting tube with Luer-Lok fittings, a 30 ml syringe filled with saline solution, a syringe containing the radiopharmaceutical dose, a lead syringe shield, a tourniquet, alcohol sponges, and dry sterile sponges.

Part of the injection set should be assembled prior to the venipuncture. The flexible connecting tube is inserted between the three-way stopcock and the syringe containing the saline flush. Air within the flexible tube and stopcock is displaced with saline solution from the syringe.

Proper steps are taken to immobilize the area where the venipuncture will be performed. A tourniquet is applied, and the injection site is swabbed with an alcohol sponge. The intravenous catheter is inserted into an antecubital vein. When the vein is successfully entered, blood will flow back into the stylette. The tourniquet is then released, the stylette removed from the catheter, and the catheter connected to the stopcock. A small volume of saline is injected to prevent possible formation of clots. The lead-shielded syringe containing the radionuclide is attached to the three-way stopcock, and the radiopharmaceutical is injected through the stopcock into the extension tube. The valve on the stopcock is opened between the catheter and the extension tube, and a rapid injection of saline propels the dose into the vein. Injection should be rapid and steady so that an intact and compact bolus may be delivered. See Fig. 11-4.

Injection of the radionuclide into a central venous catheter inserted to the level of the superior vena cava may be advantageous but is not essential.

Special considerations are important in certain circumstances. A child crying at the time of injection will perform a Valsalva maneuver, leading to increased intrathoracic pressure. Consequently the bolus may become fragmented or trapped in part at the thoracic inlet.

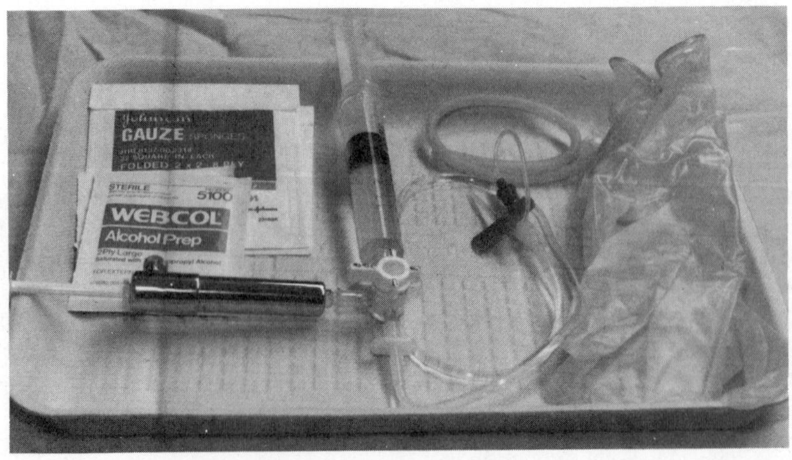

Fig. 11-4. Bolus injection set.

Sedation can be helpful but may not always be desirable clinically. The procedure requires two or more technologists—one to operate the equipment and one or more to inject and assist with the patient. It is preferable that such technologists communicate nonverbally, since sudden and loud instructions can lead to the startling of some patients and result in their performing breathholding maneuvers, which will degrade the bolus.

Utility of radionuclide angiocardiography and cardiography

Qualitative and quantitative evaluation of the central cardiopulmonary circulation may be obtained from the radionuclide angiocardiogram and cardiogram. Qualitative information concerning the gross anatomy of the central circulation such as the presence of pericardial effusion or cardiac shunts may be obtained. Quantitative analysis of time-activity curves obtained from the lung or from a cardiac chamber is based on the assumption that clearance of the bolus from such structures is monoexponential in nature. The following parameters can be quantitated:

1. Left and right ventricular ejection fraction (see first-pass method, p. 298)
2. Cardiac output (CO) (p. 304)
3. Stroke volume (SV), from the equation:

$$SV = \frac{CO/\text{minute}}{\text{Heart rate/minute}}$$

4. End-diastolic volume (EDV) from the equation:

$$EDV = \frac{SV}{\text{Ejection fraction}}$$

5. End-systolic volume (ESV) from the equation:

$$ESV = EDV - SV$$

6. Cardiac-shunt calculation (p. 305)
7. Quantitative estimation of fraction of blood regurgitated at an incompetent heart valve[47]
8. Mean transit time of right side of heart[47]
9. Mean pulmonary transit time (MPTT), which is calculated as the difference between the time of peak bolus activity in the left atrium and mean transit time through the right side of the heart or through the pulmonary artery.[47]
10. Pulmonary blood volume from the equation[47]:

$$\text{Pulmonary blood volume} = MPTT \times CO$$

EVALUATION OF LEFT VENTRICULAR FUNCTION WITH RADIONUCLIDES

Left ventricular ejection fraction, myocardial wall motion, and cardiac output

Optimal function of the left ventricle is vital in maintaining an adequate systemic arterial circulation. When the left ventricle fails as a pump, the functions of the different parts of the body suffer as a result. Evaluation of the efficiency of the pumping action of the left ventricle provides an objective criterion for the adequacy of myocardial performance.

The left ventricular ejection fraction (LVEF), left ventricular wall motion, and cardiac output provide measures for the evaluation of left ventricular performance.

The LVEF is considered one of the most sensitive indicators of left ventricular function. It is more sensitive an indicator than the cardiac output. In the compensated state of heart disease, the LVEF may decline earlier than the cardiac output, which may be maintained by compensatory mechanisms. The results of these compensatory mechanisms are an increase in the heart rate or an increase in the stroke volume or both, thus maintaining a normal range of cardiac output. At the same time, the increase in the stroke volume is accompanied by a larger increase in the end-diastolic volume of the heart, that is, dilatation, hence the decrease in LVEF and a normal cardiac output.

The determination of LVEF is useful in the evaluation of patients with myocardial infarction, ischemic heart disease, cardiomyopathy, and other cardiac disorders.

Myocardial wall motion reflects the contractile function of the heart muscle. Normally when the ventricle contracts, it does so circumferentially with decrease in the ventricular diameters in all directions along with thickening of the interventricular septum. Normal myocardial contraction requires an adequate supply of oxygen to a healthy heart muscle. If there is an imbalance between myocardial oxygen supply and demand (as in ischemic heart disease) or there is a myocardial infarct or scar, the involved area will not contract normally. By radionuclide ventriculography, it is possible to evaluate regional myocardial wall motion abnormalities.

Regional myocardial wall motion abnormalities may be classified as follows:

1. Hypokinesia—a region does contract inward during systole but with less excursion compared to other normal areas.
2. Akinesia—a region does not move at all during systole.
3. Dyskinesia—the region shows paradoxical motion; that is, as the rest of the ventricular wall contracts and moves inward, the abnormal area bulges and moves outward. This paradoxical motion is diagnostic of a ventricular aneurysm, a condition that may complicate myocardial infarction and scarring.

Generalized or diffuse hypokinesis of the entire left ventricle may occur with global ischemia or other generalized conditions such as cardiomyopathy or heart failure.

The detection of a hemodynamically significant coronary artery disease can be enhanced when rest and exercise studies of LVEF and myocardial wall motion are compared. Frequently, abnormalities are not present or are equivocal at rest but become exaggerated during exercise (stress), which induces imbalance between myocardial oxygen supply and demand.

Cardiac catheterization and contrast ventriculography are the definitive procedures for the estimation of LVEF and evaluation of myocardial wall motion. The invasiveness and expense of these procedures, however, preclude their indiscriminate use. Recently, accurate radionuclide techniques have been developed to obtain such information with the following advantages:

1. The procedures are noninvasive and safe, imparting only a small radiation hazard to the patient.
2. They can be repeated as often as may be necessary allowing the evaluation of therapeutic interventions and disease progress.
3. They can be performed on outpatients, on inpatients, and at the patient's bedside.
4. They can be used for screening and selection of patients for cardiac catheterization.
5. They can be performed on high-risk patients in whom invasive techniques cannot be otherwise performed.

METHODS

Two radionuclide techniques are available for the determination of LVEF and the study of myocardial wall motion, as follows:

1. First-pass (first-transit) method
2. Gated cardiac blood-pool methods

FIRST-PASS METHOD

Principle of the test

The first-pass method refers to radionuclide cardiac angiography in which the initial transit of an intravenously administered bolus through the heart is recorded and analyzed.

For calculation of LVEF and evaluation of myocardial wall motion, a high-frequency time-activity curve is necessary. During each cardiac cycle, the net left ventricular (LV) maximum and minimum counts and the difference between such net maximum and minimum counts are proportional to the left ventricular end-diastolic (ED), end-systolic (ES), and stroke (ejected) volumes, respectively. The LVEF can be calculated from the data points on the curve that correspond to the ED and ES phases. The following formula is applied:

$$\text{LVEF} = \frac{\text{Net LV counts at ED} - \text{Net LV counts at ES}}{\text{Net LV counts at ED}} \quad (1)$$

Myocardial wall motion can be evaluated when the ED and ES images generated by computer are compared.

Radiopharmaceutical and dosage

An adult dose of 20 to 30 mCi of ^{99m}Tc-sodium pertechnetate is routine. The radiopharmaceutical should be of a high specific activity, that is, small in volume (preferably less than 1 ml), so that a compact bolus may be delivered.

Technique

The optimal imaging view is controversial and must be decided upon by the nuclear medicine physician. The different views used include 20- to 30-degree right anterior oblique, anterior, 30-degree left anterior oblique, or 30-degree left posterior oblique projections. The overlap between the two ventricles on some of these views is not crucial, since the flow in the right ventricle precedes the flow in the left.

The recording interval selected should be long enough for statistical reliability of the counts collected in each frame, but short enough to reflect closely the heart volume at the particular interval of the frame. For example, consider a sampling time aimed at recording the end-diastolic period. If the sampling (frame) time is too long, it will include counts from a period before or after the end-diastolic period. Conversely, if the recording time is too short, the end diastole will be covered by more than one frame, each of which will contain a small number of counts and thus be statistically inadequate. The rate of 20 frames per second or higher is usually satisfactory.

The radiopharmaceutical is injected in a suitable arm vein, in the form of a compact bolus by use of the saline flush technique described on p. 296. Data recording by computer is ordinarily begun prior to arrival of the bolus into the right side of the heart and is continued until the bolus has traveled through the left ventricle. The total recording time usually lasts about 30 seconds.

To calculate the LVEF, the computer must generate the time-activity curve from the left ventricular area. This curve shows cyclic changes in the counts, with the peaks corresponding to the counts at the end-diastolic phases and the valleys to those at end systole.

Unfortunately, the recorded counts in the region of the left ventricle include the contribution from overlapping structures. Therefore these extraneous background counts must be subtracted for determination of the net counts.

The following steps are undertaken for calculation of the LVEF:

1. The dynamic images are replayed on the com-

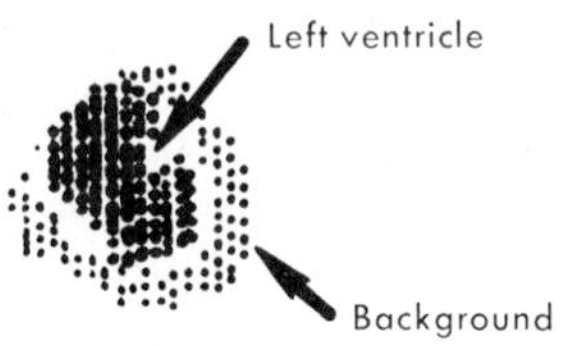

Fig. 11-5. Determination of left ventricular and background regions of interest in first-pass method.

puter screen, and the frames are displayed sequentially.

2. The frame that best visualizes the left ventricle is chosen.
3. Two regions of interest (ROI) are then selected, one corresponding precisely to the left ventricle and the other to a background area. The background is chosen as a horseshoe-shaped area immediately surrounding the left ventricular ROI (Fig. 11-5); this must not include the aortic root or other major vascular structures.
4. The counts from the selected background ROI are normalized by computer so that for each data point (frame), the normalized background counts correspond to those of an area exactly equal to that of the left ventricular ROI. For this normalization, the number of matrix elements (pixels) of the two regions of interest is determined by the computer and the following formula is applied:

$$\text{Normalized background counts} = \frac{\text{Number of LV matrix elements} \times \text{Total counts in background ROI}}{\text{Number of matrix elements in background ROI}}$$

5. Two simultaneous time-activity curves are then generated and displayed, one for the left ventricular ROI and the other for the normalized (and smoothed if smoothing was applied) background ROI. Each curve point corresponds to the counts within the particular ROI during that period. Correction for dead-time losses by the camera-computer system may also be applied, but doing so is not essential.
6. The normalized background curve is subtracted point for point from the time-activity curve originating from the left ventricular ROI. A corrected (subtracted) curve, representing the net counts within the left ventricular cavity, is then displayed by the computer (Fig. 11-6). About four to six cardiac cycles at the apex of the subtracted curve are chosen for analysis. For each beat, the net end-diastolic counts and net end-systolic counts are determined. The LVEF is calculated by use of equation (1), p. 298. The LVEF values obtained from those beats should be averaged to limit the statistical errors because of the relatively small number of counts in each frame.

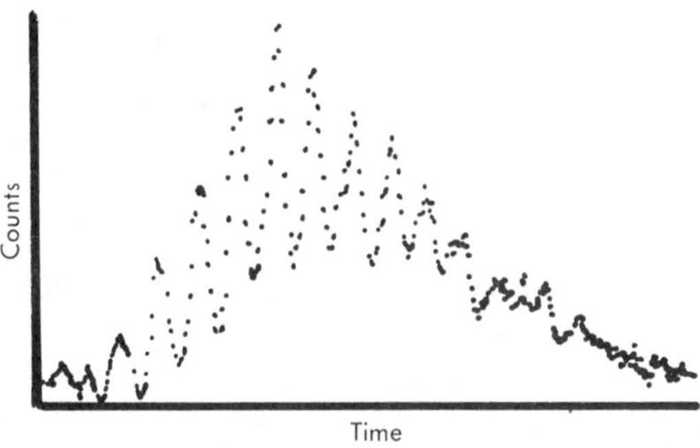

Fig. 11-6. Corrected left ventricular time-activity curve in first-pass method.

Evaluation of myocardial wall motion. Myocardial wall motion can be evaluated by aid of the computer. After subtraction of the normalized background counts, the data from multiple selected cardiac cycles are summed up in a way so as to produce a single representative cardiac cycle. This is achieved by addition of the frames of the corresponding phases of the different cardiac cycles. Repetitive ciné display of the different sequential frames of the computer-derived representative cardiac cycle will allow evaluation of myocardial wall motion.

Alternative technique

The study can be performed essentially as just indicated except that the data collection is performed at discrete time intervals corresponding to end diastole and end systole. Such intervals can be defined by the application of a physiologic cardiac gate marker (see Chapter 7, p. 207, and Fig. 7-8). The duration of recording at end diastole and at end systole ranges from 0.04 to 0.06 second. For the evaluation of LVEF, background area selection and normalization of its counts are performed as outlined above. Myocardial wall motion is evaluated from the continuous alternate replay of end-diastolic and end-systolic images produced after summation of the end-diastolic frames as well as the end-systolic frames of the selected cardiac cycles.

Reliability of the first-pass method

The first-pass method provides excellent results, which correlate well with those of x-ray contrast ventriculography and with gated radionuclide equilibrium techniques. The errors in calculation of the LVEF are mainly attributable to an improper assignment of the left ventricle and background regions of interest.

The advantage of the first-pass method is that data

collection requires only a short time. For myocardial wall motion evaluation, optimal evaluation requires multiple views. For this purpose, therefore, the technique has the disadvantage of requiring multiple studies, each with a separate injection in a different projection.

Use of first-pass method for evaluation of right ventricular function

It is possible to calculate the ejection fraction of the right ventricle and evaluate its wall motion by the same techniques described above. After administration of the radionuclide bolus, the early part of the recording showing the initial passage of the bolus through the right side of the heart is utilized for analysis. Unlike the left ventricular region, the time-activity curve of the right ventricular region is much less affected by background radioactivity, but correction is still necessary.

GATED CARDIAC BLOOD POOL–IMAGING PROCEDURES

Principle of the tests

After the intravenous administration of a blood-pool radiopharmaceutical, gated imaging of the cardiac blood pool at end diastole and end systole or at multiple sequential intervals during the cardiac cycle including the end-diastolic and end-systolic phases may be performed.

Radiopharmaceuticals and dosages

An adult dose of 20 to 30 mCi of one of the following agents is given intravenously:

1. ^{99m}Tc-labeled human serum albumin (HSA) has the disadvantage of having its radionuclide label escape to the extravascular space shortly after injection and the delayed imaging is thus degraded.
2. ^{99m}Tc-labeled autologous red blood cells (RBC), as an agent, is preferable to ^{99m}Tc-HSA if delayed studies are desired since the rate of elution of the radionuclide from the RBCs is slow. The patient's RBCs may be labeled by either in vitro[17] or in vivo[30] techniques.

Techniques

Several techniques are available for the equilibrium gated studies. The techniques used depend on whether a computer is involved.

Gated cardiac blood pool–imaging at end diastole and end systole and the area-length technique for calculation of LVEF. This technique is used when a computer is not available. The gated images are recorded on photographic film. The left ventricle is outlined on the end-diastolic and end-systolic images, and the LVEF is calculated by use of geometric parameters for the derivation of ventricular volumes. Ventricular wall motion is evaluated by superimposition of the end-diastolic and end-systolic images. The method is the simplest and least sophisticated of the radionuclide techniques for the study of LVEF and myocardial wall motion.

IMAGING TECHNIQUE. The patient is placed supine, the detector head is adjusted in the modified left anterior oblique (MLAO) position (30-degree left anterior oblique with a 10- to 15-degree caudal tilt) and gated end-diastolic and end-systolic images are obtained. Imaging is begun 10 minutes after radiopharmaceutical administration.

CALCULATION OF LEFT VENTRICULAR EJECTION FRACTION. The left ventricular outline is drawn on the end-systolic and end-diastolic images. If the images are recorded in other than life-size, either they are projected to real life-size and the outline from the projected image is traced, or a calibration factor is employed for the calculation of absolute ventricular volumes. To facilitate identification of valvular planes, the dynamic study that was performed in the same position is utilized. The frame that best shows the left ventricle and ascending aorta usually defines the valvular planes. By superimposition of this frame on the gated images, the valvular planes may be then identified.

Ventricular volumes can be derived by use of geometric parameters. The formula of an ellipsoid

$$V = \frac{\pi}{6} LM^2$$

(where V is the volume, L is the longitudinal axis, and M is the minor axis perpendicular to and bisecting L at its midpoint) is employed.[15]

Calculation of LVEF is carried out after the left ventricular area is outlined and the L and M axes on each of the gated images is drawn.

In case the study is performed in the MLAO view alone, equation (3) below is used. This equation is derived as follows:

$$\text{EF} = 1 - \frac{\text{ESV}}{\text{EDV}} \qquad (1)$$

$$= 1 - \frac{\frac{\pi}{6} L_S M_S^2}{\frac{\pi}{6} L_D M_D^2} \qquad (2)$$

$$= 1 - \frac{L_S M_S^2}{L_D M_D^2} \qquad (3)$$

(L_S and M_S are the long and minor axes of the left ventricular area at end systole, and L_D and M_D represent those axes at end diastole.)

EVALUATION OF LEFT VENTRICULAR WALL MOTION. Superimposition of the end-diastolic and end-systolic images in each projection allows for the study of left ventricular wall motion.

Multigated equilibrium cardiac blood pool–imaging for the evaluation of left ventricular function. Multigated radionuclide cardiac blood-pool imaging is a sophisticated technique that produces a dynamic pictorial representation of the beating heart. The study requires the administration of a blood-pool radiopharmaceutical that must be uniformly mixed within the intravascular compartment before data collection is started. A computer and a gating device are essential in performing the study. In principle, the cardiac cycle is temporally sliced into multiple segments and an image of the cardiac blood pool of each segment is produced. When these images are displayed sequentially and rapidly in the right temporal order, the result is a dynamic representation of a single cardiac cycle. When the computer displays the images of this cardiac cycle repeatedly, a movie-like presentation of the beating heart is produced.

Analysis of the images, both qualitatively and quantitatively, provides excellent means of evaluation of cardiac function. LVEF is calculated after determination of the net ventricular counts at end diastole and end systole. Cardiac wall motion is evaluated by observing the ciné display of the study on the computer screen.

The computer must be capable of performing certain sophisticated tasks through its hardware and software. In order to produce a sequential series of images, with each image representing the cardiac blood pool during a short time segment, the cardiac cycle is sliced into multiple sequential phases and an image (frame) of each phase is obtained. The number of frames per cardiac cycle must be determined before one starts data collection.

The counts in each frame from a single cardiac cycle are not statistically sufficient; therefore many cardiac cycles are required to achieve the required count density. With each cardiac cycle, the start of data collection is synchronized with the gating signal, and as time proceeds, the incoming counts are sorted into the different frames, with each frame being stored in a certain compartment in the computer memory. The sorting process is restarted with each new cycle; that is, with each new gating signal corresponding frames of all previously accepted cycles are added together while the temporal sequence of assembled images is preserved. each frame being stored in a certain compartment in the computer memory. The sorting process is restarted with each new cycle, that is, with each new gating signal. Corresponding frames of all previously accepted cycles are added together while the temporal sequence of assembled images is preserved.

The acquired images must have good spatial resolution. The computer must be capable of providing a dynamic display of the collected images and of replaying these images repeatedly to provide a movie-like simulation of the beating heart. The rate of display may be varied by the computer operator to make the heartbeat appear slower or faster as required to facilitate evaluation of myocardial wall moticn. Sophisticated mathematical and image-processing techniques must be available for qualitative and quantitative analysis of the images.

The maximum framing rate (frames per cycle) and matrix size are largely determined by the size of the available computer memory. A minimum acceptable requirement gives 16 64×64 pixel images per cycle.

PROCEDURE

1. *Radiopharmaceutical administration*. The patient is injected with a ^{99m}Tc-labeled blood-pool radiopharmaceutical (p. 300) and enough time is allowed for uniform intravascular mixing (at least 10 minutes).
2. *Patient positioning and views*. The study is usually performed with multiple views. However, the exact number is controversial and must be decided upon by the nuclear medicine physician. The following views can be utilized:
   a. 30- to 45-degree left anterior oblique (LAO) view: This view separates the left ventricle from the right. The angle for optimal separation of the ventricles varies in different patients, and the correct angle is chosen by aid of the monitor oscilloscope of the scintillation camera, or by the display screen of the computer. This view is *always* necessary for calculation of LVEF.
   b. Anterior view.
   c. 30- to 45-degree right anterior oblique (RAO) view.
   d. 60- to 70-degree left anterior oblique (LAO) view.
   e. Left lateral view.
   f. 45-degree left posterior oblique (LPO) view: This view gives results similar to those of the RAO, but the latter has the advantage of the heart being closer to the collimator.

   When more than one view is obtained, optimal visualization of the motion of the different myocardial walls can be observed. Reproducibility of positioning is achieved when the patient lies supine and the detector head of the scintillation camera is properly angled. However, for the left lateral projection, the patient should lie on his right side. The left arm should be raised above the patient's head when the left lateral or left anterior oblique views are recorded.

3. *Connection of gating device*. The electrocardiograph is the most common gating device and the R wave is the trigger for gating. The electrodes are placed over the patient's chest as appropriate. The ECG signal is input to the computer.
4. *Data acquisition*. The exact procedure of data acquisition varies with different computer systems or laboratories. In principle the following parameters must be decided upon:
   a. Number of frames per cardiac cycle.
   b. Total number of counts or duration of study.
   c. Matrix resolution of images.

   The R-R interval must be divided into a sufficient number of small segments to make it likely that end systole and end diastole are accurately represented without inclusion of portions of the cardiac cycle that occur before and after those phases. It appears that temporal resolution of 30-millisecond segments at a heart rate of 60 per minute is satisfactory, but in some laboratories a lower framing rate is employed.[40]

   A sufficient number of counts should be collected during the study so that each image is statistically reliable. A range of 150,000 to 250,000 counts per frame is satisfactory. The total counts required are calculated when the counts of each frame are multiplied by the number of frames per ECG cycle. The number of heartbeats required for the study can be calculated when the total number of required counts for all images are divided by the number of counts collected during one cardiac cycle. This is accomplished automatically by most computer systems.

   Difficulty in data acquisition may be encountered when the heartbeats are irregular (that is, variable in duration) as in some cases of atrial fibrillation with varying R-R intervals and also with premature ventricular beats. Some computer programs may be set to allow for the options of rejecting or accepting the heartbeats that vary in duration outside specified tolerance limits from that of the average beat. In patients with frequent premature ventricular beats exceeding 10% of the recorded beats, the results may be unreliable for the measurement of ventricular function.
5. *Data analysis*
   a. Subjective evaluation of myocardial wall motion: The result of data acquisition is a series of images reflecting the dynamics of a single cardiac cycle. A movie-like display of this cycle on the computer screen allows for evaluation of cardiac wall motion. The frequency

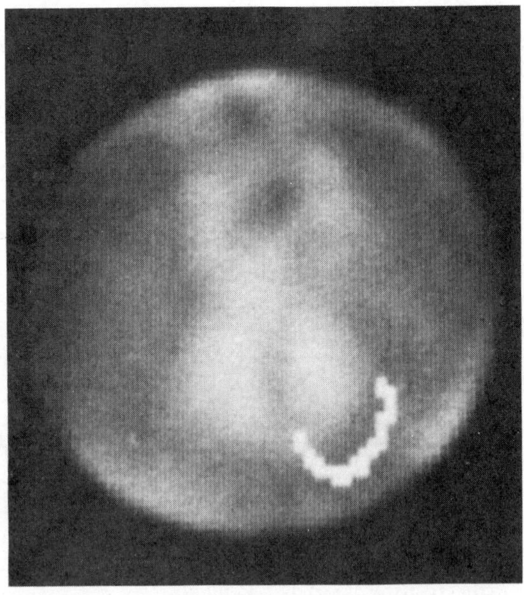

Fig. 11-7. Background region of interest selection from end-diastolic image of equilibrium gated study.

with which the cycle is displayed can be varied by the computer operator; thus the subjective interpretation is facilitated. Evaluation of the motion of the myocardial wall is best achieved by multiple views.
   b. Quantitative analysis: In principle, quantitative analysis can be carried out by identification of the left ventricle in each of the recorded frames, on the study performed at the 30- to 45-degree LAO position. Computer-operator interaction is usually necessary for the selection of the left ventricular area. Semiautomatic or automatic edge-detection computer programs are also available to facilitate the procedure and improve reproducibility.

   For determination of the net left ventricular counts in each frame, background activity must be subtracted. For this, a background region of interest is selected and one of the following methods may be utilized:
   (1) The background ROI is usually selected as a horseshoe-shaped area next to the left ventricle on the end-diastolic image, with the aortic root and other well-defined vascular structures being excluded (Fig. 11-7). In order to ensure that no vascular structures are included, a time-activity curve of the selected background ROI must be reasonably horizontal.
   (2) The background area is selected on the

end-systolic image just outside the free wall of the left ventricle. The selected area is chosen in such a way that it corresponds to a region situated between the outer borders of the left ventricle at end systole and end diastole, with the major vascular structures being avoided.

(3) A zone of the lung, usually adjacent to the posterior wall of the left ventricle, is chosen to serve as a background ROI. Similarly this area should be free of well-defined vascular structures, and a histogram of this area should appear as a horizontal line.

Normalization of background counts must also be performed for each frame (p. 299). For each frame, the normalized background counts are subtracted. The LVEF can be calculated from the net counts corresponding to the end-diastolic and end-systolic phases with the equation:

$$\text{LVEF} = \frac{\begin{matrix}\text{Net LV} \\ \text{counts at ED}\end{matrix} - \begin{matrix}\text{Net LV} \\ \text{counts at ES}\end{matrix}}{\text{Net LV counts at ED}}$$

A left ventricular time-activity curve is also generated from the net left ventricular counts of the different frames. This curve reflects the changes in left ventricular volume during the cardiac cycle (Fig. 11-8). Measurements of the rate of change in ventricular volume relative to time (that is, D_V/D_T) can also be calculated.

The multigated equilibrium study is particularly useful when multiple tests are required within a short time, such as for evaluation of therapeutic interventions and also for studying the effect of exercise on cardiac function by comparison to the status at rest. The technique is reliable and reproducible and correlates well with contrast angiography and the radionuclide first-pass method.

Evaluation of left ventricular function at rest and exercise by use of the multigated radionuclide equilibrium cardiac blood pool–imaging technique. During exercise, a person with a normal heart will show an increase in the LVEF, and the myocardial wall motion will remain normal. In patients with ischemic heart disease, the LVEF declines with exercise and abnormalities in myocardial wall motion become more exaggerated.

In some patients with ischemic heart disease, evaluation of left ventricular function at rest may not yield definitely abnormal results; abnormalities may only be demonstrable when the myocardium is stressed as a result of physical exercise. During exercise, the LVEF declines and the ischemic heart area may show a regional wall motion abnormality.

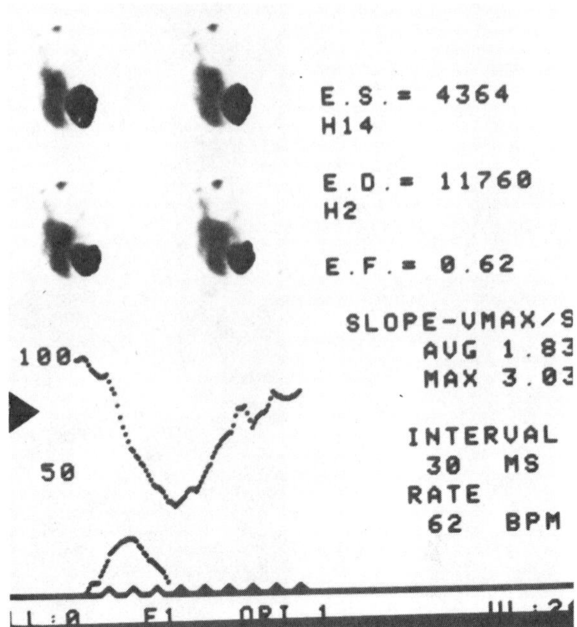

Fig. 11-8. Left ventricular time-activity curve *(arrow)* shown as part of computer display of ejection fraction (multigated equilibrium study).

PROCEDURE. The safety precautions for exercise testing are the same as those required for the exercise ^{201}Tl imaging (p. 314). The radionuclide mitigated cardiac blood-pool study is performed at rest and during exercise. The exercise feature of the test adds certain requirements to the procedure already described above.

To perform the study, one injects the patient intravenously with the blood-pool radiopharmaceutical. The patient lies on the imaging table, and his feet are placed on the ergometer pedals (Fig. 11-9). The shoulder supports are positioned to fit the patient, and the pelvis straps are placed and tightened. The ECG electrodes are placed on the chest. Base-line measurements of blood pressure and pulse rate and an ECG tracing are obtained prior to exercise. The patient should then practice pedaling briefly to make sure the position is comfortable and that he understands the procedure.

After enough time is allowed for the radionuclide to equilibrate with the blood, a base-line multigated cardiac blood pool–imaging study is performed at rest in the LAO position. After completion, the patient is instructed to begin exercising. Initially, this should be with a fairly low work load. Enough time is allowed for the heart to stabilize at a steady rate. While

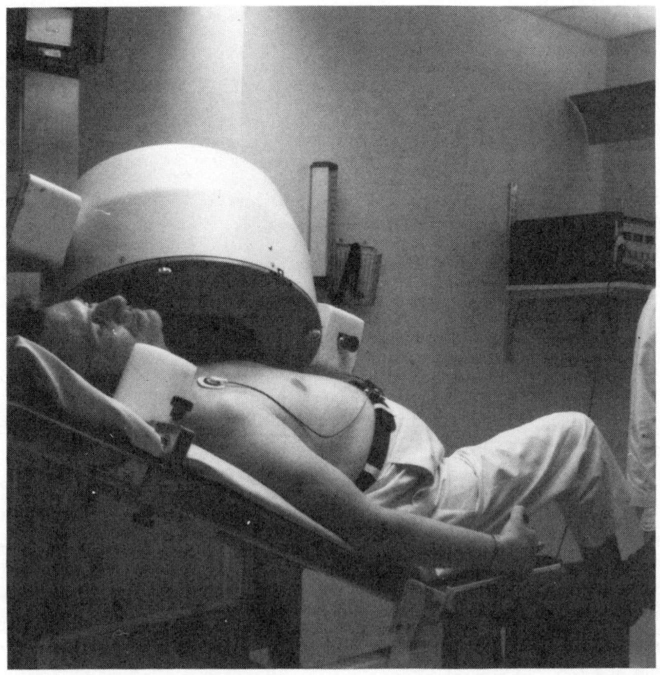

Fig. 11-9. Patient undergoing a stress multigated radionuclide cardiac blood pool study.

the patient is exercising at this steady rate, a second multigated study is recorded. After completion of data collection, the work load on the ergometer is increased and the procedure is repeated. The testing procedure continues in this manner until the maximal level of exercise is reached or the study is terminated.

The patient's blood pressure and pulse rate are monitored throughout the study. At each exercise level an ECG tracing strip is obtained. At the end of the procedure, the patient is observed closely until his heart rate, blood pressure, and ECG changes (if any) return to the preexercise status. The images are analyzed as described previously.

DETERMINATION OF CARDIAC OUTPUT (CO)

As mentioned before, the CO is the volume of blood expelled by either ventricle per unit time. The CO is usually expressed in liters per minute.

In principle, CO determination by radionuclide techniques requires an intravenous administration of a bolus of a blood-pool radiopharmaceutical. The dynamic flow of the bolus through the heart is recorded, and at a later time (at about 10 minutes after injection), without disturbing the position of the patient or scintillation detector, a record of the equilibrium counts is obtained. By selection of a region of interest (ROI) over the heart, a time-activity curve for the initial bolus and equilibrium phase can be constructed (Fig. 11-10). A linear least-squares fit to the initial bolus transit determines the area of the bolus. After subtraction of background activity from the selected ROI, the CO is calculated by use of the Stewart-Hamilton approach. The equation applied is as follows:

$$\text{CO} = \text{Blood volume} \times \frac{\text{Equilibrium counts per minute}}{\text{Total counts under bolus area}}$$

The CO can be calculated in conjunction with the first-pass method, which is performed for calculation of LVEF and evaluation of myocardial wall motion. The recording technique and equipment, as well as the background subtraction method, are the same as previously described (p. 298).

An intravenous bolus of ^{99m}Tc-HSA is usually utilized. For calculation of the blood volume, an aliquot of the radiopharmaceutical is prepared as a standard. The amount of the injected material is determined so that the total counts injected may be calculated. The counts in 1 ml of blood from a sample taken at the time of radionuclide equilibration are determined. The blood volume is calculated as follows:

$$\text{Blood volume (ml)} = \frac{\text{Total injected counts}}{\text{Counts in 1 ml of blood}}$$

Note that it is possible to calculate the CO from re-

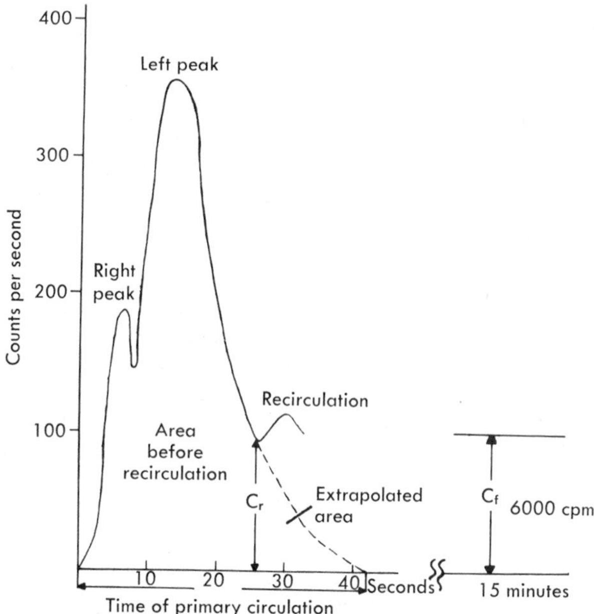

Fig. 11-10. Determination of cardiac output. C_r, Counting rate at beginning of recirculation; C_f, final counting rate after equilibration. (From Early, P. J., Razzak, M. A., and Sodee, D. B.: Textbook of nuclear medicine technology, ed. 3, St. Louis, 1979, The C. V. Mosby Co.)

cordings derived from any cardiac chamber, combination of chambers, or the entire heart. This is valid so long as the bolus recording and the equilibrium counts are derived from the same region. Obviously the same bolus travels through the different cardiac chambers. Whether the first transit and equilibrium counts are recorded from one chamber or multiple chambers makes no difference to the CO determination.

DETECTION OF INTRACARDIAC SHUNTS WITH RADIONUCLIDES

Normally the right side of the heart is concerned with the collection of the systemic venous return from the body and pumping this blood into the pulmonary arterial circulation for gaseous exchange in the lungs. The left side of the heart gathers oxygenated blood from the lungs and delivers it into the systemic arterial circulation. Intracardiac or extracardiac mixing of blood from the left-to-right circulations or vice versa does not occur in the normal individual. However, such shunting of blood may occur as a result of certain congenital abnormalities affecting the heart or great vessels.

When an abnormal communication between the left and right sides of the heart exists, the size of the opening and the pressures on either side of it will determine the direction and magnitude of the shunt flow.

Because the pressures in the left ventricle and systemic arterial circulation are higher than those in the right ventricle and pulmonary circulation, ordinarily, if an abnormal communication is present, a left-to-right shunt occurs. This may be associated with conditions such as atrial septal defect, ventricular septal defect or patent ductus arteriosus (communication between aorta and pulmonary artery).

A right-to-left shunt occurs when the communication between the two sides of the circulation is complicated by a lesion that raises the right-sided pressure above that of the left. Also an obligatory right-to-left shunt may occur with certain abnormalities such as tetralogy of Fallot. Right-to-left shunting of blood is the cause of cyanosis that is associated with congenital cyanotic heart disease.

Shunts can also be bidirectional; for example, blood may be shunted in one direction through an atrial septal defect and in the opposite direction through a ventricular septal defect. Mixing of blood in such a manner occurs in some cases of transposition of the great vessels (when there is an anatomic switch of the great vessels or cardiac chambers, or of both).

In some conditions, the patient may benefit from surgical closure of the shunt. In certain other anomalies, creation of shunts or enlarging the one already present may be indicated. For example, in certain congenital cyanotic heart diseases, the patient may benefit from the creation of a left-to-right shunt, which increases in the blood supply to the lungs thus improving oxygenation of blood.

Indications of shunt-evaluation procedures

Shunt evaluation is an important clinical problem especially in the pediatric age group. An increasing number of congenital intracardiac and extracardiac shunts are now amenable to surgical and medical treatment. Investigations are required for screening, diagnosing, and evaluation of management of patients. The objectives of investigation are as follows:

1. To diagnose the presence and location of a shunt, as well as to define any other accompanying anatomic abnormalities in the circulatory system.
2. To quantitate the magnitude of shunting and to determine the contribution of the shunting process to the overall hemodynamic abnormalities present.
3. To evaluate patients preoperatively and postoperatively.
4. To monitor improvement, deterioration, and effect of treatment.

Cardiac catheterization versus radionuclide shunt evaluation

Although cardiac catheterization is the most definitive test available for the diagnosis and quantitation of cardiac shunts, the technique is invasive and requires a skilled team, expensive equipment, the administration of contrast with possible side effects to the patients, and blood sampling for shunt quantitation. The procedure is time consuming and delivers a high radiation dose to the patient. Cardiac catheterization can be risky for the ill child and cannot be repeated as frequently as may be needed.

Because of the invasive nature of cardiac catheterization, the need for noninvasive tests is obvious. The radionuclide techniques for the detection and quantitation of cardiac shunts fulfill such a need. However, noninvasive tests do not completely replace cardiac catheterization, since such catheterization gives accurate anatomic and hemodynamic information, including shunt quantitation and pressure measurements in the different heart chambers and vessels. Such information is mandatory prior to cardiac surgery.

The radionuclide techniques have the advantages of being noninvasive, simple, rapid, and reliable. They can be performed as often as may be needed, on severely ill patients of all age groups, and on those sensitive to radiocontrast agents who cannot undergo cardiac catheterization. The radiation dose resulting from such techniques is lower than that delivered at catheterization. The procedure requires a simple intravenous bolus administration and no blood sampling.

In 1949, Prinzmetal et al. introduced the technique of precordial radiocardiography, using ^{24}Na and a Geiger-Müller tube.[31] Many radionuclide techniques were later developed for the qualitative and quantitative evaluation of intracardiac shunts. Originally such techniques were centered around the use of external precordial counting with or without catheterization involving a variety of radionuclides, administered by either intravenous injection or inhalation.

In 1962, Folse and Braunwald showed that left-to-right shunts could be diagnosed from a radionuclide pulmonary vascular dilution (time-activity) curve.[13] Several methods of curve analysis, both qualitative and quantitative have since been developed.

With the advent of the scintillation camera and new radionuclides in the early 1960s, the use of external counting by probe systems for the detection of cardiac shunts have been largely replaced by rapid visualization of the cardiopulmonary circulation along with analysis of dynamic flow information derived from selected regions of interest. Although analysis of time-activity curves derived from cardiac chambers can detect right-to-left, left-to-right, and bidirectional cardiac shunts, the pulmonary dilution curve can only detect left-to-right shunts.

In 1971, Gates et al. developed a method using ^{99m}Tc-labeled macroaggregated albumin to detect and quantitate right-to-left shunts.[14] The technique depends on determination of the counts from the particles in the lungs and those trapped in the systemic circulation that have bypassed the pulmonary circulation through an intracardiac right-to-left shunt.

In 1976, Watson et al. described a technique utilizing inhalation of ^{15}O-labeled carbon dioxide for the detection of left-to-right shunts.[43]

EVALUATION OF CARDIAC SHUNTS USING RADIONUCLIDE ANGIOCARDIOGRAPHY AND CARDIOGRAPHY

The radionuclide angiocardiogram and cardiogram provide qualitative and quantitative information about cardiac shunts. The technique depends on intravenous administration of a radionuclide bolus and generation of time-activity curves of the first pass from a cardiac chamber or chambers or pulmonary circulation.

In a normal person, as the bolus moves through the cardiopulmonary circulation, a time-activity curve of the first transit shows an initial increase of counts, and after the peak is reached, the counts decline because of the passage of the bolus away from the area of interest. The clearance of the bolus, that is, the downslope of the curve is monoexponential in nature. This monoexponential phase of the curve is ultimately obscured by rearrival of the tracer because of normal recirculation, leading to a change in the slope.

In patients with left-to-right cardiac shunts, early recirculation of the tracer through the shunt distorts the downslope of the time-activity curve. This curve must be generated from an area distal to the shunt, usually over the lungs. The change in the slope of the clearance phase of the curve begins after the peak activity is reached but earlier than the normal systemic recirculation. The magnitude and onset of curve distortion are related to the size of the shunt.

With right-to-left shunts, dynamic imaging of the flow study shows visualization of the left ventricle and aorta earlier than, or simultaneously with, the beginning of lung visualization.

EVALUATION OF LEFT-TO-RIGHT CARDIAC SHUNTS USING PULMONARY TIME-ACTIVITY CURVE GENERATED FROM RADIONUCLIDE ANGIOCARDIOGRAPHY

Radiopharmaceutical and patient preparation

Currently ^{99m}Tc-pertechnetate is the most commonly used agent. A dose of 200 μCi/kg of body weight (with a minimum of 2 to 3 mCi per dose for small infants) is administered intravenously. The radionuclide should have a high specific activity so that the injected volume remains small (p. 296).

One half hour prior to the administration of the radionuclide the patient is prepared with potassium perchlorate, 6 mg/kg of body weight in order to block the thyroid gland trapping of the radionuclide.

Technique

The radionuclide bolus is administered by use of the saline flush technique (p. 296). The quality of the bolus is of utmost importance to the success of the procedure. Prolongation or fragmentation of the bolus makes the results useless.

The passage of the bolus through the central venous circulation, right side of the heart, lungs, left side of the heart, and aorta is recorded from the camera in a digitized form by computer or videotape system. The length of the recording is usually less than 1 minute. The data is acquired by the computer on frames 0.5 second or shorter. One-second exposure sequential images of the flow study may be obtained on photographic film.

A summed image of the flow study is formed and displayed. An area of interest over a lung free from cardiac and venous activity is selected. A time-activity curve of this area is generated. A second area over the superior vena cava or innominate vein is likewise selected, and a time-activity histogram is also generated for examination of the quality of the bolus. A study is discarded if the bolus is fragmented (that is, having more than one peak) or prolonged (more than 2.5 seconds in duration). In general about 15% to 20% of studies need to be repeated because of a poor bolus. Each data point on the curve represents one frame in the case of computer-generated studies. In the case of a recording on a videotape system, the data points on the generated curve should be separated maximally by 0.5 seconds.

The pulmonary dilution (time-activity) curve can be analyzed for left-to-right shunt evaluation in three different ways, two of which are qualitative and the third (Q_P/Q_S) is quantitative, as follows:

1. *C_2/C_1 ratio:* The C_2/C_1 ratio can be determined in three different ways:
   a. Two points, C_1 and C_2, are identified on the pulmonary time-activity curve. C_1 corresponds to the peak. C_2 represents a point on the downslope of the curve occurring at end of time t_2. Time t_2 occurs at a time t_1 after the peak count rate, where t_1 represents the time between the point at which the count rate begins to exceed background and C_1 (Fig. 11-11). The ratio of the two counting rates C_2/C_1 is then expressed as a percentage. The normal value of C_2/C_1 is 26% (±5.2% standard deviation).[1]
   b. The C_2/C_1 ratio may also be calculated after one selects the start of t_1 as the first data point in which the activity on the upslope is equal to or exceeds 10% of the peak activity. C_2 is again chosen at the end of t_2. The normal value of C_2/C_1, using this method is 30% (±7.6% SD).[1]
   c. In addition, one can calculate the C_2/C_1 ratio while selecting the data points as guided by the fitted pulmonary first-transit curve, which is generated after the use of the gamma-func-

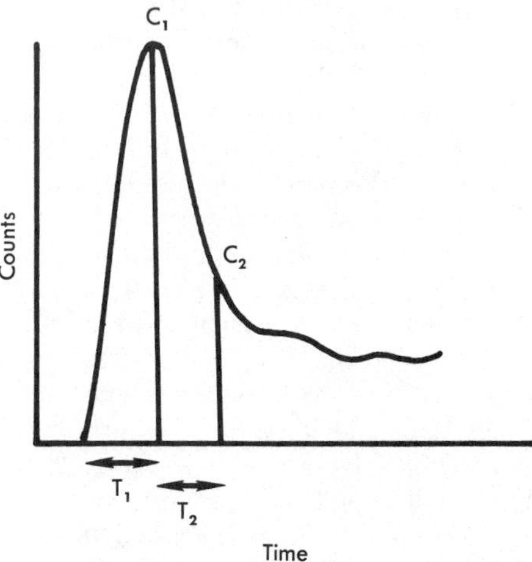

Fig. 11-11. Pulmonary time-activity curve: C_2/C_1 ratio method.

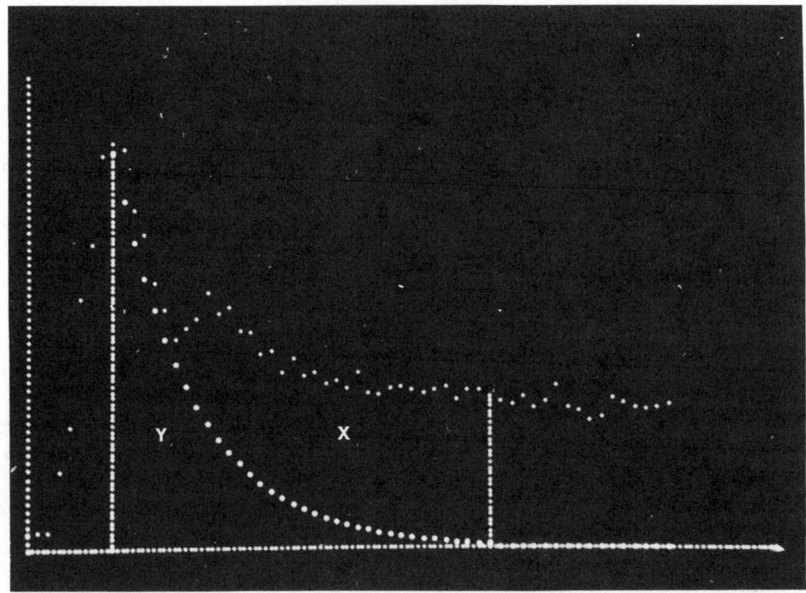

Fig. 11-12. Pulmonary time-activity curve: area-ratio method. (From Alderson, P. O., Gilday, D. L., and Wagner, H. N., Jr.: Atlas of pediatric nuclear medicine, St. Louis, 1978, The C. V. Mosby Co.)

tion computer algorithm (see below). C_1 corresponds to the real counts recorded at the time of the fitted maximum; t_1 is the time from the beginning of the fitted curve (that is, at 10% of the original maximum) to C_1; t_2 is equal to t_1, and originates at C_1; C_2 is the actual number of counts on the downslope obtained at t_2. The normal value is 26% (±7.4% SD).[1]

2. *Area-ratio calculation using regression analysis of descending portion of radionuclide pulmonary time-activity curve*[4]: This analysis is best performed by computer and is based on Stewart-Hamilton extrapolation. After generating the pulmonary radionuclide time-activity curve, the downslope is replotted on semilogarithmic coordinates. Regression analysis of the initial monoexponential portion is performed by extrapolation to 1% of the peak activity. The extrapolated portion is then redrawn on the curve. A line perpendicular to the base line is drawn at the 1% level (Fig. 11-12). Two areas *x* and *y* are now defined. Area *y* is bordered superiorly by the fitted line extrapolated to 1% peak value, inferiorly by the base line, and on its left side by a line extending perpendicularly on the base to the peak. Area *x*, which includes the recirculated (shunted) radioactivity, is bordered by the extrapolated line, the original downslope, and the line drawn perpendicularly on the base line at the point of 1% peak value. The ratio of the two areas x/y is calculated. The normal x/y ratio is less than 0.7 and the ratio in patients with left-to-right shunts is more than 0.8.[1]

   Regression analysis of the initial part of the downslope may be difficult if distortion of the curve occurs too early. The monoexponential phase may be nonexistent or too short to allow accurate analysis.

3. Q_P/Q_S *calculation using a gamma-variate computer algorithm.*[27] This method requires a computer. After the radionuclide pulmonary time-activity curve is generated (Fig. 11-13, *A*), the histogram is fitted to a gamma-variate function of the form

$$c(t_i) = K t_i^{\alpha} e^{-t_i/\beta}$$

using a least-squares technique (where K, α, and β are parameters chosen by the fitting technique, t_i is the ith time, and $c(t_i)$ is the concentration at this time). The limits of the fit are from 10% of the maximum activity on the upslope to 70% of the maximum activity on the downslope. The derived histogram is considered to represent a normal first pulmonary transit. The derived curve (Fig. 11-13, *B*) is subtracted from the remainder of the original data to obtain the difference of the original and fitted curves (Fig. 11-13, *C*). The

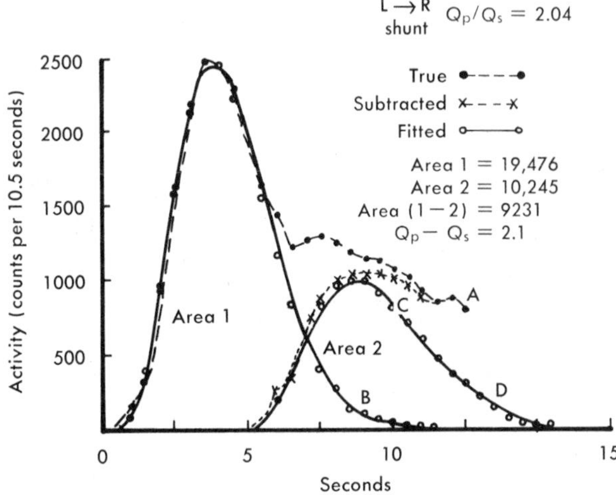

Fig. 11-13. Abnormal pulmonary time-activity histogram with area analysis. The two gamma function–determined areas and the method of determining Q_p/Q_s ratio are shown. (From Maltz, D. L., and Treves, S.: Circulation **47:**1049, 1973. By permission of the American Heart Association, Inc.)

curve representing this difference is again fitted to a gamma function; the limits of the fit are from 10% of a specially defined maximum on the upslope to one point after this maximum. This maximum is defined as the last point above which the rise of activity fails to increase to at least 105% of the previous point (Fig. 11-13, *D*). The areas of the gamma variate–fitted curves (A_1 and A_2) are calculated. The percentage of the cardiac output that is returned through the shunt is given by

$$\frac{A_2}{A_1} \times 100\%$$

A more common measure of shunt flow is the ratio of pulmonary to systemic blood flow:

$$\frac{Q_P}{Q_S} = \frac{A_1}{A_1 - A_2}$$

Interpretation of results

False-positive results may be obtained in patients with congestive failure and valvular heart disease. Patients with small shunts (less than 1.2:1) may not be detected by the above techniques.

EVALUATION OF CARDIAC SHUNTS BY DUAL-ISOTOPE RADIOCARDIOGRAPHY[16]

One can diagnose and evaluate cardiac shunts by dual-isotope radiocardiography using ^{133}Xe in saline and ^{99m}Tc-sulfur colloid. One can determine the location of the shunt by selectively obtaining time-activity curves for each radionuclide bolus from the atria and ventricles. The curves have characteristic patterns in the normal and abnormal states.

An intravenous bolus of 5 to 10 mCi ^{133}Xe in saline followed by a bolus of 2 to 4 mCi of ^{99m}Tc-sulfur colloid are administered. The techniques of bolus administration, scintigraphic recording, and generation of time-activity curves from individual cardiac chambers have been previously described.

In a normal person, the intravenous injection of a bolus of ^{133}Xe in saline results in a time-activity curve with a single peak over the right atrium or ventricle. Since ^{133}Xe is completely cleared by the lungs into air, no radioactivity will be detected in the left side of the heart. An intravenous bolus of ^{99m}Tc-sulfur colloid will produce a single peak curve over the right side of the heart and also over the left side of the heart with the left-side peak occurring later than the right; this delay is attributable to passage of the bolus through the lungs (Fig. 11-14, *A*).

In patients with right-to-left cardiac shunts, ^{133}Xe saline solution produces two simultaneous peaks, one over each side of the heart, because of shunting of some of the isotope through the septal defect. The remainder of the ^{133}Xe is cleared by the lungs. The ^{99m}Tc-sulfur colloid bolus shows a single-peak curve over the right side of the heart and dual peaks over the left side. The first peak over the left side of the heart appears simultaneously with the peak over the right side because of flow of some of the radionuclide through the shunt. The second peak over the left side of the heart occurs later and is attributable to arrival of the nonshunted part of the bolus after transit-

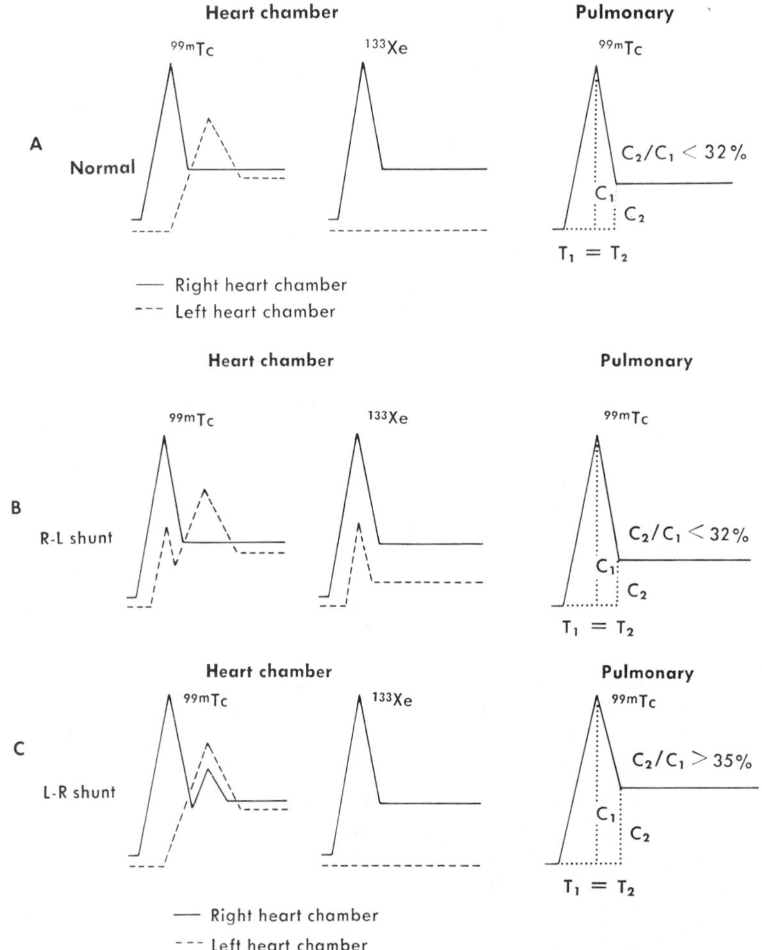

Fig. 11-14. Heart and pulmonary dilution curves. Characteristic heart chamber *(two left)* and pulmonary *(right)* dilution curves and C_2/C_1 ratio. Heart curves obtained with ^{133}Xe in saline solution and ^{99m}Tc-sulfur colloid. Pulmonary curves obtained with ^{99m}Tc. **A,** Dilution curves in normal individual. **B,** Abnormal dilution curve in patient with right-to-left shunt. Pattern of pulmonary curve and C_2/C_1 ratio are identical to those of normal individual. **C,** Curves and ratio in patient with left-to-right shunt. ^{133}Xe curve is identical to that of normal individual, but pulmonary curve is abnormal with elevated C_2/C_1 ratio. (From Greenfield, L. D., and Bennett, L. R.: Radiology **111:**359-363, May 1974.)

ing through the pulmonary circulation (Fig. 11-14, *B*).

In patients with left-to-right cardiac shunts the ^{133}Xe curves will be normal. On the other hand the ^{99m}Tc-sulfur colloid curves show a single peak over the left side of the heart and two peaks over the right side. The initial peak over the right side of the heart is caused by the initial normal bolus flow, whereas the second peak is caused by the abnormal flow of the radionuclide from the left side of the heart to the right through the abnormal shunt. The second peak over the right side of the heart occurs simultaneously with the peak over the left side of the heart (Fig. 11-14, *C*).

EVALUATION OF CARDIAC SHUNTS USING HEART CHAMBER RADIONUCLIDE TIME-ACTIVITY CURVES

After the intravenous administration of a radionuclide bolus, analysis of time-activity curves of the first transit from individual cardiac chambers can determine the anatomic location of the shunt. Qualitative as well as quantitative information about the shunt can also be derived from curve analysis. The abnormal shunt flow is detected from the curve or curves of the chambers distal to the abnormal communication.[47]

The technique of generating time-activity curves

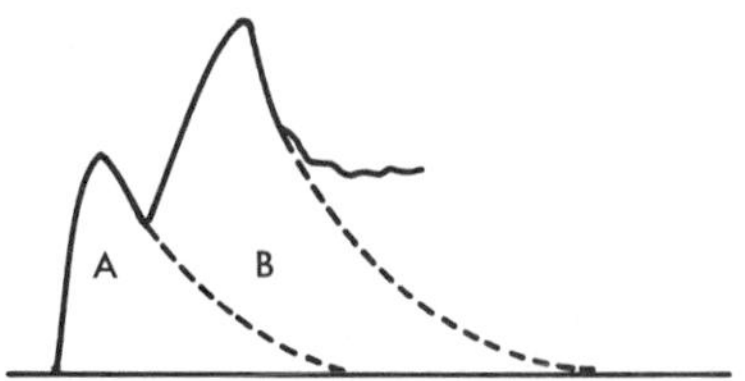

Fig. 11-15. Right-to-left shunt. In this shunt, left ventricular time-activity curve shows double peak. Downslope after each peak is extrapolated. Area *A* is attributable to shunt. Total area *(A + B)* represents area of bolus.

from individual cardiac chambers is essentially the same as that of the pulmonary time-activity curve. The only modification in the procedure is in patient positioning. For best visualization of the two ventricles as separate structures, the modified left anterior oblique view is employed. The patient lies supine, and the detector head of the scintillation camera is angled approximately 30 degrees in a left anterior oblique position and also 10 to 15 degrees caudad.

The technique, however, is difficult to perform in babies, since the size of individual cardiac chambers may be too small to be adequately selected as regions of interest from the images. Overlap between cardiac chambers and uncertainty of outlining valvular planes add to the difficulties of the procedure.

In patients with right-to-left shunts, the left ventricular time-activity curve shows a double peak. The first peak is attributable to the shunted blood, and it occurs almost at the same time as the right ventricular peak. The second peak is attributable to the arrival of the nonshunted portion of the bolus after normally passing through the pulmonary vasculature (Fig. 11-15). The downslope after the second peak is monoexponential initially, but later the slope is changed because of the arrival of the normally recirculating radionuclide. In order to determine the areas of the shunt and bolus under the curve, the downslopes after each peak are extrapolated to the base line. The area of the shunt is located under the curve before the first extrapolated line. The area of the bolus is located before the second extrapolated line (including the shunt area). The shunt flow is calculated when the shunt area is related to the total bolus area.

In patients with left-to-right shunts, a histogram from the right ventricle shows, similar to the pulmonary time-activity curve, an early change in the downslope of the curve because of superimposition of the shunted activity from the left side of the heart. Later the downslope is again altered because of normal recirculation of the tracer. Curve analysis can yield quantitative information.

In patients with bidirectional shunts, the time-activity curves from individual atria and ventricles will determine the shunts at the atrial and ventricular levels to be in opposite directions.

DETECTION OF LEFT-TO-RIGHT CARDIAC SHUNTS BY INHALATION OF $C^{15}O_2$

Oxygen 15, a positron emitter with a physical half-life of 2.05 minutes, is only available in a small number of medical centers because of the need of a cyclotron for its production. The use of $C^{15}O_2$ inhalation for the diagnosis of left-to-right shunts therefore is not common.

In principle, when CO_2 is inhaled, it dissolves in the water within the pulmonary venous blood. After the inhalation of a single bolus of $C^{15}O_2$ gas, instantaneous labeling of the pulmonary blood occurs. Subsequently, the labeled blood will flow to the left side of the heart. The clearance of radioactivity from the lungs follows a mathematically predictable pattern. In patients with left-to-right cardiac shunts, the clearance of radioactivity from the lungs is delayed because of shunt recirculation. By monitoring the pulmonary radioactivity and analyzing the pulmonary time-activity curve, one can diagnose and quantitate left-to-right cardiac shunts.[43]

DETECTION OF RIGHT-TO-LEFT CARDIAC SHUNTS USING ^{99m}Tc–HUMAN ALBUMIN MICROSPHERES OR ^{99m}Tc–MACRO-AGGREGATED ALBUMIN

After administration in a peripheral vein, the particles of radiolabeled human albumin microspheres or macroaggregated albumin are transported to the right side of the heart. The particles then enter the pulmonary circulation to be lodged into the capillary and precapillary bed of the lungs.

If a right-to-left cardiac shunt exists, part of the injected radionuclide enters the left side of the heart from the right side of the heart, bypassing the pulmonary circulation. The shunted particles enter the systemic circulation and become impacted in the capillary beds of various organs. Calculation of the shunt depends on the determination of the total body counts and those within the lungs.[14]

The total number and size of injected particles are very important. Because of the danger of embolization of the systemic circulation including the cerebral capillaries, the total number of particles must be kept to the minimum necessary to obtain the desired information (for example, 25,000 to 50,000). The particles should be in the range of 10 to 50 μm. Particles smaller than 10 μm will pass through the pulmonary capillaries to be phagocytized by the reticuloendothelial cells of the liver, spleen, and bone marrow, thus contributing to the total body counts and falsely elevating shunt estimation. Similarly, the presence of free ^{99m}Tc-pertechnetate with the injected radiopharmaceutical will contribute to the total body counts; therefore the labeling efficiency of the radiopharmaceutical must be very high.

Technique

1. The patient lies supine. The scintillation camera mounted with a parallel-hole collimator is placed beneath the patient.
2. A dose of ^{99m}Tc–macroaggregated albumin or ^{99m}Tc–human albumin microspheres is administered intravenously. The specific activity should be high to keep the injected volume small (the number of particles should be calculated prior to injection). The radioactivity varies depending on the age of the patient.
3. Imaging of the body is obtained and recorded on videotape or by computer. Multiple images with preset time may be necessary to include the entire body.
4. The net counts on the whole body are determined from the recorded images. The areas of the lungs are selected, and the pulmonary counts are also determined. The right-to-left shunt flow is calculated from the following equation:

$$\text{Percent right-to-left shunt} = \frac{\text{Total body counts} - \text{Total lung counts}}{\text{Total body counts}} \times 100$$

Remarks

1. If part of the injection is extravasated at the site of venipuncture, the infiltrated radioactivity should be isolated from the image as an area of interest and the counts subtracted from the total body counts to avoid overestimation of the shunt.
2. An increase in the amount of the shunt occurs in the crying child, and calculation may not then reflect the basal condition. This problem may be circumvented by insertion of a butterfly needle into a peripheral vein. A three-way stopcock is connected, and the vein is kept open by heparinized saline from a syringe connected to the three-way stopcock. The syringe containing the radiopharmaceutical is also connected to the three-way stopcock. When the child is calm, the radiopharmaceutical is administered and flushed with saline.
3. Precise separation of the base of the right lung from the liver dome may be difficult at times.
4. When the kidneys are visualized, the shunt is usually in excess of 15%.
5. The technique is potentially harmful because of embolization of the cerebral circulation. The procedure is kept safe when the number of particles is kept to the minimum required to give the needed information.

Common procedures used for diagnosis of cardiac shunts

From the preceding, it is clear that many techniques are available for cardiac shunt diagnosis. For left-to-right shunt determination, the radionuclide angiocardiogram with analysis of the pulmonary time-activity histogram is the procedure commonly used. For right-to-left shunts, the technique commonly used is the one that utilizes either ^{99m}Tc–human albumin microspheres or ^{99m}Tc–macroaggregated albumin.

MYOCARDIAL PERFUSION IMAGING WITH ^{201}Tl-THALLOUS CHLORIDE

Myocardial perfusion imaging is performed to detect the regional distribution of the coronary arterial blood flow. The use of thallium radionuclide for this purpose was suggested by Kawana et al.[25] in 1970. Thallous ion (Tl^+) has been shown to become distributed in tissues in a manner almost identical to that of the potassium ion.

Thallium-201 radiopharmaceutical: mechanism of localization of ^{201}thallous ion

After intravenous administration of ^{201}Tl-thallous chloride, the ^{201}Tl-thallous ion, as a potassium-ion analog, is distributed to the whole body where it is rapidly extracted in numerous organs, including the heart, kidneys, liver, spleen, and skeletal muscles. The extracted thallium is primarily located intracellularly (the extraction of thallium by the myocardium is probably caused by activation of the sodium-potassium ATPase enzyme system). Because of the high extraction efficiency of the thallous ions reaching the myocardial cells through the blood supply,[36] the initial uptake and distribution of these ions within the heart are related to the coronary blood flow.

The intravenously administered ^{201}Tl-thallous chloride clears from the blood exponentially with a biologic half-life of approximately 30 seconds. Myocardial uptake occurs rapidly and is near the maximal level in less than 2 minutes. The heart extracts only a small fraction of the injected dose (4% to 5%), and the maximal concentration in normal myocardium is reached by about 10 minutes. The blood radioactivity decreases to a range of 2% to 3% of the injected dose by approximately 10 minutes after injection. After administration, the myocardium-to-background counting ratio increases gradually and reaches a plateau at 10 to 20 minutes. Blood clearance is faster with exercise.

Thallium 201 decays by electron capture to mercury 201 with a physical half-life of 73.1 hours. The photons are emitted by the excited states of ^{201}Hg. The

Table 11-1. Radiation dose of ^{201}Tl-thallous chloride

Tissue	Rads/mCi
Heart	0.34
Small intestines	0.65
Kidneys	1.47
Liver	0.62
Red marrow	0.34
Ovaries	0.57
Testes	0.54
Thyroid	0.75
Total body	0.24

principal radiation emissions are x rays in the range of 68 to 80.3 keV (94.5% of the disintegration) and gamma rays of 167.4 keV (10% of the disintegration) as well as those of 135.3 keV (2.65% of the disintegration). ^{201}Tl is cyclotron produced and is essentially carrier free. However, contamination with minute quantities of ^{203}Pb and ^{202}Tl is present.

Thallium salts are toxic. The total amount of ^{201}thallous chloride administered for imaging in the recommended dosage contains only a few nanograms of elemental thallium. This represents a multimillion margin of safety from the reported minimal lethal dose in man. The adult dose of ^{201}Tl is 1.5 to 2 mCi given intravenously. The radiation dose is outlined in Table 11-1.

Pathophysiologic basis of ^{201}Tl-perfusion imaging at rest and exercise

Myocardial perfusion imaging is most useful in the detection of fixed perfusion abnormalities associated with prior myocardial infarction and in the diagnosis of transient focal myocardial ischemia that is induced by myocardial stress from coronary artery disease.

When the ^{201}Tl-thallous chloride is administered at rest, a perfusion defect seen on a myocardial image usually indicates a prior infarction, the age of which cannot be determined from the scan. An infarcted area of the heart contains either dead muscle in the acute phase or scar tissue after healing.

In most patients with ischemic heart disease the coronary blood flow is usually adequate for myocardial needs during rest. Transient coronary ischemia, however, is usually induced on myocardial stress, such as by exercise. With exertion, when there is a demand for increased myocardial blood supply, flow through the severely narrowed coronary arteries cannot increase to meet such a demand resulting in ischemia. The affected zone contains viable myocardial tissue, since the transient ischemia is not of sufficient magnitude or duration to cause muscle necrosis. Ischemic heart disease can be diagnosed by ^{201}Tl imaging if a perfusion defect is not seen at rest but is induced after myocardial stress. Such evaluation may be performed after one obtains two independent imaging studies separated by a few days, one with the radionuclide injection given at rest and the other at stress.

It is possible also to diagnose ischemic heart disease after a single injection of ^{201}Tl-thallous chloride given during myocardial stress. A focal abnormality seen on initial imaging, started within minutes after radionuclide administration may be caused by either stress-induced transient ischemia or a fixed perfusion defect attributable to a prior infarction. However, if the perfusion defect is caused by transient myocardial ischemia, radiothallium redistributes gradually into this perfusion defect, indicating the existence of viable myocardial tissue at the site of the abnormality. Lack of redistribution indicates a prior infarction and absence of viable tissue at the site of the abnormality. The causes of the redistribution phenomenon are not well understood, and restoration of a normal amount of blood supply is not necessary for it to happen.[39]

When the radionuclide is administered at the time of stress, evidence of redistribution may be demonstrated by a comparison of early and delayed images. The early images are started within a few minutes after the injection and the delayed, a few hours later. Stress images should be completed within 30 to 40 minutes after exercise because some redistribution begins immediately.

Since administration of the radiopharmaceutical at the time of exercise is difficult, an intravenous catheter is inserted into a suitable vein and connected to a three-way stopcock. To keep the vein open, one should connect one end of the stopcock either to a slow drip of 5% dextrose or to a syringe filled with heparinized saline with all blood in the catheter displaced by the heparinized solution to prevent clotting within the catheter. The remaining end of the stopcock is used for introducing the radionuclide.

Thallium-201 myocardial images show poor contrast between the heart and neighboring structures, particularly if the injection is administered at rest. This is caused by (1) the small differences of concentration of thallium in the heart compared to surrounding structures, (2) the low photon yield from the small dose given, (3) the tissue absorption of the low energy emissions, (4) the inherently poor resolution of the scintillation camera when low-energy photons for imaging are used, and (5) some Compton scattering in the patient as well as septal penetration of photons in the collimator. The imaging problem is further accentuated by the need to resolve small abnormalities.

To improve the myocardium-to-background counting ratios, one should inject patients in the fasting state and after they have been in an upright position (for at least 1 to 2 minutes). Fasting decreases the blood flow to the gastrointestinal organs. The upright position decreases the pulmonary blood volume and pulmonary transit time. Such measures result in decreased uptake by the gastrointestinal tract and liver, as well as by the lungs, but do not affect the myocardial blood flow or uptake. It should be noted that with injections administered during exercise the myocardium-to-background counting ratio is improved further because exercise increases the myocardial blood flow and decreases that of the viscera, since a portion of the splanchnic blood supply is diverted to skeletal muscles.

Stress test. The stress test must be performed by a qualified physician experienced in cardiology and resuscitation techniques. A defibrillator and other standard cardiopulmonary resuscitation equipment and medications must be available. The stress test is not performed on patients with recent myocardial infarction or on those with a serious disease where stress can endanger life.

Exercise can be performed on a bicycle ergometer or on a treadmill (Fig. 11-16). Prior to exercise, the intravenous catheter is inserted into a suitable vein as described above, and the patient is connected by electrodes to an ECG machine. Preexercise measurements of the pulse rate and blood pressure are obtained as a base line, and continuous ECG monitoring is begun. During exercise, the patient is observed closely by the physician, and the heart rate as well as the blood pressure are recorded every 1 to 3 minutes. The exercise level is gradually increased until the patient's maximal exercise capacity is reached. It is usually possible to judge when nearing maximal stress, and the patient should be forewarned to inform the attending physician at least 1 minute in advance before he expects the end of his ability to carry on with exercise. At this point, the radionuclide is injected, and the catheter is flushed with saline. Exercise is continued for at least 30 seconds afterwards. The radionuclide is ideally given at the time of maximal myocardial stress. However, this may be limited by the development of exercise-induced angina, dyspnea, or general fatigue. Exercise should be terminated if ventricular arrhythmia, signs of cerebrovascular insufficiency, or hypotension develops.

After exercise, the intravenous catheter should be left in place for some time in case resuscitation efforts should become necessary. Complications such as arrhythmia or postural hypotension can occur during the immediate postexercise period. The incidence of ventricular arrhythmia is, however, fortunately rare.

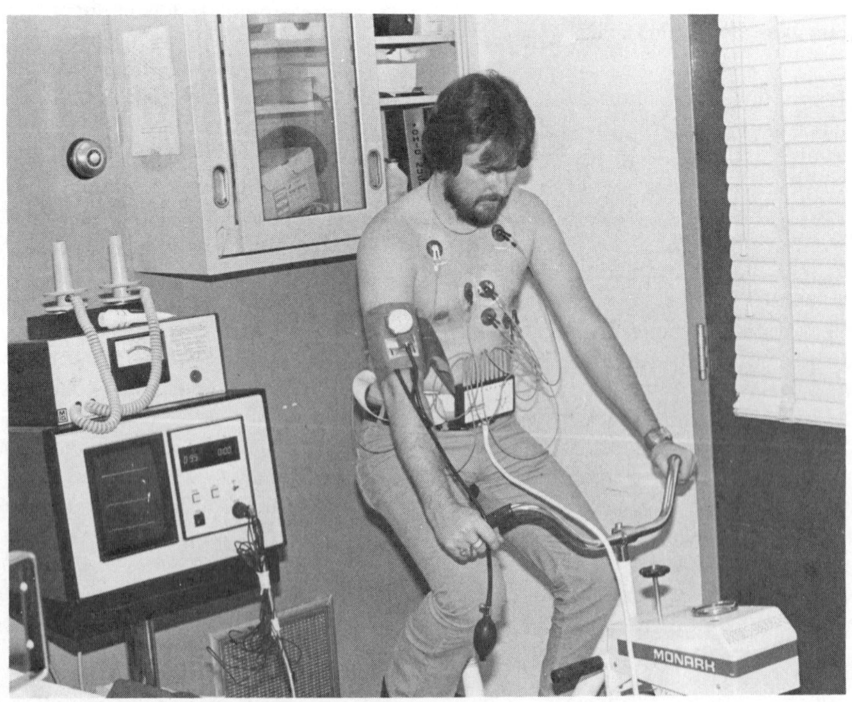

Fig. 11-16. Patient being stressed on bicycle ergometer.

ECG recording is continued during the postexercise phase until the stress-induced ECG changes and the heart rate return to the normal resting preexercise level. During this immediate postexercise phase, the physician must observe the patient closely. The intravenous catheter may be removed, and ECG monitoring may be stopped after ensuring that the patient's condition is stable and that he is out of danger from possible complications. Imaging should be started within 5 to 10 minutes after the injection.

Patient positioning and views obtained. Multiple views are required in order to visualize the heart adequately. The standard views include anterior, two left anterior oblique (such as at 30 and 60 degrees), and left lateral projections.

Precise positioning of the patient in relation to the camera is essential for comparison of the results of rest and exercise tests or of the exercise and redistribution images. This is achieved when a fixed relative position of the camera and imaging table is maintained and the patient is lying supine with the long axes of the patient and the table parallel to each other. The anterior and left anterior oblique views are obtained when the camera head is rotated to the desired position. In each view, the collimator face should just touch the skin in order to minimize the distance between the collimator and the patient and also to assure uniformity of positioning. The left lateral view is better obtained with the patient lying on the right side with the camera head parallel to the bed. In steep left anterior oblique and lateral imaging, the left arm should be raised above the head so that it would not lie between the collimator and the heart area. Care should be taken to minimize the amount of abdominal activity in the field of view because the counts recorded from this area will only detract from those recorded from the myocardium.

The scintillation camera is not capable of resolving the different photopeaks of the x rays emitted in the range of 68 to 80.3 keV. Instead these x rays appear as one peak at approximately 80 keV and account for the majority of the useful imaging emissions.

For cameras with a single spectrometer, the mercury x rays are utilized for imaging. The window is set at 20%, centered at 80 keV. If a second spectrometer is available, the photopeak at 167.4 keV may also be utilized. In the case of a third spectrometer, the 135.3 keV photons are utilized in addition, with the latter two photopeaks also incorporating 20% window widths.

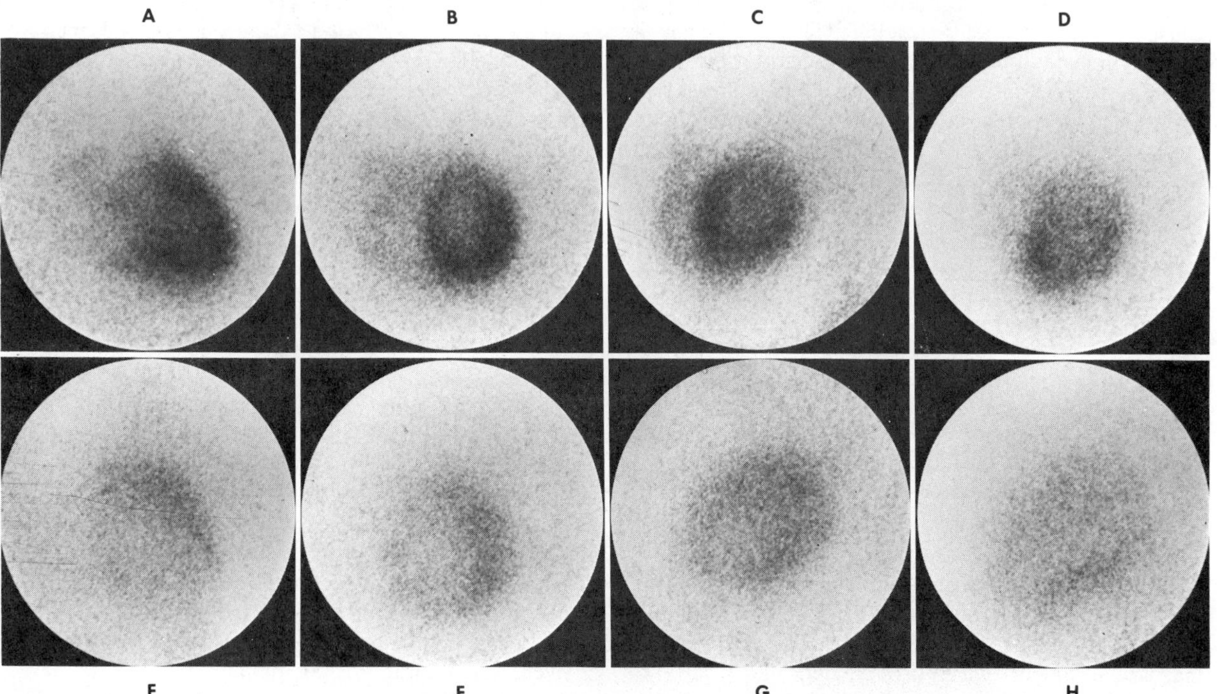

Fig. 11-17. Normal thallium-201 myocardial perfusion images: **A,** anterior; **B,** 35-degree LAO; **C,** 65-degree LAO; **D,** left lateral. Abnormal perfusion in images: **E,** anterior; **F,** 35-degree LAO; **G,** 65-degree LAO; **H,** left lateral.

Using a 10-inch scintillation camera and a low-energy, all purpose, parallel-hole collimator, an image of approximately 250,000 to 500,000 preset counts are obtained. The collection time is approximately 5 to 10 minutes.

If a region of interest over the heart is used for measurement of information density during imaging, 200,000 counts should be collected from the myocardial area.

When a computer is used for static-image collection, an acquisition matrix of 64×64 pixels or greater is employed for good spatial resolution.

Multigated imaging.[2] Static images of the heart when acquired continuously over a period of time are collected without regard to motion. Blurring from respiratory motion is negligible, but blurring from beating of the heart is significant. By the use of ECG synchronization for multigated imaging, improved resolution is achieved. The procedure is lengthy, however.

Results and interpretation

In the normal resting thallium images, only the left ventricle is visualized. The right ventricle is either not visualized at all, or very poorly seen, because of its smaller mass compared to that of the left ventricle. In normal hearts the left ventricular wall either appears like a doughnut or is U shaped with the opening at the valvular planes. The centrally decreased activity is caused by the ventricular cavity. The heart image is better delineated on exercise studies than on those obtained at rest because of the increased myocardial perfusion and decreased background activity, as previously mentioned. On exercise studies, the right ventricle is usually well visualized. If the right ventricle is visualized on a resting study, this often indicates right ventricular hypertrophy.

The significance of perfusion defects during rest-exercise or exercise-reperfusion imaging, in the diagnosis of ischemic heart disease and myocardial infarction has been described. The location of the perfusion abnormality can be defined from these studies. Fig. 11-17 shows examples of ^{201}Tl myocardial images.

DETECTION OF ACUTE MYOCARDIAL INFARCTION BY IMAGING WITH INFARCT-AVID RADIOPHARMACEUTICALS

In 1962, Carr et al. demonstrated increased uptake of ^{203}Hg-chlormerodrin in experimentally produced myocardial infarcts in dogs.[8] Several other radiopharmaceutical agents were investigated and found to localize in areas of myocardial necrosis. These agents included ^{203}Hg-mercurifluorescein derivatives, ^{99m}Tc-tetracycline, ^{67}Ga citrate, and ^{99m}Tc-glucoheptonate; however they were found unsuitable for routine clinical use.

The bone-scanning agent ^{99m}Tc–stannous pyrophosphate is presently used in the detection of acute myocardial infarction. Other bone-seeking radionuclides including other phosphate agents have been investigated, and some may be potentially useful but ^{99m}Tc–stannous pyrophosphate has been found to give the best images.

Imaging of acute myocardial infarction with ^{99m}Tc–stannous pyrophosphate demonstrates the lesion by positive (or avid) accumulation of the radionuclide at the site of the lesion[6]; the rest of the myocardium excludes the radioactivity. By contrast, other agents such as radioactive potassium (^{43}K) and its radioactive analogs of rubidium (^{86}Rb, ^{84}Rb, ^{81}Rb), cesium (^{131}Cs, ^{127}Cs, ^{129}Cs), and thallium (^{201}Tl), as well as ^{13}N-ammonia and certain radioiodinated fatty acids (such as ^{131}I–oleic acid) are taken up by the normal myocardium while the lesion is demonstrated as a cold defect.

Mechanism of localization of ^{99m}Tc–stannous pyrophosphate in acutely infarcted myocardium

The exact mechanism of localization of ^{99m}Tc–stannous pyrophosphate within an infarcted area of the heart is not clear. Calcium ions are deposited intracellularly in the form of hydroxyapatite or hydroxyapatite-like crystals within the mitochondria of acutely necrotic myocardial cells.[10,11] This deposition is associated with irreversible cell damage but only when arterial blood flow to the damaged area is present.[37,38] Similarly the uptake of ^{99m}Tc–stannous pyrophosphate occurs in areas of myocardial cell death or irreversible damage with maintained perfusion and intracellular calcification.

Residual or collateral flow is usually maintained in the peripheral zone of an infarct where such calcification takes place maximally. The central region of the infarct, which lacks perfusion, does not show calcification. These pathophysiologic parameters may explain the doughnut appearance of ^{99m}Tc–stannous pyrophosphate accumulation in the large transmural infarcts and the diffuse scintigraphic pattern seen with the subendocardial type.

Time of scan abnormalities relative to disease onset

Myocardial-infarct scans with ^{99m}Tc–stannous pyrophosphate become positive 10 to 12 hours after infarction. The intensity of uptake is maximal 2 to 3 days after the onset. The affinity of the infarct for the radiopharmaceutical rapidly decreases after 1 week. However, some infarcts may remain positive for several weeks or months.

Indications for myocardial infarct scanning

Acute myocardial infarct scanning is not required in all patients, since the diagnosis is usually made from the symptoms, signs, ECG findings, and changes in serum enzymes. However, in certain situations the scan may be the only way of establishing the diagnosis. The presence of left bundle branch block masks the infarct pattern on the ECG, and the presence of an old infarct, nonspecific ECG changes, permanent pacemaker, and drug intake may make ECG interpretation difficult. Enzyme changes are usually helpful in making the diagnosis of acute myocardial infarction when determinations are obtained at the right time but the levels are frequently elevated because of intramuscular injections or other factors. Serum determination of the specific MB-CK isoenzyme level is not routinely available in many hospitals. After heart surgery, the different serum-enzyme levels, including MB-CK as well as ECG findings, are abnormal and may not allow the diagnosis of intraoperative or postoperative infarction; in such circumstances the myocardial infarct scan is of an immense value in localizing the infarct. Myocardial contusion and right ventricular infarcts are difficult to diagnose without scanning. Myocardial infarct scanning may also be utilized for the documentation of reinfarction or extension of an existing infarct. However, such are only possible with serial scanning, documenting that the initial infarct had been receding or had disappeared prior to the revisualization of a new lesion on a recent scan.

Radiopharmaceutical dosage and administration

The adult dose is 15 to 20 mCi of ^{99m}Tc–stannous pyrophosphate, given intravenously. The radiopharmaceutical is a bone-seeking agent, of which the kinetics and radiation dose are mentioned on p. 388.

Imaging is begun 2 hours after the administration of the radiopharmaceutical. Images showing diffuse uptake in the heart region may be repeated later (4 hours after injection) to exclude the possibility of blood-pool visualization.

A scintillation camera with a low-energy parallel-hole collimator, preferably a high-resolution one, is used for imaging.

Computer processing is not essential for scan interpretation, but simple background subtraction and contrast enhancement or removal of the rib structures from the images can be helpful.

Patients who are hemodynamically unstable or have cardiac arrhythmias should be continuously monitored in the coronary care unit. If the myocardial-infarct imaging is needed, it is most desirable to use a mobile scintillation camera at the bedside. If the patient is to be moved to the nuclear medicine facility, continuous cardiac monitoring by portable equipment should be instituted during transportation and while in the nuclear medicine laboratory, and the patient should be attended at all times by personnel experienced in cardiopulmonary monitoring and resuscitation.

Imaging is obtained in the anterior, 45-degree left anterior oblique, and left lateral projections. A 45-degree right anterior oblique view is occasionally performed in some laboratories. In some other laboratories, instead of a single left anterior oblique view, two images are obtained at different degrees of obliquity, such as at 30 to 40 degrees and at 60 to 70 degress. Imaging is performed with the patient supine. Lateral views in the supine position require the patient to be positioned at the edge of the bed. The left arm should be positioned above the head out of the field of view when the lateral and left anterior oblique views are performed, so that the collimator can be placed as close as possible to the patient's chest.

The patient should be positioned so that the sternum is located half-way down the field of view and somewhat off center so that the entire left side of the chest is included. Care should be taken to avoid including the left kidney in the image, since the counts derived from it will detract from the myocardial counts. When the lateral view is being taken, the sternum should be positioned at the edge of the image.

For adequate statistics, when a scintillation camera with a standard size field of view is being used, 300,000 to 500,000 counts should be accumulated for each image. In the case of the large-field-of-view camera, 500,000 to 600,000 counts should be collected.

The results of the myocardial infarct scan are graded 0 to 4+ depending on the intensity of activity seen over the heart area. Zero (0) uptake represents no activity, and 1+ uptake means a questionable faint activity. Definite uptake that is less than, equal to, or greater than bone uptake is classified as 2+, 3+, or 4+ respectively. The abnormality can be further classified as focal, involving one area of the heart, or diffuse, involving the entire region of the heart. Diffuse 1+ uptake is usually not associated with an infarct, whereas diffuse 2+ is equivocal. More intense diffuse myocardial uptake is considered abnormal. All focal uptake is also considered abnormal. Fig. 11-18 illustrates an abnormal scan indicating an acute myocardial infarction.

Focal abnormalities are seen in patients with recent myocardial infarction. Other causes reported include old infarction with or without ventricular aneurysm, continuing low-grade myocardial necrosis, valvular calcification, invasion of the left ventricle by cancer, myocardial contusion, and electrical cardioversion. It is likely that other conditions associated with myocardial necrosis such as myocarditis, myocardial abscess, penetrating heart trauma, and aneurysmectomy may also yield focal abnormalities on the scan. Diffuse uptake is seen with subendocardial infarction and has been reported with other conditions, including delayed clearance of radionuclide from the blood pool or with scans obtained soon after radionuclide administration.

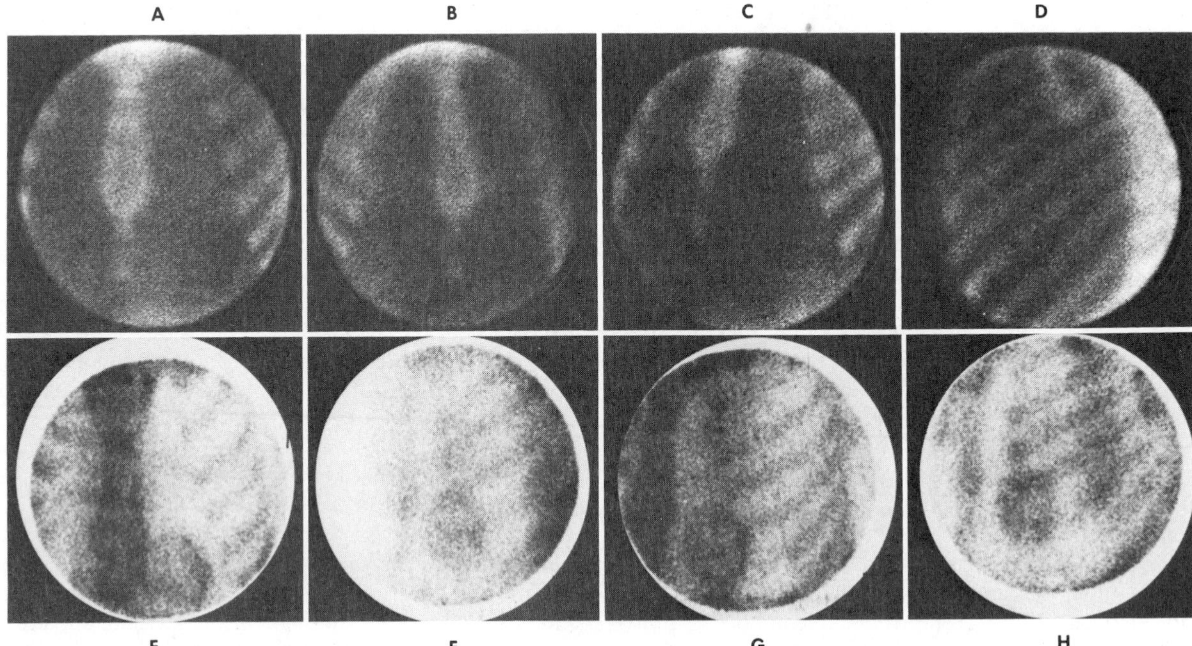

Fig. 11-18. Normal ^{99m}Tc-pyrophosphate myocardial images: **A,** anterior; **B,** RAO; **C,** LAO; **D,** left lateral. Abnormal concentration of radiopharmaceutical in **E,** anterior; **F,** left lateral; **G,** 40-degree LAO; **H,** 70-degree LAO.

The sensitivity and specificity of the scan for diagnosing or excluding the presence of acute myocardial infarction are better than 90%.

CARDIAC BLOOD-POOL IMAGING FOR DETECTION OF PERICARDIAL EFFUSION

Cardiac blood-pool imaging can be used for the diagnosis of pericardial effusion. Although the radionuclide techniques are highly sensitive for the detection of clinically significant pericardial effusions, the tests are less sensitive than is ultrasound examination. Ultrasound techniques also have the advantage of not using ionizing radiation.

Originally the radionuclide imaging technique involved rectilinear scanning of the chest after the intravenous injection of a blood pool–imaging agent such as ^{131}I–human serum albumin (HSA) or ^{99m}Tc-HSA.

Emission-transmission imaging techniques were also used for the diagnosis of pericardial effusion, however, with the advent of the scintillation camera, the methods have changed somewhat. Generally a radionuclide angiocardiogram with a bolus of ^{99m}Tc-HSA, ^{99m}Tc-pertechnetate, or ^{113m}In chloride is performed in the manner previously described. Dynamic imaging of the central circulation is recorded, followed by a static scan. The latter image shows the cardiac, pulmonary, and hepatic blood pools. Normally these three blood pools are contiguous with one another. If these organs are separated by spaces void of activity, the presence of pericardial effusion is considered highly likely. Another sign is an abnormally small cardiac blood-pool image when compared to heart size on the chest x-ray film.

With standard-sized scintillation cameras, the image should contain at least 400,000 counts. With large-field-of-view cameras 600,000 counts should be collected. The high-resolution parallel-hole collimator should be employed.

Dosages of radiopharmaceuticals

The radiopharmaceutical dosage for ^{99m}Tc-pertechnetate is approximately 200 μCi/kg of body weight. For ^{99m}Tc-HSA the adult dose is 1 to 5 mCi. For ^{113m}In chloride the adult dose is 5 to 15 mCi. The use of ^{99m}Tc-HSA or ^{113m}In chloride (the indium ion becomes bound to plasma transferrin after intravenous injection) is preferable to ^{99m}Tc-pertechnetate because those agents remain within the circulating blood pool much longer than does the radiopertechnetate.

Radiation dose

If ^{99m}Tc-pertechnetate is used, the total body radiation dose is 0.01 to 0.02 rad/mCi. When ^{99m}Tc-HSA or ^{113m}In chloride is used, the total body dose per millicurie is still 0.01 to 0.02 rad.

THROMBOSIS DETECTION

There are three factors that may lead to thrombogenesis: stasis of blood, vessel-wall abnormalities, and blood hypercoagulability. A blood clot is formed when fibrinogen in the plasma is converted to insoluble strands of fibrin, which trap blood cells. This conversion is achieved through the action of the enzyme, thrombin. Thrombin is formed from prothrombin, which is normally present in plasma through the interaction of tissue and platelet factors with other plasma factors. Calcium ions are essential for the reactions leading to the generation of thrombin and fibrin.

Thrombosis of the deep veins of the lower extremities, particularly of the illiofemoral veins, is the most common source of pulmonary emboli. Another frequent source of pulmonary emboli is thrombosis in the pelvic veins. Since pulmonary embolization can be fatal, thrombosis of the deep veins of the lower extremities or in the pelvis is considered a serious condition. Superficial vein thrombosis does not usually cause such embolization.

Risk factors associated with venous thrombosis in the lower extremities include prolonged bed rest, severe illness, immobilization, malignancy, estrogen intake including oral contraceptives, the postoperative and postpartum states, orthopedic trauma and surgery, congestive heart failure, polycythemia rubra vera, and disseminated intravascular coagulation.

To prevent the hazard of pulmonary thromboembolism, it is important that one promptly recognizes and treats deep vein thrombosis. Unfortunately such thrombosis may be silent in more than half of the patients, and when symptoms and signs are present, they are variable and nonspecific. Frequently pulmonary embolism is the initial clinical event that indicates the presence of deep vein thrombosis.

Several tests are currently available to aid in the diagnosis of deep vein thrombosis of the lower extremities. Radiographic contrast venography is the most specific test and provides the standard by which other diagnostic techniques are judged. Unfortunately, contrast venography is invasive, causes discomfort to the patient and can be risky. It cannot be repeated as often as may be indicated and by itself may lead to thrombosis in some patients. Noninvasive screening procedures are available such as Doppler ultrasound, plethysmographic techniques, ^{125}I-fibrinogen-uptake test. ^{123}I-fibrinogen scanning, and radionuclide venography.

^{125}I-FIBRINOGEN-UPTAKE TEST

The concept of using radiolabeled fibrinogen in the detection of venous thrombosis was introduced in 1957 by Ambrus et al.[3] ^{131}I-fibrinogen was used clinically for the detection of thrombi by Palko et al. in 1964.[29] In 1965, Atkins and Hawkins introduced ^{125}I-fibrinogen.[5] The ^{125}I-fibrinogen-uptake test was later developed for screening of patients and for use at bedside by Kakkar et al.[23,24]

The test is useful as a screening procedure for the detection of deep vein thrombosis of the legs in high-risk patients such as those undergoing major orthopedic or other surgical procedures, obstetrical-patient myocardial infarction, pulmonary disease, malignancies, and other medical conditions known to be associated with a high incidence of thromboembolism. It is also used for the diagnosis of deep vein thrombosis in patients with signs or symptoms suggestive of this condition with or without associated pulmonary embolism. The test can also be performed in patients with pulmonary embolism to look for evidence of peripheral deep vein thrombosis in the lower extremities.

Mechanism of localization of radiolabeled fibrinogen and pathophysiologic considerations. Intravenously administered radiolabeled fibrinogen behaves in the same way as endogenous fibrinogen; both are converted to fibrin, which is laid down in an active thrombus.[22,28] Experimental evidence in dogs suggests that incorporation may also occur in preformed thrombi and that net thrombus propagation is not necessary for labeled fibrinogen uptake.[9] However, metabolically inactive thrombi, such as some established or old clots, may not take up the radiopharmaceutical or the uptake may not be sufficient to allow detection.

Choice of radioactive label. Compared to the use of ^{131}I, ^{125}I labeling of fibrinogen results in a lower radiation dose to the patient and an increased shelf life. The major disadvantage of ^{125}I is its soft photon emissions, which are readily attenuated by thick tissue, making the diagnosis of thrombosis in the veins of the upper thighs and pelvis difficult or impossible. Although ^{131}I-fibrinogen could provide imaging capability, the associated high radiation dose to the patient precludes the use of an adequate scanning dose. The use of ^{123}I for labeling fibrinogen is ideal for imaging, but ^{123}I is expensive and not widely available, and because of its short physical half-life, labeling must be performed shortly before the administration of the radiopharmaceutical. These factors limit the use of ^{123}I-fibrinogen to only a few centers at the present time.

^{125}I-fibrinogen is commercially available and is currently the most commonly used agent for clinical practice.

The recommended dose for a 70 kg man is 100 μCi of ^{125}I-fibrinogen, given intravenously.

The clearance of radioiodinated fibrinogen from the blood is slow, allowing continuation of the test for several days. During the period of study, the count rate over the areas of interest will decline with time mainly because of the metabolism of ^{125}I-fibrinogen, which leads to breakdown of the molecule and excretion of the radioactivity. Blood clearance may be accelerated in certain conditions, such as in the postoperative states. If continuation of the test is indicated after the counting statistics become unreliable, a second dose of the radiopharmaceutical may then be administered.

Patient preparation and important considerations. Activity from other radionuclide studies will interfere with counting because of the low-energy photons of ^{125}I. ^{125}I-fibrinogen should not be injected before one ensures that the background activity in the lower extremities (measured by the ^{125}I-fibrinogen-uptake probe) is negligible; additional nuclear medicine procedures should be deferred until the test is completed.

Before the intravenous injection of ^{125}I-fibrinogen, radioiodine uptake by the patient's thyroid gland must be blocked. Oral administration of an inorganic iodide preparation such as Lugol's iodine solution or saturated solution of potassium iodide, 10 to 15 drops daily, is given, begun approximately 24 hours before the injection and continued for 10 days afterward. If repeated injections are administered within days of each other, thyroid blockage should be continued for 3 weeks after the last injection. Iodides should not be given to patients with known sensitivity to iodine compounds. If the patient is allergic to iodine preparations, thyroid uptake can be blocked instead by potassium perchlorate.

Lactating mothers should substitute formula feeding because of the possibility of excreting radioiodine in the milk, leading to irradiation of the infant's thyroid.

The patient's legs should not be used for routine injections or for obtainment of blood samples so that production of inflammation or hematomas is avoided.

An efficient scintillation probe system for counting ^{125}I is required, preferably portable for use at the patient's bedside. Several types are available. The readout can be a digital scaler indicating counts or a rate meter showing percentages of full scale, or both.

Procedure of ^{125}I-fibrinogen uptake for detection of venous thrombosis in lower extremities. The radiopharmaceutical is injected intravenously. The lower extremities and precordium are marked with a waterproof marker. Markings should not be removed during the period of the test. The precordial mark is placed over the left fourth intercostal space, just lateral to the sternum. The markings on the lower extremities are separated by 2-inch segments; they start from the femoral vein at the middle of the inguinal ligament, follow a line to the abductor tubercle, and then descend the calf following a line from the middle of the popliteal fossa to the medioposterior aspect of the medial malleolus of the ankle. Additional markings are placed on the inside and outside of the calf (Fig. 11-19).

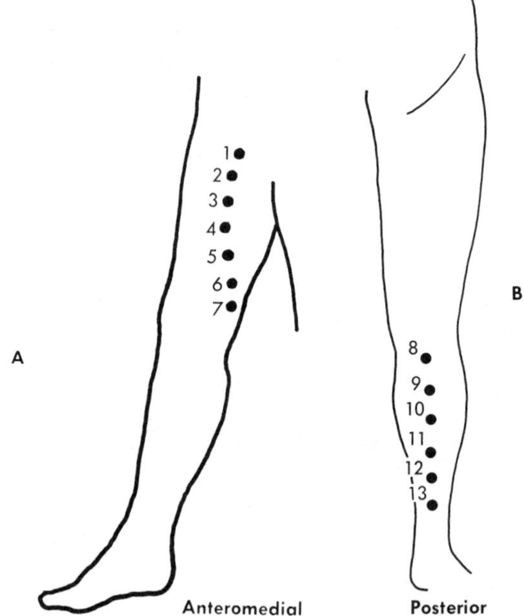

Fig. 11-19. Leg markings for ^{125}I-fibrinogen–uptake counting.

Counting procedure and schedule:

1. Calibrate the probe system to assure proper function before each counting session by counting a standard radioactive source. Protect the monitor probe by a thin cover such as a plastic wrap to prevent radioactive contamination by body fluids.
2. The patient should void immediately prior to starting each monitoring session to decrease the count contribution from ^{125}I in the urinary bladder. Skin contamination by urine should be avoided.
3. To decrease venous pooling in the lower extremities and to allow easy access to the calf, position the patient supine with the legs elevated above the heart level. The heels are placed on a stand so that both legs are elevated symmetrically.
4. Determine the precordial activity. This measured radioactivity is used as the 100% reference.
5. Then measure the radioactivity at the site of markings on the lower extremities. It is preferable to start at the thighs since ^{125}I may accumulate in the urinary bladder during the monitoring period. Each site is measured for 5 to 10 seconds, but monitoring should extend to 30 seconds in case of poor counting statistics. During counting,

place the probe on the leg without excessive pressure. Care should be given to assure the reproducibility of positioning of the probe at different monitoring sessions. Read measurements directly from the percent scale in the case of a rate meter. In the case of a scaler, read the counts and then determine the percentage values relative to the heart counts.

Initial monitoring can be performed 1 to 3 hours after radiopharmaceutical administration. Subsequently, it is performed at 24-hour intervals. The diagnosis is usually clear within 24 to 72 hours after the test is started and may be strongly suggestive from the first reading.

Depending on the clinical situation, the intervals between uptake measurements may be shortened or lengthened. When the test is performed prospectively on patients not known to have thrombosis but known to have a high risk of developing thrombosis, for example, surgical patients, monitoring can be performed every 24 or 48 hours after the initial reading (in the case of surgical patients a base-line preoperative measurement should also be obtained). With strong suspicion of thrombosis or when the measurements are suggestive of such a diagnosis, testing is performed at shorter intervals. The test can be continued for as long as there are statistically valid counts. However a second radiopharmaceutical dose may be required when the counting statistics become unreliable and continuation of the test is desired (see patient preparation, p. 320).

Interpretation of results. An area is considered abnormal when the uptake is 20% or greater than adjacent areas of the same leg or the contralateral position. A transient increase of uptake of this magnitude not confirmed on repeat monitoring is not considered abnormal. However, abnormally increased uptake attributable to active thrombosis can be seen within 1 hour after radiopharmaceutical administration. Although, in such circumstances, the diagnosis of venous thrombosis may be strongly suspected, confirmation of abnormal results depend on persistence of increased uptake obtained over a period of 24 hours or more.

The status of the legs should be known at the time of each counting session, since the existence or development of one of several conditions may lead to abnormal results. Abnormal results unrelated to thrombosis are seen with ulcers, wounds, cellulitis, abscess, hematoma, cysts, active arthritis, active psoriasis, trauma, and tissue masses and after venography, lymphangiography, or arthrography. However, the presence of one of these conditions should not preclude performing the test, since the pattern and degree of uptake may indicate the development of thrombosis. For example, at sites of orthopedic surgery, the counts may initially increase because of the postoperative changes, stabilize, and then decline; a change in this pattern with an increase in the size of the area of abnormal uptake or sudden rise in ^{125}I-fibrinogen concentration after an initial decline may indicate development of venous thrombosis.

Radiation dose. The absorbed radiation dose to the whole body for 100 μCi of ^{125}I-fibrinogen is 0.02 rad. If the thyroid gland is blocked, the highest radiation dose is delivered to the gastric wall with 0.13 rad per 100 μCi. If the thyroid uptake is not blocked, the radiation dose to the gland is 1.3 rads per 100 μCi.

RADIONUCLIDE VENOGRAPHY USING PARTICULATE RADIOPHARMACEUTICALS

Weber et al. were the first to note localized punctate uptake of radioactive macroaggregates of albumin (MAA) in the axillary region of some patients.[46] These patients were previously subjected to placement of indwelling intravenous catheters. The uptake was seen when the injection was made through the catheter and even several weeks after removal of the catheter if the injection was made on the same side. The intravenous retention of the MAA was attributed to trapping of the particles as they passed in areas of endothelial injury with associated clot deposits. This observation, in part, contributed to the present utilization of radioactive lung scanning agents for radionuclide venography.

Principle of test and mechanism of thrombus localization

The venous system to be studied is injected upstream with radioactive particles, followed by dynamic as well as delayed static imaging. The dynamic phase of the study is aimed at demonstrating abnormalities of venous blood flow such as obstruction, stasis, or collateral drainage.[45] Static imaging is directed toward detection of uptake by thrombi.

The mechanism of uptake of radioactive particles by a thrombus is not clear. More than one factor may be operative. Several theories have been proposed, but none of them, by itself, is sufficient to explain the entire phenomenon.[45] These theories are as follows[45]:

1. Adhesion of particles to the surface in areas of vascular endothelial damage or on clots that have not yet become endothelialized.
2. Electrostatic attraction between the unlike surface electrical charges of the thrombus and the particles. Such electrostatic forces are weak, however.
3. Mechanical entrapment of particles either by entanglement in microfibrils, which may extend

outward from the clot like a net, or by stasis of blood occurring as a result of venous thrombosis. The former might account for uptake in the case of fresh thrombi but fails to explain localization of old clots where such microfibrils are lacking. Stasis may lead to prolonged contact between particles and thrombus, thus aiding adhesion.

It is therefore believed that thrombus localization by radioactive particles may be related to a combination of adhesion, possibly electrostatic forces, and to a lesser extent actual mechanical entrapment.

Radioactive particles have been routinely used in many nuclear medicine laboratories for the diagnosis of venous thrombosis in the legs, pelvis, and upper extremities. Some investigators have reported results that correlate well with the more definitive study of contrast venography.[21,35,41] However, the varying degrees of success reported in the literature by different authors may be partly attributable to variations in methodology and interpretive criteria.[33,35] Standardization of an optimal test procedure will yield the most accurate results.

Radiopharmaceutical and dosage. The agents used are 3 to 6 mCi of ^{99m}Tc-labeled macroaggregated albumin (MAA) or human albumin microspheres (HAM). The number of particles injected must not violate the safety standards employed for lung scanning.

Imaging instruments. A scintillation camera, with or without whole body–imaging capability, is used. A low-energy high-sensitivity parallel-hole collimator is employed. A low-energy diverging collimator may be preferable at times.

Patient preparation

1. The patient lies supine.
2. Tourniquets are placed above the ankles, and a butterfly needle is placed in the dorsal vein of each foot. A three-way stopcock is attached to each needle, and a syringe containing saline is connected for flushing.
3. The tourniquets above the ankles are left in place. Other tourniquets applied above or below the knees are optional depending on the physician's preference. Some physicians place double tourniquets at such sites, whereas others also like to wrap bandages firmly around each leg from ankle to knee, prior to applying tourniquets.[21,48] Tourniquets and bandages are used for promoting deep-vein flow by obstructing superficial veins.
4. Radioactive markers are placed at the levels of the greater trochanters and knees.

Injection and imaging techniques. Imaging is performed from the anterior projection while the patient is supine. The collimator is placed as close to the body as possible. The details of the injection and imaging techniques published in the literature by different authors are variable.[20,21,32,35,41,45] However, the procedures to be described below are largely based on those published recently.[18,19,45] These are as follows:

Procedure when whole body–imaging capability is not available. When whole body–imaging capability is not available, the study is performed with multiple injections, so that all the desired areas are imaged. On the average, seven images are required, one for the lower abdomen and pelvis, and three for each lower extremity. Four radionuclide injections are made on each side.

Imaging is started with the camera detector being placed over the lower part of the inferior vena cava and iliac regions. For this view, an injection of 1 to 1.5 mCi of ^{99m}Tc-labeled MAA or HAM is administered simultaneously into each leg, followed by 3 to 5 ml of saline flush. The saphenofemoral junctions and midthighs are then imaged, with each side requiring an injection of 0.5 to 0.75 mCi. The popliteal veins and then the calves are subsequently imaged with again 0.5 to 0.75 mCi for each side. All injections are made with the tourniquets in place, with equal amounts of radioactivity being administered on both sides for corresponding fields and followed by saline flush. All areas are imaged for a period of 5 seconds. After each injection, the appropriate time for starting the image exposure varies in different patients and for different regions and should be guided by the monitoring oscilloscope (for example, after about 10 seconds for the region of the inferior vena cava and external iliac veins, 7 seconds for the thighs and popliteal areas, and 5 seconds for the calves).

After the dynamic phase of the procedure is completed, the needles are removed. The patient's feet are then slightly lifted from the table, and while holding an alcohol swab over the injection site, the patient exercises the feet as vigorously as possible against plantar pressure. Some physicians require 1 minute of exercise, whereas others stipulate 5 minutes. In some laboratories, the tourniquets (and bandages if applied) are removed after exercise, and in others, prior to exercise. Postexercise images of the same anatomic areas are then obtained in the same imaging sequence as in the dynamic phase. A preset imaging time (approximately 5 minutes) for each field is usually chosen. The count rates from each area may vary and require the intensity setting to be adjusted accordingly. The exercise procedure clears the venous system of radioactive particles not actually tagged to clots. Labeled thrombi will appear as "hot spots" on the static images. Lung imaging is then performed.

Procedure when whole body–imaging capability is available. When whole body imaging with the scintillation camera is available, the tediousness of the above described technique is overcome. The technique utilizes a single injection for each side, administered simultaneously in each foot. The procedure is as follows:

1. For each limb, the radiopharmaceutical is drawn in a syringe suitable for placement in a lymphangiographic injector (for example, Cordis or Harvard pump injector). The volume of the radionuclide should be sufficient to allow for a constant rate of administration over the planned injection period. The radioactive dose and injection volume should be equal for both limbs. A small amount of methylene blue (sterile and pyrogen free) could be added and mixed into the syringe, which is then placed in the lymphangiographic injector. The syringes are connected to the butterfly needles. The injector is adjusted so that the colored radionuclide just enters the needle prior to injecting. This is to provide uniform starting time for the injections on either side.
2. Imaging can be performed either retrograde or antegrade to the flow of blood. The retrograde technique, starting by the lower abdomen and moving downward is preferable. This offers better delineation of the pelvic veins, since in the antegrade method there is interference on the pelvic image from scattered photons originating from the radionuclide that already has reached the lungs. The field width of the camera is adjusted so that both lower limbs are viewed simultaneously. The motion is set at different speeds for the different regions, being slowest for the pelvis and lower abdomen (for example, 16 to 32 cm/min), faster for the thighs (48 to 64 cm/min), and fastest for the lower legs (64 to 96 cm/min). The exact speeds should be decided upon and standardized in individual laboratories. The purpose of the variable speed is to maintain a somewhat constant information density in the different regions to compensate for dilution of the radionuclide as it flows with blood. The setup of the imaging intensity is kept constant. The overall dynamic imaging time should be suitably matched with the total injection time (about 4 minutes). However, the exact timing with the continuous injection and whole body–imaging mode does not appear to be critical. The flow of radionuclide in the lower extremities is slow and the imaging procedure provides a relatively long exposure to each area; the study, in effect, represents a technique somewhere between dynamic and static blood-pool imaging.
3. Removal of tourniquets and exercise are then performed as described above, followed by a postexercise imaging pass. The postexercise imaging can be performed with a fast speed (for example, 96 to 120 cm/min).
4. Lung imaging is then performed.

The whole body–imaging technique has the following advantages over the multiple-imaging procedure:

1. The technique is simplified, obviating multiple injections and multiple-imaging setups.
2. The time of the study is shortened.
3. The shortened handling time of radioactivity by technologist or physician minimizes the occupational radiation exposure, particularly to the fingers.
4. The venous system under study is imaged on one film, a method that facilitates anatomic localization.

REMARKS

1. Prior to injection, the radiopharmaceutical in the syringe should be well mixed so that the particles are evenly suspended.
2. One should avoid drawing back blood into the syringe containing the radiopharmaceutical to prevent blood clotting in the syringe.
3. Air bubbles should not be injected with the radionuclide, no matter how small. Air bubbles may be trapped at valves in the veins to cause apparent "hot spots."
4. Between injections, it is preferable not to use a heparinized saline flush because heparin may interfere with clot tagging. Systemic heparinization of patients appears also to interfere with clot tagging, but other anticoagulant therapy does not seem to affect the study.[19]
5. If the patient is to have contrast venography immediately after the radionuclide procedure, the needles should be left in place.

Criteria for an abnormal study

1. There is evidence of venous occlusion, stasis, or collateral flow, seen during the dynamic phase of the study.[45]
2. There is a definite uptake on postexercise static images in the thighs or pelvis. Radioactivity may be seen within the urinary bladder on the delayed images of the pelvis and ought not to be confused with thrombosis (comparison of images before and after voiding may be helpful). The abnormal uptake in the thighs or pelvis is usually punctate and multiple, but occasionally it is solitary.[45] The size of the "hot spot" does not indicate the size or anatomic extent of the thrombus.
3. When an occluding thrombus is present, interruption of the normal flow and evidence of collateral drainage should be seen during the dynamic phase, along with a "hot spot" on the postexercise image. If the thrombus is nonocclud-

ing, flow may be normal on the image or show evidence of partial stasis, but delayed imaging may show an intense "hot spot." The normal venous flow is described in references 21 and 34.

4. General uptake of the linear course of the venous flow, even if more noticeable on one side, does not indicate thrombosis, unless it is limited to a certain area or is very pronounced.[45]
5. Uptake in the calf regions, punctate or linear, is indeterminate for thrombosis unless it is very striking or accompanied by collateral flow.[45]
6. Some authors consider the test as a screening procedure, and if positive, the results should be followed by other confirmation.

REFERENCES

1. Alderson, P. O., Jost, R. G., Strauss, A. W., Boonvisut, S., and Markham, J.: Radionuclide angiocardiography, improved diagnosis and quantitation of left-to-right shunts using area ratio techniques in children, Circulation **51:**1136, 1975.
2. Alderson, P. O., Wagner, H. N., Jr., Gómez-Moeiras, J. J., et al.: Simultaneous detection of myocardial perfusion and wall motion abnormalities by cinematic ^{201}Tl imaging, Radiology **127:**531, 1978.
3. Ambrus, J. L., Ambrus, C. M., Back, M., et al.: Radio-labeled thrombi, Ann. N.Y. Acad. Sci. **68:**97, 1957.
4. Anderson, P. A. W., Jones, R. H., and Sabiston, D. C.: Quantitation of left-to-right cardiac shunts with radionuclide angiography, Circulation **49:**512, 1974.
5. Atkins, P., and Hawkins, L. A.: Detection of venous thrombosis in the legs, Lancet **2:**1217, 1965.
6. Bonte, F. J., Parkey, R. W., Graham, K. D., Moore, J., and Stokely, E. M.: A new method for radionuclide imaging of myocardial infarcts, Radiology **110:**473, 1974.
7. Bradley-Moore, P. R., Lebowitz, E., Greene, M. W., Atkins, H. L., and Ansari, A. N.: Thallium-201 for medical use. II. Biologic behaviour, J. Nucl. Med. **16:**156, 1975.
8. Carr, E. A., Jr., Beierwaltes, W. H., Patno, M. E., Bartlett, J. D., Jr., and Wegst, A. V.: The detection of experimental myocardial infarcts by photoscanning, Am. Heart J. **64:**650, 1962.
9. Coleman, R. E., Harwig, S. S. L., and Harwig, J. F.: Fibrinogen uptake by thrombi: effect of thrombus age, J. Nucl. Med. **16:**370, 1975.
10. D'Agostino, A. W.: An electron microscopic study of cardiac necrosis produced by 9α-fluorocortisol and sodium phosphate, Am. J. Pathol. **45:**633, 1964.
11. D'Agostino, A. W., and Chiga, M.: Mitochondrial mineralization in human myocardium, Am. J. Clin. Pathol. **53:**820, 1970.
12. Feller, P. A., and Sodd, V. J.: Dosimetry of four heart-imaging radionuclides: ^{43}K, ^{81}Rb, ^{129}Cs, and ^{201}Tl, J. Nucl. Med. **16:** 1070, 1975.
13. Folse, R., and Braunwald, E.: Pulmonary vascular dilution curves recorded by external detection in the diagnosis of left-to-right shunts, Br. Heart J. **24:**166, 1962.
14. Gates, G. F., Orme, H. W., and Dore, E. K.: Measurement of cardiac shunting with technetium-labeled albumin aggregates, J. Nucl. Med. **12:**746, 1971.
15. Greene, D. G., Carlisle, R., Grant, C., and Bunnell, I. L.: Estimation of left ventricular volume by one plane cineangiography, Circulation **35:**61, 1967.
16. Greenfield, L. D., and Bennett, L. R.: Comparison of heart chamber and pulmonary dilution curves for the diagnosis of cardiac shunts, Radiology **111:**359, 1974.
17. Harwig, J. F., Alderson, P. O., Primeau, J. L., Boonvisut, S., and Welch, M. J.: Development and evaluation of a rapid and efficient electrolytic preparation of ^{99m}Tc-labeled red blood cells, Intern. J. Appl. Radiat. Isot. **28:**113, 1977.
18. Hayt, D. B., Blatt, C. J., and Freeman, L. M.: Radionuclide venography: its place as a modality for the investigation of thromboembolic phenomena, Semin. Nucl. Med. **7:**263, 1977.
19. Hayt, D. B., Blatt, C. J., Reddy, K., Patel, H., and Freeman, L. M.: Radionuclide venography by antegrade and retrograde whole body gamma camera imaging methods, Clin. Nucl. Med. **1:**198, 1976.
20. Hayt, D. B., Reddy, K., Patel, H., and Freeman, L. M.: Radionuclide venography of the lower extremities and inferior vena cava by continuous injection and moving bed gamma camera technique, Radiology **121:**748, 1976.
21. Henkin, R. E., Yao, J. S. T., Quinn, J. L., III, and Bergan, J. J.: Radionuclide venography (RNV) in lower extremity venous disease, J. Nucl. Med. **15:**171, 1974.
22. Hobb, J. T., and Davies, J. W. L.: Detection of venous thrombosis with ^{131}I-labeled fibrinogen in the rabbit, Lancet **2:**134, 1960.
23. Kakkar, V. V.: The diagnosis of deep vein thrombosis using the ^{125}I-labeled fibrinogen test, Arch. Surg. **104:**152, 1972.
24. Kakkar, V. V., Nicolaides, A. N., Penney, J. T. G., Friend, J. R., and Clarke, M. B.: ^{125}I-labeled fibrinogen test adapted for routine screening for deep vein thrombosis, Lancet **1:**540, 1970.
25. Kawana, M., Krizek, H., Porter, J., Lathrop, K. A., Charleston, D., and Harper, P. V.: Use of 199-thallium as a potassium analog in scanning, J. Nucl. Med. **11:**333, 1970. (Abstract.)
26. Lane, S. D., Patton, D. D., Staab, E. V., and Baglan, R. J.: Simple technique for rapid bolus injection, J. Nucl. Med. **13:**118, 1972.
27. Maltz, D. L., and Treves, S.: Quantitative radionuclide angiocardiography: determination of $Q_p:Q_s$ in children, Circulation **47:**1049, 1973.
28. McFarlane, A. S.: Labeling of plasma proteins with radioactive iodine, Biochem. J. **62:**135, 1956.
29. Palko, P. D., Mansen, E. M., and Fedoruk, S. O.: The early detection of deep vein thrombosis using ^{131}I-tagged human fibrinogen, Can. J. Surg. **7:**215, 1964.
30. Pavel, D. G., Zimmer, A. M., and Patterson, V. N.: In vivo labeling of red blood cells with ^{99m}Tc: a new approach to blood pool visualization, J. Nucl. Med. **18:**305, 1977.
31. Prinzmetal, M., Corday, E., Spritzler, R. J., and Flieg, W.: Radiocardiography and its clinical application, J.A.M.A. **139:** 617, 1949.
32. Rosenthall, L.: Combined inferior vena cavography, iliac venography and lung imaging with ^{99m}Tc albumin macroaggregates, Radiology **98:**623, 1971.
33. Rosenthall, L., and Greyson, N. D.: Observations on the use of ^{99m}Tc albumin macroaggregates for detection of thrombophlebitis, Radiology **94:**413, 1970.
34. Ryo, U. Y., Colombetti, L. G., Polin. S. G., and Pinsky, S. M.: Radionuclide venography significance of delayed washout; visualization of the saphenous system, J. Nucl. Med. **17:**590, 1976.
35. Ryo, U. Y., Qazi, M., Srikantaswamy, S., and Pinsky, S.: Radionuclide venography: correlation with contrast venography, J. Nucl. Med. **18:**11, 1977.
36. Sapirstein, L. A.: Regional blood flow by fractional distribution of indicators, Am. J. Physiol. **193:**161, 1958.
37. Shen, A. C., and Jennings, R. B.: Kinetics of calcium accumulation in acute myocardial ischemic injury, Am. J. Pathol. **67:**441, 1972.
38. Shen, A. C., and Jenning, R. B.: Myocardial calcium and magnesium in acute ischemic injury, Am. J. Pathol. **67:**417, 1972.
39. Strauss, H. W., and Pitt, B.: Thallium-201 as a myocardial imaging agent, Semin. Nucl. Med. **7:**49, 1977.

40. Strauss, H. W., and Pitt, B.: Gated cardiac blood-pool scans: use in patients with coronary heart disease. In Holman, B. L., Sonnenblick, E. H., and Lesch, M., editors: Principles of cardiovascular nuclear medicine, New York, 1978, Grune & Stratton, Inc.
41. Van Kirk, O. C., Burry, M. T., Jansen, A. A., Barnett, D., and Larson, S.: A simplified approach to radionuclide venography: concise communication, J. Nucl. Med. **17:**969, 1976.
42. Vogel, R. A., Kirch, D. L., LeFree, M. T., and Steele, P. A.: Improved diagnostic results of myocardial perfusion tomography using a new rapid inexpensive technique, J. Nucl. Med. **19:**730, 1978. (Abstract.)
43. Watson, D. D., Kenny, P. J., Gelband, H., Tamer, D. R., Janowitz, W. R., and Sankey, R. R.: A non-invasive technique for the study of cardiac hemodynamics utilizing $C^{15}O_2$ inhalation, Radiology **119:**615, 1976.
44. Watson, E. E., and Coffey, J. L.: Radiation dose to the liver from ^{201}Tl, J. Nucl. Med. **16:**1089, 1975.
45. Weber, M. M., Labeled albumin aggregates for detection of clots, Semin. Nucl. Med. **7:**253, 1977.
46. Weber, M. M., Bennett, L. R., Cragin, M., and Webb, R.: Thrombophlebitis—demonstration by scintiscanning, Radiology **92:**620, 1969.
47. Weber, P. M., dos Remedios, L. V., and Jasko, I. A.: Quantitative radioisotopic angiocardiography, J. Nucl. Med. **13:**815, 1972.

Chapter 12

THE GASTROINTESTINAL SYSTEM

Donald R. Bernier and Gaellan McIlmoyle

The gastrointestinal system consists of the alimentary canal and several accessory organs. The alimentary canal originates at the mouth, and its ensuing components are the pharynx, esophagus, stomach, and small and large intestines (Fig. 12-1).

The purpose of the alimentary canal is to provide a route of intake for nourishment, to digest and absorb nutrients, and to eliminate waste products. For the purpose of this chapter, the accessory organs involved are the liver, gallbladder, pancreas, and salivary glands. Although not a part of the gastrointestinal system, the spleen is mentioned, but only its morphology is considered.

LIVER AND SPLEEN

Prior to the advent of radionuclide studies, the liver was a difficult organ to evaluate morphologically. Radiographs of the abdomen were often quite accurate in determining enlargement of the liver and spleen; additionally, the position and size of the gallbladder could be accurately assessed by oral or intravenous contrast studies. In most cases, however, the internal structure of the liver could only be visualized by contrast angiography with its attendant discomfort and occasional more serious vascular complications and hypersensitivity reactions. Various contrast agents that failed to concentrate well in bile did increase the radiographic density of the liver. These agents were rejected for clinical use, since visualization was poor by existing techniques but are now being resurrected for use with computerized tomography.[1]

Since the liver is a frequent site for the metastatic spread of disease, visualization of the internal structure of the liver is desirable. The size, shape, and position of the liver and its relation to upper abdominal masses is valuable information for the clinician. Ideally, scintigraphic agents should concentrate at the site or sites of intrahepatic disease, but to date abnormal tissue is detected only by reduction of radionuclide accumulation compared with surrounding normal tissue. This increases slightly the minimum size of a lesion that can be resolved.

The recent development of gray-scale ultrasonography and computer-assisted tomography has added new dimensions to the evaluation of tissue consistency and the investigation of the internal structure of the liver and spleen. These modalities are at present complimentary with radionuclide scintigraphy in the evaluation of hepatobiliary disease.[6]

ANATOMY, PHYSIOLOGY, AND PATHOPHYSIOLOGY

The liver is the major organ in the upper abdomen where it occupies most of the right upper quadrant (Fig. 12-2). It extends across the midline and may normally be palpable in the epigastrium. The largest organ of the body, the liver, weighs 1400 to 1600 g in the adult male and slightly less in the adult female. Normally, the inferior liver margin is palpable slightly below the costal margin. The lungs cap the dome of the liver separated only by the diaphragm. The right kidney lies against the posterior aspect of the right lobe and the transverse colon abuts the posterior inferior margin. The stomach lies directly behind the thin irregular left lobe, and the fifth to eleventh ribs protect the liver laterally.

The configuration of the normal liver varies widely; however, the right lobe is generally larger than the left. Most of the volume of the liver lies in the anterosuperior abdomen.

The liver thins peripherally; hence, distribution of radioactivity may normally be slightly irregular over the left lobe and along the inferior right lobe. Scintigraphically, this can be mistaken for pathologic involvement. The subdiaphragmatic portion of the liver curves smoothly in the absence of adjacent disease in the subphrenic space, the diaphragm, or the lung base (for example, pleural effusion, emphysema, and pneumonia). An impression is made on the superior medial aspect of the right lobe by the heart; consequently enlargement of the heart may result in a more impressive "cardiac fossa."

The left and right lobes of the liver receive a separate hepatic arterial and portal venous blood supply. At the

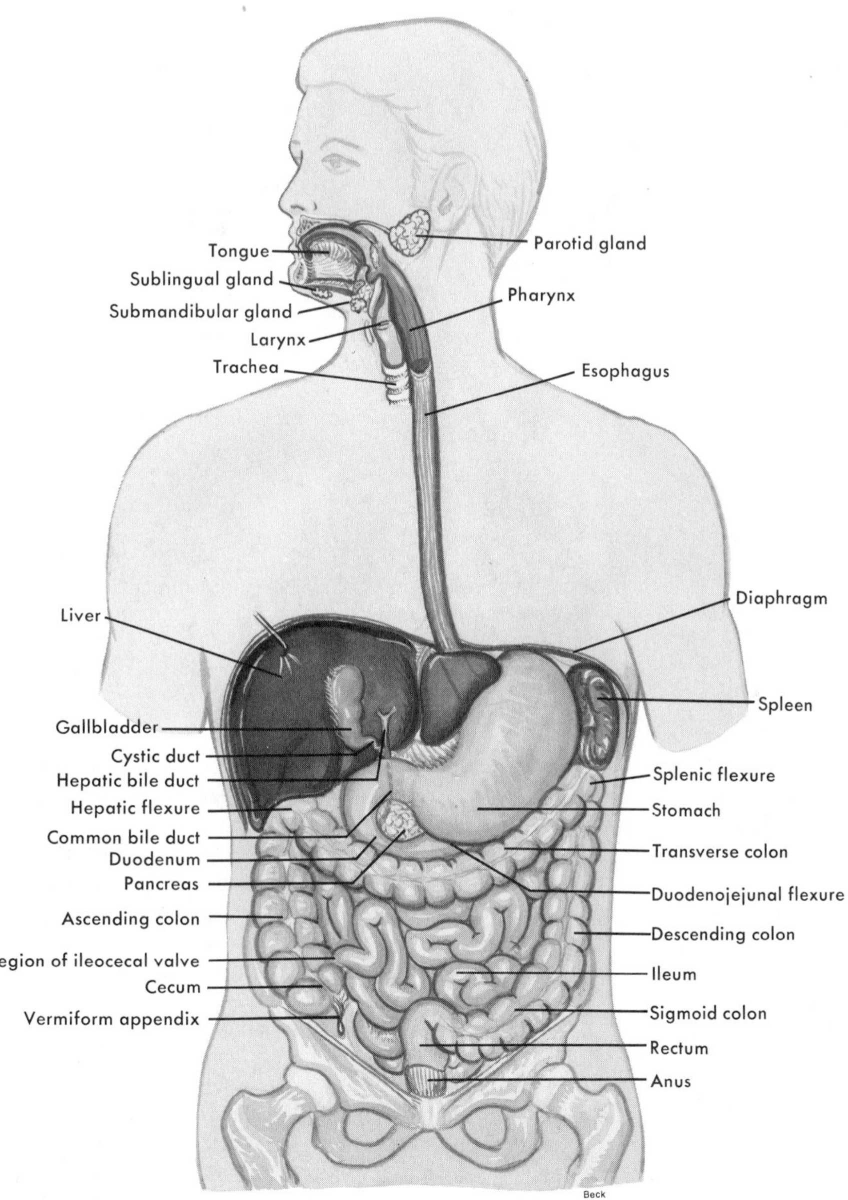

Fig. 12-1. Location of gastrointestinal system organs. (From Anthony, C. A., and Thibodeau, G. A.: Textbook of anatomy and physiology, ed. 10, St. Louis, 1979, The C. V. Mosby Co.)

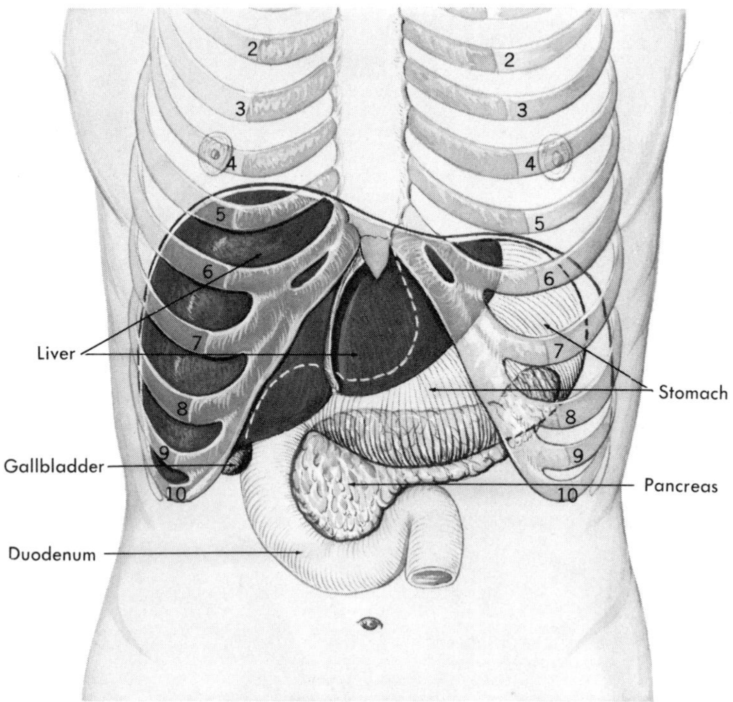

Fig. 12-2. Liver in its normal position relative to rib cage, diaphragm, stomach, and pancreas. (From Anthony, C. P., and Thibodeau, G. A.: Textbook of anatomy and physiology, ed. 10, St. Louis, 1979, The C. V. Mosby Co.)

watershed area a zone of division may exist, and slightly reduced radionuclide concentration may be present between the smaller left lobe and the right. Focally decreased tissue mass may be apparent in the porta hepatis, that is, in the area where blood vessels enter and leave the liver and from which the bile ducts proceed. This region lies on the posterior aspect in the midvertical plane within the zone of separation between the right and left lobes (Fig. 12-3). Because the left lobe is of smaller mass and more anterior in position, scintigraphic visualization from the posterior may be suboptimal. Attenuation of radioactivity by the spine may also cause an apparent vertical defect on that same view. An extension of normal tissue from the inferior aspect of the right lobe (referred to as ''Riedel's lobe'') may angle anteriorly under the costal margin. This is a variant in liver shape. The normal liver rarely, however, despite alterations in shape, exceeds 20 cm in its greatest longitudinal diameter.[38]

The liver consists of an irregular cellular mass of functioning liver cells (hepatocytes or polygonal cells) excavated by lacunae, which are communicating cavities that contain the blood capillaries of the liver in the walls of which reside the reticuloendothelial (Kupffer) cells (Fig. 12-4). These act as phagocytes or filters for particulate matter (such as ^{99m}Tc-sulfur colloid) in the blood. These capillaries deliver oxygenated blood from the hepatic artery and nutritiously rich blood from the portal vein. The portal vein obtains its blood supply from the spleen and the capillary bed of the bowel. It furnishes approximately 75% of the liver's blood, and, under normal circumstances, a total interruption of the hepatic artery supply will not result in hepatic necrosis. The hepatic veins, which drain blood from the liver to the heart by way of the inferior vena cava, travel separately and unite superiorly to the right lobe under or in the diaphragm.

At regular intervals tiny bile ductules drain waste products and bile from the hepatocytes. Bile canaliculi, hepatic arterioles, and portal venules all travel together in a connective tissue sheath. Larger and larger divisions join together to penetrate the liver parenchyma at a common site called the porta hepatis (gate of the liver). The bile ducts converge and unite into a common hepatic duct from which the cystic duct directs bile into the gallbladder where, by reabsorption of water, bile is concentrated. At the next meal, fat in the upper gastrointestinal tract stimulates the gall-

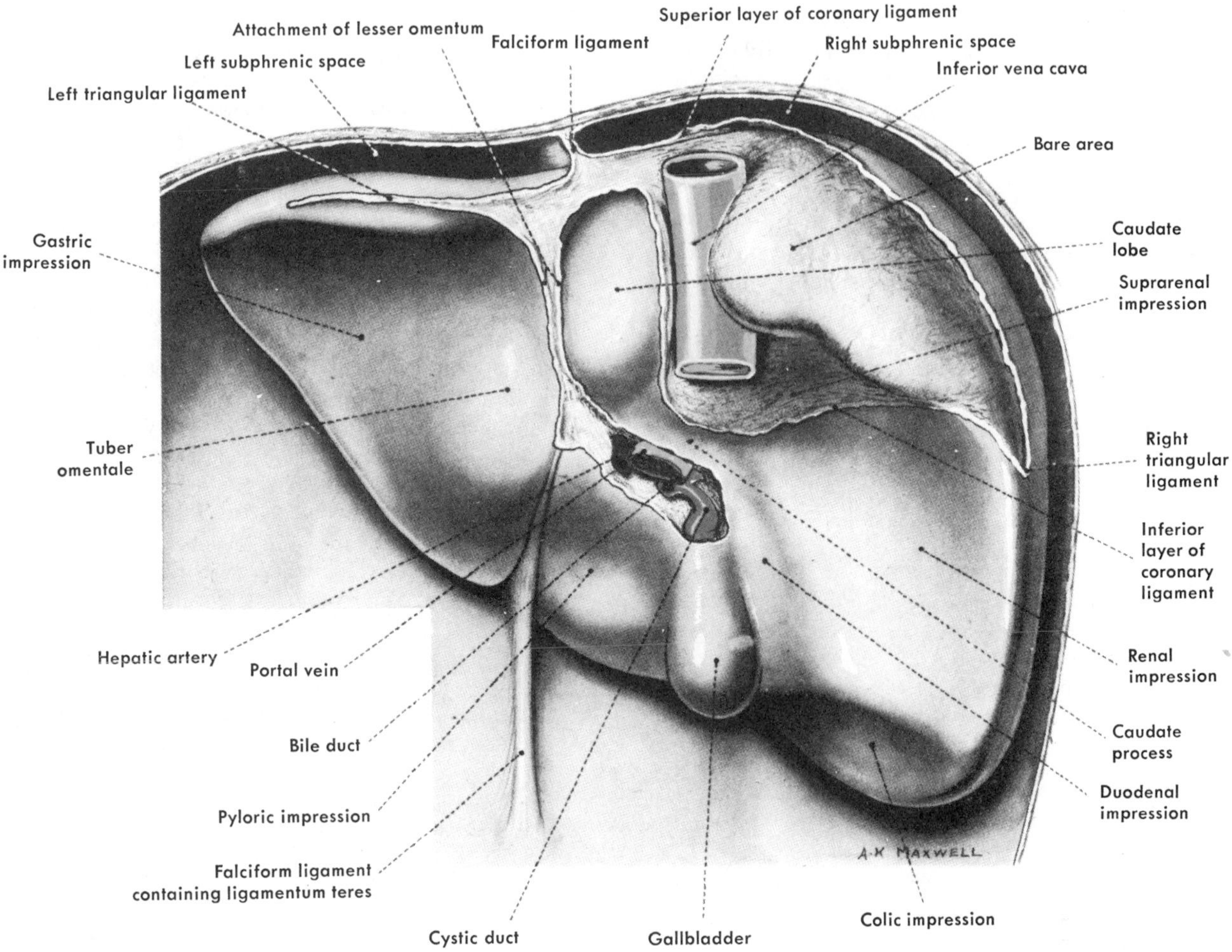

Superior layer of coronary ligament
Attachment of lesser omentum
Falciform ligament
Right subphrenic space
Left subphrenic space
Inferior vena cava
Left triangular ligament
Bare area
Gastric impression
Caudate lobe
Suprarenal impression
Tuber omentale
Right triangular ligament
Inferior layer of coronary ligament
Hepatic artery
Portal vein
Renal impression
Bile duct
Caudate process
Duodenal impression
Pyloric impression
A·K MAXWELL
Falciform ligament containing ligamentum teres
Colic impression
Cystic duct
Gallbladder

Fig. 12-3. Posterior view of liver. (From Hamilton, W. J.: Textbook of human anatomy, ed. 2, St. Louis, 1976, The C. V. Mosby Co.; courtesy The Macmillan Press Ltd., Houndsmill Basingstoke, Hampshire, England.)

Endothelial cell
Bile canaliculus
Perisinusoidal space
Hepatocyte
Sinusoid
Frank B. Price

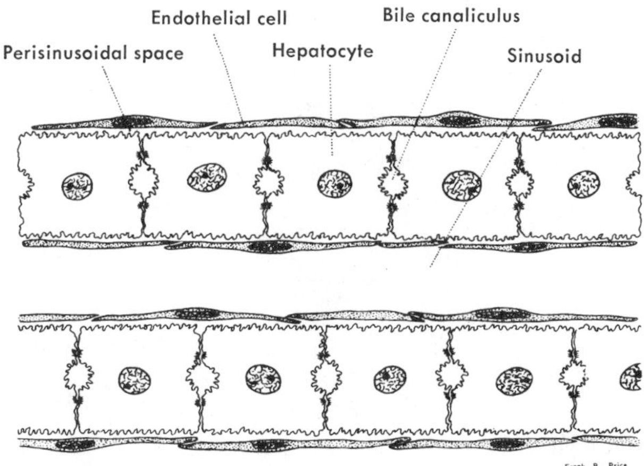

Fig. 12-4. Schematic representation of liver sinusoid with its lining of endothelial cells. (From Hamilton, W. J.: Textbook of human anatomy, ed. 2, St. Louis, 1976, The C. V. Mosby Co.; courtesy The Macmillan Press Ltd., Houndsmill Basingstoke, Hampshire, England.)

bladder to contract, and bile is delivered to the duodenum through the common bile duct. Bile aids in breakdown and absorption of fats and fatty acids.

The common bile duct enters the duodenum at the papilla. At the same site the pancreas empties its secretions, consisting of enzymes, which assist in the breakdown and absorption of protein (Fig. 12-5).

The polygonal cells (hepatocytes) constitute 85% of the normal cell population in the liver and perform the metabolic functions of the liver, including protein synthesis, carbohydrate metabolism, fatty acid kinetics, vitamin and mineral storage and regulation, hormone and toxin degradation, secretion of bile salts necessary for absorption of fats, and the production of coagulation factors and carrier proteins for the blood.

Since polygonal cells handle certain intravenously injected dyes such as phenolphthalein, Congo red, and indocyanin green by the same mechanism used to conjugate bilirubin, the liver has been visualized using ^{131}I-labeled rose bengal (a derivative of phenolphthalein).[18] In addition, these agents are excreted into the bile and allow visualization of the bile duct. Passage into the duodenum ensures elimination without resorption in the gastrointestinal tract. This class of agents has been used to (1) evaluate liver parenchyma, (2) determine patency of the bile ducts, and (3) identify the normally functioning gallbladder. In addition, they will be pooled in choledochal cysts, which are abnormally dilated segments of the extrahepatic biliary tree, believed to be either developmental in origin or associated with birth trauma.

Although a fatty meal administered at the completion of the study should cause contraction of the gallbladder and subsequent expression of the radiopharmaceutical, the choledochal cyst with no smooth muscle in its walls will not respond to lipid stimuli.[34,50] Currently, ultrasound and computed axial tomography with better anatomic resolution have largely replaced this study in the investigation of childhood right upper quadrant masses and pain. However, the newer ^{99m}Tc-labeled hepatobiliary agents[37] may prove useful as a means for visualizing the liver and assessing its function especially in the differentiation of right upper quadrant accumulations.

Fifteen percent of the cells in the liver are phagocytic Kupffer cells, which clear foreign particulate matter such as damaged cells, bacteria, and proteins from the bloodstream. Colloids are cleared from the bloodstream by these cells, and hence radiolabeled colloids are concentrated within the liver.

Reticuloendothelial (RE) cells are not, however, restricted to the liver but exist in the spleen and bone

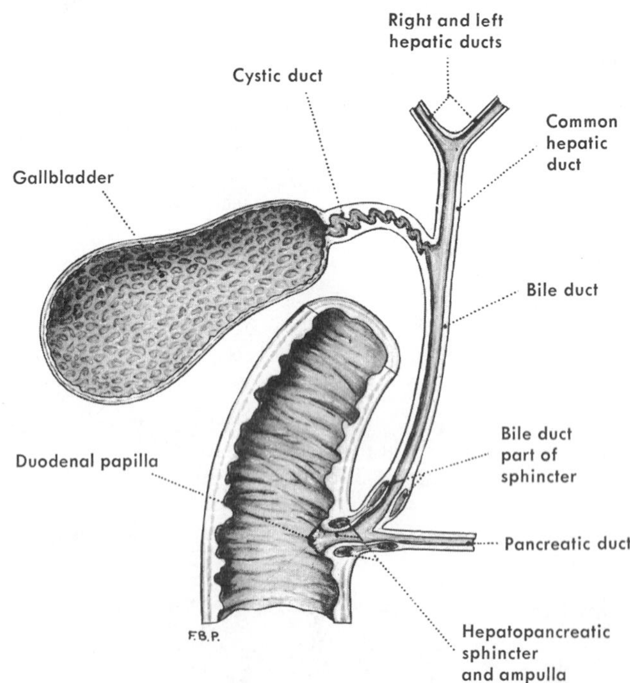

Fig. 12-5. Schematic representation of extrahepatic biliary apparatus. (From Hamilton, W. J.: Textbook of human anatomy, ed. 2, St. Louis, 1976, The C. V. Mosby Co.; courtesy The Macmillan Press Ltd., Houndsmill Basingstoke, Hampshire, England.)

marrow and in lesser concentrations in the lungs, kidneys, and other body tissues. In the normal individual 85% of injected ^{99m}Tc-sulfur colloid will be deposited in the liver, with another 10% in the spleen. The remaining 5% extracted by the bone marrow normally does not allow scintigraphic visualization because it is such a low proportion of the total counts and is spread over a large area when compared to the liver and spleen.

If liver tissue is damaged, both polygonal and reticuloendothelial cells suffer.

Subtle changes in the distribution of radiocolloids, such as patchy uptake in the liver or a shift of concentration to the spleen or bone marrow, are used as evidence of hepatic function and integrity.[31] Blood clearance may be assessed by computer analysis of both types of agents after injection. A 1-minute image in an anterior projection made 10 minutes after colloid injection is a rough guide to liver function, since little activity should be present in the bloodstream (heart pool). In most institutions, static views are not begun before 10 to 15 minutes after injection.

^{99m}Tc-sulfur colloid is the most widely used agent at the present time. Because of the short physical half-life (6 hours) and the absence of particulate radiation, 3 to 10 mCi doses may be administered with an acceptable absorbed radiation dose to the liver (0.4 rads/mCi). In this way, high count density can be obtained in a short time. With the large-field cameras, breath-holding images may be obtained. The size of the colloid determines in part its concentration at various sites. Most suspensions include particles between 0.3 and 0.5 μm in size.[13] However, the colloid may be more finely dispersed for bone marrow or lymph-node imaging.[13,14]

Other agents that are concentrated by the RE cells but that are not used so widely are ^{99m}Tc–microaggregated albumin[3,4] and ^{113m}In-colloid.[20]

Of the hepatobiliary agents, ^{123}I–rose bengal yields elegant images and a good pictorial display of hepatic physiology.[44] The 159 keV photopeak is an acceptable energy for scintillation-camera imaging and the 13-hour half-life is a considerable improvement over the 8 days of ^{131}I. However, ^{123}I is cyclotron produced and expensive at the present time. For this reason, hepatobiliary agents that can be labeled with ^{99m}Tc, which is inexpensive and readily available,[37] have been developed. These compounds are of molecular weights between 300 and 1000. Below 300, renal excretion predominates.[52]

Radiopharmaceutical doses

Two to 10 mCi of ^{99m}Tc-sulfur colloid are injected intravenously, and a dose of 50 μCi/kg is used in children. The higher dose may be useful where poor liver function makes it difficult to assess intrahepatic integrity.

Higher doses of hepatobiliary agents may be used, since the biologic half-life of the isotope in the liver lies between 20 and 40 minutes.[52]

Dosimetry

Dosimetry has in the past been calculated for standard man with the expectation of normal blood clearance and organ distribution. However, both hepatobiliary and Kupffer cell agents have altered distribution during disease. In the former, greater radiation is delivered to the gastrointestinal system during biliary obstruction, and in the latter the spleen and bone marrow are the recipients of shifted radioisotope concentration. In both instances the total body dose delivered through the vascular pool is greater when a pathologic condition in the liver is present.[31]

Imaging time after injection

A 100,000-count image made 5 to 10 minutes after injection of ^{99m}Tc-sulfur colloid gives information about blood clearance. This is a gross test of liver function, but a large amount of activity still present in the cardiac blood pool is abnormal. Static imaging is usually begun 10 to 15 minutes after injection to allow full clearance from the bloodstream.

Since hepatobiliary agents deliver dynamic information about hepatocyte kinetics, imaging from the anterior begins at once and continues through the next 45 to 60 minutes,[15,16] with additional projections included whenever doubt exists concerning the localization of radioisotope in the genitourinary versus gastrointestinal system (Fig. 12-6). Further delayed imaging with rose bengal may occasionally be of value if incomplete obstruction or severe parenchymal disease is present. Clearance of the ^{99m}Tc-labeled radiopharmaceuticals is, however, generally much more rapid.

Technique variation

1. Hepatic blood flow
2. Computer uptake studies
3. Breath-holding
4. Liver-lung scans
5. Comparison studies
   a. Two types of agents
   b. Gallium
   c. Bone-seeking radiopharmaceuticals

Hepatic blood flow

Once focal disease in the liver has been detected, the process may be evaluated by biopsy without interim angiography, ultrasound, or computed axial tomography in some cases. Prudence on the part of the physician suggests that information about vascu-

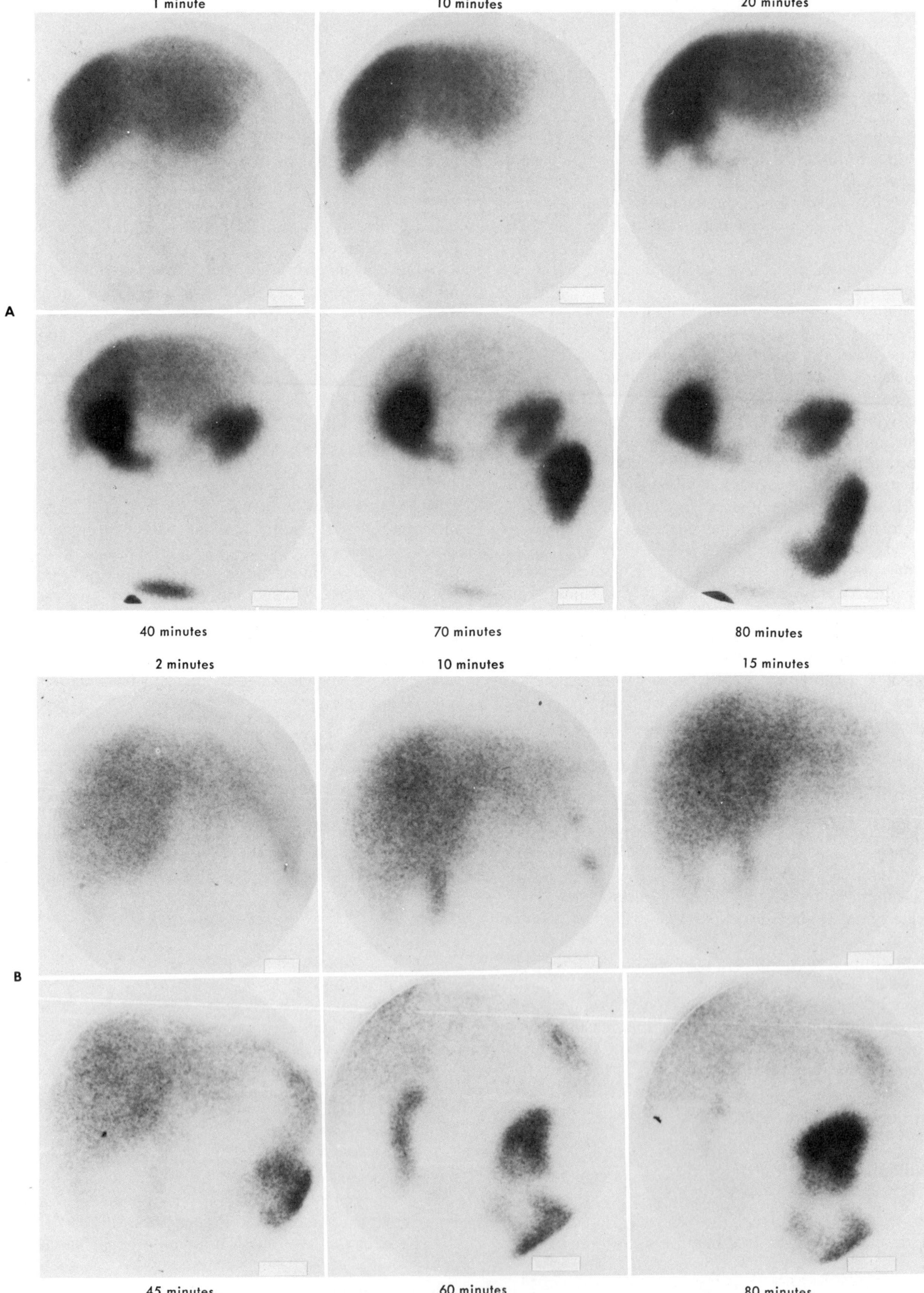

Fig. 12-6. For legend see opposite page.

larity of the lesion would be helpful. First-pass studies prior to static imaging using ^{99m}Tc-sulfur colloid have been employed.[12,49] Flow through vascular lesions may not, however, be rapid. Equilibrium images with blood-pool agents are more likely to reflect the tissue vascularity, which may be pooled and stagnant. Various patterns of perfusion have been reported,[12,49] arteriovenous malformations frequently have hepatic arterial supply. Capillary hemangiomas, however, may not become evident until the portal venous phase of perfusion. Hepatoblastomas and hepatic adenoma are also frequently vascular as compared to some metastases and areas of focal regeneration associated with hepatic necrosis. Cysts and abscesses are hypovascular. Metastases frequently have vascularity equivalent to normal parenchyma.

Computer uptake studies

Mundschenk et al.[32] have made attempts at quantitating extraction of ^{99m}Tc-sulfur colloid from the bloodstream by collecting over the liver from the time of injection and plotting a time-activity histogram. Although this potentially allows sensitive comparison of efficiency of hepatic function with time, abnormal patterns appear nonspecific. Although accurate information about hepatocyte function can be obtained from similar studies using hepatobiliary agents, it is not clear that the data obtained are of greater clinical value than existing biochemical tests.[5]

Breath-holding techniques

With large crystal cameras and slightly higher doses of radioactivity, 100,000-count images can sometimes be obtained within 20 seconds with breath holding. Alternatively, the patient is instructed to take a deep breath, hold it as long as possible, and then indicate to the technologist when to interrupt counting. After a period of normal breathing the process is repeated until at least 500,000 counts are collected. Elimination of respiratory movement may significantly improve resolution confirming the presence of focal defects where doubt exists.[24] Inspiration and expiration views of the liver have been used to identify defects produced by extrinsic compression of liver tissue by ribs or sternum.[33] Although the liver will clearly change position on alternate views, the artifact will retain a constant relation to the bony thorax. If the defect moves with the liver, the source most likely is intrinsic disease.

When the liver has been infiltrated by fibrous tissue or tumor (usually lymphoma or leukemic cells), it loses pliability.[24] Although focal disease is not present, the lack of change in the shape of the liver with respiration suggests a widespread infiltrative process. Adhesions from inflammatory or metastatic disease also cause this effect.

Liver-lung scans

Combined imaging of the liver and lung has been used to evaluate the presence of subphrenic abscess[43] (infection between the diaphragm and the liver often arising from perforation of a duodenal ulcer, the appendix, or a diverticulum of the colon).

Comparison of agents

The usual dose of ^{99m}Tc-sulfur colloid lies between 3 and 6 mCi. For hepatobiliary agents 5 mCi is the standard adult dose.[16,17] Obviously, the statistical information is superior when hepatic parenchyma is visualized with the latter agents. In addition, they reflect functional capability of the liver. Additional information concerning patency of the biliary tract and gallbladder is available. Although most institutions continue to use RE cell agents, there may be a distinct indication for the substitution of hepatocyte agents in liver damage from cirrhosis to assess regeneration, in damage where radiation portals have included the liver, in congenital anomalies, and in the need for clear definition of the liver from the spleen.

Gallium

In the past gallium has been used as a secondary agent in the identification of hepatoma and amebic abscess.[27] In both conditions, there is a pronounced gallium accumulation in most cases where a defect has been present by ^{99m}Tc-sulfur colloid scan. By contrast, regenerating liver tissue and metastases have variable uptake but usually do not concentrate radiogallium above normal background. Gallium, however, will also accumulate in bacterial abscesses and in subphrenic inflammatory tissue.[25]

Today with computerized tomography and gray-

Fig. 12-6. A, Normal visualization of liver at 1 minute. At 20 minutes gallbladder and part of duodenum are visualized as well. There is activity within jejunum at 40 minutes and thereafter. **B,** There is prompt visualization of liver and excretion into common bile duct by 5 minutes. Duodenojejunal loops are seen at 10 minutes. There is progression of activity seen throughout small bowel. At no time is gallbladder visualized. Nonvisualization of gallbladder, despite visualization of liver, common duct, and duodenum, suggests acute or chronic cholecystitis with obstruction of cystic duct.

scale ultrasound, the use of gallium in hepatic disease has been decreasing.[6]

Bone-seeking radiopharmaceuticals

The ^{99m}Tc-labeled phosphates will occasionally accumulate in abnormal liver tissue. Frequently, this is seen in calcium-containing metastases from the bowel or breast.[19,46] Diffuse phosphate accumulation is more likely related to colloid formation associated with alumina breakthrough from the generator.

Counts collected

The anterior, posterior, and both lateral views constitute the basic examination. Multiple anterior and posterior views are usually necessary to accommodate both the liver and spleen if a standard-field-of-view camera (11-inch crystal) is used. A minimum of 500,000 counts per image is statistically acceptable. If separate posterior views of the spleen and liver are necessary, the spleen image should be taken for the same length of time as the liver image.

With wide-field cameras (15-inch crystal) 1 million counts are collected for the anterior view and the other views are done with the same time interval being used as that obtained from the anterior view.

Collimation

High-resolution parallel-hole collimators are the ideal, since they do not introduce distortion with depth. However, in small babies the magnification afforded by the use of a converging collimator may significantly improve resolution. It should be emphasized that a parallel-hole collimator on a 15-inch crystal camera will deliver better resolution than a diverging collimator on an 11-inch crystal camera despite the similarity of images. It is esthetically pleasing to include both liver and spleen in the same image, but the quality of the image will be degraded by use of the diverging collimator.

Positioning

Four standard views contain a minimum of information to assess anatomy and function of the liver. Anterior, posterior, and right and left lateral views will survey all of the organ (Fig. 12-7). With the 11-inch crystal two images made anteriorly and posteriorly may be necessary to include the whole liver and spleen. With very large patients or with organomegaly, two images may again be necessary to cover the whole vertical span of the organ.

An additional anterior view may be obtained for evaluation of liver size and position. A lead strip is placed on the costal margin to outline this landmark, and a calibrated lead ruler is positioned over the liver. Since this is a reference image, the counts accumulated from the liver do not need to exceed 100,000.

There is considerable controversy concerning the direction of the imaging of the lateral views.[11,51] Those who image the "up" side affirm that there is less respiratory motion and hence better resolution of the

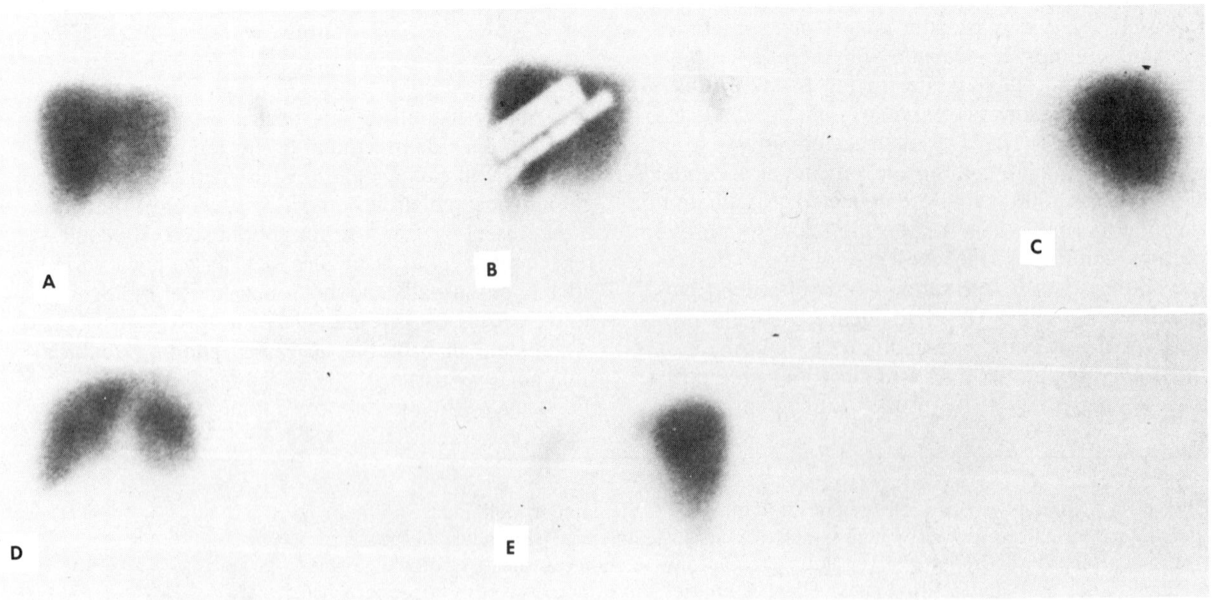

Fig. 12-7. Normal liver-spleen scan. **A,** Anterior. **B,** Anterior with marker. **C,** Right lateral. **D,** Left lateral. **E,** Posterior.

elevated organ. Those who image the dependent lateral claim that it is closer to the collimator face, since it is immediately adjacent to the costal margin. Cross-table laterals may be necessary if the patient cannot turn because of pain or recent surgery.

Forty-five-degree oblique views of the liver and spleen may be requested by the physician to confirm or better delineate a defect detected on the routine views. If necessary, additional 30- and 60-degree oblique views may be added to the examination to probe tangentially an ill-defined peripheral abnormality. The left anterior oblique is most helpful in clearly separating the left lobe of the liver from the spleen. Occasionally, a photon-deficient, crescent-shaped artifact will appear over the superior portion of the right lobe of the liver on the anterior image. This is caused by overlying breast tissue, which attenuates the ^{99m}Tc photons. The problem is easily solved when the image is repeated with breast held up and away from the field of view. Right anterior and posterior obliques may be used routinely in hepatic trauma to increase the sensitivity of detection of hematoma. At least three views of the spleen should also be included if hepatic trauma is suspected, since splenic rupture or hematoma may accompany any abdominal accident. Should an abdominal mass be present, an anterior view with the mass outlined by radioactive marker may help differentiate internal from extrahepatic disease.

PANCREAS

Scintigraphy of the pancreas has been directed historically at the early detection of tumors. In the light of current technology this study is infrequently indicated today.[2]

Anatomy. The pancreas is a yellow-orange retroperitoneal organ 10 to 15 cm long extending transversely in the upper abdomen from the concavity of the duodenum to the splenic hilum (Fig. 12-8). It is found at the first and second lumbar vertebral body behind the stomach and transverse colon. The inferior vena cava and aorta lie posteriorly and the superior mesenteric vessels pass over the anterior surface. The organ is pistol shaped, with the head lying adjacent to the duodenum, the tail projecting into the splenic pedicle, and the body lying between. The splenic artery runs along its superior surface. The common bile duct passes over the head or through the substance of the pancreas to enter the duodenum with the main pancreatic duct at a common orifice (the ampulla of Vater).

Physiology. The pancreas is both an endocrine and exocrine gland. It delivers insulin from the beta cells in the islets of Langerhans into the bloodstream and produces glucagon from the alpha cells. Both hormones regulate carbohydrate synthesis and determine blood glucose levels. The exocrine functions of the organ include bicarbonate, fluid, and electrolyte secretion to the bowel and the secretion of enzymes, which break down food substances for absorption through the gastrointestinal tract. Amylase reduces starch to dextrins, lipase breaks fat down into glycerol and fatty acids, and trypsin acts on protein to release peptides and amino acids.

Pathophysiology. Tumors of the pancreas can thus arise from alpha cells, beta cells, or glandular elements

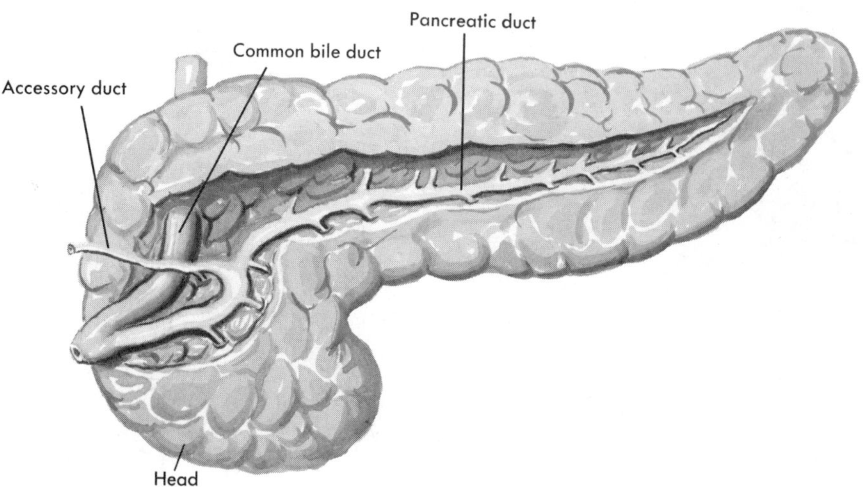

Fig. 12-8. Pancreas dissected to show main and accessory ducts. (From Anthony, C. P., and Thibodeau, G. A.: Textbook of anatomy and physiology, ed. 10, St. Louis, 1979, The C. V. Mosby Co.)

and can easily produce bile duct obstruction when they arise in the head of the gland. Diabetes mellitus is caused by failure of function of the islets of Langerhans, but the exact etiology of this process is unknown. Acute inflammatory disease may be the result of infection (such as mumps virus) or trauma. Chronic pancreatitis is associated with chronic alcoholism though the exact mechanism is unclear.

The search for an early accurate method of diagnosing pancreatic tumors when they are still small and potentially curable included imaging by radionuclides. Since the pancreas is retroperitoneal, conventional radiography could not visualize the organ, and displacement by a neoplasm of the gastrointestinal tract did not become evident by barium until late in the course of disease.

The pancreas may be visualized after intravenous injection of ^{75}Se-selenomethionine, which is a gamma-emitting radioactive analog of the amino acid methionine in which ^{75}Se has been substituted for the sulfur atom. Although amino acids localize in many tissues, high concentrations of ^{75}Se are achieved in the pancreas because there is a rapid synthesis of digestive enzymes in that organ. (The pancreas secretes 10 to 45 g of protein per day.)

Patient preparation with a high-protein meal just prior to injection or a fat-free sugar-rich breakfast has been used to enhance isotope uptake.[15,36] However, many institutions report acceptable results without special techniques.[22,26] Fasting, however, is discouraged, since it favors uptake by the liver attributable to the biologic priority of plasma protein synthesis.

Although the half-life of ^{75}Se is 120 days, the biologic turnover is in fact more rapid; after intravenous injection, the blood radioactivity falls to a minimum between 30 and 45 minutes. It rises to 75% of the post-injection level where it remains stable, descending to 35% over 7 days. The early fall in blood level reflects uptake by the pancreas and liver; the rise reflects a release of proteins synthesized in the liver back into the bloodstream. Sixty-eight percent of the administered dose concentrates in the pancreas, where there is approximately seven times the concentration per gram found in the liver. However, by weight, there is three times more agent in the liver releasing a target dose of 25 mrad/μCi of ^{75}Se than in the pancreas with a

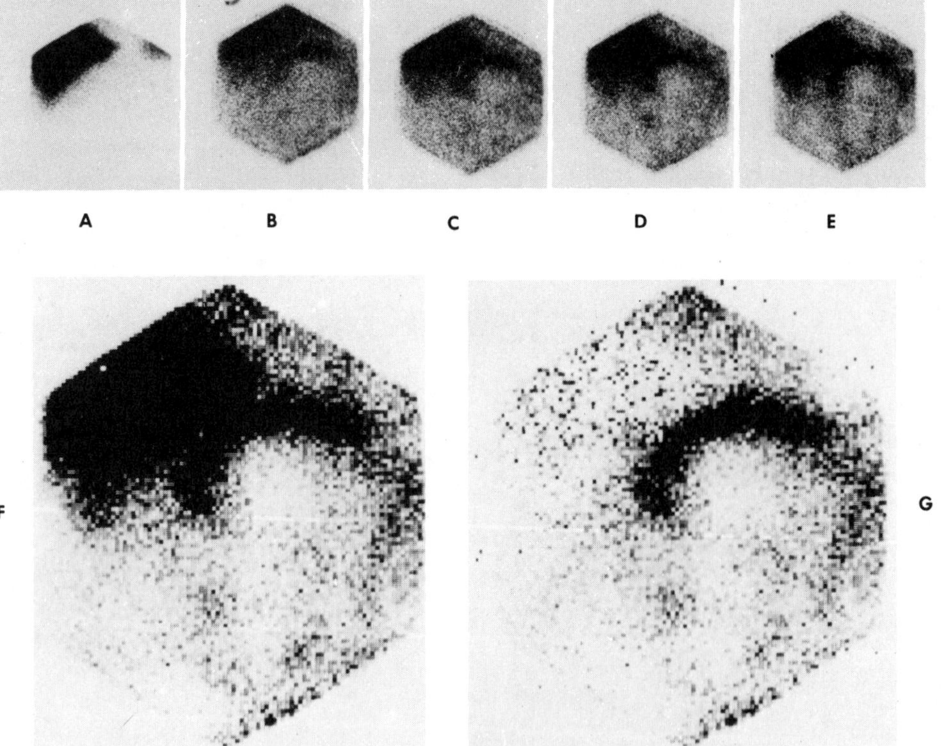

Fig. 12-9. ^{75}Se-selenomethionine pancreas scan without, **F**, and with, **G**, computer subtraction. (From Early, P. J., Razzak, M. A., and Sodee, D. B.: Textbook of nuclear medicine technology, ed. 3, St. Louis, 1979, The C. V. Mosby Co.)

total body dose of 8 mrad/μCi. Eighty percent of the dose will subsequently clear in the urine and 15% in the feces.[30]

The usual dose is 250 μCi for an adult. Although several photopeaks are available, 265 keV is commonly used for imaging with the medium-energy collimator.

Anterior images are done with the camera angled 10 to 15 degrees to the patient's right and 10 degrees to the head. In most instances the normal pancreas will be visualized within an hour of injection as a broad band of activity beneath the inferior margin of the liver. Variability in pancreatic shape and overlapping of pancreas by the liver contribute to difficulty in interpretation. Computer-assisted subtraction of the liver image at the conclusion of the study may be performed by injection of the patient with ^{99m}Tc-sulfur colloid while the patient is in the same position used for pancreatic imaging[47] (Fig. 12-9). A flow study performed during injection of the ^{99m}Tc-sulfur colloid can also be used to confirm the position of the aorta, which may thin a portion of the neck of the overlying pancreas.

The finding of a normal pancreatic image indicates with 90% accuracy that the pancreas is normal. Abnormal scan findings in patients with pancreatitis or pancreatic tumors include diffuse poor uptake of tracer and focal areas of diminished activity. The accuracy of detection of tumors cannot compare with information currently available from computerized axial tomography and ultrasound.[2]

Pancreas scanning may, however, still provide some information concerning the functional status of the pancreas that may be of supportive value when duodenal aspiration of secretions suggest a deficiency. Scintigraphy may also be of some assistance when surgery has been performed for tumor or trauma and the presence or position of functioning pancreatic tissue is in question.

SALIVARY GLANDS

The salivary glands consist of three paired glands that empty their contents into the mouth. The sublingual and submandibular are located beneath the tongue. The parotid glands are located below and to the front of the ears (Fig. 12-10). Radiographic studies of the salivary glands provide information about integrity and displacement of the duct system only. Functional capacity of tumor cells can be estimated by use of ^{99m}Tc-pertechnetate. Both Warthin's tumors and oncocytomas show hyperconcentration of radiopertechnetate (Fig. 12-11). Other tumors, including carcinoma, mixed tumors, and lymphoma are either "warm" or show decreased uptake.[41]

^{99m}Tc-pertechnetate is handled by the body in a fashion similar to iodine. It is concentrated in salivary duct cells but not in acinar cells. No patient preparation is necessary. A dose of ^{99m}Tc-pertechnetate (15 to 20 mCi) is administered intravenously. Perchlorate may be given at the end of the study to wash activity out of the gland but is withheld during the study, since it will reduce salivary gland uptake. An initial flow study with images made every 1 to 2 seconds from the anterior is followed at 10 minutes by 100,000-count images made with the pinhole collimator centered on a point just anterior to the earlobe. If a mass is present, an additional image is made with a radioactive marker over the mass. A final anterior view with the parallel-hole collimator to include both glands is made, and occasionally a posterior view may be required (Fig. 12-11). Benign tumors will show hyperconcentration and may be surgically removed through a small incision. Masses showing decreased uptake or nondelineated lesions have malignant potential, and surgery may include a much larger incision with dissection of neck nodes if cancer is present.

Occasionally, salivary scans are performed for an estimation of the production of saliva. After the initial flow study, images are collected anteriorly (to compare uptake in the glands and evaluate transit time to the mouth) using a scintillation camera interfaced to a computer. Prolonged clearance of isotope from the glands determines how severely impaired salivary production is.[40] Decreased function of one or both salivary glands may be attributable to aplasia, surgical removal, injury, or radiation. Bilateral decrease may be associated with rheumatoid arthritis.

The salivary study is useful in planning treatment of patients with mass lesions. It may be used to evaluate size, position, and function of the gland.

ESOPHAGUS

The function of the esophagus is to transport food and liquids from the mouth to the stomach (Fig. 12-1). Equally important is preventing reflux of gastric contents. The symptoms of gastroesophageal reflux include heartburn and postural regurgitation of gastric contents. Complications include esophagitis, esophageal ulceration, and stricture formation.

Techniques currently employed to evaluate gastroesophageal reflux include barium esophagography, barium ciné-swallows, endoscopy, mucosal biopsy, manometry, and acid-perfusion, clearance, and reflux testing. Barium studies and acid-reflux testing alone detect reflux directly. Other tests diagnose the consequences of reflux.

Isotope techniques were introduced in the hope of improving sensitivity of detection of reflux and also of quantitating the same.[28]

One hundred microcuries of ^{99m}Tc-sulfur colloid in

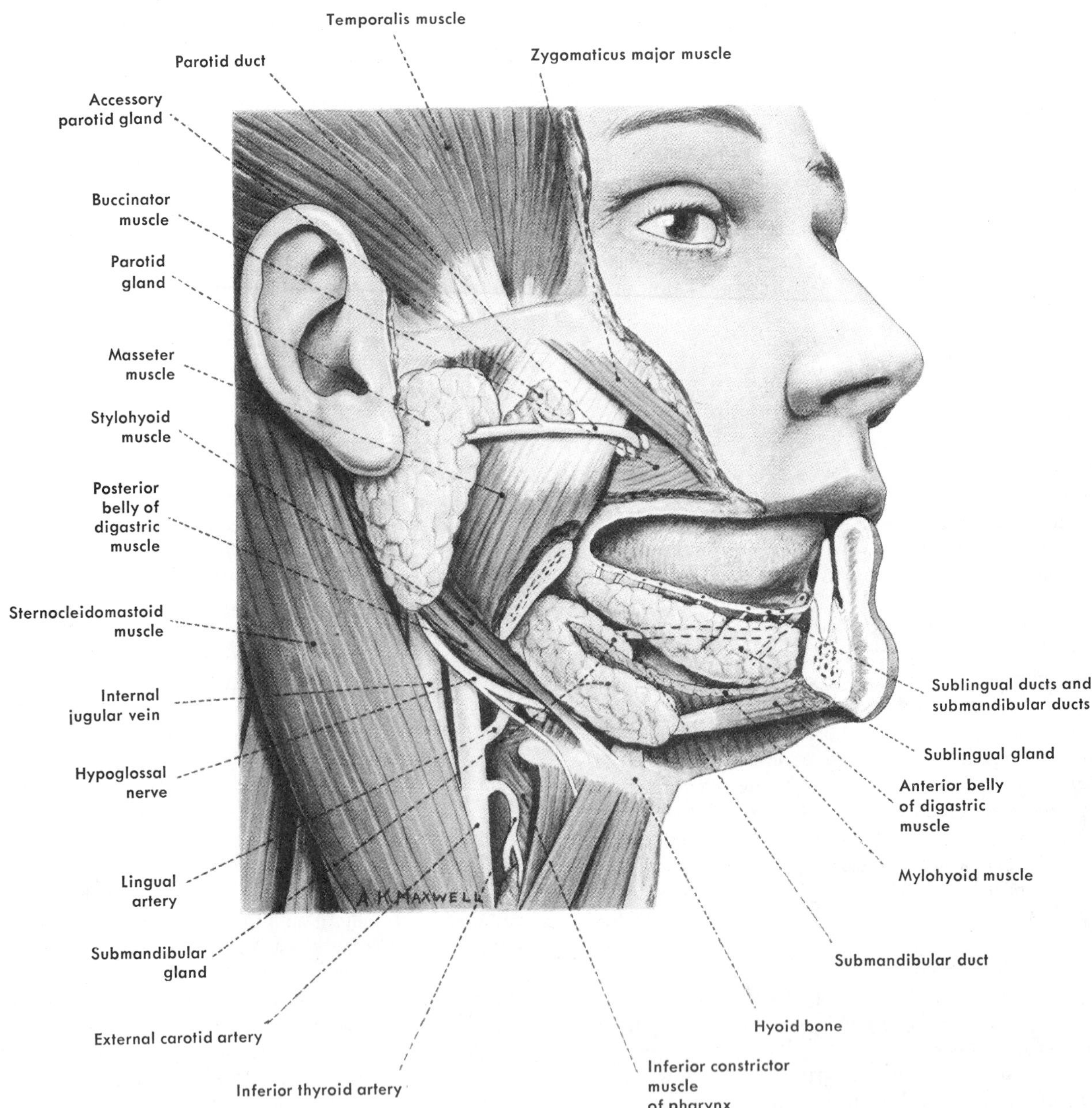

Fig. 12-10. Lateral view of glands in relationship with floor of mouth. Portion of mandible has been removed. (From Hamilton, W. J.: Textbook of human anatomy, ed. 2, St. Louis, 1976, The C. V. Mosby Co.; courtesy The Macmillan Press Ltd., Houndsmill Basingstoke, Hampshire, England.)

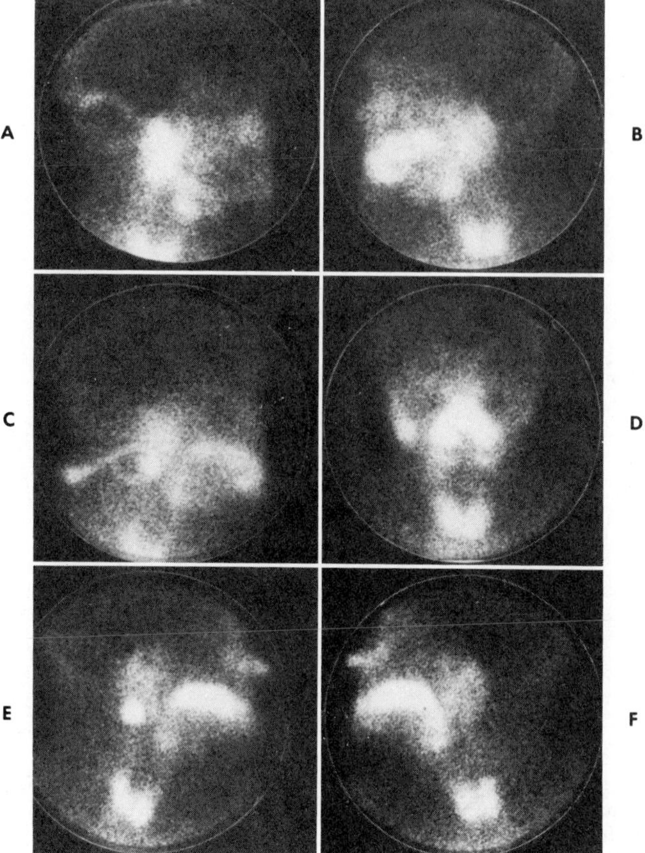

Fig. 12-11. Warthin's tumor of right parotid gland. Immediate right, **A,** and left lateral, **B,** views. Delayed right lateral view with radioactive string marker around palpable nodule, **C.** One-hour delayed views taken in the anterior **(D),** right **(E),** and left lateral **(F)** positions.

300 ml of isotonic saline at room temperature is instilled into the stomach through a nasogastric tube with the patient supine under a scintillation camera directed at the thorax. Using a double-lumen tube, one increases the pressure on the gastroesophageal junction by 5 mm Hg increments from 10 to 35 mm. Thirty-second exposures at each pressure are made. Counts in the esophagus may be compared to counts in the stomach by use of a computer. If no reflux is demonstrated, the test may be repeated using 300 ml of ^{99m}Tc-sulfur colloid in weak acid.

The test is positive if counts are observed at any point in the esophagus and the percentage of gastric contents refluxed acts as a quantitation of severity of the process.

The clinical significance of minimal degrees of esophageal reflux is questionable at best. It has been suggested recently that diminished muscle tone in the lower esophagus rather than hiatus hernia is the cause of most reflux.[35] Simple inexpensive regimens such as the use of antacids and changes in the diet to include more protein may resolve symptoms in most patients (only 5% of whom may eventually require surgery). Small degrees of reflux are hardly grounds for surgery, and a trial of therapy (known to be innocuous) may satisfy both patient and referring physician much more than the results of complicated diagnostic tests.[7]

STOMACH

The stomach is a crescent-shaped pouchlike organ that lies just below the diaphragm (Fig. 12-12). Proximally, it is linked to the esophagus and distally to the small intestine. It is usually described as having three parts: the fundus into which the esophagus empties, the body with its greater and lesser curvatures, and the pylorus. The cardiac sphincter muscle envelopes the junction of the esophagus and fundus, and the pyloric sphincter joins the pylorus and small intestine.

Interest in normal rates of gastric (stomach) empty-

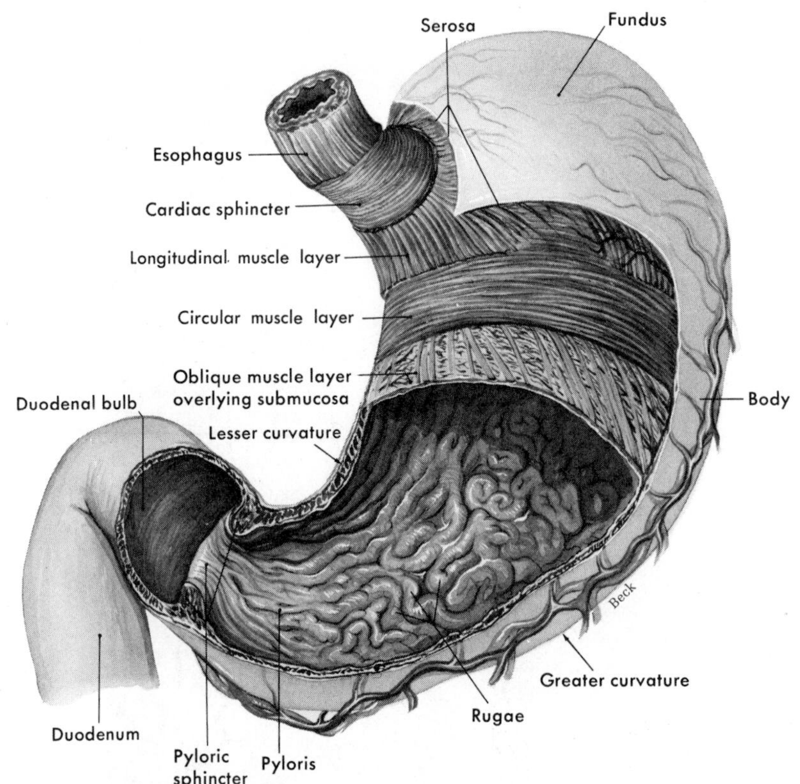

Fig. 12-12. Stomach. (From Anthony, C. P., and Thibodeau, G. A.: Textbook of anatomy and physiology, ed. 10, St. Louis, 1979, The C. V. Mosby Co.)

ing has resulted in a variety of methods of study, including intubation tests, contrast radiography, and isotopic imaging.[10] Operations for duodenal ulcer may result in alteration of motility and emptying. Diabetes, degenerative diseases, and infiltrative processes in the stomach wall may all prolong gastric emptying time. Since medical therapy in addition to surgery is now available to treat these conditions, interest both in normal emptying times and in base-line pretreatment assessment has now become more intense.

The proximal part of the stomach normally serves a reservoir function. A pacemaker located one third of the way from the esophagus to the duodenum on the greater curvature initiates contractions that propel food out of the stomach when the pyloris is open. The rate of gastric emptying is dependent on resistance of the pyloric sphincter. Nearly all hormones (for example, gastrin, secretin, and cholecystokinin) that arise in or act on the alimentary tract delay gastric emptying. Volume receptors in gastric muscle sensitive to distension trigger gastric contraction. Osmoreceptors in the duodenum may inhibit emptying to slow passage of foodstuffs. Acid receptors in the first part of the duodenum inhibit gastric contractions. Both fats and amino acids present in the duodenum will delay contractions until the concentration of foodstuffs again falls to a threshold level.

A variety of isotopes, including chromium, cesium, iodine, indium, and technetium,[10] have been used. The ideal tracer should not be absorbed through or adsorb to the gastric mucosa, should have no effect on gastric emptying, and should mix evenly with ingested food.

When a liquid meal is used, 500 ml of normal saline with 0.5 mCi of ^{99m}Tc-sulfur colloid is administered and sequential images of 500,000 counts each are made of the abdomen while continuous monitoring is performed by a computer.[10] The study is usually complete by 30 minutes but may continue if prolonged retention is present.

Various solid meals including chicken liver (from a chicken previously injected with ^{99m}Tc-sulfur colloid),[29] cornflakes and milk,[8,23] soft boiled eggs, and ham and cheese sandwiches have been used.[21,48]

Normal values are expressed as the half-time of gastric emptying and are on the order of 37 ± 5 minutes for ^{99m}Tc–cornflakes and milk and 12 minutes for ^{99m}Tc-sulfur colloid saline.[10]

At present there are few clinical applications of the test, but physiologic information gained about gastric emptying and pharmacokinetics make this a useful laboratory tool.

ABSORPTION OF PROTEIN, FAT, AND GASTROINTESTINAL PROTEIN LOSS

In pancreatic disease, insufficiency of enzyme production may lead to diminished gastrointestinal (GI) absorption of proteins, fats, and other nutrients. An additional group of diseases, the protein-losing gastroenteropathies, lead to hypoproteinemia by excess loss of plasma proteins, primarily albumin, from the blood into the gastrointestinal tract. A variety of approaches utilizing radiolabeled substances have been attempted for diagnosis and evaluation of this series of disorders.

Absorption of protein

In the past, absorption tests utilizing ^{131}I-labeled albumin have been used.[9] Blood and fecal levels were studied after ingestion of a measured amount of this labeled protein. Because of interfering factors such as small-bowel disease, bacterial decomposition of protein in the large intestine, and the evolution of better tests, the use of ^{131}I-labeled albumin has no practicality today.[42]

Gastrointestinal protein loss

The loss of protein, particularly albumin, into the gastrointestinal tract may be attributable to a number of gastrointestinal disorders. Several radioisotopic agents have been used to study this disease. To date chromium 51–labeled albumin remains as the agent of choice.[42]

The test is performed in two parts. After intravenous injection of 75 μCi of ^{51}Cr-labeled albumin, the patient is instructed to collect all stools, free of urine contamination, for 96 hours in 24-hour aliquots. A diluted standard of the injectate is retained for later comparison. Daily blood samples are collected as well, and appropriate samples of plasma are prepared for counting.

At the end of the collection period, the stools are homogenized and aliquots of each 24-hour sample are counted. The amount of the administered dose recovered in stool is determined by the following formula:

$$\% \text{ recovered} = \frac{\text{Net cpm (counts per minute) of all stool samples} \times 100}{\text{Net CPM of injectate standard} \times \text{Dilution factor}}$$

Normal values are Less than 2% of the administered dose recovered in 96 hours of stool collection.[42]

The second part of the test is the measure of the amount of plasma (in milliliters) that is lost in the gastrointestinal tract per day. This is determined by the following:

$$\text{Plasma lost (ml)} = \frac{\text{Net CPM in 24-hour stool collection}}{\text{Net CPM per ml of plasma on day preceding collection period}}$$

Normal values are 5 to 35 ml per day.[42]

Fat absorption—^{131}I-triolein test

The gastrointestinal tract's inability to absorb fat, proteins, vitamins, and minerals often is reflected as steatorrhea (large, bulky, fatty stools). Fat (lipid) is normally digested in the small bowel by the action of lipase, an enzyme excreted by the pancreas. Steatorrhea may also occur because of many other conditions not related to pancreatic exocrine insufficiency.

^{131}I-labeled triolein, a neutral fat, was investigated in the early 1950s[39] in the hope of providing an esthetic method of studying fat absorption by the determination of radioactivity levels in blood. Unfortunately, this method did not prove to be so accurate as the measurement of fecal activity after an adequate collection period (72 to 96 hours).[42]

Although ^{131}I-triolein has been available commercially for a number of years, this test is not popular today, primarily because of its poor reliability and the necessity to collect and process multiple stool samples. Upon our recent inquiry, a large commercial supplier informed us that it was likely the product would be discontinued in the near future.

^{131}I–oleic acid test

The ^{131}I–oleic acid test came into prominence because it was believed that steatorrhea from lack of lipase secretion by the pancreas could be differentiated from that resulting from small-bowel disease. This did not prove to be the case, and as a result the oleic acid test is of no clinical value today.

CO_2 breath analysis test

The analysis of breath exhalation after the oral administration of $^{14}CO_2$-labeled fats is probably the most definitive isotopic test of fat absorption. Unfortunately, this test has not become popular partly because not many nuclear medicine departments have liquid scintillation counters. For more information on breath analysis testing, the reader is referred to the review by Shreeve.[45]

REFERENCES

1. Alfidi, R. J., Haaga, J., Meaney, T. F., et al.: Computed tomography of the thorax and abdomen: a preliminary report, Radiology **117**:257, 1975.
2. Barkin, J., Vining, D., Miale, A. J., Jr., et al.: Computerized tomography, diagnostic ultrasound and radionuclide scanning.

Comparison of efficacy in diagnosis of pancreatic carcinoma, J.A.M.A. **238**(19):2040, 1977.

3. Benacerraf, B., Biozzi, G., Halpern, B. N., et al.: Phagocytosis of heat denatured human serum albumin labeled with I-131 and its use as a means of investigating liver blood flow, Br. J. Exp. Pathol. **38:**35, 1957.
4. Biozzi, G., Benacerraf, B., Halpern, B. N., et al.: Exploration of the phagocytic function of the reticuloendothelial system with heat denatured human serum albumin labeled with I-131 and application to the measurement of liver blood flow in normal man in some pathologic conditions, J. Lab. Clin. Med. **51:** 238, 1958.
5. Bradley, E. L., III: Measurement of hepatic blood flow in man, Surgery **75:**783, 1974.
6. Bryan, P. J., Dunn, W. M., and Grossman, Z. D.: Correlation of computerized tomography, gray scale ultrasonography and radionuclide imaging of the liver in detecting space-occupying processes, Radiology **124:**387, 1977.
7. Castell, D. O.: The lower esophageal sphincter: physiologic and clinical aspects, Ann. Intern. Med. **83:**390, 1975.
8. Chaudhuri, T. K., Heading, R. C., Greenwald, A., et al.: Measurement of gastric emptying (GET) of solid meal using ^{99m}Tc DTPA, J. Nucl. Med. **15:**483, 1974.
9. Chinn, A. B., Lavik, P. S., Stitt, R. M., et al.: Use of ^{131}I-labeled protein in the diagnosis of pancreatic insufficiency, N. Engl. J. Med. **247:**877, 1952.
10. Cooperman, A. M., and Cook, S. A.: Gastric emptying—physiology and measurements, Surg. Clin. N. Am. **56**(6):1277, 1976.
11. Crandell, D. C., Boyd, M., Wennemark, J. R., et al.: Liver-spleen scanning: the left lateral decubitus position is best for lateral views, J. Nucl. Med. **13:**720, 1972.
12. DeNardo, G. L., Stadalnik, R. C., DeNardo, S. J., et al.: Hepatic scintiangiographic patterns, Radiology **111:**135, 1974.
13. Dunson, G. L., Thrall, J. H., Stevenson, J. S., et al.: ^{99m}Tc minicolloid for radionuclide lymphography, Radiology **109:**387, 1973.
14. Dunson, G., Chandler, R., Pinsky, S., et al.: ^{99m}Technetium minicolloid for RES bone marrow imaging, 1972, Mid-Eastern Society of Nuclear Medicine.
15. Espiritu, C. R., and Rolfs, H. E.: Diagnostic accuracy of pancreatic scanning, Am. J. Dig. Dis. **17:**539, 1972.
16. Fonseca, C., Greenberg, D., Rosenthall, L., et al.: Assessment of the utility of gallbladder imaging with ^{99m}Tc-IDA, Clin. Nucl. Med. **3:**437, 1978.
17. Fonseca, C., Rosenthall, L., Greenberg, D., et al.: Differential diagnosis of jaundice by ^{99m}Tc-IDA hepatobiliary imaging, Clin. Nucl. Med. **4:**135, 1979.
18. Friedell, H. L., MacIntyre, W. J., and Rejali, A. M.: A method for visualization of the configuration and structure of the liver, Am. J. Roentgenol. **77:**455, 1957.
19. Garcia, A. C., Yeh, S. D. J., and Benua, R. S.: Accumulation of bone-seeking radionuclides in liver metastasis from colon carcinoma, Clin. Nucl. Med. **2:**265, 1977.
20. Goodwin, D. A., Stern, H. S., Wagner, H. N., Jr., et al.: Indium-113m: a new radiopharmaceutical for liver scanning, Nucleonics **24:**65, 1966.
21. Griffith, G. H., Owen, G. M., and Shields, R.: The rate of gastric emptying in gastroduodenal disease, Br. J. Surg. **53:** 995, 1966.
22. Hatchette, J. B., Shuler, S. E., and Murison, P. J.: Scintiphotos of the pancreas: analysis of 134 studies, J. Nucl. Med. **13:**51, 1972.
23. Heading, R. C., Tothill, P., Laidlaw, A. J., et al.: An evaluation of ^{113m}indium DTPA chelate in the measurement of gastric emptying by scintiscanning, Gut **12:**611, 1975.
24. Kranzler, J. K., Vollert, J. M., Harper, P. V., et al.: The diagnostic value of hepatic pliability as assessed from inspiration and expiration views on the gamma camera, Radiology **97:**323, 1976.
25. Kumar, B., Coleman, R. E., and Alderson, P. O.: Gallium citrate Ga-67 imaging in patients with suspected inflammatory processes, Arch. Surg. **110:**1237, 1975.
26. Landman, S., Polcyn, R. E., and Gottschalk, A.: Pancreas imaging—Is it worth it? Radiology **100:**631, 1971.
27. Lomas, F., Dibos, P. E., and Wagner, H. N., Jr.: Increased specificity of liver scanning with the use of ^{67}gallium citrate, N. Engl. J. Med. **286:**1323, 1972.
28. Malmud, L. S., and Fisher, R. S.: Quantitation of gastroesophageal reflux before and after therapy using the gastroesophageal scintiscan, South. Med. J. **71**(Suppl. 1):10, 1978.
29. Meyer, J. H., MacGregor, I. L., Gueller, R., et al.: ^{99m}Tc-tagged chicken liver as a marker of solid food in the human stomach, Am. J. Dig. Dis. **21:**296, 1976.
30. Medical internal radiation dose (MIRD): dose estimate report no. 1: Summary of current radiation dose estimates to humans from ^{75}Se-L-selenomethionine, J. Nucl. Med. **14**(1):49, 1973.
31. Medical internal radiation dose (MIRD): dose estimate report no. 3: Summary of current radiation dose estimates to humans with various liver conditions from ^{99m}Tc-sulfur colloid, J. Nucl. Med. **16**(1):108A, 1975.
32. Mundschenk, H., Hromec, A., and Fischer, J.: Phagocytic activity of the liver as a measure of hepatic circulation—a comparative study using ^{198}Au and ^{99m}Tc-sulfur colloid, J. Nucl. Med. **12:**711, 1971.
33. Oppenheimer, B. E., Hoffer, P. B., Gottschalk, A.: The use of inspiration-expiration scintiphotographs to determine the intrinsic or extrinsic nature of liver defects, J. Nucl. Med. **13** (7):554, 1972.
34. Park, C. H., Garafola, J. H., and O'Hara, A. E.: Preoperative diagnosis of asymptomatic choledochal cyst by rose bengal liver scan, J. Nucl. Med. **15:**310, 1974.
35. Pope, C. E., II: Pathophysiology and diagnosis of reflux esophagitis, Gastroenterology **70:**445, 1976.
36. Rodríguez-Antúnez, A.: Photoscanning of the pancreas, J.A.M.A. **205:**347, 1968.
37. Ronai, P. M.: Hepatobiliary radiopharmaceuticals: defining their clinical role will be a galling experience, J. Nucl. Med. **18:**488, 1977.
38. Rosenfield, A. T., Schneider, P. B.: Rapid evaluation of hepatic size on radioisotope scan, J. Nucl. Med. **15:**237, 1974.
39. Ruffin, J. M., Shingelton, W. W., Baylin, G. J., et al.: ^{131}I labeled fat in the study of intestinal absorption, N. Engl. J. Med. **255:**594, 1956.
40. Schall, G. L., Anderson, L. G., Wolf, R. O., et al.: Xerostomia in Sjögren's syndrome: evaluation by sequential salivary scintigraphy, J.A.M.A. **216:**2109, 1971.
41. Schmitt, G., Lehmann, G., Strötges, W., et al.: The diagnostic value of sialography and scintigraphy in salivary gland diseases, Br. J. Radiol. **49:**326, 1976.
42. Schwabe, A. D.: Gastrointestinal tract function and disease. In Blahd, W. H., editor: Nuclear medicine, New York, 1971, McGraw-Hill Book Co.
43. Selby, J. B.: Radiological examination of subphrenic disease process, CRC Crit. Rev. Diagn. Imaging **9**(3):229, 1977.
44. Serafini, A. N., Smoak, W. M., Hupf, H. B., et al.: Iodine-123 rose bengal: an improved hepatobiliary imaging agent, J. Nucl. Med. **16:**629, 1975.
45. Shreeve, W. W.: Labeled carbon breath analysis. In Rocha, A. F. G., and Harbert, J. C., editors: Textbook of nuclear medicine: basic science, Philadelphia, 1978, Lea & Febiger.
46. Shultz, M. M., Morales, J. D., Fishbein, P. G., et al.: Bilateral breast uptake of ^{99m}Tc polyphosphate in a patient with metastatic adenocarcinoma, Radiology **118:**377, 1976.

47. Staab, E. V., Babb, O. A., Klatte, E. C., et al.: Pancreatic radionuclide imaging using electronic subtraction technique, Radiology **99:**633, 1971.
48. van Dam, A. P. M.: The gamma camera in clinical evaluation of gastric emptying, Radiology **110:**155, 1974.
49. Waxman, A. D., Apaw, R., and Siemsen, J. K.: Rapid sequential liver imaging, J. Nucl. Med. **13:**522, 1972.
50. Williams, L. E., Fisher, J. H., Courtney, R. A., et al.: Preoperative diagnosis of choledochal cyst by hepatoscintography, N. Engl. J. Med. **283:**85, 1970.
51. Winston, M. A., Karelitz, J., Weiss, E. R., et al.: Variation in the appearance of the lateral liver scan with patient position, Radiology **102:**665, 1972.
52. Wistow, B. W., Subramanian, G., Van Heertum, R. L., et al.: An evaluation of ^{99m}Tc-labeled hepatobiliary agents, J. Nucl. Med. **18:**455, 1977.

Chapter 13

THE GENITOURINARY SYSTEM

Richard J. Beschi, Eva Dubovsky, and Frances N. Kontzen

Renal imaging and functional studies are recognized as reliable means to evaluate the structure and location of the anatomic components of the urinary tract as well as to determine the total and differential performance of the kidneys. This can be accomplished without danger of allergic reactions, unpleasant side effects, or excessive radiation dose to the organs involved. However, a thorough knowledge of physiology and pathology of the genitourinary tract is important for optimizing the technique and understanding the results. The dynamic approach, which incorporates in vitro work, scintigraphy, data processing and analysis, though complex, is neither beyond the comprehension of the competent technologist nor beyond the capabilities of today's average nuclear medicine laboratory.

Complemented by other imaging modalities, radionuclide renal imaging has emerged as an important diagnostic tool in nephrology, urology, and renal transplantation.

ANATOMY AND PHYSIOLOGY

Renal circulation

The kidneys regulate the volume and composition of the body's extracellular fluid through their excretory function. They also play an important role in circulatory dynamics because under normal conditions they receive one fourth of the cardiac output.[19] Blood is supplied to the kidneys (Fig. 13-1) by the renal artery, which enters the renal hilum and divides into four or five lobar branches, which in turn give rise to the interlobar arteries in the renal columns of the medulla. At the medulla-cortex junction the interlobar arteries branch out into the arcuate arteries, which at intervals give rise to interlobular arteries penetrating upward into the renal cortex.

Nephron circulation

After entering the cortex (Fig. 13-2), the interlobular arteries branch out into the afferent arterioles, which terminate as tufts of capillaries, the glomeruli, numbering over 1 million per kidney. These capillary beds do not reform into venules but into efferent arterioles, which leave the glomeruli and ramify into a network of capillaries (peritubular capillaries and vasa recta) enmeshing the entire tubular system of the nephron. It is from this second capillary bed that the venules unite to initiate the venous return with the interlobular veins and complete it through the arcuate veins, interlobar veins, and renal veins, which leave the renal hilum and empty into the inferior vena cava.

The nephron

The functional unit of the kidney, the nephron (Fig. 13-3), consists of a glomerulus and a renal tubule, and lies for the most part in the renal cortex. The glomerulus is a tuft of capillaries enclosed by a capsule (Bowman's), which is actually an expanded, invaginated portion of a renal tubule. As it arises from the Bowman's capsule, the tubule follows a tortuous course and hence is termed the proximal convoluted tubule; then it proceeds straight, dips downward into the medulla, makes a hairpin turn (Henle's loop) upward, and returns to the vicinity of the glomerulus where again it assumes a winding course named the distal convoluted tubule and finally ends in a collecting tubule. The collecting tubule passes downward through the medulla as a component of a renal pyramid, joins larger tubules, which converge to form one tube that opens at a renal papilla into one of the minor calyces; these converge in the major calyces, which compose the renal pelvis and funnel into the ureter.[1]

Clearance

Renal clearance may be considered to represent the volume of blood or plasma that is completely cleared of any substance per unit time. The values needed to calculate plasma clearance, C, are (1) the concentration of a substance in the urine, U, in milligrams per milliliter, (2) the concentration of the same substance

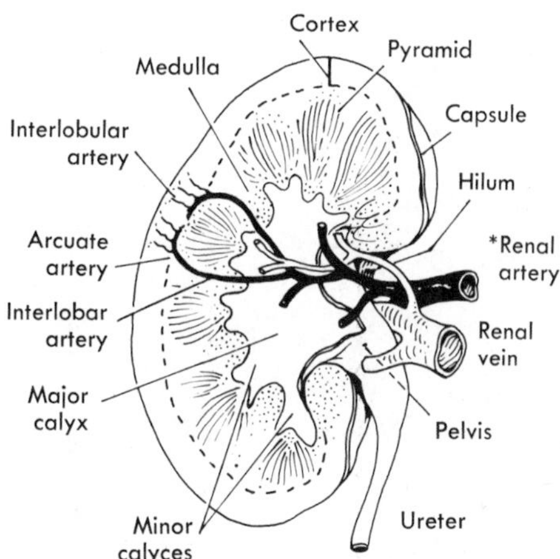

Fig. 13-1. Diagram of coronal section of right kidney. *Vascular distribution of renal artery *(black)* is magnified for clarity.

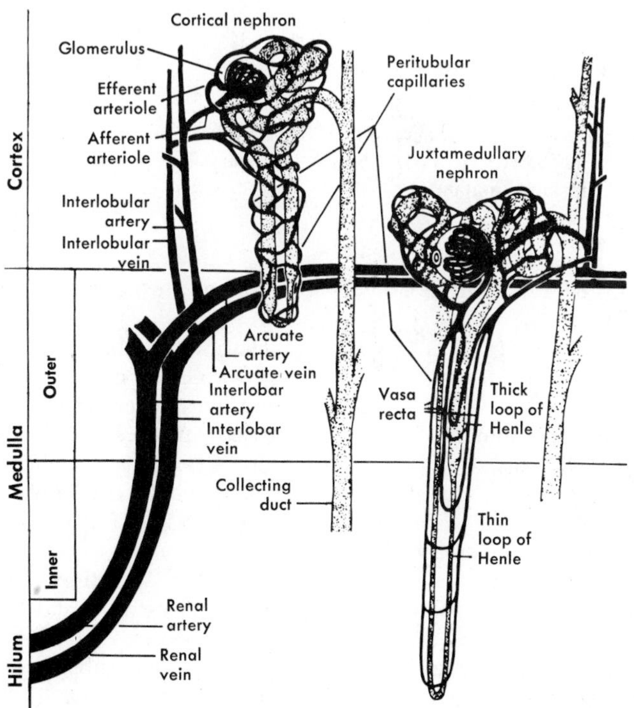

Fig. 13-2. Schematic representation of nephron, circulation, and respective location in kidney structure. (From Hamilton, W. J.: Textbook of human anatomy, ed. 2, St. Louis, 1976, The C. V. Mosby Co.; courtesy The Macmillan Press Ltd., Houndsmill Basingstoke, Hampshire, England.)

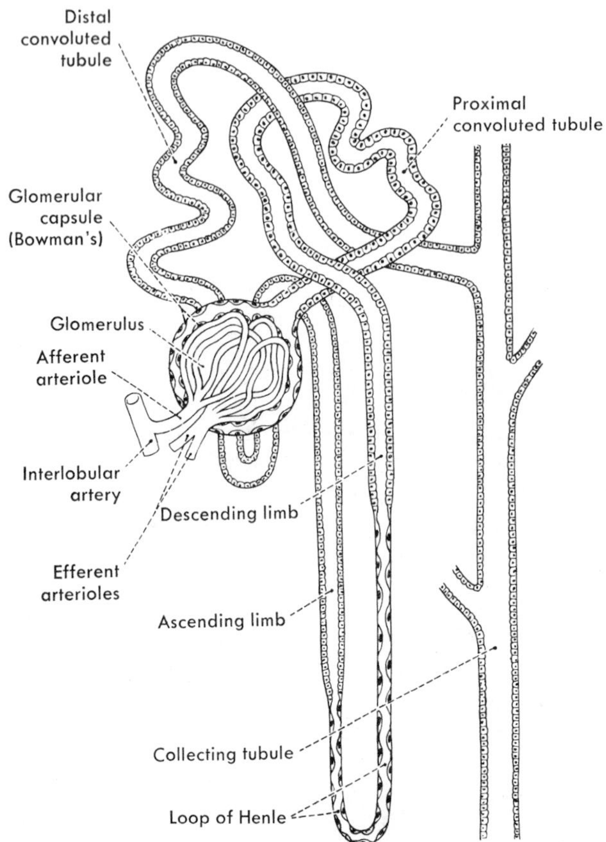

Fig. 13-3. Simplified diagram of nephron. (From Hamilton, W. J.: Textbook of human anatomy, ed. 2, St. Louis, 1976, The C. V. Mosby Co.; courtesy The Macmillan Press Ltd., Houndsmill Basingstoke, Hampshire, England.)

in plasma, P, (mg/ml), and (3) the rate of urine flow, V, in milliliters per minute. Thus:

$$C = \frac{UV}{P}$$

where C is expressed in milliliters per minute.

Excretion

Three processes are involved in urine formation (Fig. 13-3): glomerular filtration, tubular reabsorption, and tubular excretion.

Glomerular filtration. Water and solutes filter out of the glomeruli into Bowman's capsule because a pressure gradient exists between the two areas. This gradient is normally determined by the glomerular hydrostatic pressure of 70 mm Hg, which tends to move fluid out of the glomeruli. The blood colloidal osmotic pressure of 30 mm Hg combined with the capsular hydrostatic pressure of 20 mm Hg exert their force in the opposite direction. The net or effective filtration pressure is then 70 − (30 + 20), or 20 mm Hg.

Tubular reabsorption. The second process is the reabsorption of most of the water and part of the solutes from the glomerular filtrate back into the blood. It is carried out by cells in the walls of convoluted tubules, loop of Henle, and collecting tubules that absorb substances vitally needed by the body, such as water, glucose, Na^+, Cl^-, HCO_3^-, amino acids, and other nutrients.

Tubular secretion. In addition to reabsorption, tubular cells extract and excrete certain substances out of the blood into the filtrate. In both reabsorption and excretion, some substances are moved by active transport and some by passive mechanisms such as diffusion and osmosis. Ions and glucose are reabsorbed, and potassium and hydrogen ions are excreted by active-transport mechanisms, while water is reabsorbed by osmosis and ammonia is excreted by diffusion, both passive mechanisms. Of clinical importance is the

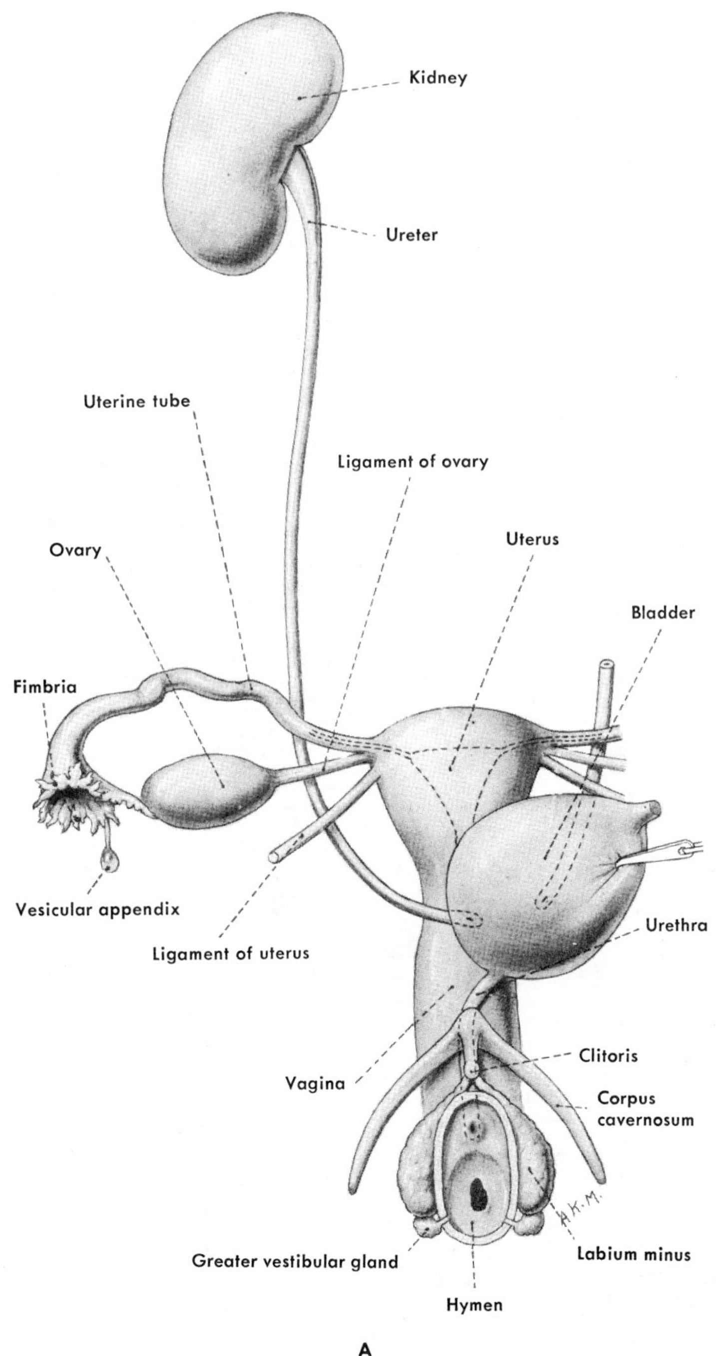

Continued.

Fig. 13-4. Schematic representation of urogenital organs in the female, **A,** and male, **B.** (From Hamilton, W. J.: Textbook of human anatomy, ed. 2, St. Louis, 1976, The C. V. Mosby Co.; courtesy The Macmillan Press Ltd., Houndsmill Basingstoke, Hampshire, England.)

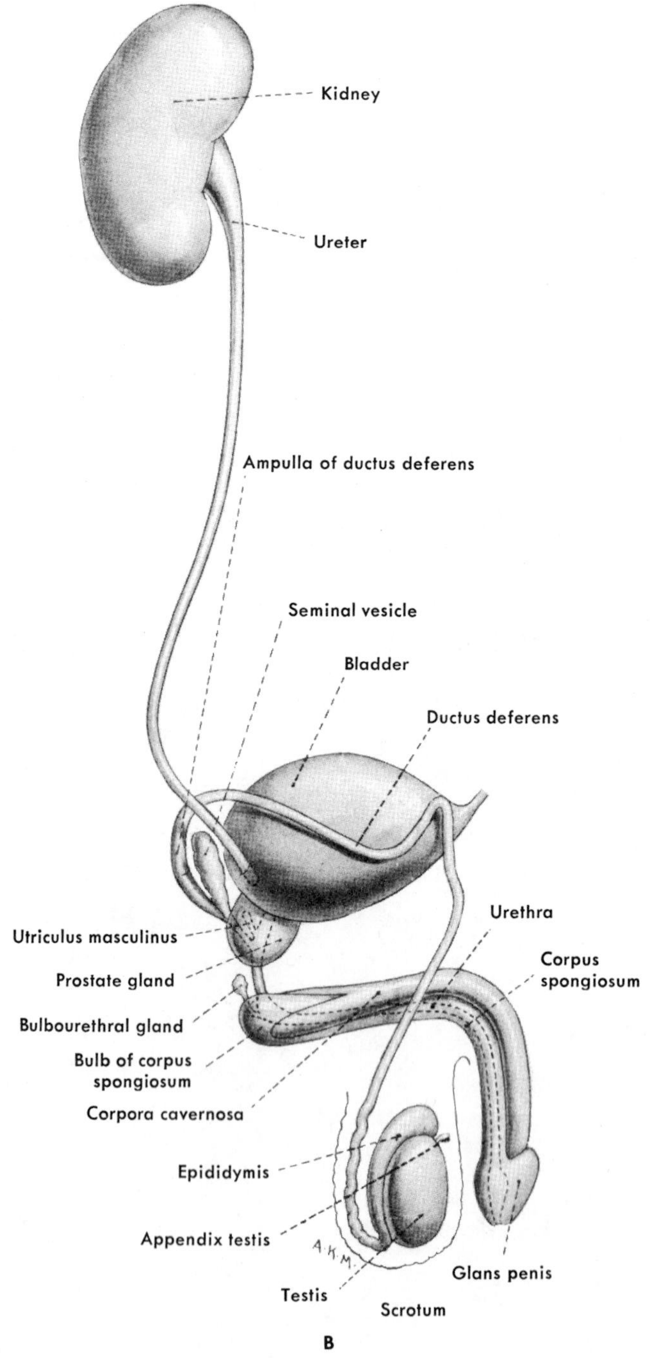

Fig. 13-4, cont'd. For legend see p. 347.

excretion of certain substances and drugs, such as para-aminohippuric acid (PAH),[1] by the tubular cells.

Drainage

As the urine is excreted, it flows from the collecting tubules into the calyces, to the pelvis, then down the ureters into the bladder, and finally out of the urethra (Fig. 13-4).

Ureters. These tubular structures, 24 to 30 cm long, approximately 0.9 cm in diameter, have walls lined by a mucous membrane covered by a two-layer muscular coat: the outer layer being circular, the inner longitudinal. The function of the ureters is to drain the urine into the urinary bladder. The muscular layers contract in peristaltic waves (1 to 5 per minute), forcing the urine into the bladder.

Urinary bladder. A collapsible bag, located directly behind the pubic symphysis, whose wall is composed of three smooth muscle layers and lined by a mucous membrane arranged in prominent folds or rugae. Because of its elastic structure, the bladder can distend considerably to a capacity that varies greatly with individuals (100 to 500 ml). Its function is to retain urine and, aided by the urethra, to expel it from the body. Distension of the bladder, as it fills with urine, triggers reflex contractions of the bladder wall. Simultaneous relaxation of the internal and external sphincters of the urethra will cause the bladder to empty. Contraction of the bladder and relaxation of the internal sphincter (neck of the bladder) are involuntary, whereas contraction of the external sphincter (at the urogenital diaphragm) to prevent or terminate urination is learned.

Urethra. The urethra is the tube extending from the floor of the bladder to the exterior. In the female it is 2.5 to 3 cm long, in the male 10 to 12 cm. Its function is to eliminate the urine from the body. In the male it also serves as a passageway for the seminal fluid.

Scrotum. In the male the scrotum is a pouchlike structure covered by corrugated skin suspended from the perineal region; it contains the testes, epididymis, and the first part of the seminal ducts (ductus deferens). The function of the scrotum is the maintenance of the optimal temperature of the testes; this is accomplished by adjustment of the scrotal walls to the external temperature by contraction and relaxation of the dartos muscle in cold and warm temperatures respectively. The blood is supplied to the scrotum, epididymis, and testes by branches of the internal pudendal arteries, by the inferior epigastric artery, and by the internal spermatic and seminal duct arteries, which anastomose in a network enveloping the epididymis and testes. The veins are usually paired with the arteries.

RADIONUCLIDE RENAL PROCEDURES

Glomerular filtration rate measurement

The inulin clearance test,[22,23] long recognized as the best measure of glomerular filtration rate (GFR), presents difficulties such as the availability of constant infusion apparatus and laborious blood and urine analysis not easily available in clinical laboratories. This led to the search for simpler, reliable tests of renal function. The use of chelates seemed to solve the problem.

Chelating agents are detoxifying substances forming complexes with radioactive or stable metals, which are eliminated primarily by the kidneys. The chelates most widely tested for the measurement of the glomerular filtration rate are edetic acid (ethylenediaminetetraacetic acid, EDTA), labeled with ^{51}Cr, and pentetic acid (diethylenetriaminepentaacetic acid, DTPA), labeled with ^{111}In, ^{99m}Tc, or other radionuclides (Table 13-1). At the present time, no single radiopharmaceutical has emerged as the ideal agent for measurement of glomerular filtration rate.

Effective renal plasma flow

Sodium *ortho*-iodohippurate (OIH) labeled with ^{131}I is cleared both by glomerular filtration (20%) and tubular secretion (80%).

It gives sharper accumulation peaks and more rapid clearance times than agents cleared only by glomerular filtration. Most importantly, its secretion by the tubular cell emphasizes renal function differences more distinctly than do agents cleared by filtration alone.

The availability of ^{131}I-OIH of high radionuclidic purity and current nuclear instrumentation allow clinically satisfactory determination of the effective renal plasma flow (ERPF) from ^{131}I-OIH plasma clearance curves obtained from a simple IV injection.[24] The term "effective" specifically refers to the portion of the renal blood that is presented to renal secretory tissue as opposed to the small fraction of blood perfusing nonsecretory renal tissues such as perirenal fat, the capsule, and the pelvis.[13]

Table 13-1. Radiopharmaceuticals used for measurement of glomerular filtration rate

Inulin	^{14}C, ^{125}I, ^{131}I, ^{51}Cr
Diatrizoate sodium (Hypaque, Renografin)	^{131}I
Iothalamate sodium	^{125}I, ^{131}I
Edetic acid (ethylenediaminetetraacetic acid, EDTA)	^{51}Cr
Pentetic acid (diethylenetriaminepentaacetic acid, DTPA)	^{99m}Tc, ^{111}In, ^{169}Yb

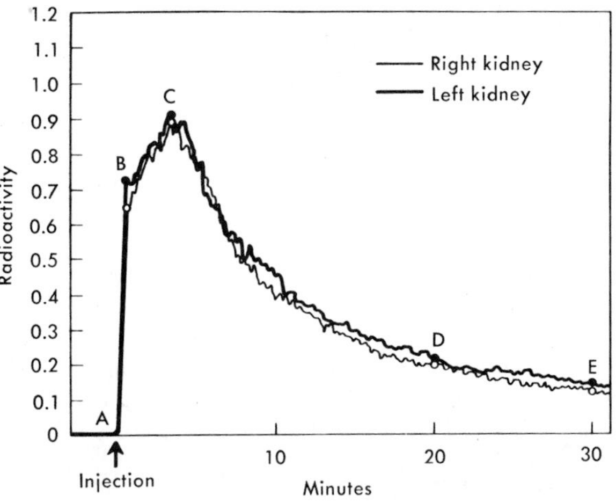

Fig. 13-5. Normal renogram recordings display equal curves bilaterally as illustrated in this study.

^{131}I-OIH renal function study (renogram)

The renogram is a graphic expression of the flow of a radiopharmaceutical through the kidneys. This procedure may be performed with collimated scintillation detectors connected to rate meters and the information is recorded on strip chart recorders, or with a scintillation camera with graphic-output capabilities.

Renograms with use of ^{131}I-OIH in a normal subject with adequate hydration (Fig. 13-5) have three parts: initial rise *(A-B),* ascending limb *(B-C),* and descending limb (*C* to *E*). The first portion, *A-B,* reflects arrival of the labeled blood under the detector. The second portion, *B-C,* is an expression of more activity arriving and being concentrated by the kidney than is leaving the region of the kidney. The third portion, *C* to *E,* reflects the drainage process. The peak time shows accurately when the accumulation trend is reversed.

Patients are positioned so that the probes may be accurately placed over the kidneys. As little as 30 μCi of ^{131}I-OIH is administered intravenously. If a standard-field-of-view camera with a parallel-hole collimator is used, both kidneys can be included in the field of view in at least 85% of all patients, otherwise a diverging collimator is required.

With the large-field-of-view camera (such as one with a 15-inch crystal) proper positioning is accomplished with little difficulty. The recommended doses of ^{131}I-OIH for camera renography in the various age levels are as follows:

1 year old and under	50 μCi
1 to 6 years old	100 μCi
6 to 15 years old	200 μCi*
15 years old and over	300 μCi*

*The dose for a patient with a transplanted kidney or a postnephrectomy patient is reduced by one half, thus 100 and 150 μCi, respectively.

The base-line study should be performed on a patient in a normal hydrated state (Fig. 13-6). This is accomplished by having the patient drink approximately 0.5 liter of liquid during the hour preceding the study. Sometimes a repeat study in a dehydrated state is required (for detection of renal vascular disease). Urine specific gravity is determined to monitor the degree of hydration.[19] On a camera equipped with a tape system, the data may be stored and played back, and the regions of interest (ROI) defined. The curves generated from these ROIs are more representative of renal function. Where a computer is available, body background subtraction, isointensity-line ROI selection, and other technical refinements add to the overall quality of the procedure.

Comprehensive renal function study

A comprehensive nuclear medicine renal function study (CRFS) using radioiodinated *ortho*-iodohippurate (OIH) has proved to be a very sensitive test in the diagnosis of both bilateral and unilateral disease before it is evident by other means.[18] The CRFS includes:

1. Complete evaluation of total and differential function of kidneys
2. Evaluation of renal pelvises, ureters, and urinary bladder (residual urine)
3. Estimation of effective renal plasma flow (ERPF)
4. Evaluation of sequential scintigraphic images
5. Calculation of excretory indices
6. Renographic curves (Figs. 13-7 and 13-8)

Total excretion of an agent by the kidney, or complete clearance of an agent during one circulation through the kidney, determines renal plasma flow. No agent meets this criterion, but para-aminohippuric acid (PAH) comes close. Approximately 90% of PAH is cleared by the normal kidneys in one pass. The remaining 10% is found in the venous blood. No suitable

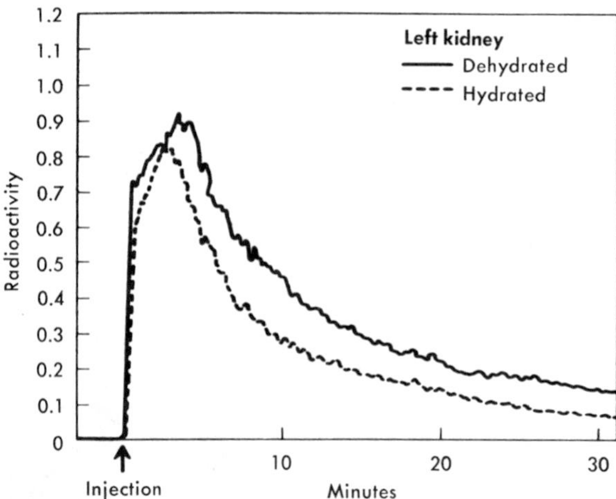

Fig. 13-6. This study demonstrates effect of hydration and dehydration on renogram curves. Second portion of curve, which reflects transit time, is prolonged; therefore peak is also delayed.

gamma emitter has been found to label PAH; consequently, when ^{131}I-OIH became available, it proved to be a valuable substitute for the measurement of the ERPF. When OIH and PAH were compared by Burbank et al.,[3] the average value for the clearance ratio was 0.87. Two of the reasons suggested for the lack of correlation of OIH compared to PAH are free iodide content of the ^{131}I-OIH and plasma protein binding.

Since the early 1960s, radionuclide renal studies have been utilized; however, because of inadequate instrumentation and the overestimation of only one parameter (for example, the renogram), nuclear medicine was unable to offer the urologists and nephrologists consistently reliable information that could be acquired by already established clinical procedures. With the advent of large-field-of-view cameras, relatively low-cost data systems, minicomputers, and chemically pure OIH with an acceptable quantity of free iodide, urologists and nephrologists have found the CRFS to be helpful in making the diagnosis, maintaining the medically treated patient, and keeping under observation the postsurgical patient.[8]

The single injection–single sample method used in the CRFS has proved to be both accurate and reproducible. The equipment necessary is available in most nuclear medicine departments and the technologist's time has been shortened considerably. The patient's radiation exposure is minimal, as seen in Table 13-2.

Only recently has ^{123}I-OIH with a 13-hour half-life, a 159 keV gamma radiation, and an absence of beta radiation been available in areas near cyclotrons. With its purification the future looks even brighter for this most useful urologic study.

For a more comprehensive discussion of CRFS refer to reference 18.

Table 13-2. Dosimetry*

Condition	Radiation dose to kidneys	
	Rads/μCi	**Rads/300 μCi**
Normal	1.6×10^{-4}	0.048
Ureteral obstruction	1.0×10^{-3}	0.3
Glomerulonephritis	6.9×10^{-4}	0.207
Lower perfusion (renal artery stenosis)	2.4×10^{-4}	0.072
	Rads/μCi	**Rads/150 μCi**
Transplant		
Acute tubular necrosis (ATN)	1.7×10^{-4}	0.0255
Acute rejection	4.4×10^{-4}	0.066
Normal	1.8×10^{-4}	0.027

*From Radiopharmaceutical Internal Dosimetry Information Center, Oak Ridge, Tennessee.

Static imaging

Static renal imaging is performed for evaluation of position, size, and shape of the kidneys. Radiopharmaceuticals used for this purpose are transported to the nephrons through the renal arterial circulation. After being filtered through glomeruli, they are reabsorbed to a different degree by the tubular cells and localized there. Tumors, cysts, and abscesses, which do not contain tubular cells, or parts of the kidneys deprived of their blood supply (infarction), or are injured (hematoma), will appear as cold areas. The amount of activity in each kidney is directly proportional to the amount delivered to the kidney and therefore reflects the degree of perfusion. This fact can be used to evaluate differential function of the kidneys.

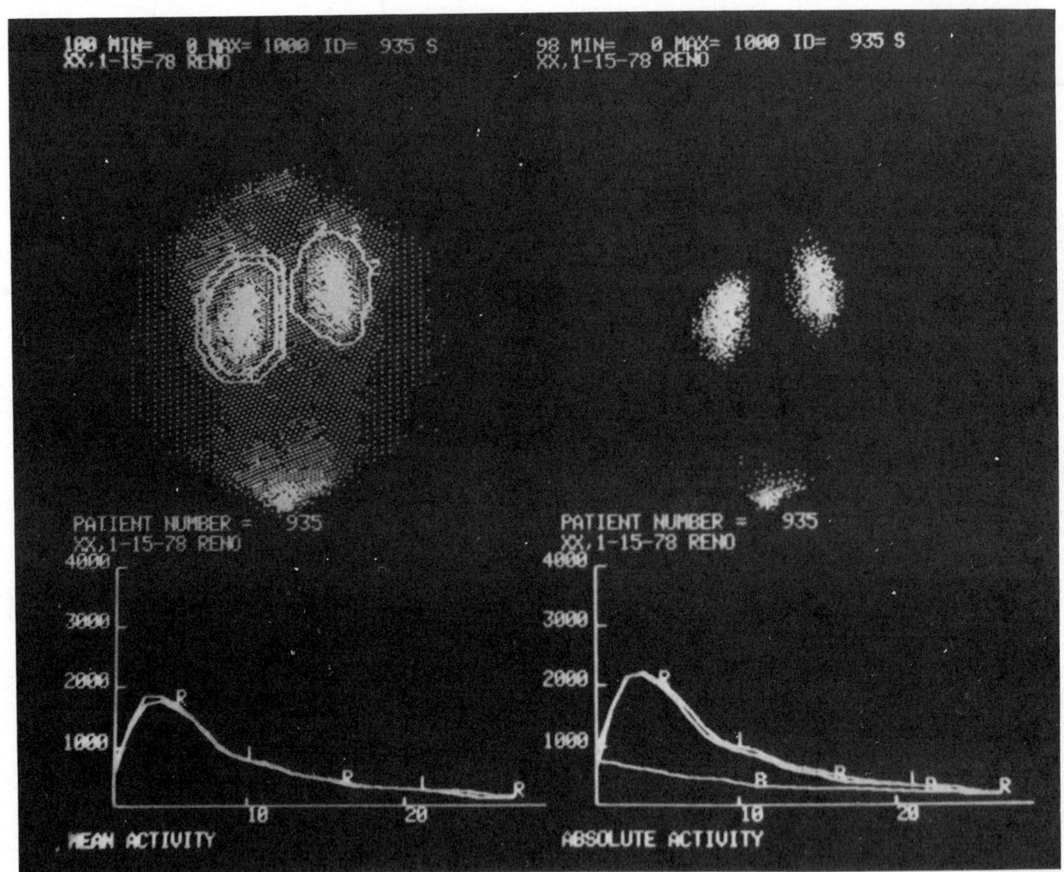

Fig. 13-7. Scintigrams and activity curves in normal patient. *Upper left quadrant* shows a 27-minute added image with ROI's chosen over both kidneys and one for background subtraction. Background-subtracted image is depicted in *right upper quadrant*. Absolute activity curves and background curves generated from corresponding ROI's are displayed in *right lower quadrant*, and curves are corrected for size of kidney in *left*.

```
                         V.A. HOSPITAL
                    NUCLEAR MEDICINE SERVICE
                     BIRMINGHAM, ALABAMA

                     ***RENOGRAPHIC DATA***

NAME:XX
PT NO:  935
AGE:54    SEX:M
HEIGHT(IN): 68.0      WEIGHT(LBS):165.0       SURFACE AREA(M2): 1.88
LEFT KIDNEY AREA(CM2):  66.(53.%)        RIGHT KIDNEY AREA(CM2):  58.(47.%)
                                         URINE
     LT KIDNEY          RT KIDNEY         SPECIFIC GRAVITY:          1.009
MIN    NT CT      %       NT CT     %     VOLUME(ML):                134.
0-1      605     57        463     43              *****
1-2     1611     51       1579     49
2-3     2157     50       2159     50    OIH DOSE(UCI):             300.
3-4     2244     51       2188     49    TOTAL ERPF(ML/MIN)@44 MIN: 551.4
4-5     2157     51       2072     49      RIGHT:264.5   LEFT:287.0
10-11    959     52        874     48    CORR ERPF(ML/MIN/1.73 M2): 506.3
15-16    560     54        474     46    EXPECTED EXCRETION:         77.2%
25-26    241     48        256     52    ACTUAL VOID:                66.4%
                                            AT 33. MIN
PEAK TIME LEFT:   4 MIN                  RESIDUAL URINE(ML):          4.3
PEAK TIME RIGHT:  4 MIN                  TOTAL EXCRETION:            68.6%
                                         EXCRETORY INDEX:             .89
                   ***********************


IMPRESSION:
```

Fig. 13-8. Computer-generated report includes all important data about patient. This consists of values needed for total functional evaluation of urinary tract (effective renal plasma flow [ERPF], residual urine, and excretory index), and differential function (net counts over kidneys throughout study and peak activity times).

Table 13-3. Commonly used renal radiopharmaceutical agents for static imaging

Radiopharmaceutical	Recommended dose	Injected dose in both kidneys (%)	Best imaging time (hours)	Radiation dose to kidneys using maximum recommended dose (rads)	
				Kidneys	Bladder
^{197}Hg-chlormerodrin	100 to 150 μCi	10	1 to 3	1.2 to 1.8	
^{99m}Tc–pentetic acid (^{99m}Tc-DTPA)	5 to 10 mCi	8	1	0.4	6
^{99m}Tc-glucoheptonate (^{99m}Tc-GH)	10 mCi	13	2 to 6	1.7	8
^{99m}Tc–iron ascorbate	5 to 10 mCi	20	2 to 6	2.7	
^{99m}Tc-2,3-dimercaptosuccinic acid (^{99m}Tc-DMSA)	1 to 5 mCi	42	3 to 6	7	0.6

Radiopharmaceuticals and some of their properties are summarized in Table 13-3.[2]

Because of its physical properties (beta radiation, low gamma energy), *^{197}Hg-chlormerodrin* has been almost completely replaced by ^{99m}Tc-labeled complexes.

^{99m}Tc–pentetic acid (^{99m}Tc-DTPA) is a complex of diethylenetriaminepentaacetic acid and reduced technetium 99m. Because of its rapid clearance, it is not an ideal agent for demonstrating lesions within the kidney. However, recent improvements in commercially available kits have increased its stability and made it useful in assessing the glomerular filtration rate.

^{99m}Tc-glucoheptonate (or *^{99m}Tc-GH*),[2] commercially available, is a simple carbohydrate, easily labeled with ^{99m}Tc in the presence of stannous ion. This is a very stable complex that may be used up to 5 hours after preparation and is quickly cleared from the circulation. Only about 13% of the injected dose is retained in the kidneys; the rest is cleared in the urine (40% at 1 hour, 80% at 24 hours). Early camera images demonstrate the renal cortex and the collecting system (Fig. 13-9). In delayed images at 2 to 4 hours, there is excellent visualization of the parenchyma (Fig. 13-10), primarily because of the high kidney-to-background ratio. Posterior and both posterior oblique views should be obtained routinely. The anterior view is optional depending on the nature of the lesion. Early voiding should be encouraged to decrease the radiation to the bladder wall. The liver uptake may be significant in patients with poorly functioning kidneys.

^{99m}Tc–iron ascorbate has a slightly higher uptake in the kidneys (20% of the injected dose) than ^{99m}Tc-glucoheptonate has, but the excretion rates are not significantly different. The same timing and positioning is used as with ^{99m}Tc-glucoheptonate.

^{99m}Tc-DMSA[2] is a complex of 2,3-dimercaptosuccinic acid and technetium in a low oxidation state. DMSA is available commercially and is easily labeled with pertechnetate. ^{99m}Tc-DMSA is slowly cleared from the blood and reaches high concentration in the renal cortex (42% of the injected dose at 6 hours). The urinary clearance is low (10% of the dose is excreted at 1 hour, 40% at 24 hours). Images are obtained with an accumulation of a minimum of 300,000 counts at 3 to 6 hours after administration of the dose (1 to 5 mCi). It is important to obtain scintigrams with low intensity settings so that deep-seated lesions may be seen (Fig. 13-11). A relatively high radiation dose is delivered to the kidneys (up to 7 rads) because of a high uptake and a long effective half-life of the radiopharmaceutical.

Perfusion study or renal scintiangiogram

A perfusion study is performed either as the first phase of static imaging or after completion of the static scintigrams. The main indication is to evaluate vascularity of renal masses. Cystic lesions and abscesses are usually avascular, and tumors are usually moderately or highly vascular. Uncommonly occurring arteriovenous (A-V) malformations show high vascularity.

The patient is injected with a bolus (10 to 15 mCi) of ^{99m}Tc-pertechnetate, ^{99m}Tc-DTPA, and ^{99m}Tc-GH, and sequential scintiphotos of a duration of 2 to 5 seconds are obtained during the angiographic phase of the study. Immediately after completion of the angiographic phase, a single static image reflecting the vascular pool is obtained (Fig. 13-12). If a data processor is available, the study may be acquired on tape or disk in 0.5- to 1-second frames, and after the frames are added together, a region of interest (ROI) over the aorta and both kidneys is chosen, with activity curves then being generated. This is sometimes helpful in the evaluation of bilateral renal disease.

Radionuclide cystography

Radionuclide cystography has been available for many years,[3,4] but only recently has there been renewed interest in its routine use. ^{99m}Tc compounds and the scintillation camera are primarily responsible

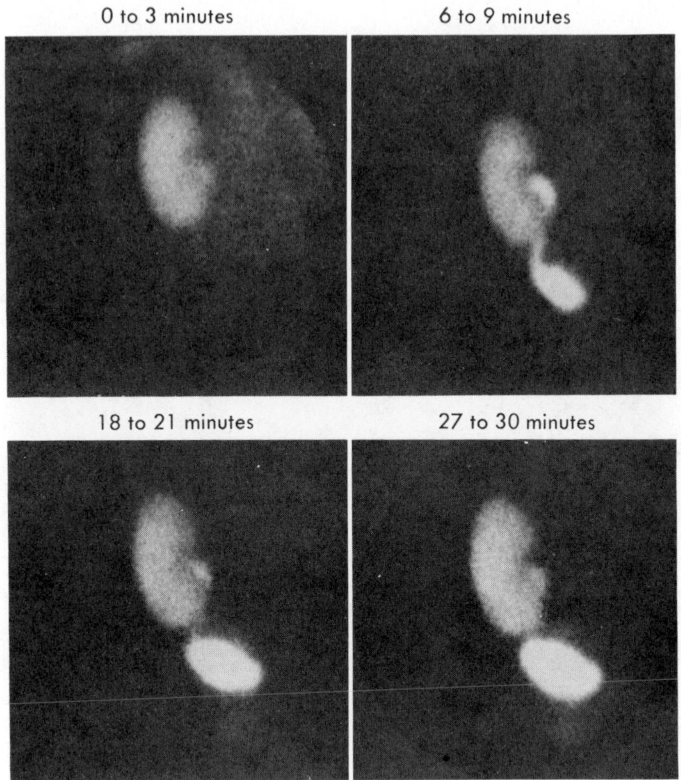

Fig. 13-9. Normal kidney allograft. Three-minute exposures, obtained at any time between 5 and 15 minutes after injection of 10 mCi of ^{99m}Tc-glucoheptonate, demonstrate both cortex and collecting system.

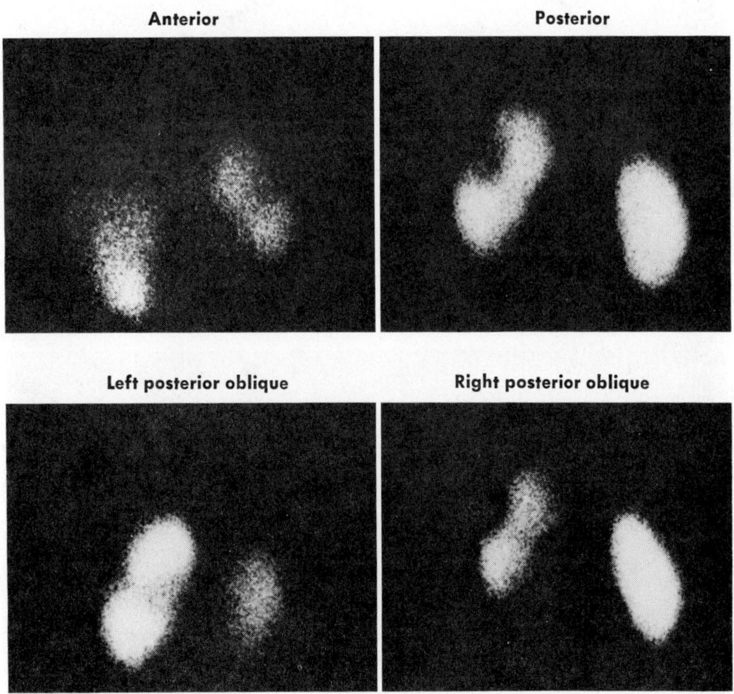

Fig. 13-10. Abnormal scintigram demonstrating space-occupying lesion in cortical portion of left kidney. Images were obtained 3 hours after injection of 10 mCi of ^{99m}Tc-glucoheptonate. (Courtesy Dr. James DeLong, Lloyd Noland Hospital, Birmingham, Alabama.)

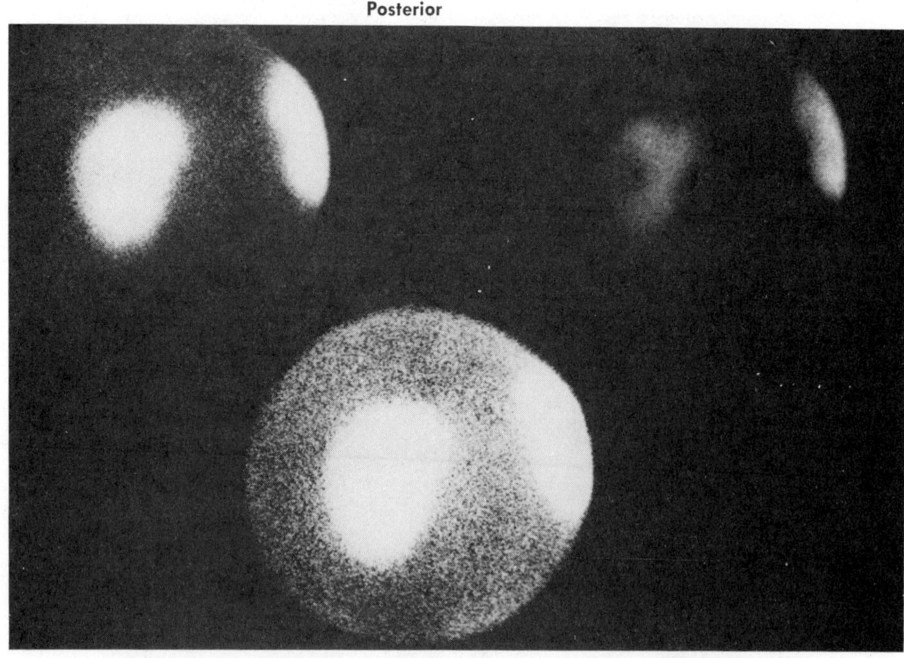

Fig. 13-11. Posterior view of left kidney with two space-occupying lesions. Lesions are seen only on low-intensity exposure. (300,000 counts at 3 hours with 5 mCi of ^{99m}Tc-DMSA).

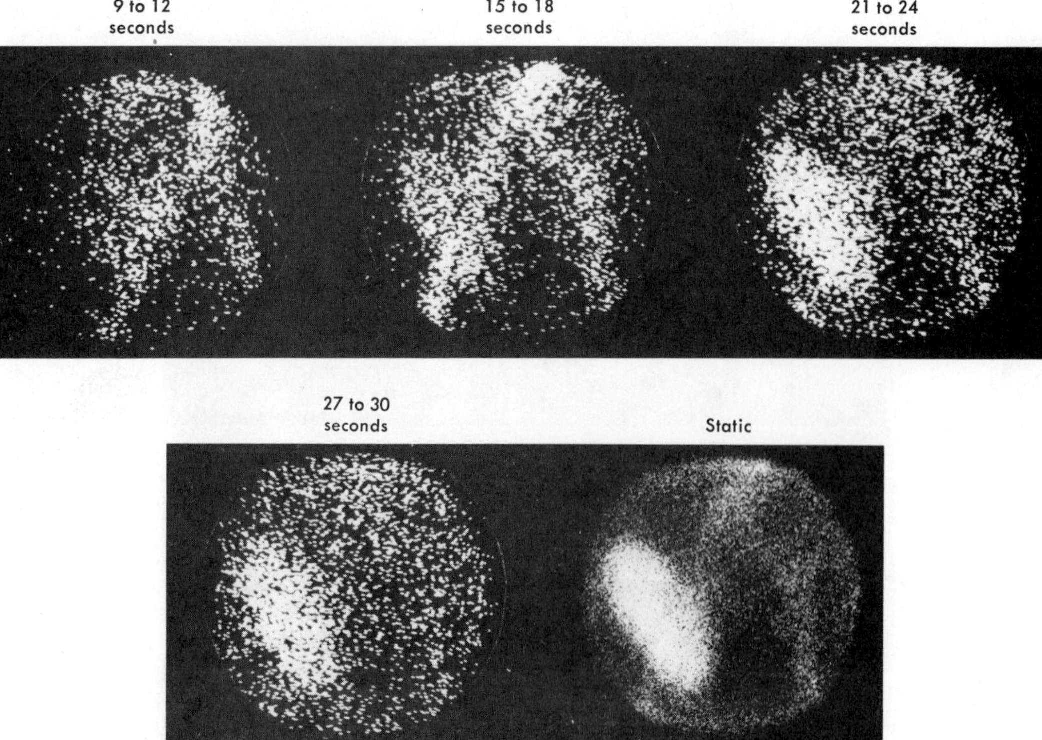

Fig. 13-12. Perfusion study depicting transplanted kidney in chronic rejection. Sequential pictures were exposed for 3 seconds each. (300,000 counts were collected for a static scintigram at 1 minute.)

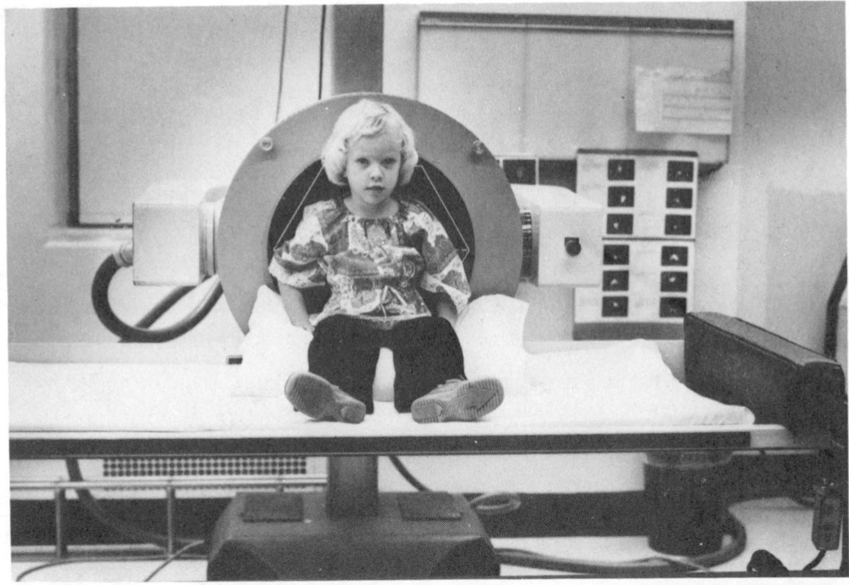

Fig. 13-13. Position of patient for voiding phase of cystogram both direct and indirect.

for its wide acceptance as a practical test with not only functional but also prognostic value.[5,6,25,26]

The single most important indication is the evaluation of the vesicoureteral reflux, a relatively common problem in children. This condition is often responsible for recurrent infection of the urinary tract, which is potentially damaging to the kidneys.

Two methods can be used to detect reflux: indirect and direct.

Indirect cystography. Indirect cystography is used less often. It relies upon the rapid and complete clearance of the intravenously injected ^{131}I-*ortho*-iodohippurate or ^{99m}Tc-DTPA. When the radionuclide is accumulated in the bladder and the residual activity in the kidney region is low, the patient is positioned with his back to the camera and is asked to void (Fig. 13-13). Sudden appearance of activity in the region of the ureter or ureters is suggestive of reflux.

Advantages of the indirect approach include (1) the elimination of the bladder catheterization and (2) the evaluation of the function of the kidneys in the first phase of the study.

The drawbacks and requirements limiting the usefulness of this method include the following:

1. The cooperation of the patient is required; the patient must be able to hold the urine sometimes for 1 to 2 hours and then to void on command after the activity has cleared completely from the kidney region.
2. The reflux is sometimes not evident during voiding but is present only during the filling phase (Fig. 13-14).

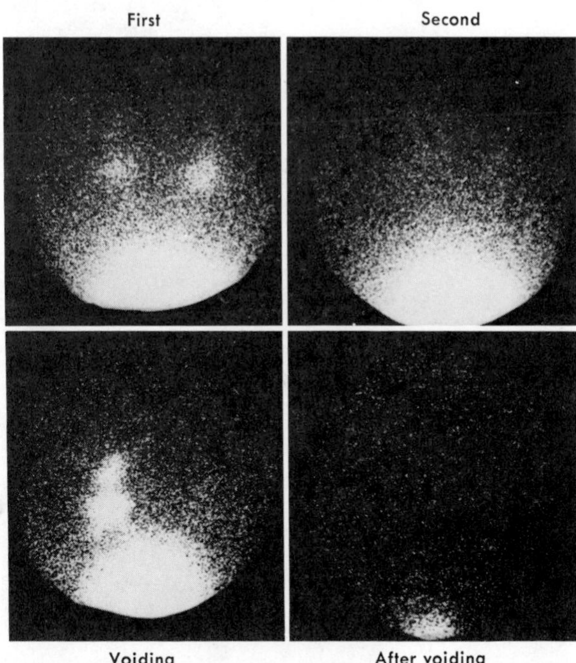

Fig. 13-14. This series of images demonstrates dynamic nature of reflux in this patient. Bilateral reflux was initially visualized; minutes later reflux has disappeared. Pronounced reflux was seen on left while patient was voiding, but it disappeared within seconds. (By permission of Conway, J. J., Belman, A. B., and King, L. R., Semin. Nucl. Med. **4:**209, 1974.)

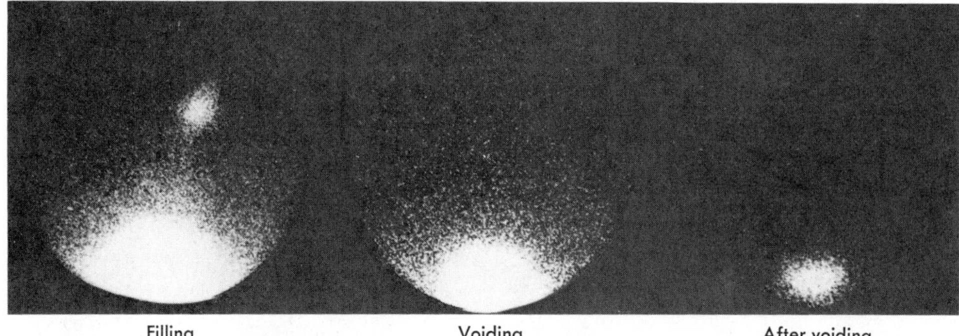

Fig. 13-15. Reflux detected only during the filling phase. Such reflux would be missed by indirect cystography. (From Conway, J. J., and Kruglik, G. D.: J. Nucl. Med. **17**:82, 1976.)

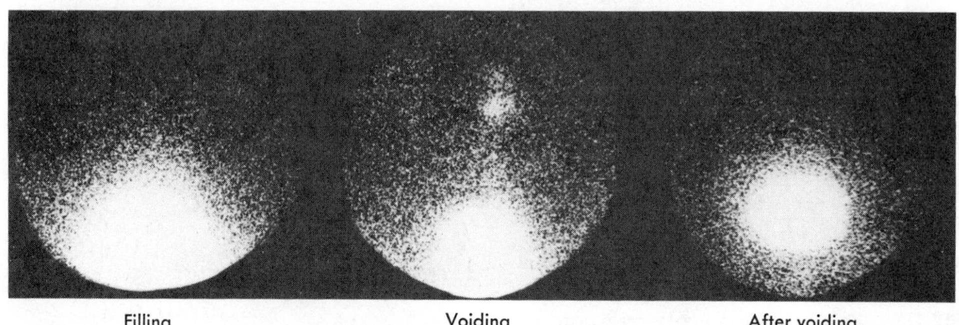

Fig. 13-16. Reflux detected only during voiding phase. (From Conway, J. J., and Kruglik, G. D.: J. Nucl. Med. **17**:82, 1976.)

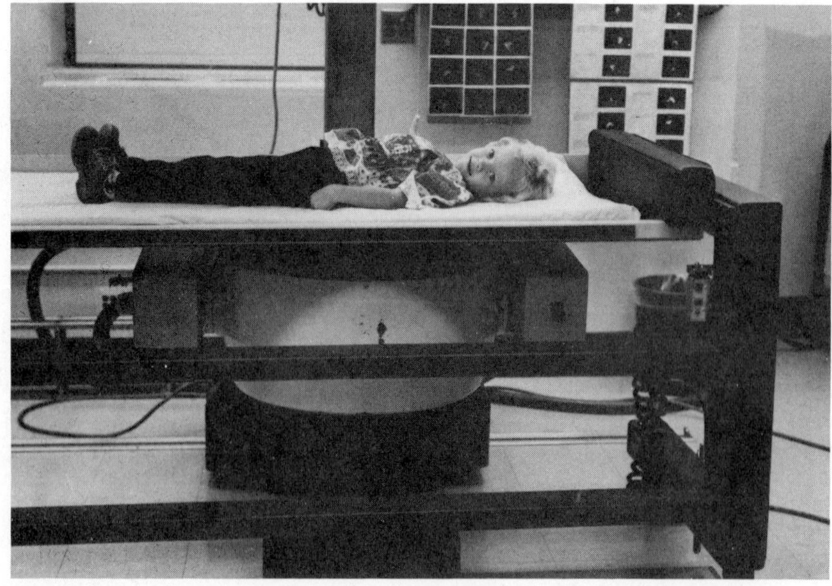

Fig. 13-17. Patient position for filling phase of radionuclide cystography.

3. Impaired function of the kidneys or retention in the collecting system prevents reliable assessment of the reflux.

Direct cystography. Direct cystography is rapidly becoming the method of choice for the detection of vesicoureteral reflux. The advantages of this technique over radiographic methods are a significant reduction in radiation dose (mrads versus rads) and quantification of various functional parameters.

Direct cystography, however, requires catheterization of the patient.

After catheterization and drainage of the bladder, the patient is placed on the imaging table and the catheter is connected to a bottle of normal saline. After a free flow of saline into the bladder is established, 1 mCi of ^{99m}Tc-pertechnetate is injected into the injection section of the catheter. ^{99m}Tc-DTPA or ^{99m}Tc-sulfur colloid may be used. During the filling phase the patient is in a supine position with the upper half of the bladder visualized at the bottom of the imaging field (Figs. 13-14 to 13-16) with the detector underneath the table (Fig. 13-17). The upper urinary tract is closely monitored on the persistence oscilloscope as the saline infusion continues. The appearance of the reflux is registered on a data sheet (Fig. 13-18) indicating the instilled volume of saline. Sequential imaging begins after sufficient bladder filling (Figs. 13-14 to 13-16). Scintigrams of 300,000 counts require approximately 5 minutes. Supine posterior and both left and right posterior oblique projections are recorded with a high intensity setting so that one may visualize a small reflux into the upper urinary tracts.

A 2-minute posterior image with a low intensity setting is obtained and a total abdominal count is recorded on the data sheet before initiation of the voiding phase.

During the voiding phase the patient is seated with his back to the camera (Fig. 13-13). The catheter is removed, and the patient is asked to void. The voiding phase can be recorded on videotape or on computer-compatible magnetic tape for further processing. Sequential images are obtained directly or from playback of the videotape with again a high-intensity setting being used.

The volume of the collected urine is measured and recorded. The 2-minute postvoid image and counts are obtained for residual urine calculation. Other functional indices such as actual volume of the urine, which refluxed into the pelvises, can be derived from the recorded data (Fig. 13-18). A technically important step is to recognize adequate filling of the bladder before initiation of the voiding. This is indicated by increased protestations by the patient, leakage of the urine around the catheter, cessation of flow from the bottle, or excessive volume of instilled saline solution. The usual bladder capacity for children is approximately 250 ml. Contamination by radioactive urine, which may simulate reflux, is a common difficulty with uncooperative patients. A similar problem may arise if larger quantities of ^{99m}Tc-pertechnetate are absorbed through bladder mucosa and are secreted by the gastric mucosa. Oblique and lateral projections are helpful.

Scrotal imaging

Scrotal imaging using ^{99m}Tc-pertechnetate was introduced in 1974.[20] Since then it has become an important tool in the evaluation of acute and chronic testicular pain and scrotal swelling.[7,15,21]

Both dynamic perfusion and static imaging are essential parts of the test. Two clinical entities can be diagnosed with a high degree of accuracy: (1) acute testicular torsion where perfusion and tissue uptake are decreased (Fig. 13-19) and (2) acute inflammation, especially acute epididymo-orchitis where both parts are increased (Fig. 13-20).

Scintigraphic findings showing decreased uptake have to be closely correlated with clinical findings to consider other possibilities such as torsion of the appendix testis, infected hematoma, hydrocele, or inguinal hernia. Normal findings are consistent with chronic inflammation and some mass lesions (carcinoma). Diffusely increased uptake is sometimes seen in seminomas. Increased uptake around a cold area is noted in chronic testicular torsion, where inflamed tissue surrounds a necrotic testis (Fig. 13-21).

Scrotal imaging is performed with 10 to 15 mCi of ^{99m}Tc-pertechnetate in adult patients, 5 to 10 mCi in patients 5 to 10 years of age, and less than 5 mCi in younger children (200 μCi/kg). No special preparation is necessary. The patient is in a supine position, the penis is taped to the abdomen, and the scrotum is supported by a flexible lead shield or a tape cradle. A scintillation camera with a low-energy collimator is positioned over the groin with the scrotum in the lower half of the field. After a bolus injection of the pertechnetate is given, sequential images are obtained at 3- to 5-second intervals until the angiographic phase is complete, followed by a static scintiphoto.

The study should be considered an emergency procedure if the indication is to rule out testicular torsion.

Evaluation of transplanted kidney

The implantation site of choice for the transplanted kidney is the right iliac fossa extraperitoneally (Fig. 13-22). The donor renal artery is anastomosed to the recipient's hypogastric artery; the renal vein is joined to the external iliac vein of the recipient; the ureter is joined to the recipient's ureter or directly to the bladder. Although vulnerable to trauma such a superficial implant allows palpation, assessment of change

RADIONUCLIDE CYSTOGRAM

Name:____________________

Hospital
number:____________________

Date:____________________

Dose:____________________

Right reflux at____________ml

Left reflux at____________ml

Total instilled____________ml

Urinary bladder:________Before voiding________After voiding

Voided volume of urine:____________ml

$$\text{Residual volume} = \frac{\text{Voided volume} \times \text{Residual count}}{\text{Initial count} - \text{Residual count}}$$

$$\text{Residual volume} = \frac{\qquad \times \qquad}{\qquad - \qquad}$$

Residual volume =

Reflux bladder volume
Total volume = Voided volume + Residual volume

Total volume = ________ + ________ = ________

Initial volume = Total − Total instilled

Initial volume = ________ − ________ = ________

Reflux volume = Initial + Bottle volume

Reflux volume = R________ + ________ = ________

L________ + ________ = ________

Fig. 13-18. Cystogram data sheet. (Courtesy Dr. J. J. Conway, Children's Memorial Hospital, Chicago, Ill.)

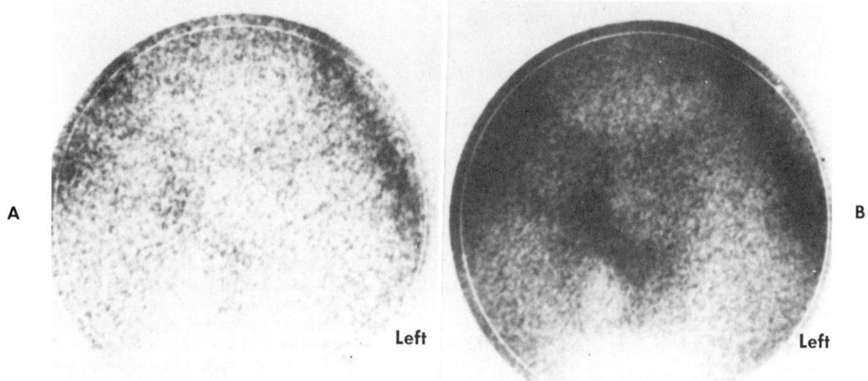

Fig. 13-19. Testicular torsion early stage. **A,** Perfusion phase shows iliac arteries and spermatic cord on right, but no scrotal activity. **B,** Tissue phase shows diminished activity in right testis and prominent right spermatic cord. (From Datta, N. J., and Mishkin, F. S.: J.A.M.A. **231:**1060, 1975. Copyright 1975, American Medical Association.)

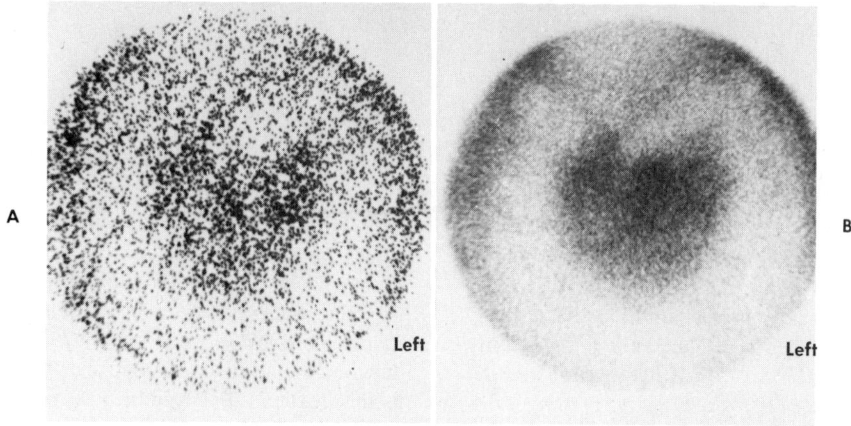

Fig. 13-20. Bilateral epididymo-orchitis. **A,** Perfusion phase shows bilaterally increased flow to scrotal contents. **B,** Tissue phase shows bilateral increase of scrotal activity. (From Datta, N. S., and Mishkin, F. S.: J.A.M.A. **231:**1060, 1975. Copyright 1975, American Medical Association.)

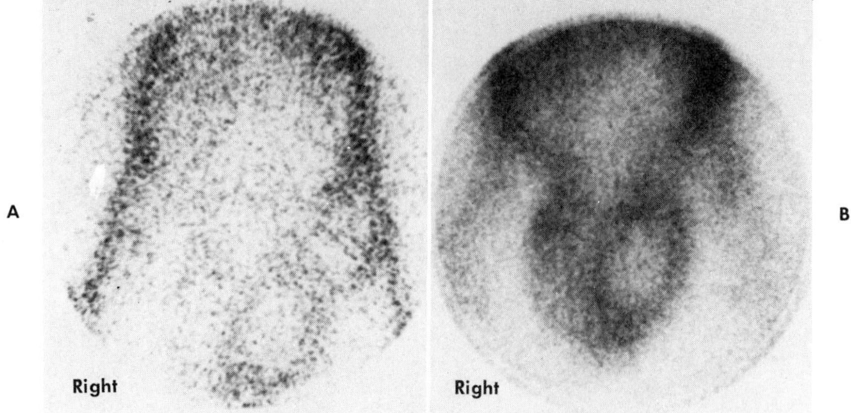

Fig. 13-21. Testicular torsion, late stage. **A,** Perfusion phase shows iliac arteries bilaterally, left spermatic cord area, and left pudendal artery. **B,** Tissue phase shows reduced content of left testicle. Increased rim of activity reflects reactive inflammation around necrosis. (From Datta, N. S., and Mishkin, F. S.: J.A.M.A. **231:**1060, 1975. Copyright 1975, American Medical Association.)

of volume, and easy access for biopsy or surgical repair.

The transplanted kidney is subjected to a variety of immunologic, vascular, and obstructive processes, each of which may require a different form of specific therapy. Most conventional diagnostic procedures do not adequately identify these processes at an early stage. Although nuclear medicine procedures are widely accepted as the best way to evaluate renal transplant performance, there is no universally accepted protocol. However, most of the studies are designed to assess:

1. Renal artery patency
2. Level of graft function
3. Patency of urinary tract
4. Various complications occurring after transplantation

A variety of nuclear medicine instruments ranging from scintillation cameras with strip chart recorders to cameras with highly sophisticated on-line computer systems have been used. Various radiopharmaceuticals have been recommended, but the most commonly used ones are ^{99m}Tc-DTPA, ^{99m}Tc-glucoheptonate, and ^{131}I-*ortho*-iodohippurate (or recently ^{123}I-*ortho*-iodohippurate).

Whatever approach is used, the following considerations apply: (1) Good performance of the graft depends on many factors. Functional changes may develop rapidly. Good practice, therefore, requires that serial studies be performed more often in the early posttransplant period and at longer intervals thereafter. (2) Because of the anatomic location of the graft (Fig. 13-22), the studies are performed with the patient in the supine position and the scintillation-camera detector positioned anteriorly to the bifurcation of the aorta, the iliac arteries, the urinary bladder, and the kidney in the field of view (Fig. 13-23). (3) A quantitative approach is advisable because comparison of one study to the next is more reliable.

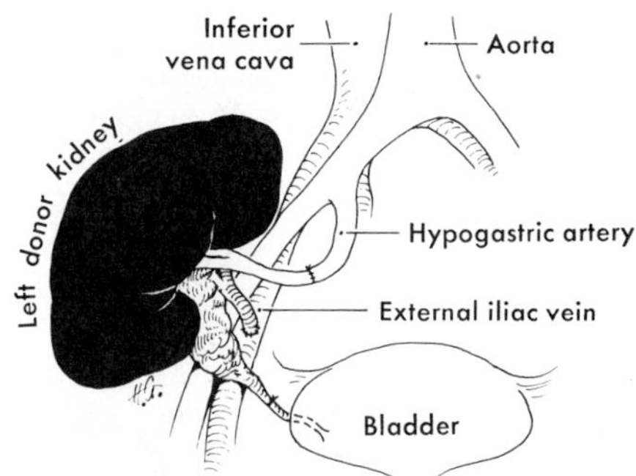

Fig. 13-22. Left kidney implant in right iliac fossa showing anastamosis of renal artery to hypogastric artery, and renal vein to recipient's external iliac vein.

Methods using ^{99m}Tc-DTPA or ^{99m}Tc-glucoheptonate

A 10 to 15 mCi bolus of activity is injected IV and 3- to 10-second scintiphotos are begun upon visualization of the radionuclide on the persistence oscilloscope. These allow excellent delineation and dynamic evaluation of the studied structures. After completion of the angiographic phase, a static image provides morphologic information (Fig. 13-12). Scintigrams acquired

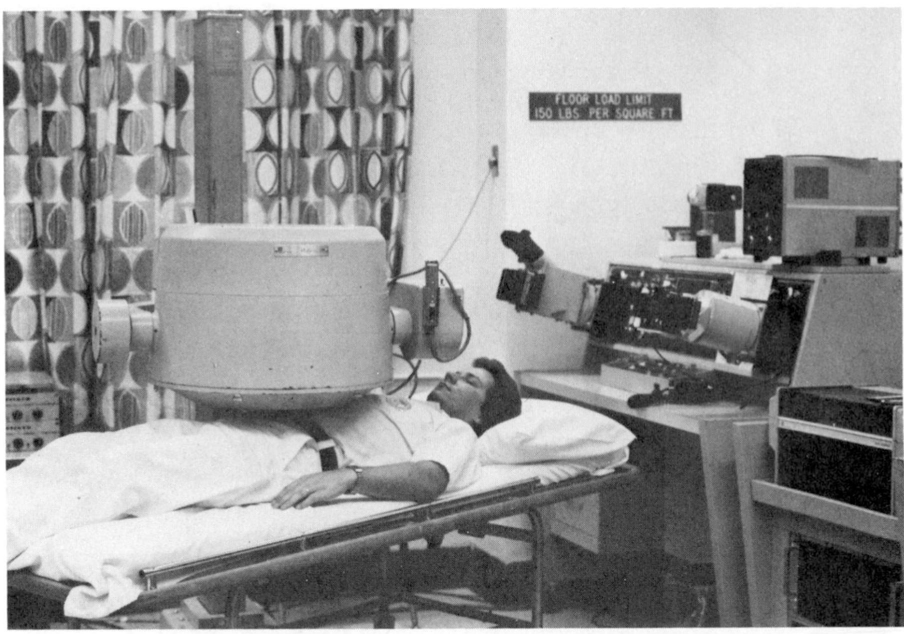

Fig. 13-23. Usual position for renal transplant study.

at various times after injection reflect the functional state of the graft. This approach yields only information regarding the morphology of the abdominal vascular structures, the transplanted kidney, and the bladder but cannot detect with confidence minor functional changes. Recent improvements in instrumentation and processing capabilities allow construction of the activity curves from the ROI and calculation of aorta-kidney, kidney-bladder or kidney-background ratios[17] (Fig. 13-24). Some very sophisticated approaches using newer background subtraction techniques and curves drawn from the cortical or medullar portion of the kidney have been recommended, resulting in great improvement in diagnostic accuracy.[4,16]

High concentration of ^{99m}Tc-glucoheptonate in the urine allows detection of abnormalities of the collecting system (obstruction, urinoma) (Fig. 13-25).

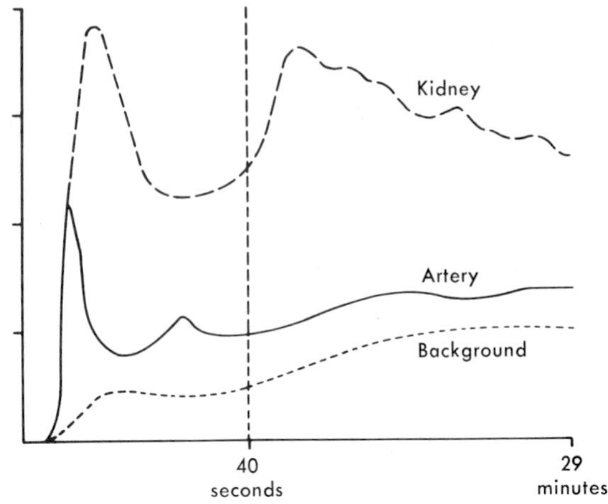

Fig. 13-24. Curves obtained from region of interest over kidney iliac artery and background in normal kidney, plotted as counts per cell against frame number. Note change of time scale. Relationship and shape of curve change in a rejecting transplant, obstructed kidney, or patient with acute tubular necrosis. (Courtesy Dr. A. J. W. Hilson, London, England.)

Methods using ^{131}I-*ortho*-iodohippurate

^{131}I-*ortho*-iodohippurate (or recently ^{123}I-*ortho*-iodohippurate) is still the best radiopharmaceutical for functional evaluation of the transplanted kidney. As discussed in the previous section, a comprehensive renal function study combining imaging, activity-curve analysis, and clearance technique using 50 to 150 μCi of ^{131}I-OIH not only supplies quantitative data, but also differentiates with reasonable accuracy between various complications[9] and the degree of impairment.[10,11] The effective renal plasma flow (ERPF) and excretion index (EI) are especially helpful in differentiating acute and chronic graft rejection as well as acute renal failure (acute tubular necrosis) (Fig. 13-26). Examples of such a study are depicted on Figs. 13-27 and 13-28.

Other methods have been recommended mainly for

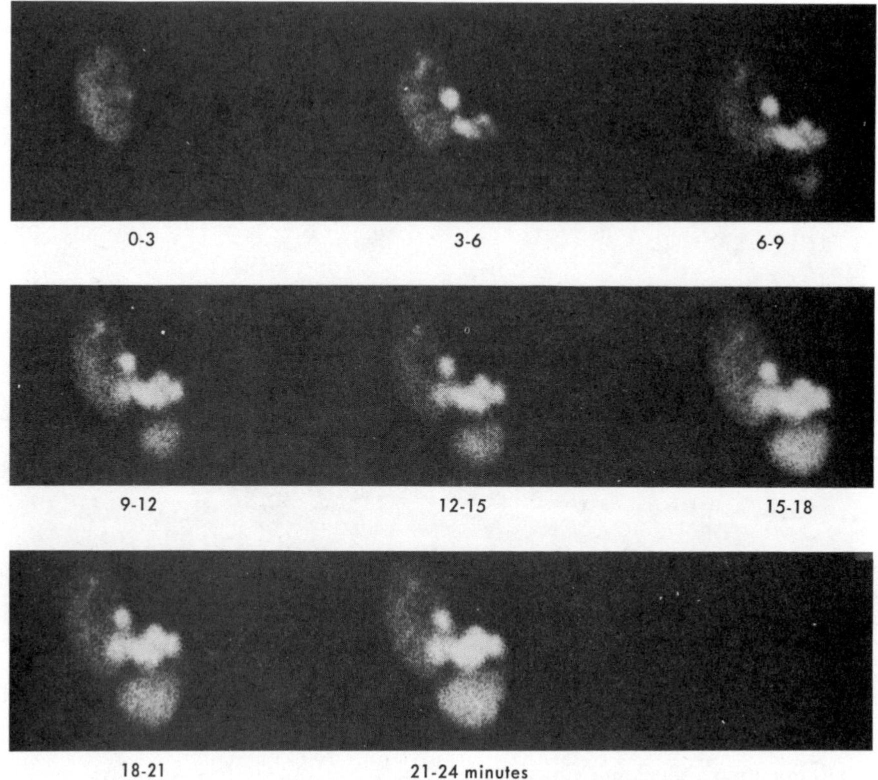

Fig. 13-25. Sequential images obtained after injection of 3 mCi of ^{99m}Tc-glucoheptonate demonstrating urinoma.

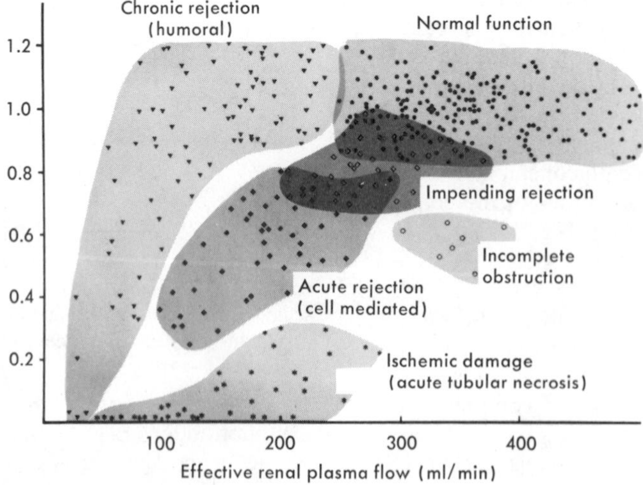

Fig. 13-26. Graph of excretion index (EI) plotted against effective renal plasma flow (ERPF) in renal transplantees. Normal EI, or total excretion versus expected excretion, indicates a normal transit time through entire renourinary pathway.

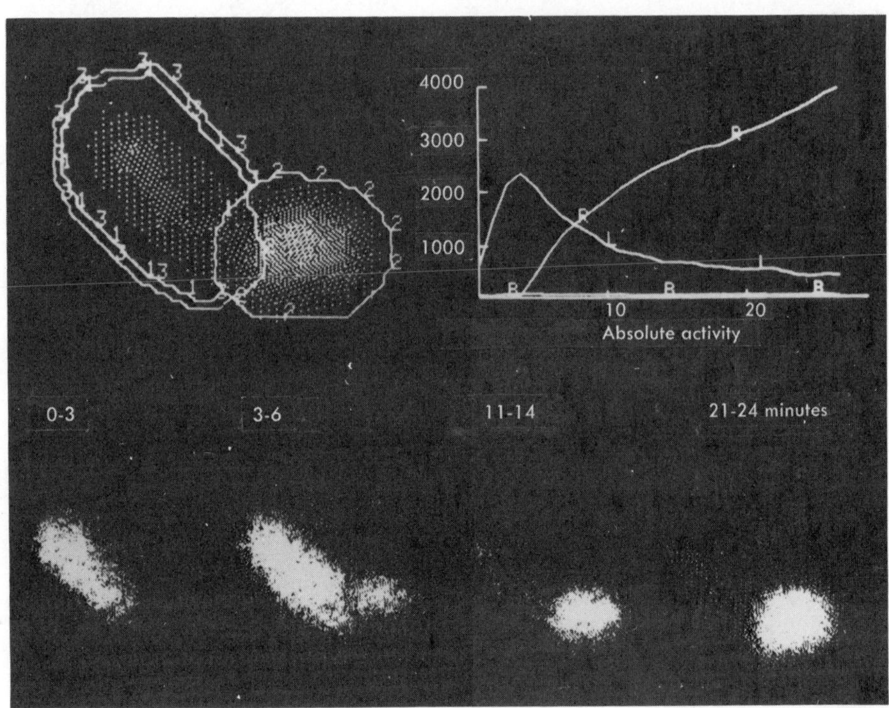

Fig. 13-27. Scintigrams and activity curves in patient with normally functioning kidney graft. Display of 27-minute added image with regions of interest over kidney *(L)*, bladder *(R)*, and background *(B)*. Absolute activity curves generated from kidney and bladder regions of interest are corrected for overlap of respective areas.

V.A. HOSPITAL
NUCLEAR MEDICINE SERVICE
BIRMINGHAM, ALABAMA

RENOGRAPHIC DATA
2/28/77

NAME:
PT NO: 235
AGE:41 SEX:M
HEIGHT(IN): 69.0 WEIGHT(LBS):198.0 SURFACE AREA(M2): 2.06
LEFT KIDNEY AREA(CM2): 107.(10*%) RIGHT KIDNEY AREA(CM2): 0.(0.%)

	LT KIDNEY		RT KIDNEY	
MIN	NT CT	%	NT CT	%
0-1	728	1*	0	0
1-2	1706	1*	0	0
2-3	2423	1*	0	0
3-4	2645	1*	0	0
4-5	2385	1*	0	0
10-11	1006	1*	0	0
15-16	729	1*	0	0
25-26	378	1*	0	0

PEAK TIME LEFT: 4 MIN
PEAK TIME RIGHT: 0 MIN

URINE

SPECIFIC GRAVITY:	1.040
VOLUME(ML):	234.

*****

OIH DOSE(MCI):	150.
TOTAL ERPF(ML/45 MIN):	341.4
RIGHT: 0.0 LEFT:341.4	
CORR ERPF(ML/MIN/1.73 M2):	287.0
EXPECTED EXCRETION:	65.2%
ACTUAL VOID: AT 40. MIN	60.6%
RESIDUAL URINE(ML):	19.0
TOTAL EXCRETION:	65.5%
EXCRETORY INDEX:	1.01

****

Fig. 13-28. Computer-generated report of patient's data: Effective renal plasma flow of 341.4 ml/min (normal value 250 ml/min or more) and excretion index of 1.01 (normal value 0.88 to 1.12) are both within normal limits.

early detection of the rejection process and its differentiation from other complications, mainly acute tubular necrosis.[12]

1. ^{99m}Tc-sulfur colloid uptake has been observed in rejecting grafts (both acute and chronic) significantly more often than in acute renal failure. Scintigrams are obtained after a 3 mCi dose with the camera positioned over the kidney.
2. ^{125}I- or ^{131}I-labeled fibrinogen uptake has been observed early in acute rejection. Both uptake quantification and imaging with this material have provided useful clinical data.
3. Gallium-67 accumulation in the graft has been observed during the rejection process. However, significant bowel activity and uptake by the infected kidney decrease the diagnostic value of the test.

REFERENCES

1. Anthony, C. P., and Thibodeau, G. A.: Textbook of anatomy and physiology, ed. 10, St. Louis, 1979, The C. V. Mosby Co.
2. Arnold, R. W., Subramanian, G., McAfee, J., et al.: Comparison of ^{99m}Tc complexes for renal imaging, J. Nucl. Med. **16**:357, 1975.
3. Burbank, M. K., Tauxe, W. N., Maher, F. T., et al.: Evaluation of radioiodinated Hippuran for the estimation of renal plasma flow, Mayo Clin. Proc. **36**:372, 1961.
4. Cahill, P. T., Ho, S.-L., Jacobstein, T. G., et al.: Evaluation of edge detection algorithms for the delineation of myocardial infarcts with ^{99m}Tc-glucoheptonate, Proceedings of Seventh Symposium on Sharing of Computer Programs and Technology in Nuclear Medicine: Computer-Assisted Data Processing, Atlanta, Ga., 1977, Springfield, Va., 1977, U.S. Department of Commerce, Technical Information Center, p. 150.
5. Conway, J. J., Belman, A. B., and King, L. R.: Direct and indirect radionuclide cystography, Semin. Nucl. Med. **4**:197, 1974.
6. Conway, J. J., and Kuglik, G. D.: Effectiveness of direct and indirect radionuclide cystography in detecting vesicoureteral reflux, J. Nucl. Med. **17**:81, 1976.
7. Datta, N. S., and Mishkin, F. S.: Radionuclide imaging in intrascrotal lesions, J.A.M.A. **231**:231, 1975.
8. Dubovsky, E. V., Bueschen, A. J., Tobin, M., et al.: A comprehensive computer assisted renal function study: a routine procedure in clinical practice. In Hollenberg, N., and Lange, S., editors: Radionuclides in nephrology, Proceedings of the Fourth International Symposium, Boston, New York, 1980, Grune & Stratton, Inc., pp. 52-58.

9. Dubovsky, E. V., Logic, J. R., Diethelm, A. G., et al.: Comprehensive evaluation of renal function in the transplanted kidney, J. Nucl. Med. **16:**1115, 1975.
10. Dubovsky, E. V., Diethelm, A. G., and Tauxe, W. N.: Differentiation of cell-mediated and humoral rejection by ortho-iodohippurate kinetics, Arch. Intern. Med. **137:**738, 1977.
11. Dubovsky, E. V., Diethelm, A. G., and Tauxe, W. N.: Early recognition of chronic humoral rejection of long-term follow-up of kidney recipients by a comprehensive renal radionuclide study, Transplant Proc. **9:**43, 1977.
12. George, E., Codd, J. E., Newton, W. T., et al.: Comparative evaluation of renal transplant rejection with radioiodinated fibrinogen, ^{99m}Tc-sulfur colloid and ^{67}Ga-citrate, J. Nucl. Med. **17:**175, 1976.
13. Goldring, W., Clarke, R. W., and Smith, H. W.: The phenol-red clearance in normal man, J. Clin. Invest. **15:**221, 1936.
14. Hamburger, J., Crosnier, J., Dormont, J., and Bach, J.-F.: Renal transplantation: theory and practice, Baltimore, 1972, The Williams & Wilkins Co.
15. Heck, L. L., Coles, J. L., Van Hove, E. D., and Riley, T. W.: Value of ^{99m}Tc-pertechnetate imaging in evaluation of testicular torsion, J. Nucl. Med. **15:**501, 1974.
16. Hilson, A. J. W., Maisey, M. N., Ogg, C. S., Bewich, M., and Brown, C.: Quantitative assessment of renal transplant perfusion in the post-operative period. Proceedings of Seventh Symposium on Sharing of Computer Programs and Technology in Nuclear Medicine: Computer Assisted Data Processing, Atlanta, Ga., 1977, Springfield, Va., 1977, U.S. Department of Commerce, Technical Information Center, p. 106.
17. Kirschner, P. T., Goldman, M., Leapman, S., and Keipfer, R. F.: Accuracy of the kidney aortic blood flow index (K/A ratio) for assessing renal transplant function, J. Nucl. Med. **18:**595, 1977.
18. Kontzen, F. N., Tobin, M., Dubovsky, E. V., et al.: Comprehensive renal function studies: technical aspects, J. Nucl. Med. Technol. **5:**81, 1977.
19. Langley, L. L., Telford, I. R., and Christensen, J. B.: Dynamic anatomy and physiology, New York, 1974, McGraw-Hill Book Co.
20. Lawrence, D., and Mishkin, F. S.: Radionuclide imaging in scrotal abnormalities, J. Nucl. Med. **15:**518, 1974.
21. Lutzker, L. G., Novich, O., Periz, L. A., et al.: Radionuclide scrotal imaging, Appl. Radiol., p. 184, Jan.-Feb. 1977.
22. Richards, A. N., Westfall, B. B., and Bott, P. A.: Renal excretion of inulin, creatinine and xylose in normal dogs, Proc. Soc. Exp. Biol. Med. **32:**73, 1934.
23. Shannon, J. A., and Smith, H. W.: The excretion of inulin, xylose, and urea by normal and phlorhizinized man, J. Clin. Invest. **14:**393, 1935.
24. Tauxe, W. N., Maher, F. T., and Taylor, W. F.: Effective renal plasma flow estimation from theoretical volumes of distribution of intravenously injected ^{131}I-orthoiodohippurate, Mayo Clin. Proc. **46:**524, 1971.
25. Winter, C. C.: New test for vesicoureteral reflux: an external technique using radioisotopes, J. Urol. **81:**105, 1959.
26. Weiss, S., and Conway, J. J.: The technique of direct radionuclide cystography, Appl. Radionucl. Med., May-June 1975.

Chapter 14

THE SKELETAL SYSTEM

Paul E. Christian and R. Edward Coleman

The skeleton performs several functions for the body including support, protection, movement, and blood formation. Bone, like other connective tissues, consists of living cells and a predominant amount of nonliving intercellular substance that is calcified. It is a metabolically active tissue with large amounts of nutrients being exchanged in the blood supplying the bone. Thus the skeleton and body fluids are in an equilibrium. Tracer techniques have been used for many years to study the exchange between bone and blood.[4] Radionuclides have played an important role in understanding normal bone metabolism, in addition to the metabolic effects of pathologic involvement of bone.

Radionuclide imaging of the skeleton is being used with increasing frequency in the evaluation of abnormalities involving bones and joints.[6] Several studies have demonstrated that different information can be obtained by radionuclide bone imaging compared to radiography and blood chemistry analysis.[16,20,26,32,38] Radionuclide joint imaging has been utilized for a shorter period of time than has bone imaging and is still being evaluated in many diseases involving the joints.[13,28,33,34,46,47]

The anatomy and physiology of bones and joints must be well known for full understanding of the technical and clinical aspects of radionuclide imaging of the skeletal system. The first portion of this chapter reviews skeletal anatomy and physiology. The remainder of the chapter discusses radionuclide imaging of the bones and joints with an emphasis on the technical aspects and applications of the imaging procedure.

COMPOSITION OF BONE

Bone is no different from other tissues in the body in that it is maintained by living cells in addition to having amorphous ground substance and fibers like other connective tissue. The main difference between bone and other connective tissue is that it is calcified; thus it is harder. Bone matrix, the other major constituent of bone, consists of collagen, amorphous ground substance, and mineral.

The composition by weight of normal adult cortical bone is approximately 5% to 10% water, 25% to 30% organic matter (collagen, ground substance, and cellular elements), and 65% to 70% inorganic matter (bone mineral). Collagen is the main protein constituent and accounts for 90% to 95% of the organic matter of bone. Collagen is present in the form of fibrils bunched together into bundles of fibers. The ground substance is the interfibrillar cement substance in which the fibrils are embedded.

The bone salt mineral (inorganic matter) has the crystalline form of an apatite, and chemical analysis reveals the following ions: calcium, phosphate, hydroxyl, carbonate, and citrate with lesser amounts of sodium, magnesium, potassium, chloride, and fluoride. Approximately 27% of the weight of cortical bone is calcium. The main anion constituent of bone is phosphorus (as phosphate), contributing approximately 12% of the weight of cortical bone. The bone mineral consists of individual crystals so small that the electron microscope is needed for visualization of the crystals. The crystalline structure is hydroxyapatite, $Ca_{10}(PO_4)_6(OH)_2$. This formula represents the ratio of the constituent elements and is not necessarily the molecular formula.

GROSS STRUCTURE OF BONE

Bones have obvious differences in size and shape but also have certain features in common. They have a cortex (compact bone) surrounding various amounts of cancellous (spongy or trabecular bone), which contains blood-forming (myeloid) elements or fatty marrow (Figs. 14-1 and 14-2). In the adult, most of the myeloid marrow is in the bones of the trunk, with some in the calvarium and upper ends of the humeri and femora. Bones are also similar in that they are covered by periosteum, except in areas of articulation or where tendons and ligaments connect them. The gross structure of bones are discussed in respect to

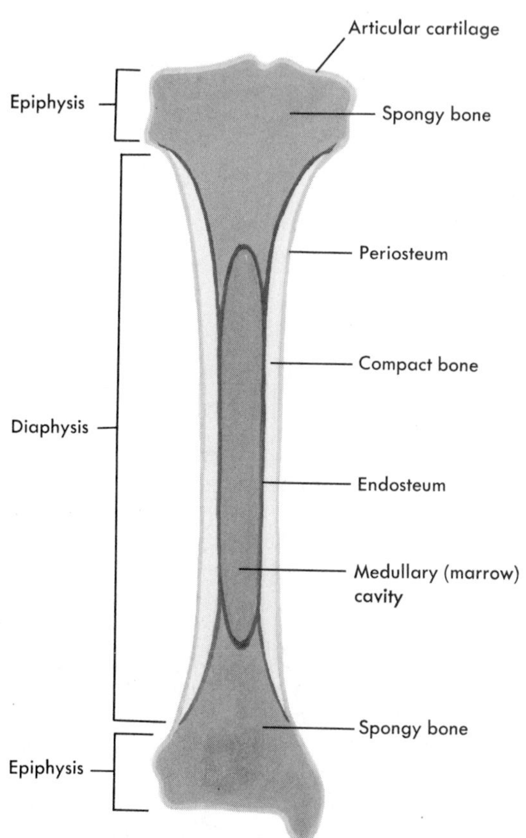

Fig. 14-1. Structure of long bone in longitudinal section. (From Anthony, C. P., and Thibodeau, G. A.: Textbook of anatomy and physiology, ed. 10, St. Louis, 1979, The C. V. Mosby Co.)

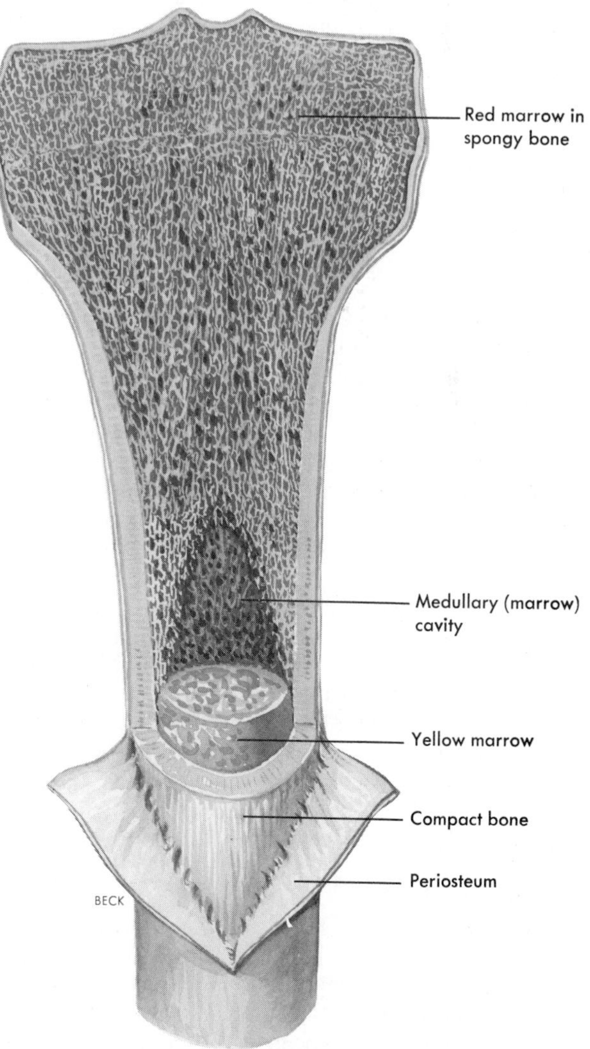

Fig. 14-2. Cutaway section of long bone. (From Anthony, C. P., and Thibodeau, G. A.: Textbook of anatomy and physiology, ed. 10, St. Louis, 1979, The C. V. Mosby Co.)

their general architecture into the following groups: tubular, short, flat, and irregular.

Tubular bones

The long tubular bones include the humerus, radius, ulna, femur, tibia, and fibula. The short tubular bones include the metacarpals, metatarsals, and phalanges. Often the tubular bones are all classified as long bones. The tubular bones have a shaft (diaphysis) consisting of a cortex of compact bone surrounding a cavity (medullary cavity) that contains bone marrow (Fig. 14-1). In the adult, this is mainly yellow, or fatty, marrow except for the proximal humerus and femur where it is red (blood-forming) marrow (Fig. 14-2). The cortex is thickest at the midshaft and tapers toward the ends of the shaft. The end of a bone that previously had an epiphysis is known as an epiphyseal bone end. The juncture of the cancellous bone of the epiphyseal bone end and the spongy bone of the diaphysis is called the metaphysis.

Short bones

The short bones include the wrist (carpals), ankle (tarsals), sesamoids (small bones forming in a tendon or joint capsule), and other anomalous or extra bones. These bones are generally cubic and have spongy osseous tissue covered by a shell of compact bone.

Flat bones

The flat bones include the ribs, sternum, scapulae, and several of the skull bones. These bones are thin and have little spongy bone between two layers of compact bone. The flat bones of the skull consist of an inner and outer table (layers of cortical bone) separated by a thin layer of spongy bone (diploë). The spongy layer of the ribs and sternum contains considerable red marrow.

Irregular bones

The irregular bones include the bones of the spine, pelvis, and some of the skull. A part of an irregular bone may fit into one of the other categories, but the entire bone does not fit into any of the previous categories. The largest part of these bones often consists of large amounts of spongy osseous tissue with the surrounding cortex being very thin, whereas another part of the same bone may have no spongy tissue and be composed of two layers of compact bone.

THE SKELETON

The skeletal system (Figs. 14-3 and 14-4) usually contains 206 bones and provides a supporting framework for the body, as well as forming protective chambers such as the skull and thorax. The skeleton is divided into two main parts: the axial and appendicular parts (Table 14-1). The axial skeleton is composed of the bones of the skull, thorax, and vertebral column, which form the axis of the body. The appendicular skeleton is composed of the bones of the shoulder, upper extremities, hips, and lower extremities.

Table 14-1. Skeletal system

Skeletal parts	Number of bones	
Axial skeleton		
Skull and hyoid	29	
Vertebrae	26	
Ribs and sternum	25	
		80
Appendicular skeleton		
Upper limbs	64	
Lower limbs	62	
		126
TOTAL		206

Axial skeleton

The skull consists of 28 distinct bones, including several flat bones united by sutures and irregular bones forming the framework of the face and base of the cranium, which is the bony cavity containing the brain. The cranium consists of 8 bones, the face consists of 14 bones, and the middle ear 6 bones. The bones of the ear are tiny, and 3 are located in the middle ear cavity of both temporal bones. The middle ear bones are not discussed further, since there is no relevance to nuclear medicine. The 8 cranial bones are one frontal, one occipital, two parietal, one sphenoid, two temporal, and one ethmoid (Figs. 14-5 to 14-7). The frontal bone forms the forehead and is the anterior part of the skull, as well as part of the orbit and nasal cavity. Superciliary arches (superior orbital ridges) are rims projecting from the frontal bone above the orbits. The frontal sinuses, which are air-filled cavities, are within the frontal bone and communicate with the nasal cavities. The parietal bones form the top and sides of the skull separated by the midline sagittal suture. Posteriorly, the parietal bones join with the occipital bone at the lambdoidal suture. The occipital bone forms the back and a large portion of the base of the skull. The foramen magnum, a large opening through which the spinal cord enters the skull, is within the occipital bone. The external occipital protuberance is a prominent projection on the posterior aspect of the occipital bone in the midline and can be felt beneath the skin. The temporal bones form a portion of the sides and base of the skull. Each temporal bone consists of four parts, which are the squamous, tympanic, mastoid, and petrous portions. The squamous portion is thin, located at the side of the skull and has a projection

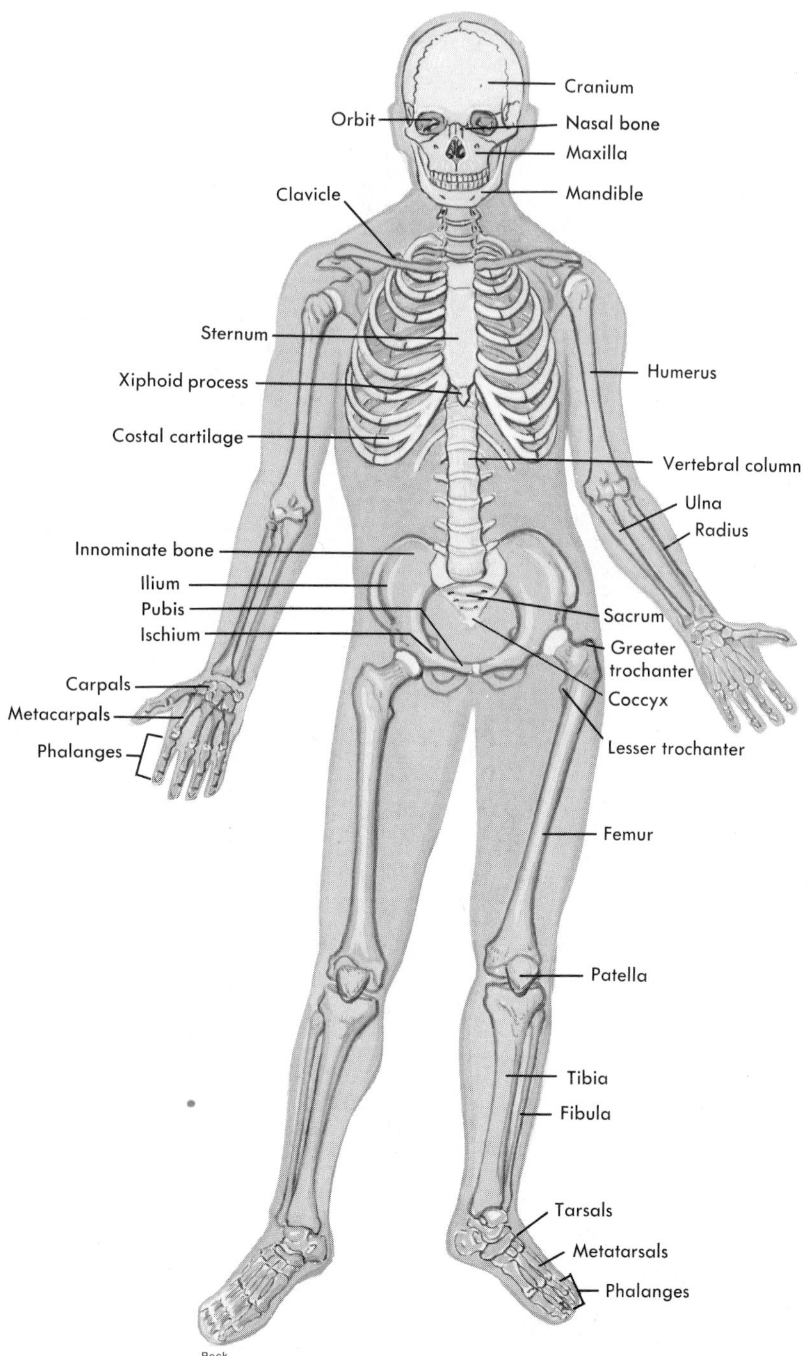

Fig. 14-3. Skeleton, anterior view. (From Anthony, C. P., and Thibodeau, G. A.: Textbook of anatomy and physiology, ed. 10, St. Louis, 1979, The C. V. Mosby Co.)

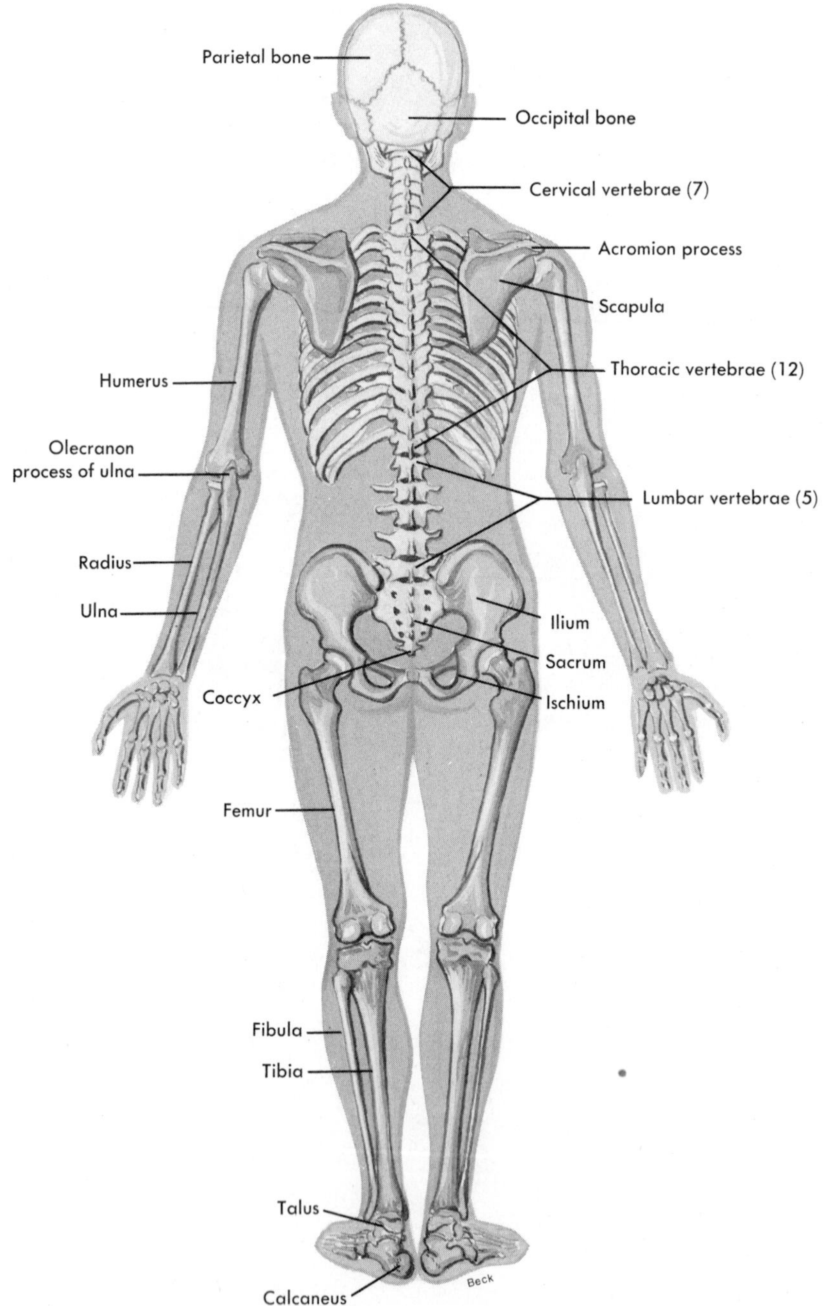

Fig. 14-4. Skeleton, posterior view. (From Anthony, C. P., and Thibodeau, G. A.: Textbook of anatomy and physiology, ed. 10, St. Louis, 1979, The C. V. Mosby Co.)

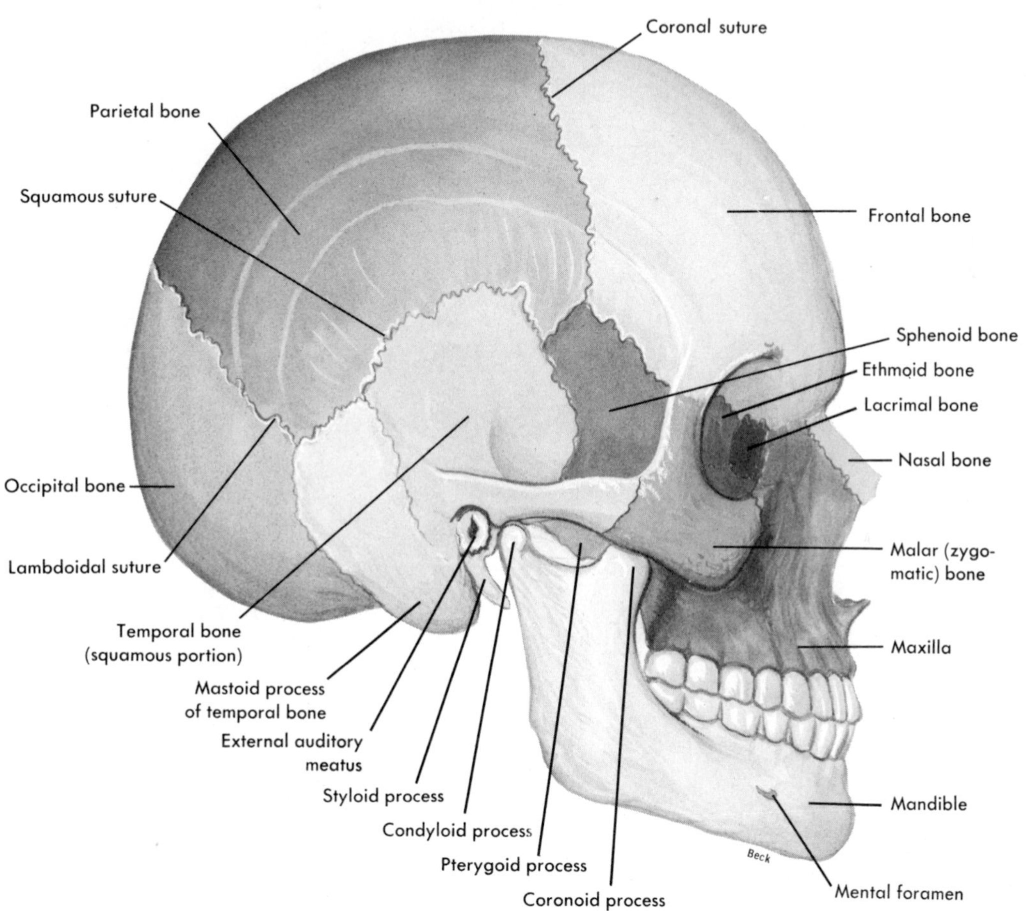

Fig. 14-5. Skull viewed from right side. (From Anthony, C. P., and Thibodeau, G. A.: Textbook of anatomy and physiology, ed. 10, St. Louis, 1979, The C. V. Mosby Co.)

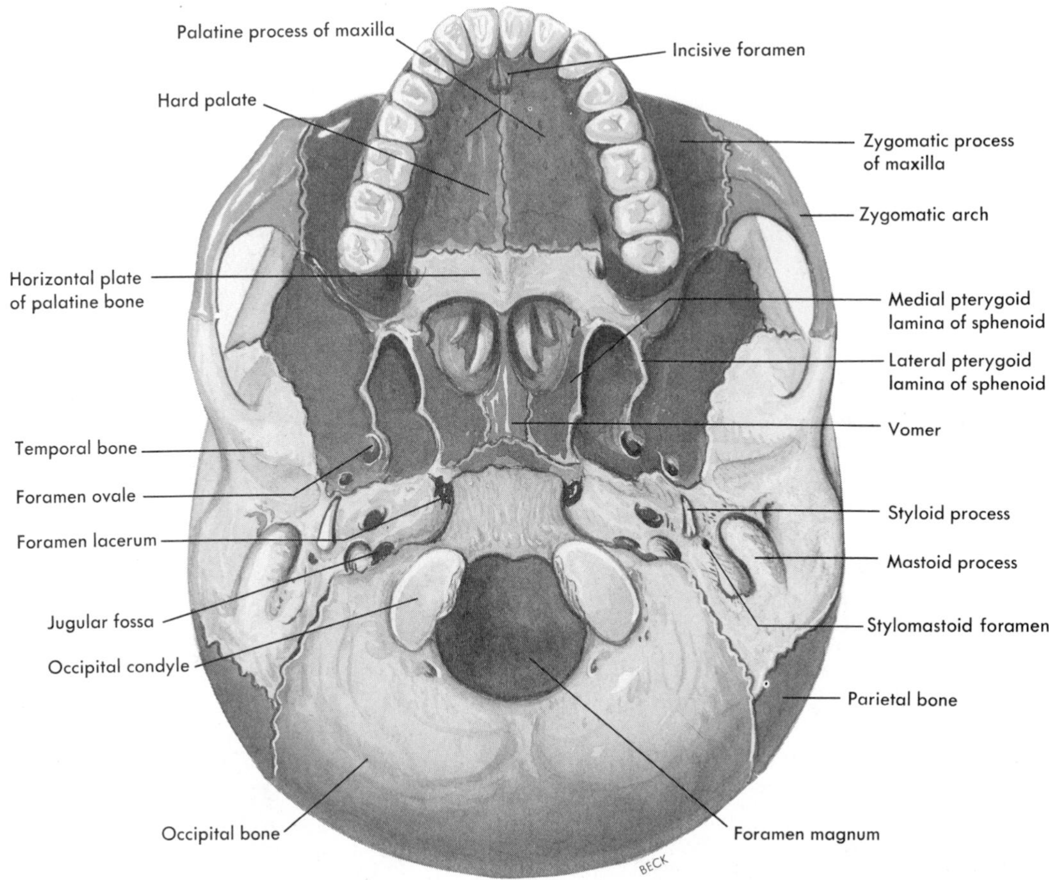

Fig. 14-6. Skull view from below. (From Anthony, C. P., and Thibodeau, G. A.: Textbook of anatomy and physiology, ed. 10, St. Louis, 1979, The C. V. Mosby Co.)

known as the zygomatic process, which connects with the temporal process of the malar or zygomatic bone (cheekbone) to form the zygomatic arch (Figs. 14-5 and 14-6). The inferior surface of the squamous portion articulates with the mandible in an area known as the mandibular fossa. The tympanic portion is inferior to the squamous portion and forms part of the wall of the external auditory meatus. Posterior to the squamous and tympanic portions is the mastoid portion, which has the mastoid process projecting downward behind the external meatus. Air cells within the mastoid communicate with the middle ear. The petrous portion of the temporal bone constitutes part of the base of the skull and contains the organs of hearing and position sense.

The sphenoid bone has a central location in the base of the cranium and articulates with most of the other bones of the cranium (Figs. 14-5 to 14-7). Anteriorly it joins with the frontal bone, laterally with the temporal bones, and posteriorly with the occipital bone. The middle portion of the sphenoid contains air cells—the sphenoid sinuses, which communicate with the nasal cavity. The superior surface of the sphenoid has a saddle-shaped depression known as the sella turcica, in which the pituitary gland is located. Two greater wings extend laterally from the body of the sphenoid, with two lesser wings above them.

The ethmoid (Fig. 14-7) is a cancellous bone between the orbital cavities and consists of a horizontal cribriform plate, a crista galli (cock's comb) extending from the upper surface of the plate, a perpendicular plate forming the upper part of the nasal septum, two lateral masses containing the ethmoid sinuses, and two ridges of bone known as the superior and middle turbinates, which serve to increase the total surface area of the nasal cavities. There are multiple openings

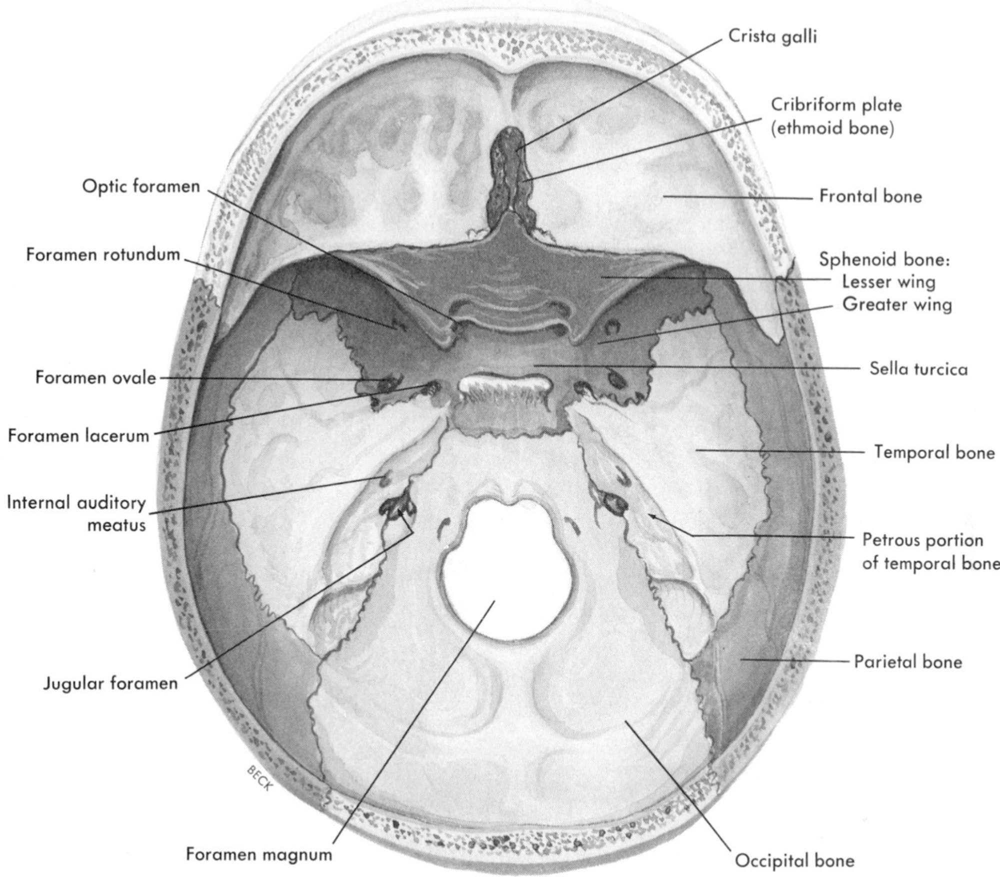

Fig. 14-7. Floor of cranial cavity. (From Anthony, C. P., and Thibodeau, G. A.: Textbook of anatomy and physiology, ed. 10, St. Louis, 1979, The C. V. Mosby Co.)

known as olfactory foramina in the cribriform plate through which the nerves of smell course on their way to the brain.

The bones of the face consist of the superficial and deep bones (Figs. 14-5 and 14-6). The superficial bones include two nasal, two maxillae, two malar, and one mandible. The deep bones include two lacrimal, two palatine, one vomer, and two inferior conchae.

The nasal bones are small bones that unite in the midline to form the bridge of the nose. Superiorly, they articulate with the frontal bone.

Each malar bone forms the prominence of the cheek and articulates posteriorly with the zygomatic process of the temporal bone to form the zygomatic arch. The malar bone also forms part of the lateral wall and base of the orbit.

The two maxillae are fused in the midline to form the upper jaw (Figs. 14-5 and 14-6). The maxillae form part of the floor of the orbit, the hard palate, and the bony structure of the face from the eyes to the teeth with processes containing sockets for the teeth. The medial aspect forms part of the lateral wall of the nasal cavity. The body of the maxilla contains a large air space known as the maxillary sinus.

The mandible is the lower jaw and is the largest bone of the face. The body of the mandible is horseshoe-shaped with rami extending from the posterior portion of the body (Fig. 14-5). On top of each ramus are two processes, the condyloid process, which extends posteriorly and articulates with the temporal bone to form the temporomandibular joint, and an anterior coronoid process, which provides for muscle attachments that move the mandible.

The lacrimal bones are thin bones in the front part of the medial wall of the orbit lateral and posterior to the nasal bones. The tear duct passes through the lacrimal canal, which is a groove in the bone.

The vomer is a thin bone forming the posterior part of the nasal septum (Fig. 14-6). The palatine bones are in the back of the nasal cavity (Fig. 14-6). The horizontal portion of each palatine bone forms the posterior part of the hard palate and the floor of the nasal cavity, whereas the vertical portion forms part of the floor of the orbit and part of the lateral wall of the nasal cavity. The inferior conchae, also known as turbinates, extend horizontally along the lateral nasal wall.

The hyoid bone is a small, horseshoe-shaped bone in the anterior neck, located just above the larynx. Posteriorly the hyoid is joined with the styloid processes of the temporal bones. The hyoid serves for muscle attachments used in moving the tongue.

The vertebral column consists of 26 separate bony fragments (Figs. 14-8 and 14-9) in adults and 33 or 34 vertebrae in children. Starting from the neck vertebrae and going down, we find 7 cervical vertebrae, 12 thoracic vertebrae, 5 lumbar vertebrae, a sacrum, which results from the fusion of 5 separate vertebrae, and a coccyx, which results from the fusion of 4 or 5 vertebrae. There are strong similarities in structure among the vertebrae. Each vertebra, except for the first two cervical ones, has an anterior body that is separated from the body above and below it by a fibrous cartilage known as the intervertebral disk. Two short projections known as the pedicles extend posteriorly from the body to meet with the laminae, which are fused in the midline posteriorly. The posterior portion of the vertebral body, the pedicles, and the laminae form the vertebral foramen containing the spinal cord and its coverings. Projecting posteriorly and downward from the junction of the laminae is the spinous process. Extending laterally from the junction of the pedicle and lamina on either side is the trans-

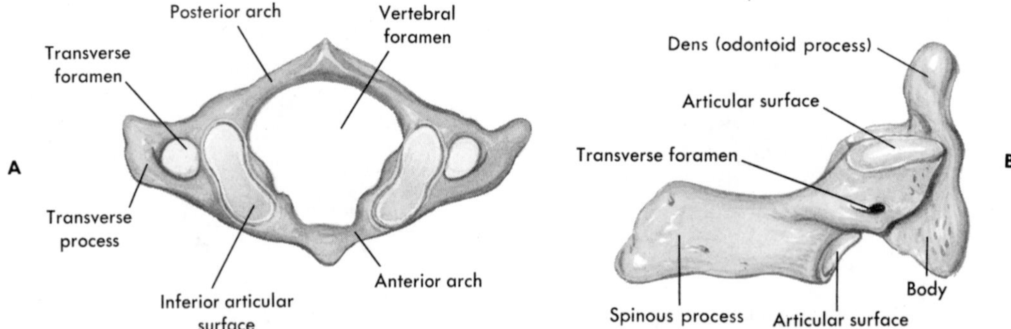

Fig. 14-8. Cervical vertebrae viewed from, **A,** below and, **B,** side. (From Anthony, C. P., and Thibodeau, G. A.: Textbook of anatomy and physiology, ed. 10, St. Louis, 1979, The C. V. Mosby Co.)

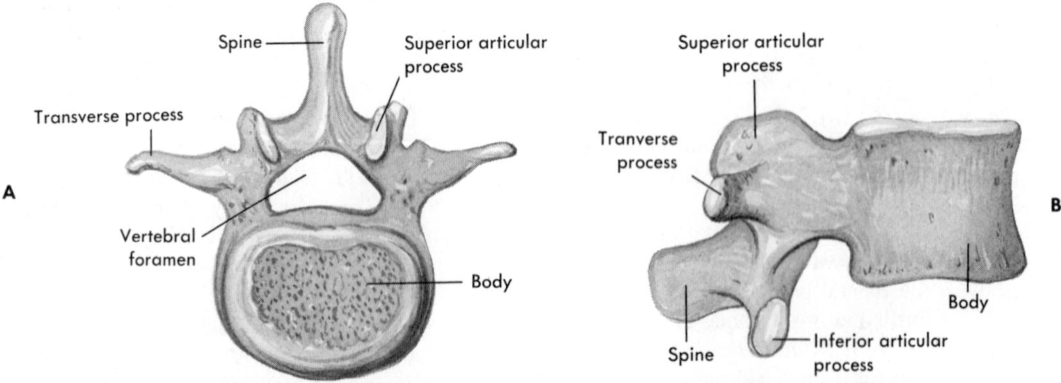

Fig. 14-9. Third lumbar vertebra viewed from, **A,** above and, **B,** side. (From Anthony, C. P., and Thibodeau, G. A.: Textbook of anatomy and physiology, ed. 10, St. Louis, 1979, The C. V. Mosby Co.)

verse process. Two superior and two inferior articular processes facilitate movement of the vertebrae on one another. Spinal nerves leave the vertebral foramen by passing in front of the joints connecting the vertebrae.

The cervical vertebrae are smaller than the other vertebrae and form a column, which permits motion of the neck (Fig. 14-10). In each transverse process of the cervical vertebrae is an additional foramen through which the vertebral arteries course on their way to the brain. As mentioned above, the first two cervical vertebrae are different from the other vertebrae. The first cervical vertebra articulates superiorly with the skull and is known as the atlas. The second cervical vertebra, the axis, has a large projection known as the odontoid process, which projects superiorly into the anterior atlas.

The distinctive feature of the thoracic vertebrae is the presence of articular surfaces for the ribs known as facets. The lumbar vertebrae are larger than the thoracic vertebrae and have neither transverse foramina nor facets. The sacrum resembles a concave triangle with the base articulating with the fifth lumbar vertebra (Figs. 14-3 and 14-4). The sacrum forms the posterior portion of the pelvis and articulates with the iliac bones. The coccyx is a small, fused bone articulating with the distal sacrum.

The vertebral column generally ranges 72 to 75 cm in length. Approximately one fourth of this length is accounted for by the intervertebral disks. There are four curvatures to the adult vertebral column—anterior convexity in the cervical region, anterior concavity in the thoracic region, anterior convexity in the lumbar region, and an anterior convexity in the sacrococcygeal region. The curvature of the spine makes it a flexible support.

The thorax is a bony cage, narrow at the top and broad at the base, and consists of the 12 pairs of ribs, the sternum anteriorly, and the 12 thoracic vertebrae posteriorly (Figs. 14-3 to 14-4). The thorax is covered with muscles and skin, and the inferior boundary is formed by the muscular diaphragm. The thorax functions both for protection and respiration. The sternum is a flat, narrow bone composed of a central body, a manubrium, which lies above the body, and a xiphoid process, which lies below the body. The clavicle and first rib articulate with the manubrium. The second rib articulates at the sternal angle, the junction of the manubrium and the body. The ribs are all attached posteriorly to the thoracic vertebrae and have variable anterior attachments. Costal cartilages join the top 10 pairs of ribs to the sternum. The bottom two pairs of ribs have no anterior attachment.

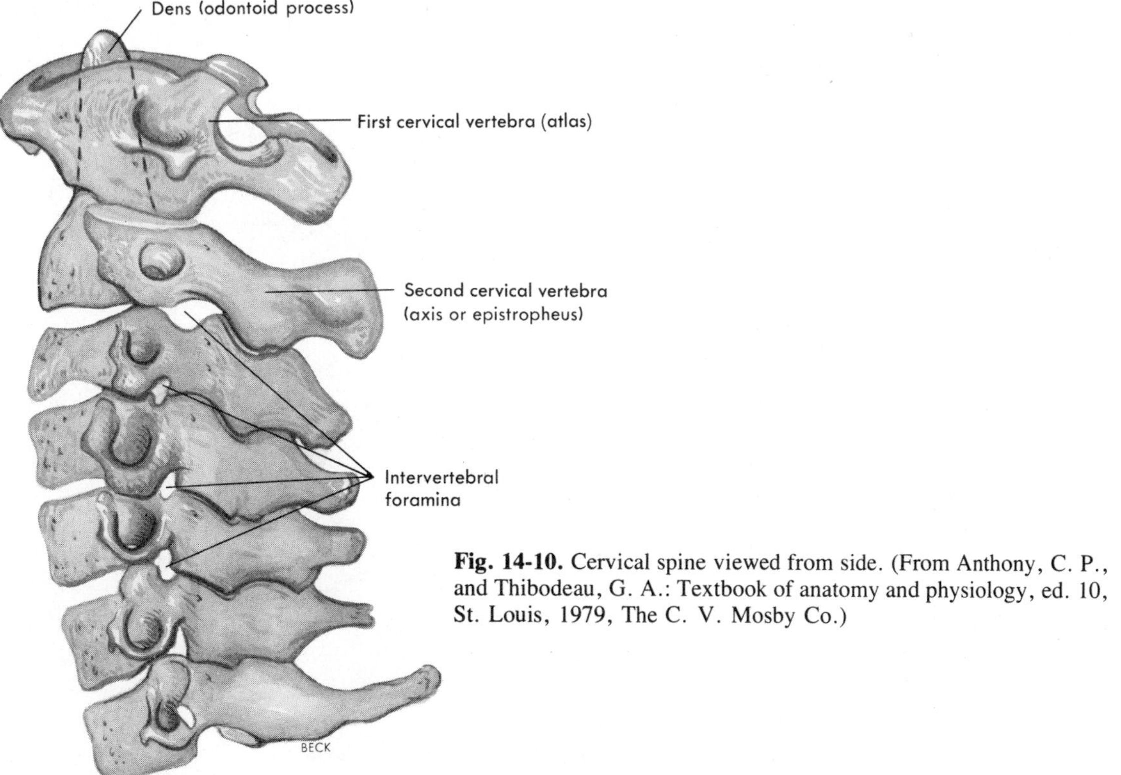

Fig. 14-10. Cervical spine viewed from side. (From Anthony, C. P., and Thibodeau, G. A.: Textbook of anatomy and physiology, ed. 10, St. Louis, 1979, The C. V. Mosby Co.)

Appendicular skeleton

The appendicular skeleton is divided into the bones of the upper extremity, pelvis, and the lower extremity.

The bones of the upper extremity consist of the clavicle, scapula, humerus, ulna, radius, 8 carpals, 5 metacarpals, and 14 phalanges. The clavicle (collarbone) lies horizontally at the base of the neck, articulating medially with the sternum to form the sternoclavicular joint and laterally with the acromion process of the scapula to form the acromioclavicular joint. The clavicle functions as a support for the shoulder. The scapula (shoulderblade) is a triangular bone at the posterior aspect of the thorax overlying the upper ribs (Fig. 14-11). The spine of the scapula is a prominent process that traverses the upper surface and ends in a large acromion process, which forms the point of the shoulder. The glenoid cavity is the smooth socket that receives the humeral head. The coracoid process, like a beak, projects above the glenoid and beneath the clavicle.

The humerus is the largest bone of the upper extremity and extends from the shoulder to the elbow. It consists of a shaft and two articular ends (Fig. 14-12). The upper end (head) articulates with the glenoid cavity. The anatomic neck is a slight narrowing at the margin of the head where the articular capsule attaches. Near the anatomic neck are two bony projections, the greater and lesser tubercles, for muscle attachments. The area just below the tubercles is the surgical neck, a frequent site of fractures. The lower portion of the bone is widened mediolaterally by the medial and lateral epicondyles. Beneath the lateral epicondyle is the capitulum, the surface articulating with the radius. The trochlea is the medial area for articulation with the ulna. The coronoid and olecranon fossae accommodate the respective processes of the ulna.

The ulna, the medial bone of the forearm, is attached more securely to the humerus but less securely to the wrist than the radius (Fig. 14-13). The proximal portion of the ulna forms a hook, with the open portion forming the trochlear (semilunar) notch and the back part forming the olecranon process (the elbow prominence). The other processes are located proximally on the ulna for muscle insertion. The small distal portion has an enlarged area known as the head and a small downward projection, the styloid process. The distal surface of the head forms part of the radioulnar joint.

The radius is the shorter, more laterally placed fore-

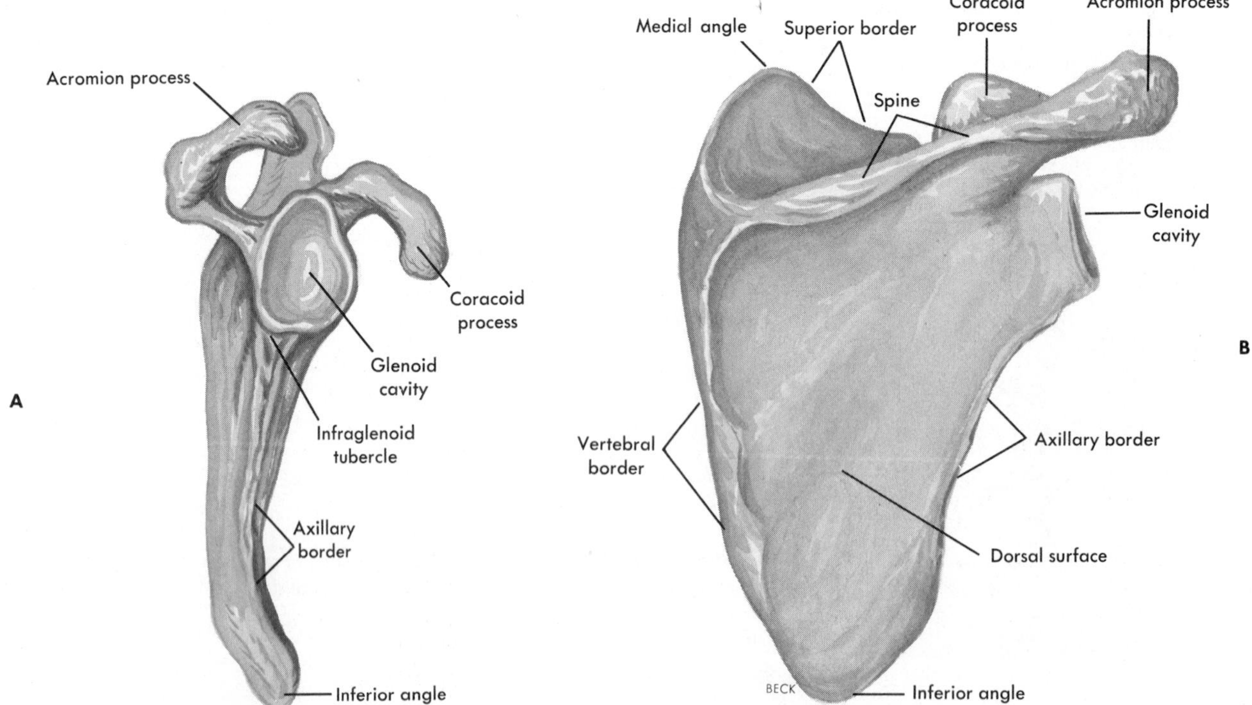

Fig. 14-11. Right scapula: **A,** lateral and, **B,** posterior views. (From Anthony, C. P., and Thibodeau, G. A.: Textbook of anatomy and physiology, ed. 10, St. Louis, 1979, The C. V. Mosby Co.)

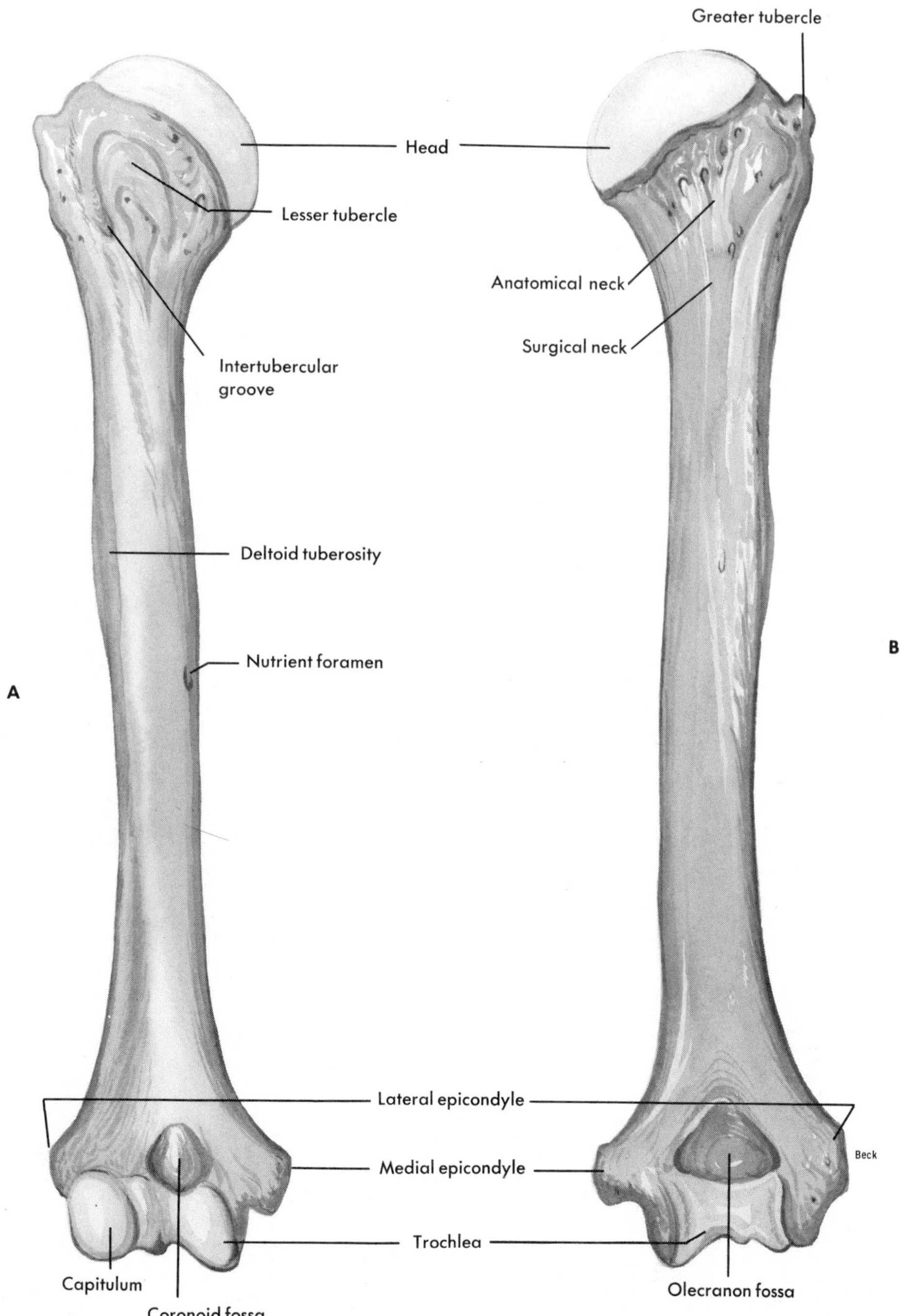

Fig. 14-12. Right humerus: **A,** anterior and, **B,** posterior views. (From Anthony, C. P., and Thibodeau, G. A.: Textbook of anatomy and physiology, ed. 10, St. Louis, 1979, The C. V. Mosby Co.)

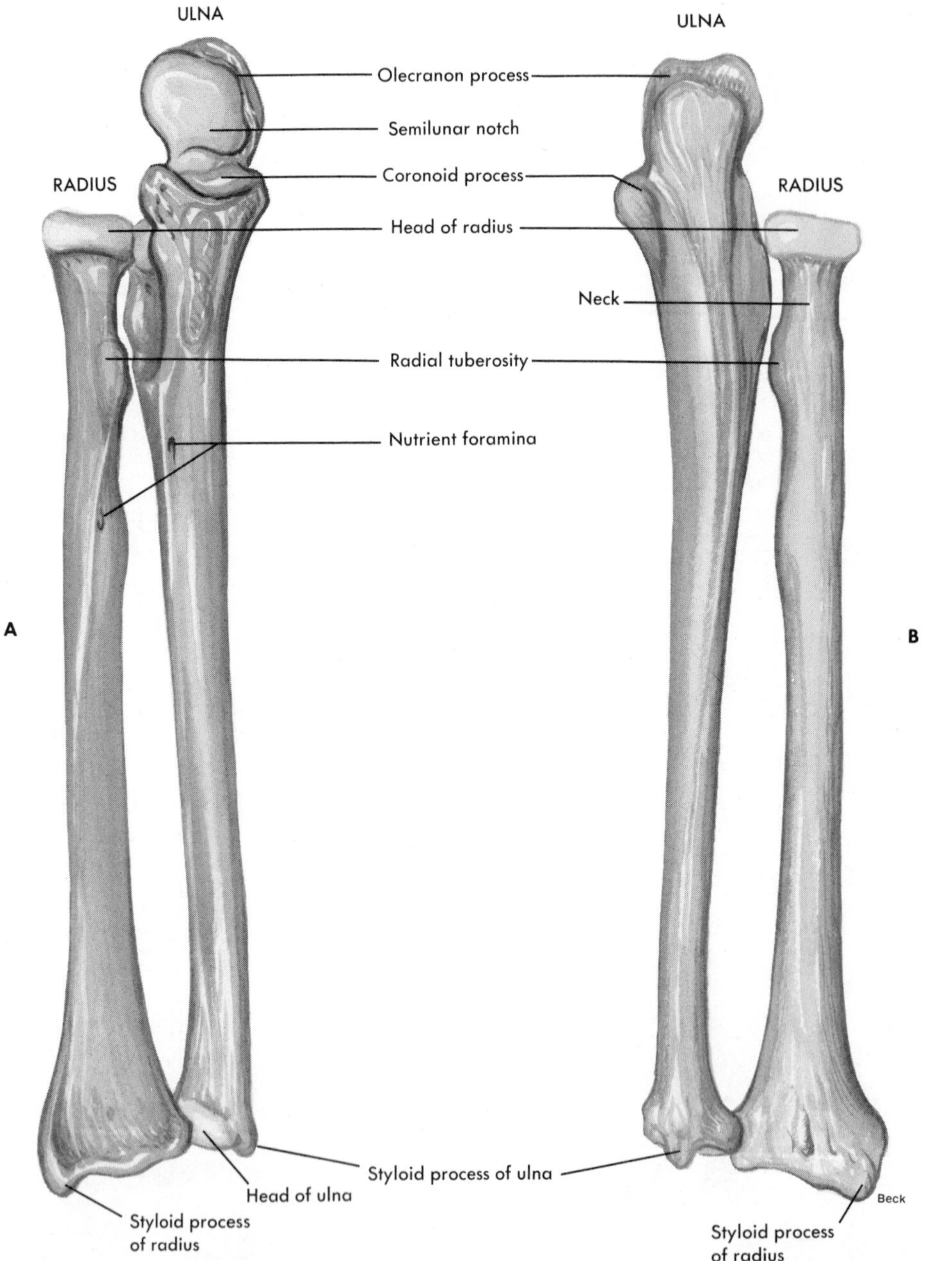

Fig. 14-13. Right radius and ulna: **A,** anterior and, **B,** posterior surfaces. (From Anthony, C. P., and Thibodeau, G. A.: Textbook of anatomy and physiology, ed. 10, St. Louis, 1979, The C. V. Mosby Co.)

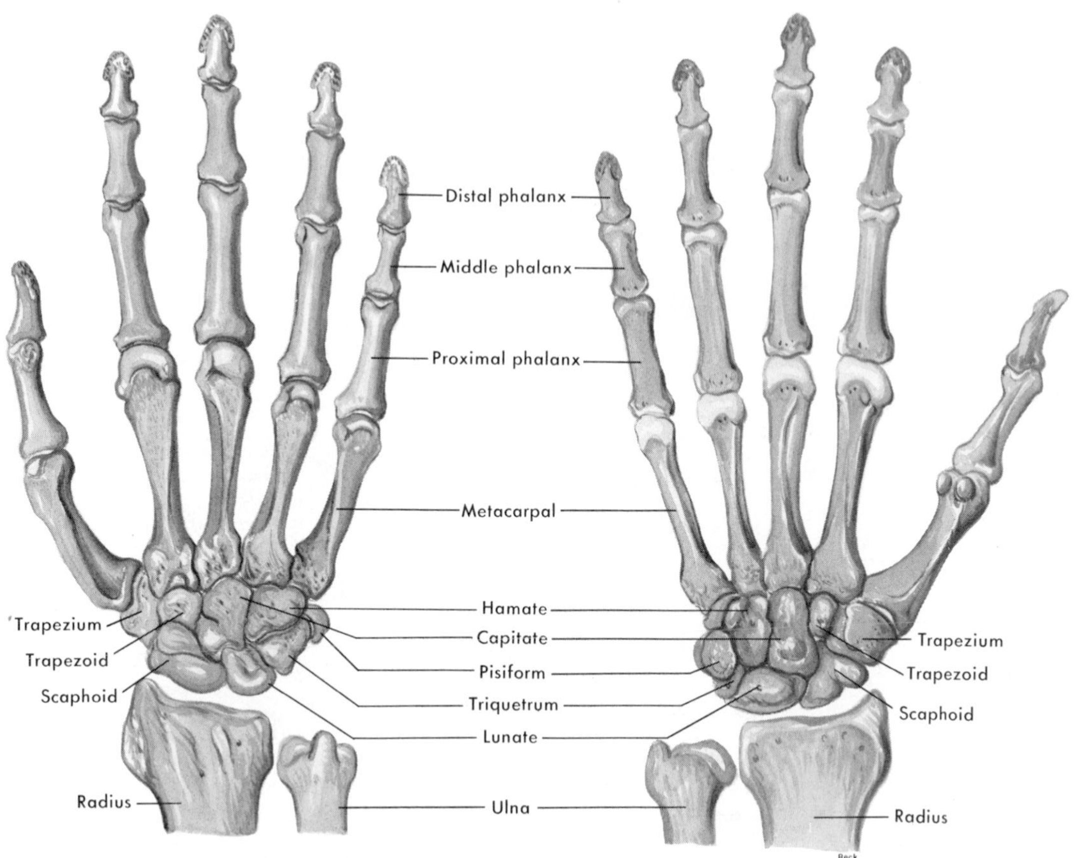

Fig. 14-14. Bones of right hand and wrist: **A,** dorsal and, **B,** palmar surfaces. (From Anthony, C. P., and Thibodeau, G. A.: Textbook of anatomy and physiology, ed. 10, St. Louis, 1979, The C. V. Mosby Co.)

arm bone. The proximal portion, the head, articulates with the humeral capitulum and the ulna. The shaft has an interosseous border connecting with an interosseous membrane between the radius and ulna. The prominent distal end has a smooth surface for articulation with the wrist and lateral styloid process.

The wrist consists of 8 small carpal bones in two rows of four each (Fig. 14-14). The proximal row, starting on the thumb side, are the scaphoid (navicular), lunate, triquetrum, and pisiform. The distal row consists of the trapezium (greater multangular), trapezoid (lesser multangular), capitate, and hamate. The 5 metacarpals form the skeleton of the hand. Proximally, the metacarpals articulate with the wristbones and distally with the phalanges. There are 14 bones of the fingers, known as phalanges, of which 3 are located within each of the four fingers and two in the thumb.

The pelvis consists of the two hipbones (also referred to as ossa coxae [sing., os coxae], or innominate bones), which are joined together anteriorly at the pubic symphysis and posteriorly to the sacrum, forming a protective ring of bone and uniting the trunk to the lower extremities (Figs. 14-15 and 14-16). Each hipbone is large and irregular and is formed from three separate parts including the ilium, ischium, and pubis, which fuse during the midteen years. The ilium is the large, fan-shaped portion forming the prominence of the hip with the curved upper rim called the iliac crest. The bony projections at each end of the iliac crest are the anterior and posterior superior iliac spines. The posterior articulation with the sacrum forms the sacroiliac joints. The ischium is the lower and most posterior portion of the pelvis, and while one is sitting, the weight of the body is on the ischial tuberosities. The anterior portion of the hipbone is the pubis, consisting of two rami. The superior ramus unites with the superior ramus of the other hipbone forming the pubic symphysis. The inferior ramus unites with the ischial ramus forming the medial border of the obturator

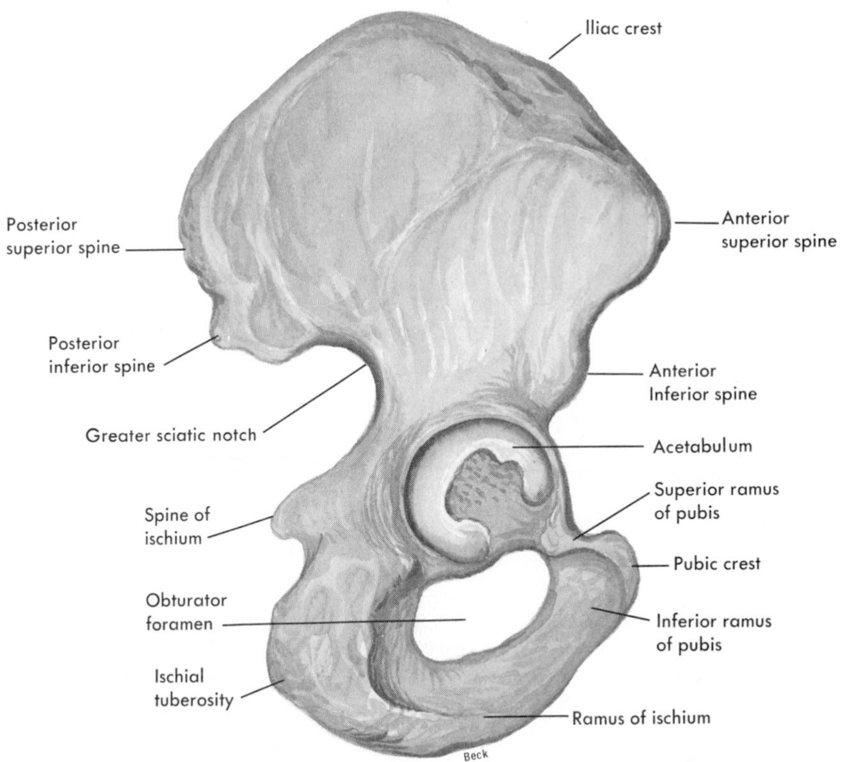

Fig. 14-15. Disarticulated right hip bone viewed from side and directly into acetabulum. (From Anthony, C. P., and Thibodeau, G. A.: Textbook of anatomy and physiology, ed. 10, St. Louis, 1979, The C. V. Mosby Co.)

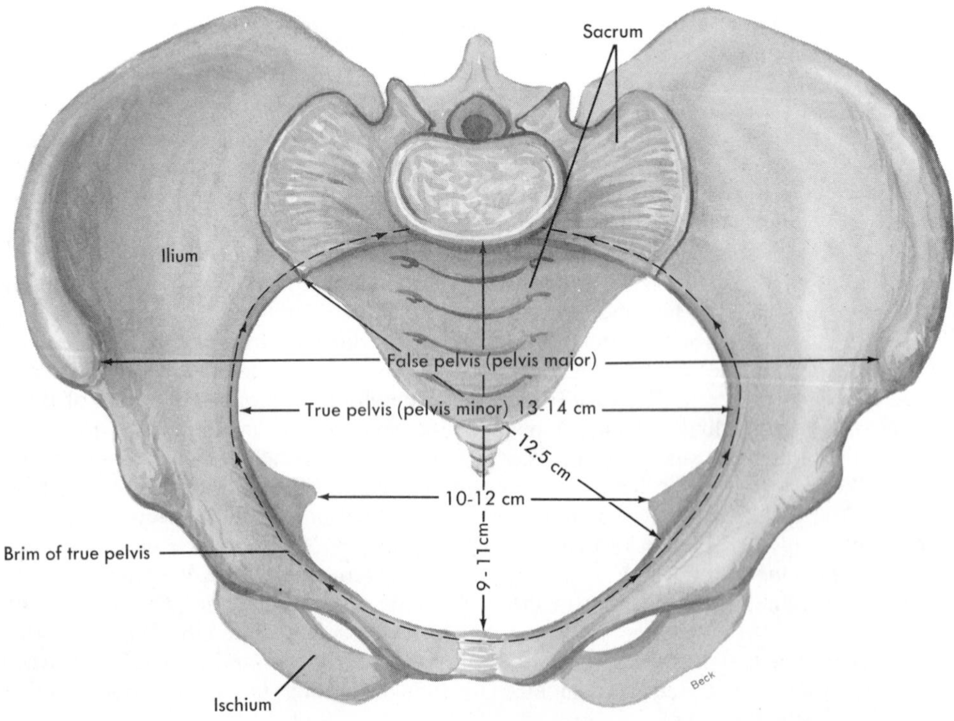

Fig. 14-16. Female pelvis viewed from above. (From Anthony, C. P., and Thibodeau, G. A.: Textbook of anatomy and physiology, ed. 10, St. Louis, 1979, The C. V. Mosby Co.)

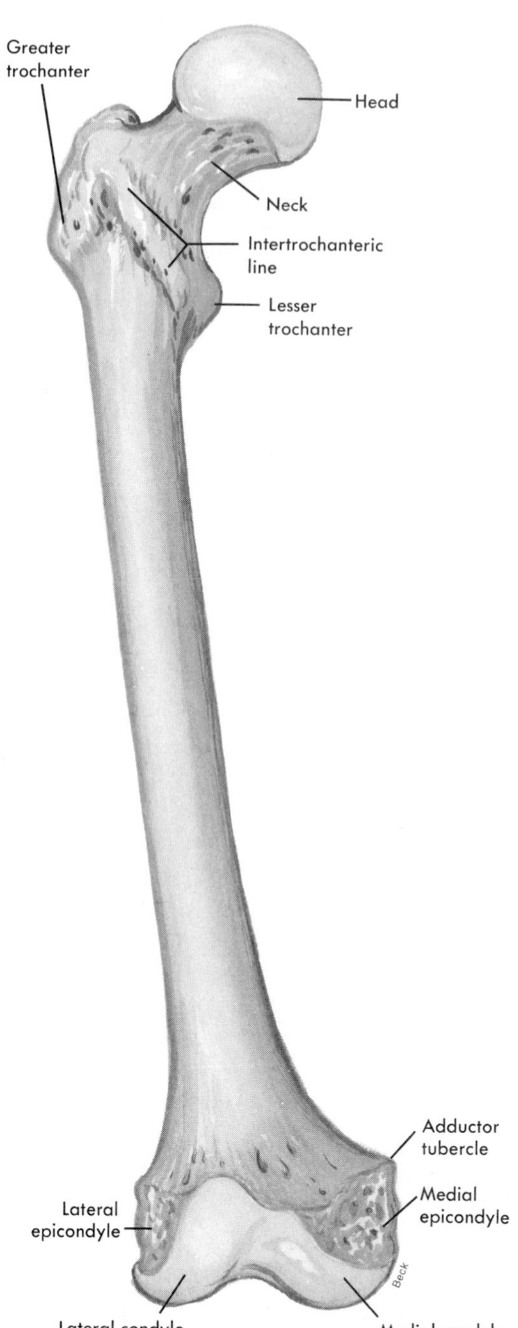

Fig. 14-17. Right femur, anterior surface. (From Anthony, C. P., and Thibodeau, G. A.: Textbook of anatomy and physiology, ed. 10, St. Louis, 1979, The C. V. Mosby Co.)

foramen. The acetabulum is the deep, cuplike socket on the lateral aspect of the hipbone for the articulation with the femoral head. The acetabulum is formed from parts of the pubis, ischium, and ilium.

The bones of the lower extremity consist of the femur, patella, tibia, fibula, 7 tarsals, 5 metatarsals, and 14 phalanges.

The bone of the thigh is the femur, the longest and strongest bone in the body, which has a long, uniform shaft with irregular ends (Fig. 14-17). The proximal end forms a rounded head with a narrower neck joining the shaft at an angle. The head articulates with the hipbone and the long neck enables free movement. The superior border of the neck leads to the greater trochanter, a prominent projection on the lateral surface of the femur. The inferior border of the neck leads to a smaller projection on the medial side, the lesser trochanter. The distal end of the femur consists of two large bulges, the medial and lateral condyles, which articulate with the tibia.

The patella, or kneecap, is a sesamoid bone that lies anterior to the distal femur and develops in the tendon of the large quadriceps femoris muscle (Fig. 14-3). The patella forms the prominence of the knee and serves to protect the knee joint anteriorly.

The leg bones consists of the tibia and fibula (Fig. 14-18). The tibia is the medial and larger bone and bears the weight. The proximal portion is expanded to accept the femoral condyles. The bony masses on the proximal surfaces are the medial and lateral condyles. The tibial tuberosity is the anterior projection just below the condyles. The shaft of the tibia is fairly uniform in size. There is an interosseous border for attachments of the interosseous membrane between the tibia and fibula. The distal portion of the tibia is somewhat widened for articulation with the ankle and fibula. A projection from the tibia, the medial malleolus, forms the prominence on the inner aspect of the ankle.

The fibula is a thin bone lying next to the tibia and does not support any weight. The proximal head articulates with the tibia. The lower end has a projection, the lateral malleolus, which forms the lateral side of the joint with the talus.

The 7 tarsal bones are the talus, calcaneus, navicular, 3 cuneiforms, and the cuboid (Fig. 14-19). The talus articulates with many bones including the tibia and fibula and receives the weight of the body from the tibia. The calcaneus, or heel bone, is the largest and strongest bone of the foot. The navicular is a flattened bone located between the talus and the 3 cuneiforms. The 3 cuneiforms articulate with the first 3 metatarsals. The cuboid lies on the lateral side of the foot and articulates posteriorly with the calcaneus and anteriorly with the fourth and fifth metatarsals.

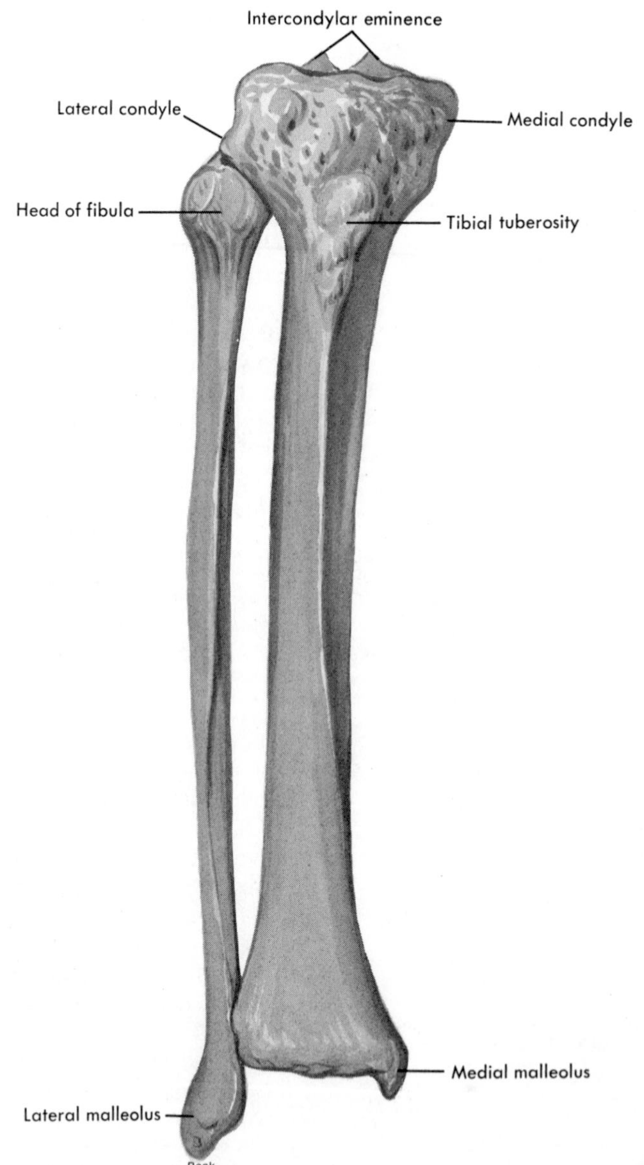

Fig. 14-18. Right tibia and fibula, anterior surface. (From Anthony, C. P., and Thibodeau, G. A.: Textbook of anatomy and physiology, ed. 10, St. Louis, 1979, The C. V. Mosby Co.)

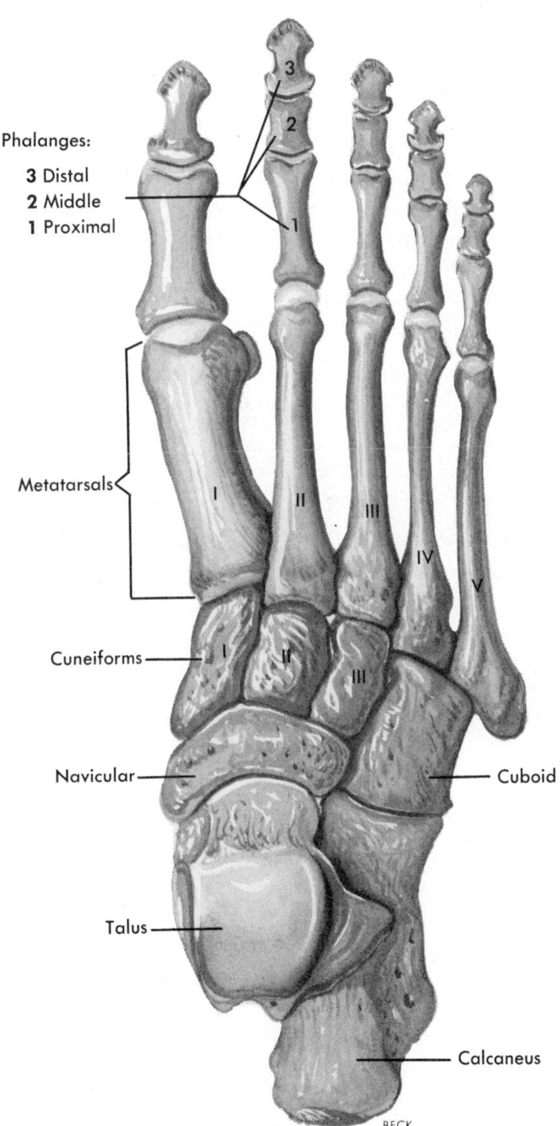

Fig. 14-19. Right foot viewed from above. (From Anthony, C. P., and Thibodeau, G. A.: Textbook of anatomy and physiology, ed. 10, St. Louis, 1979, The C. V. Mosby Co.)

The five metatarsals lie anteriorly to the tarsals. The 14 phalanges are distributed with 2 in the great toe and 3 in each of the other toes.

Joints

Joints (articulations) are spaces where bones come into contact and are bridged in some manner. The articulations have variable amounts of movement and have been classified into two main types according to the amount of movement: rigid (synarthroses) or freely movable (diarthroses).

With a synarthrosis there is absence of a joint space with little or no movement allowed. In the formation of a synarthrosis the tissue connecting the bones is replaced by the ends of the bone growing together. The sutures of the skull are examples of synarthroses with only a thin fibrous membrane separating the ends of the bones (Fig. 14-20, *A*). In some synarthroses cartilage grows between the articular surfaces of the bones and may allow some motion. Examples of the cartilaginous synarthroses are the symphysis pubis and the joints between the vertebral bodies (Fig. 14-20, *B* and *C*).

A diarthrosis permits freedom of movement and is the most common type of joint in the body. There is a well-defined articular cavity containing fluid (synovia) and lined by a synovial membrane (Fig. 14-20, *D* and *E*). Intra-articular structures such as ligaments and menisci may be present. There is a thin layer of hyaline cartilage, known as articular cartilage, that cushions the ends of each bone in the joint. The synovial joint develops from undifferentiated mesenchyme between the bone rudiments. Part of the undifferentiated mesenchyme differentiates into synovial mesenchyme and subsequently into synovial membrane, menisci, and ligaments. The outer portion of

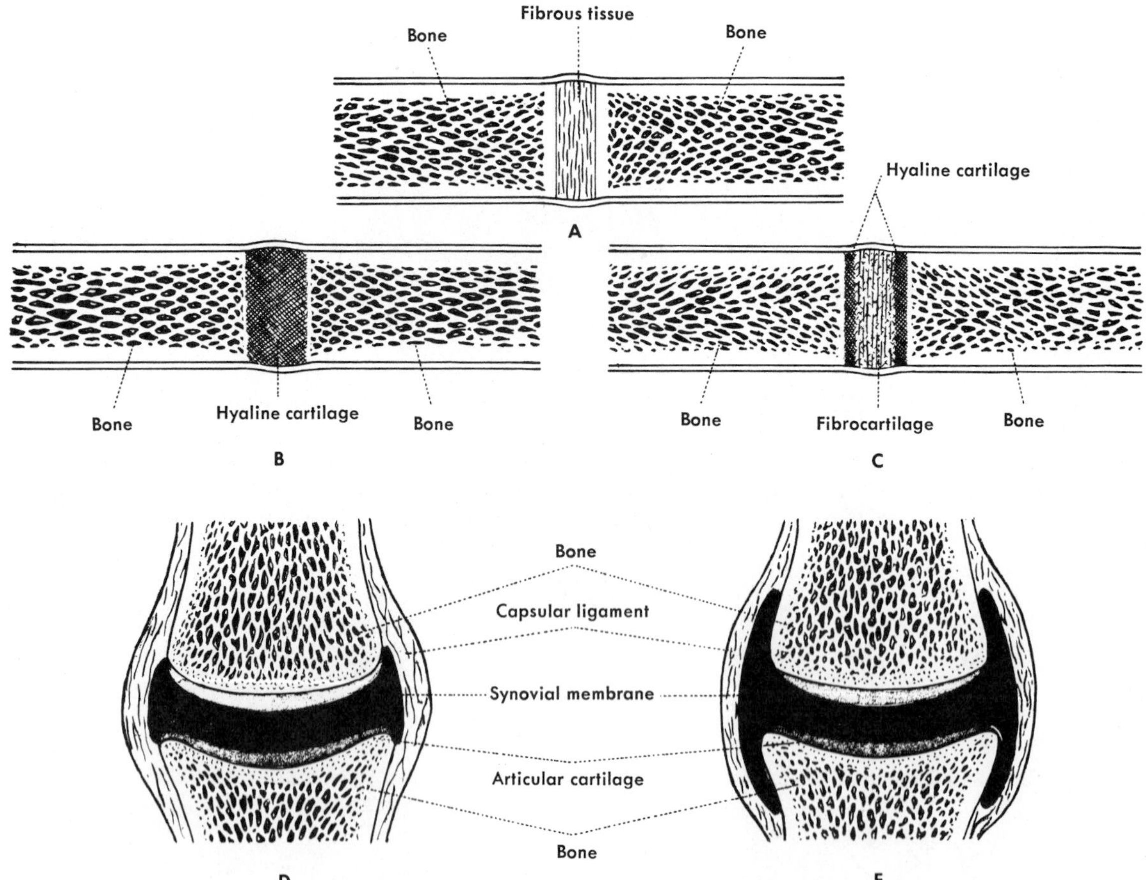

Fig. 14-20. Classification of joints. **A,** Fibrous synarthrosis. **B** and **C,** Cartilaginous synarthroses. **D** and **E,** Synovial diarthrosis. (From Hamilton, W. J.: Textbook of human anatomy, ed. 2, St. Louis, 1976, The C. V. Mosby Co.; courtesy The Macmillan Press Ltd., Houndsmill Basingstoke, Hampshire, England.)

the undifferentiated mesenchyme condenses and forms the joint capsule, which attaches to the bone ends of the joints beyond their articular cartilages.

RADIONUCLIDE IMAGING

Of the many different imaging procedures performed in clinical nuclear medicine, radionuclide bone and joint studies require a thorough knowledge of anatomy and imaging techniques by the technologist so that excellent images of the radiopharmaceutical distribution can be obtained. Since early disease involvement of bone may initially be subtle, improper positioning of the patient for imaging or improper exposure of the film may lead to an inaccurate interpretation. Furthermore, since these studies are frequently used to follow therapy, the technique used must be reproducible to allow careful comparison with a previous study.

Several different types of radionuclide studies can be performed in the evaluation of bone and joint disorders. The most commonly performed procedure is radionuclide bone imaging with a technetium-99m phosphate compound. Joint imaging is being used in the evaluation of suspected inflammatory processes involving bones and joints.

PAST AND PRESENT RADIOPHARMACEUTICALS

The earliest applications of radionuclides to the study of bone were performed with phosphorus 32 and calcium 45 for observation of bone structure and function.[2,35] These radionuclides are pure beta-particle emitters and accumulate in regions of increased bone mineral deposition, but their lack of gamma radiation limits external measurement. Clinical application was not made possible until the use of strontium 85, a calcium analog, whose gamma rays could be detected externally[3,11] (Table 14-2). The introduction of the rectilinear scanner and strontium 85 in the early 1960s made bone scanning possible, but because of the high radiation dose, its use was limited to patients with documented malignancy. Strontium 85 has a half-life of 65 days and emits a gamma ray at 513 keV. The long effective half-life of this radionuclide limits the amount of activity injected to 100 μCi. With this small amount of activity, scanning time was extensive and the information density of the image was extremely low. Although the accumulation of strontium in bone is rapid, the blood and gastrointestinal clearance are slow; thus a 2- to 7-day interval between the times of injection and scan was needed.

Another isotope of strontium used for bone scanning is strontium 87m, which has a 2.9-hour half-life and a gamma-ray energy of 388 keV.[43] The short half-life allows the administered dose to be increased to a range of 1 to 4 mCi, and scans can be performed 2 to 3 hours after injection. Strontium 87m is a generator-produced isotope from a parent product of yttrium 87, which has an 80-hour half-life. This generator-produced radionuclide was rather expensive.

Fluorine 18 was the first bone-seeking radiopharmaceutical that gave an acceptable radiation dose to the patient and provided a higher quality scan than did the

Table 14-2. Radionuclides used for bone imaging

Characteristic	^{85}Sr	^{87m}Sr	^{18}F	^{99m}Tc
Decay mode	Electron capture	Isomeric transition	Positron	Isomeric transition
Energy (keV)	513	388	511 (annihilation)	140
Physical $T_{\frac{1}{2}}$	64 days	2.8 hours	1.8 hours	6 hours
Effective $T_{\frac{1}{2}}$	2 days (50%) 60 days (15%)	2.8 hours	1.8 hours	6 hours
Lesion-nonlesion uptake	Moderate	Moderate	Moderate	High
Usual adult dose	100 μCi	1 to 4 mCi	1 to 4 mCi	15 mCi
Radiation dose (rads) for adult dose				
Whole body	0.42	0.08	0.16	0.13
Bone	3.60	0.32	0.60	0.59
Bone marrow	1.10	0.40	0.16	0.41
Kidney			0.31	2.10
Bladder			8.00	3.20
Time from injection to imaging	2 to 7 days	2 to 3 hours	2 to 4 hours	2 to 4 hours
Chemical form	Nitrate or chloride	Nitrate or chloride	Sodium fluoride	Polyphosphate, pyrophosphate, ethylenehydroxydiphosphonate (EHDP), methylenediphosphonate (MDP)

isotopes of strontium, thus permitting a wider application of bone imaging in the late 1960s and early 1970s.[9] The rapid blood clearance of fluorine 18 is advantageous for the performance of bone scans, since the blood and tissue activity levels are low compared to that of bone at the time of imaging and therefore give a high ratio of bone to soft tissue. The disadvantage of using fluorine 18 is its half-life of 1.87 hours, which makes it very expensive to manufacture and deliver to a large number of hospitals at any great distance from the production facility. The annihilation radiation (511 keV) from its positron emission is suitable for imaging with a rectilinear scanner but not a scintillation camera because of the high-energy photons.

The development of technetium 99m–labeled phosphate complexes for bone imaging was introduced by Subramanian in 1971.[44,45] Technetium 99m in the form of pertechnetate does not localize to any useful extent in bone. Technetium 99m has excellent physical properties for nuclear medicine imaging because of its ideal characteristics for use with the Anger scintillation camera. The short half-life of ^{99m}Tc allows the administration of several millicuries of activity to be injected; thus images with high information density can be obtained.

Mechanism of accumulation

The accumulation of radionuclides in bone is related to both vascularity and rate of bone production.[17,45] Increased blood supply to an area of bone will result in a blood-pool image (obtained immediately after radiopharmaceutical administration) with increased activity.

The localization of various bone-imaging agents is related to exchange with ions in the bone. The process of exchange of an ion native to bone for a labeled, bone-seeking ion is termed "heterionic exchange."[10,25] Calcium phosphate is the main inorganic constituent of bone; however, calcium is also found in the form of carbonate and fluoride. Calcium is located in microcrystals of hydroxyapatite, $Ca_{10}(PO_4)_6(OH)_2$.[36] Analog elements of calcium, such as strontium, are believed to exchange with the calcium. Fluorine 18 exchanges with the hydroxyl (OH) ion in the hydroxyapatite. The accumulation of labeled phosphate compounds is probably related to the exchange of the phosphorus groups onto the calcium of hydroxyapatite. Although these mechanisms are not completely understood, the principle of bone imaging is fairly basic. Calcium analogs or phosphate compounds have a low concentration in blood and tissue.

Radiopharmaceuticals used for bone imaging can localize in soft-tissue areas demonstrating not only calcification but also infarction, inflammation, trauma, and tumor. The portion of any radiopharmaceutical that does not accumulate in bone and tissue or stays in the circulation is eliminated from the body by various routes, depending on the radiopharmaceutical. Strontium 85 has some concentration in the gastrointestinal tract for several days. Fluorine 18 and phosphate scans labeled with technetium 99m demonstrate activity in the kidneys and bladder, since these agents are excreted through the urinary tract.

Technical considerations

The physical characteristics of the radionuclides that have been used for bone imaging present several important factors in radiopharmaceutical selection (Table 14-2). These factors relate primarily to the amount of activity that may be administered to the patient, the gamma-ray energy, and the amount of accumulation of radiopharmaceutical in the bone.

Prior to the introduction of ^{18}F- and ^{99m}Tc-phosphate compounds, bone imaging was a time-consuming procedure associated with a high radiation dose to the patient and poor information content in the images. The subsequent development of better radiopharmaceuticals and improved instrumentation produced images of higher quality with better information concerning bone physiology. In conjunction with the improved information in the images, the need for carefully controlling the technical aspects of the procedure became apparent.

Choosing the best radionuclide for bone imaging is currently a simple choice based on the physical characteristics. The strontium and fluorine isotopes have high-energy gamma rays and require the use of coarse-resolution collimators with thick lead septa. The high-energy gamma rays have a low attenuation coefficient resulting in such poor detection efficiency in a one-half-inch-thick sodium iodide crystal that the use of the Anger scintillation camera is nearly excluded. Also, these radionuclides must be administered in amounts of activity smaller than those of ^{99m}Tc, yielding lower information-density images. Fluorine 18 is an excellent agent for bone imaging, but its short half-life and high cost limit its general availability. Technetium 99m–labeled compounds allow larger quantities of activity to be administered with a resultant lower radiation dose than do the other radionuclides. The monoenergetic gamma-ray emission of 140 keV and the absence of particulate radiation make ^{99m}Tc well suited for use with all types of imaging instruments, particularly the scintillation camera. Technetium 99m is also readily available to all laboratories at a very low cost, unlike other radionuclides for bone imaging.

Radiopharmaceuticals

Since ^{99m}Tc is the present radionuclide of choice, the phosphate compound that produces the best image

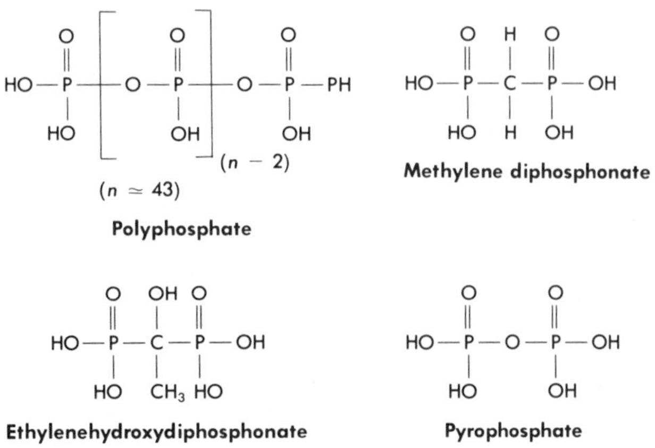

$(n - 2)$

$(n \simeq 43)$

Polyphosphate

Methylene diphosphonate

Ethylenehydroxydiphosphonate

Pyrophosphate

Fig. 14-21. Structural formulas of various phosphate pharmaceuticals in acid form.

needs to be determined. Fig. 14-21 shows the structure of four phosphate compounds that have been utilized in routine clinical use for bone imaging. To evaluate these various phosphate compounds, their distribution in the body relative to the rate and amount of accumulation in various organ systems and bone must be determined.

Polyphosphate was the first commercially available ^{99m}Tc-labeled compound for bone imaging. As seen in Fig. 14-21, the structural formula of polyphosphate includes a group of phosphates with a chain length of approximately 40 to 55. Phosphate chains that are extremely long can result in the formation of a radiocolloid in the bloodstream, causing hepatic localization of the pharmaceutical. Further development of this agent moved from longer phosphate chains toward shorter, more stable phosphate complexes. Among these were pyrophosphate and EHDP (ethylenehydroxydiphosphonate). Pyrophosphate is a naturally occurring compound in the body and its P—O—P bond is subject to breakdown by phosphatase enzymes. The carbon-carbon bond of EHDP is believed to offer greater stability than pyrophosphate. Both pyrophosphate and EHDP have a faster blood and tissue clearance than does polyphosphate. MDP (methylenediphosphonate) is a similar complex to pyrophosphate and EHDP but has a faster blood clearance. The blood clearance of MDP in the initial 3 to 4 hours after administration is very similar to fluorine. MDP labeled with ^{99m}Tc provides, however, a better image of the bones, since the lower blood and tissue concentration gives a higher ratio of bone to tissue.

Patient preparation

The preparation of the patient for bone imaging is minimal when any of the ^{99m}Tc-labeled agents are used, but several factors must be taken into consideration. The patient needs to have a complete understanding of the procedure, especially the reason for the delay between radiopharmaceutical administration and imaging. A delay of approximately 3 hours is generally an adequate time for good bone accumulation and a low soft-tissue level of the radiopharmaceutical. Radiopharmaceuticals with fast blood and tissue clearance, such as MDP, allow imaging as early as 2 hours after administration.

Unless contraindicated, patients should be hydrated to aid in clearance of the radiopharmaceutical from the body. The administration of four to six glasses of liquid during the delay period is adequate, with the patient being encouraged to void frequently to decrease the radiation dose. Patients must also void immediately before imaging begins so that the image of the pelvis is not obscured by a large amount of radioactivity in the bladder. Because of the high concentration of radioactivity in the urine, care must be taken to avoid contamination of the patient, the patient's clothing, or the bed sheets, which may lead to a false-positive study.

INSTRUMENTATION

Several types of instruments have been used for bone imaging. Wider application of this procedure has been responsible for the design of new instruments and accessories. In this section, application of the Anger scintillation camera, with whole body–imaging capability and the multiplane tomographic scanner are discussed.

Anger scintillation camera

The Anger scintillation camera is currently the most versatile and most commonly utilized imaging device for use with ^{99m}Tc-labeled compounds. Since the skeleton is one of the most extensive organ systems in the body, the application of the standard stationary camera with an approximately 10-inch field of view requires 25 to 30 separate views for complete imaging (Fig. 14-22). Performing bone imaging by this technique requires a large amount of the technologist's time and effort in positioning the patient for all these views. High-resolution or medium-resolution (140 keV) collimators are well suited for bone imaging with a standard-field camera (high-sensitivity collimators should not be used). However, a 140 keV diverging collimator would maintain good resolution and allow reduction of the total number of images because of the larger effective field of view. The presently used diverging collimators result in slight spatial distortion and loss of resolution at the image edges. The use of a large (11.5- to 15-inch) crystal scintillation camera with a parallel-hole collimator allows inclusion of a larger area of the body in each view, reducing the total number of images to approximately 13 views (Figs. 14-22, *A*, and 14-23).

The bone area and activity in the field of the camera can be highly variable for different portions of the body, and some images may require a long imaging time to achieve high information density. Commonly, multiple individual images are taken for an equal amount of time. This equal-time technique allows the film density in one image to be compared to the density

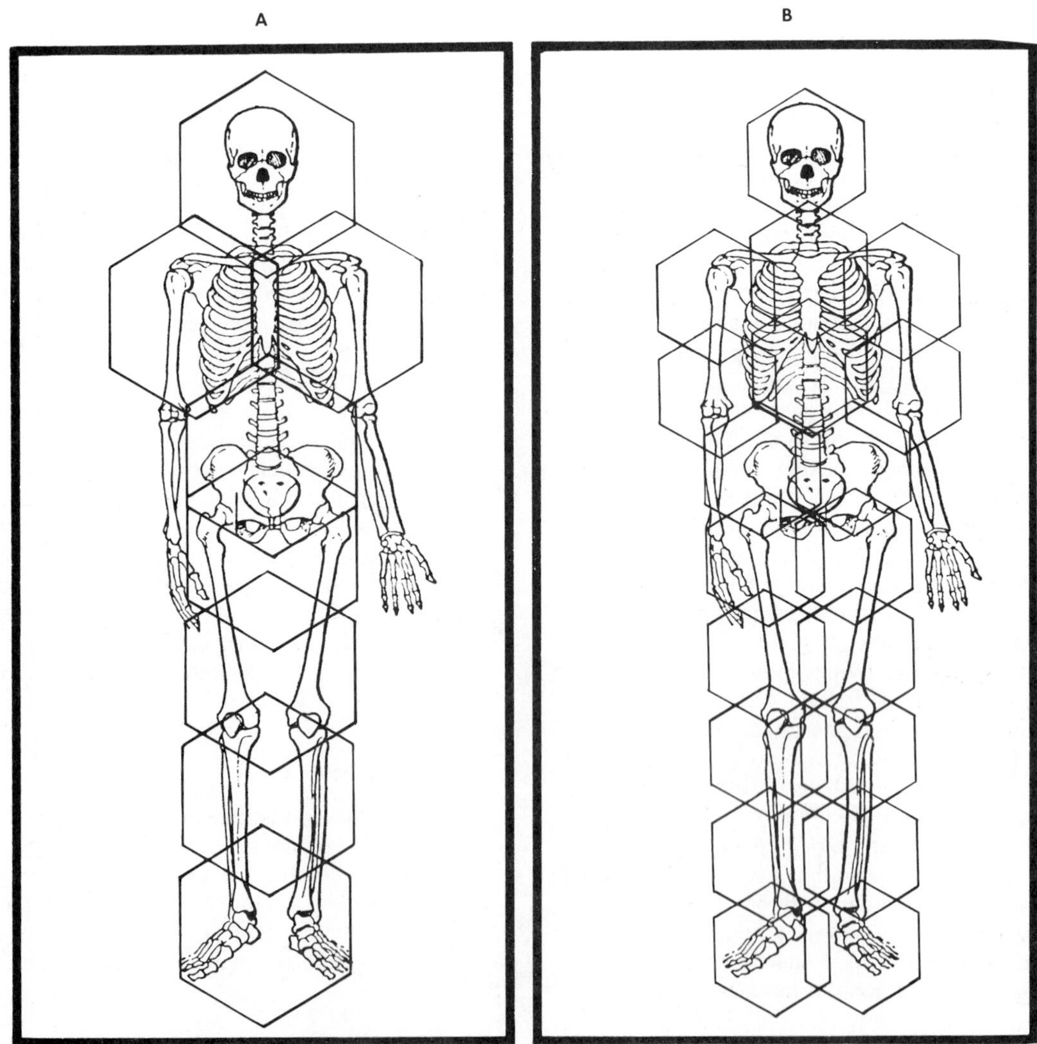

Fig. 14-22. Views necessary for imaging whole body with, **A,** individual images with large-crystal camera and, **B,** individual images with standard-field-of-view camera. (Courtesy Ohio-Nuclear, Inc., Solon, Ohio.)

in another image, since the exposure is made for an equal amount of time. This method is effective so long as adequate statistics are achieved. First, one area of the body (such as the anterior or posterior view of the chest) is imaged for a preset number of counts. Between 400,000 and 600,000 counts are accumulated for a standard-field camera and 500,000 to 1 million for a large-crystal camera. After this first exposure, all subsequent images are taken for the same interval of time. An alternative method of performing equal-time imaging is to use the information-density feature available on some scintillation cameras. An area of normal bone as found in the sternum or spine is selected with the information density (ID) marker, and an

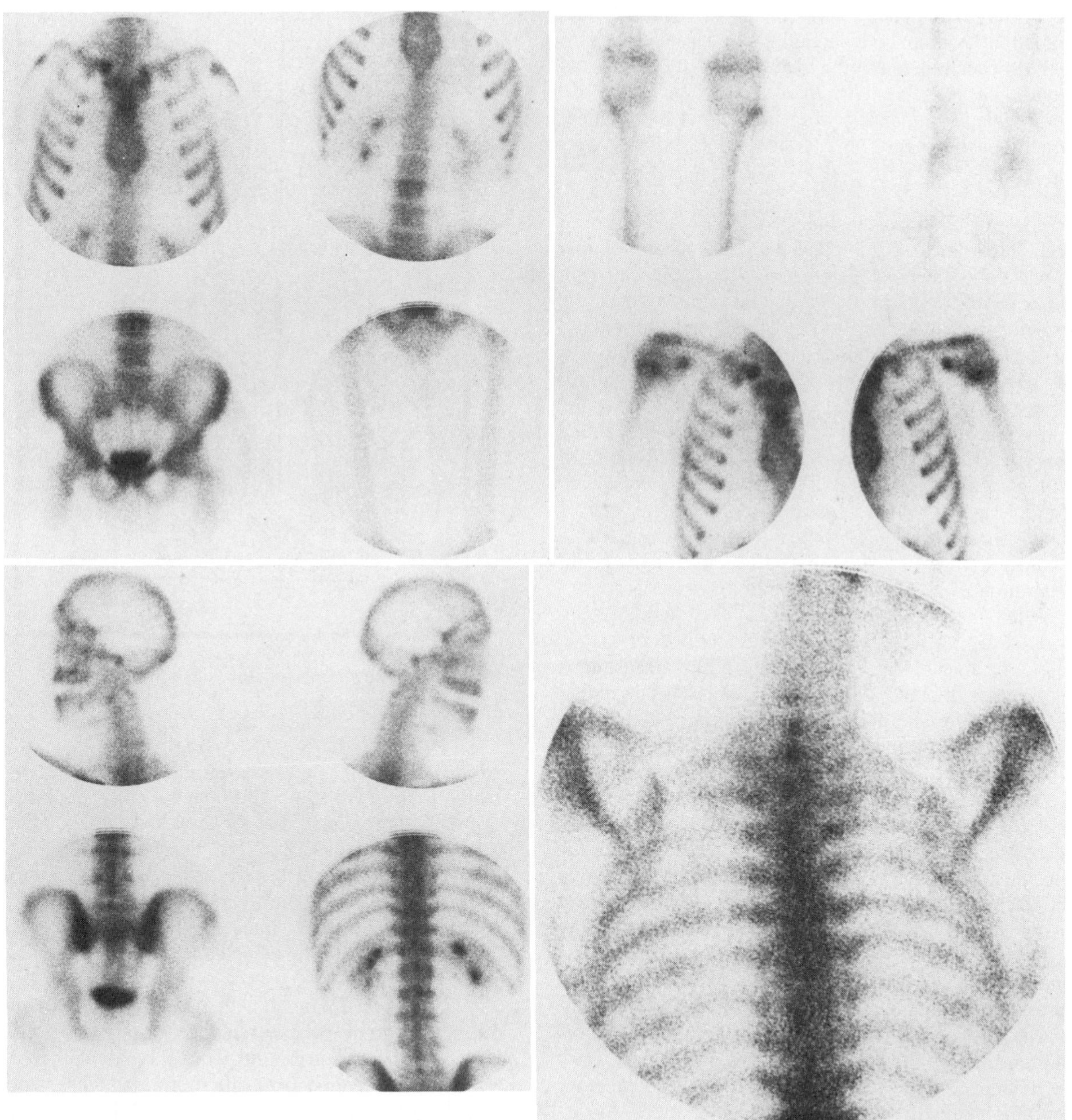

Fig. 14-23. Thirteen images necessary to cover whole body with large-crystal camera. Forearms and hands are still omitted with these images.

exposure is made until the ID in this region reaches a range of 2500 to 4000 counts. The time for this exposure is then used to obtain the other images.

Individual images of certain areas may be obtained with the scintillation camera after the initial image of the total skeleton on another type of instrument is performed. The spot films provide detailed images of areas that were not well visualized on the whole body–imaging instruments or provide additional views aiding in the determination for presence (or absence) of abnormality. A detailed view of the pelvis can be degraded by whole body–imaging devices because of activity accumulated in the bladder before the imaging device reaches the pelvis. Images of the pelvis should be obtained immediately after the patient has voided, which can be before or after the whole body image.

TOTAL BODY IMAGING

The production of an image of the total body area onto one film is accomplished by an accessory that moves either the camera detector or the patient through the camera field of view. As the body moves past the detector, the area seen by the camera is minified and advances across the film at a speed proportional to that of the patient. A standard-field-of-view camera will require two to three passes over the patient to cover the entire body width (Fig. 14-24). A large-crystal camera can cover the body in two passes or, when equipped with a special diverging collimator, in one pass. When multiple passes are required to produce the image, faint longitudinal lines appear on the image. This "zipper" (Fig. 14-25) is created because of the slight separation of each pass over the body.

When a scintillation camera is used with a total body–imaging accessory, a portion of the crystal is masked either electronically or by collimation into a rectangular field of view. It is essential that this region of the detector be proportional in its speed over the patient compared to the motion of the minified image area that moves across the cathode-ray tube.

One determines the technique for establishing imaging parameters by monitoring of the count rate or information density from the patient. A region for measuring the count rate is usually selected anteriorly over the chest or posteriorly over the spine. The same scan speed should be used for both the anterior and the posterior images. The scan speed is determined by one of several techniques. Most camera manufacturers supply a table, chart, or nomogram for determining the proper scan speed, based on the desired information density in the image and the count rate from the patient. Some systems may have a microcomputer for automatically calculating the scan speed, determined from monitoring the count rate from the patient. All these methods are basically the same, but some additional variations from the manufacturer's method may give improved image quality.

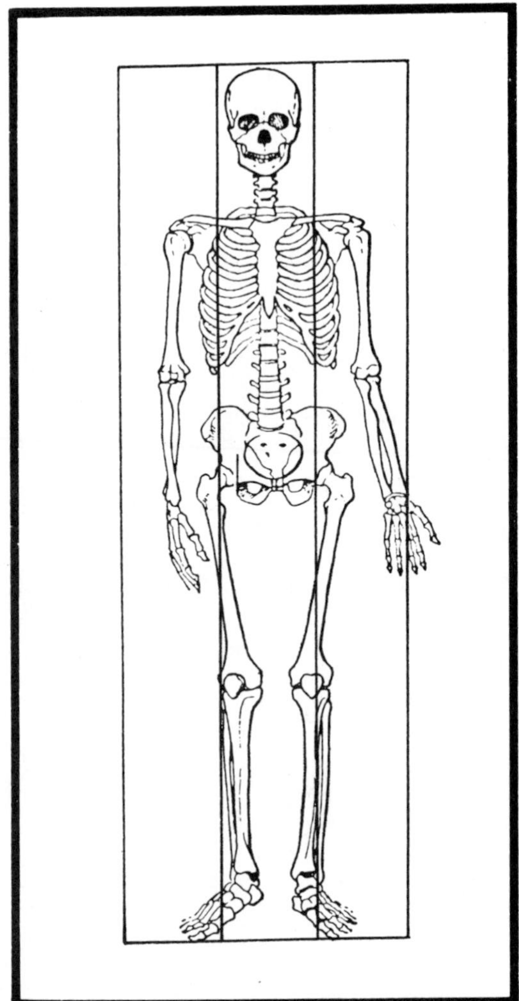

Fig. 14-24. View necessary for imaging whole body in three scans.

It is recommended that the total body image include greater than 1 million counts. The best positioning of the patient is to have the detector under the table and have the patient lie prone and supine to produce the anterior and posterior images respectively. By using this technique, the detector can be nearer the patient during imaging.

Whole body imaging with the scintillation camera provides a good esthetic relationship of overall radiopharmaceutical distribution with only a small loss in resolution generated from the motion synchronization of the table and the CRT recording. Patients are manipulated less and little effort is required of the technologist during the imaging procedure.

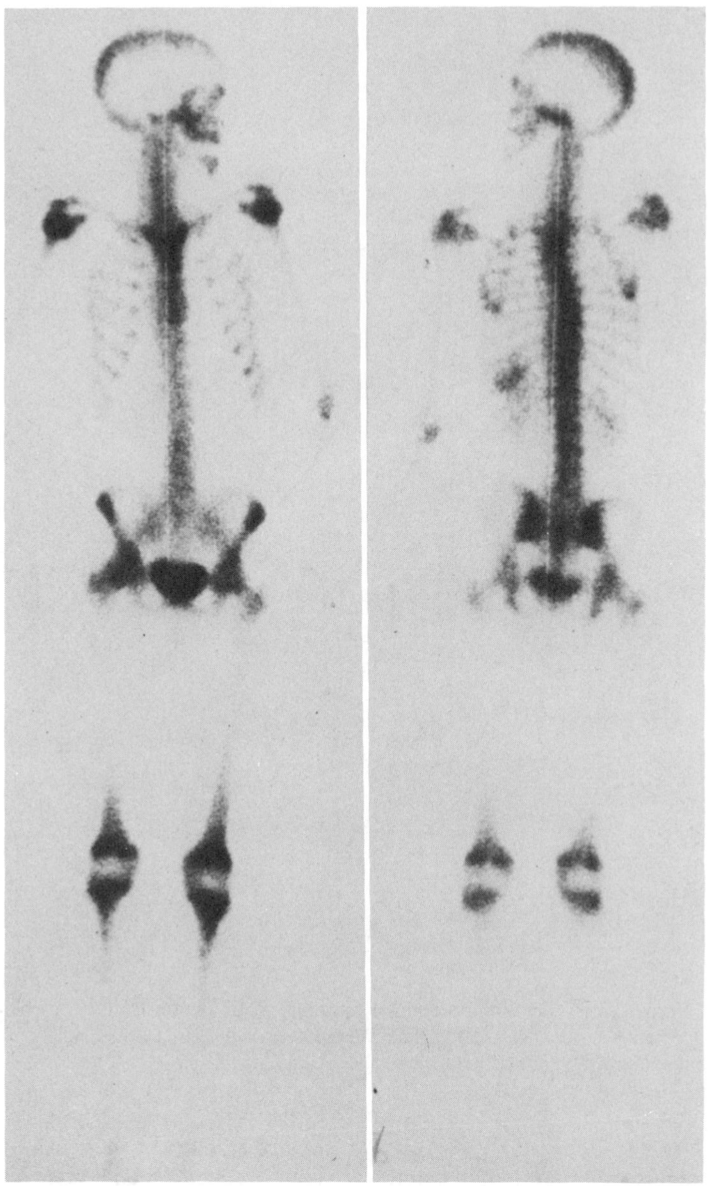

Fig. 14-25. Normal whole-body bone scan with large-crystal camera and moving table. Note "zipper" in center of both anterior and posterior images. Activity in shoulder and knee areas relate to epiphyseal growth still occurring.

Three other types of instrumentation may also be used to produce total body images. The rectilinear scanner may be used, but its resolution leaves a great deal to be desired. Another device, the multiplane longitudinal tomographic scanner, provides a unique visualization of the skeletal system. This device (as described in the instrumentation chapter) can produce 12 image slices through the body from a single scan. These images may be of additional diagnostic value when one is evaluating the extent of bone involvement in disease states. An example of a tomographic scan is shown in Fig. 14-26. A third device, a multidetector hybrid scanner, utilizes 10 crystals per detector head. This device has proved to be useful in whole body bone imaging and provides excellent images in a relatively short period of time (approximately two times faster than a camera and three times faster than a rectilinear scanner).

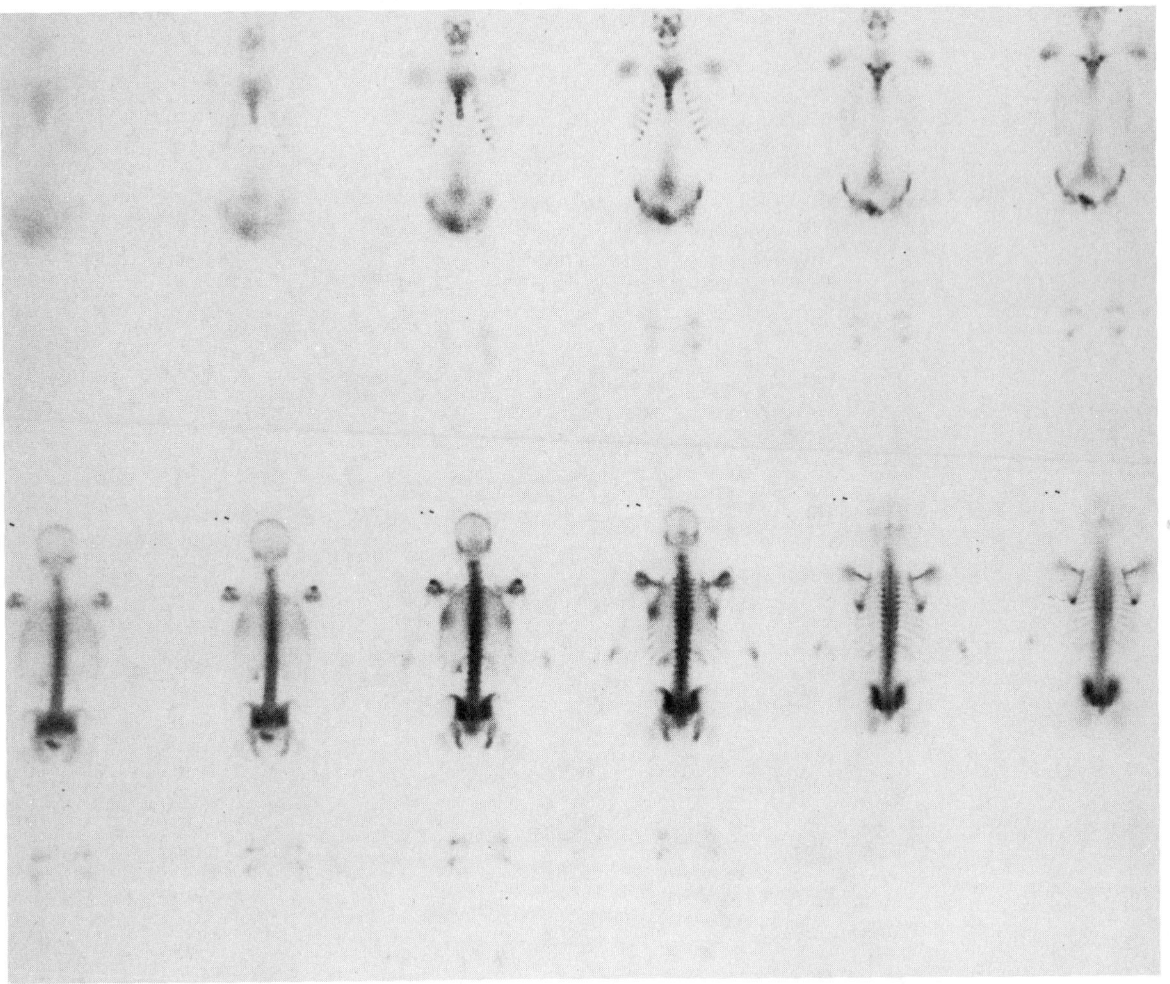

Fig. 14-26. Normal multiplane longitudinal tomography scan demonstrating 12 images, with most anterior image being in upper left corner and most posterior image in lower right corner. (Courtesy Toussant Battison and Dr. Philip Frederick, Salt Lake City, Utah.)

CLINICAL ASPECTS

The skeleton is a complex organ system subjected to many different types of adversities. Bone disease can be generally classified into two broad categories, congenital and acquired. Of the congenital bone diseases, radionuclide imaging has essentially no role, since most of the diseases have characteristic radiographic appearances. Radionuclide bone imaging, however, is important in the evaluation of several acquired bone diseases. The acquired bone diseases can be classified as traumatic, neoplastic, inflammatory, metabolic, degenerative, vascular, and other bone diseases not fitting into these listed categories.

The localization of the bone-seeking radiopharmaceuticals is mainly dependent on two factors: bone blood flow and bone production. The relative importance of each of these parameters is not well defined, but frequently both are increased. Increased radiopharmaceutical deposition accompanying increased bone production is well exemplified by the epiphyseal growth plate in bone imaging in children (Fig. 14-25). Occasionally an abnormality will be detected as a focal area of decreased pharmaceutical accumulation (Fig. 14-27). This decreased accumulation may be related to impaired blood flow or to complete destruction or replacement of bone by tumor, inflammatory mass, or radiation.

The indications for bone imaging are listed below:

1. Staging of malignant disease
   a. Screening of high-risk patients
   b. Localization of biopsy sites
2. Evaluation of primary bone neoplasms

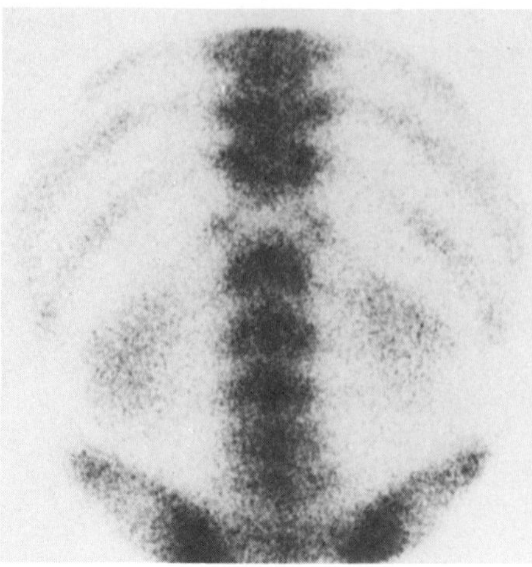

Fig. 14-27. Absent accumulation of radiopharmaceutical in vertebral body.

3. Diagnosis of early skeletal inflammatory disease
4. Evaluation of skeletal pain of undetermined etiology
5. Evaluation of elevated alkaline phosphase of undetermined etiology
6. Determination of bone viability
7. Evaluation of painful total joint prostheses

The most frequent reason for ordering a bone scan is staging of malignant disease by determining if spread to bone has occurred. The other indications are used less frequently, but they are important reasons for bone imaging.

Anterior and posterior images of the whole body are generally obtained (Fig. 14-23). The anterior skull, facial bones, mandible, clavicle, sternum, anterior ribs, anterior iliac spine, and pubic rami are best visualized on the anterior images. The posterior skull, spine, posterior ribs, scapulae, sacroiliac joints, and ischia are best visualized on the posterior images. Shoulders, hips, and extremities are commonly seen well on both views, primarily dependent on patient positioning.[12] The activity within the skeleton is usually symmetric from side to side. However, some asymmetry may be seen in the skull, shoulders, sternoclavicular joints, and anterior ends of the ribs without a pathologic condition present.[48] The activity within the kidneys is variable. With ^{99m}Tc-MDP, the kidney activity is usually less than the surrounding bone activity. Kidney disease may be associated with pronounced asymmetry of renal activity, a focal area of absent activity (cyst or tumor), or ureteral visualization suggesting ureteral obstruction.[8,31]

In most institutions, radionuclide bone imaging has replaced the radiographic skeletal survey for the evaluation of skeletal metastatic disease. Metastases to bone are common in several primary malignancies including lung, breast, and prostate carcinomas. Metastases to the spine are difficult to detect radiographically, since loss of approximately 50% of the mineral content of the bone must occur before lytic lesions are detected.[14] Whereas 10% to 40% of the adult patients with metastatic bone disease and an abnormal bone scan may have normal radiographs, less than 5% of bone scans are negative when the radiograph demonstrates metastatic disease.[27,42] In the pediatric population one study has demonstrated 68% of metastases are identified by radionuclide imaging alone.[21] False-negative scans have been related to several factors. If the skeleton is diffusely involved with metastatic disease, the focal nature of the lesions may not be apparent.[15] The diffusely abnormal scan may be difficult to differentiate from the normal scan, but with quality images from the scintillation camera, irregularities of radiopharmaceutical deposition can generally be noted. Metastatic lesions may have no associated osteoblastic activity and thus may not be detected by bone scan or may be detected as a photon-deficient area.[22] An example of a disease in which the lesions may not produce an abnormality on the bone scan is multiple myeloma, which has a high false-negative rate. After the bone images are performed, radiographs of the abnormal areas are often recommended for a more definitive diagnosis and to exclude other etiologies of an abnormal scan in the patient with suspected metastatic disease.

The usual pattern of skeletal metastatic disease is multiple focal lesions throughout the skeleton with the greatest involvement generally in the axial skeleton[24,26] (Figs. 14-28 and 14-29). The area of abnormal radiopharmaceutical deposition represents the edge of the metastatic deposit where osteoblastic repair is attempted. However, a few bone-producing metastatic lesions do occur, such as those attributable to osteogenic sarcoma (Fig. 14-30). Accumulation of the agent in soft-tissue metastases may prove helpful in detecting extraskeletal involvement.[39]

The malignancies in which bone imaging has demonstrated importance for the staging of the disease are breast, lung, and prostatic carcinomas.[26,32,38] These are common malignancies with a high incidence of bony metastatic disease. Other malignancies are now being evaluated with bone imaging, and a higher incidence of bony metastases is being found than previously suspected. Therefore, most patients with malignancies now have a bone scan as part of their evaluation.

Bone scanning is also used for the evaluation of primary bone neoplasms. Usually the patient has already had radiographs of the primary tumor, and the bone

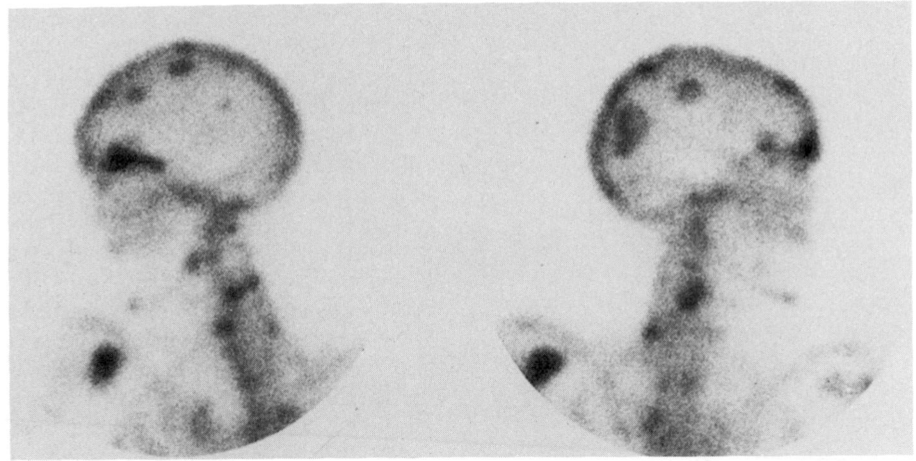

Fig. 14-28. Multiple metastases in bone of patient with breast carcinoma.

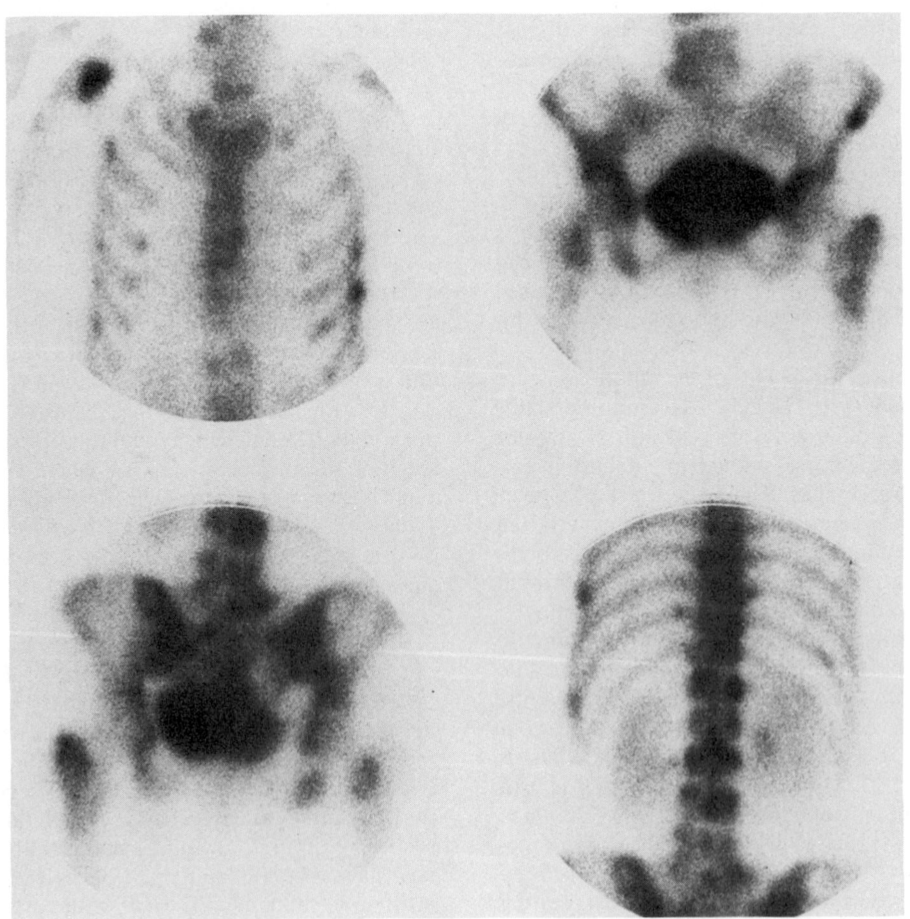

Fig. 14-29. Multiple focal lesions in bone of patient with breast carcinoma.

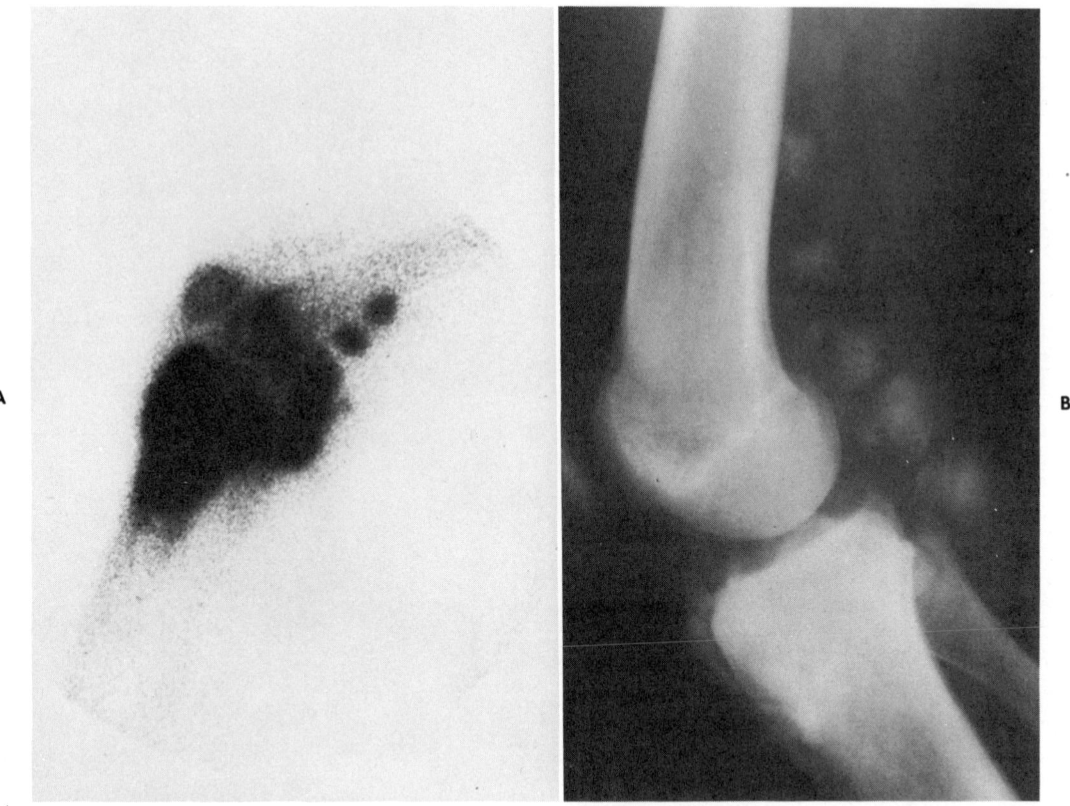

Fig. 14-30. Osteogenic sarcoma of proximal tibia. **A,** Lateral bone images reveals abnormal accumulation in proximal tibia with activity posterior to normal bone representing accumulation in lymph nodes. **B,** Lateral knee radiograph reveals destructive changes in proximal tibia and bone deposition in lymph nodes behind knee.

scan does offer no additional information of that area. The extent of the abnormality on the bone scan is generally not much different from the radiographically apparent lesion. The value of bone scanning in patients with primary bone malignancy lies in the detection of the disease elsewhere.[21] As many as 30% of the patients with Ewing's sarcoma may have lesions in other bones, a finding that significantly alters the therapy of the disease.[7,21,49] Metastatic deposits in soft tissue from osteogenic sarcoma can be detected by scan prior to the appearance of radiographic abnormalities.[39]

In addition to being used in the evaluation of malignant disease involving the skeleton, radionuclide bone imaging is used in the evaluation of several other nonmalignant processes. Bone imaging has been demonstrated to be useful in the evaluation of patients with suspected osteomyelitis.[18,29,40,50] The bone scan may be positive within 24 hours after the onset of symptoms, whereas the radiographic changes are not apparent for 10 to 14 days. Early blood-pool images of the area of interest are important in the evaluation of possible inflammatory bone disease (Fig. 14-31). With cellulitis, there may be increased blood-pool activity diffusely throughout the area of involvement, as well as some diffusely increased activity on the regular bone images obtained 2 to 3 hours after injection. Osteomyelitis, however, will demonstrate focally increased activity in the involved bone on both the blood-pool and routine images (Fig. 14-31). Since the use of bone imaging for detecting osteomyelitis, it has been found that several patients do not subsequently develop the typical radiographic changes because the early treatment prevents the development of radiographic abnormalities.

In some instances trauma is being evaluated with bone scanning.[37] Immediately after a fracture, for the first day or two, there may be decreased activity visualized at the site. After day 3, there is generally diffusely increased activity in the area of fracture, which becomes focally increased by day 10. Depending on angulation of fracture, stress, and so forth,

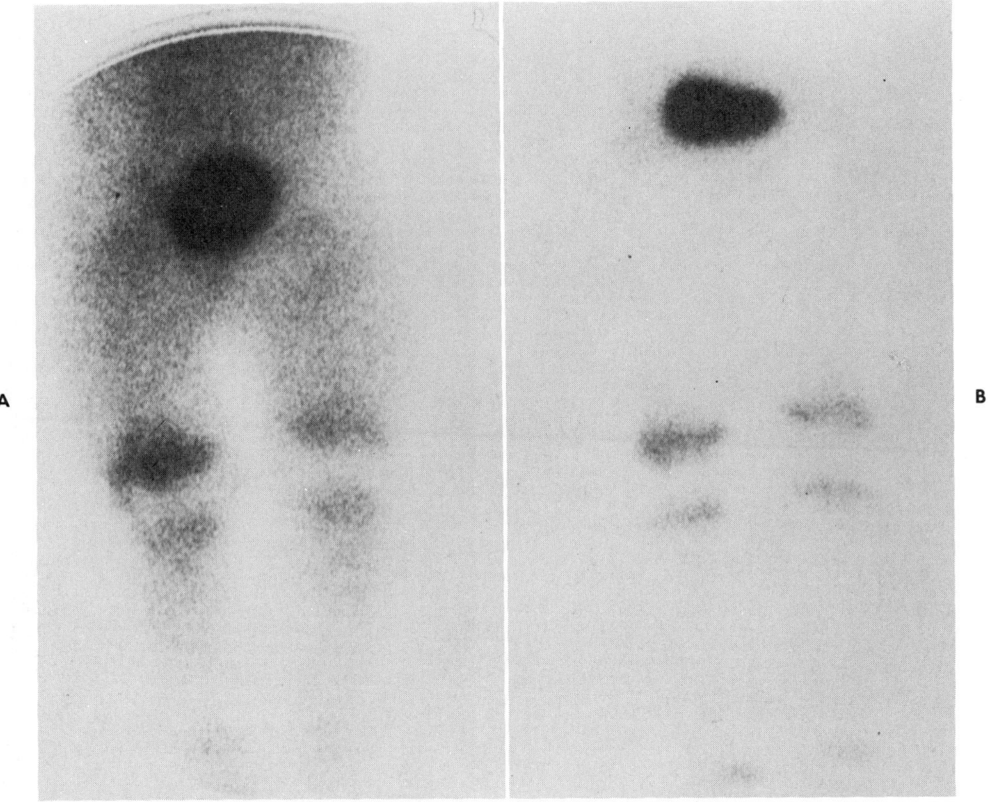

Fig. 14-31. Osteomyelitis of right distal femur. **A,** Blood-pool image reveals abnormal accumulation in right distal femur. **B,** Bone image 2½ hours after injection demonstrates only slight increase in activity in right distal femur.

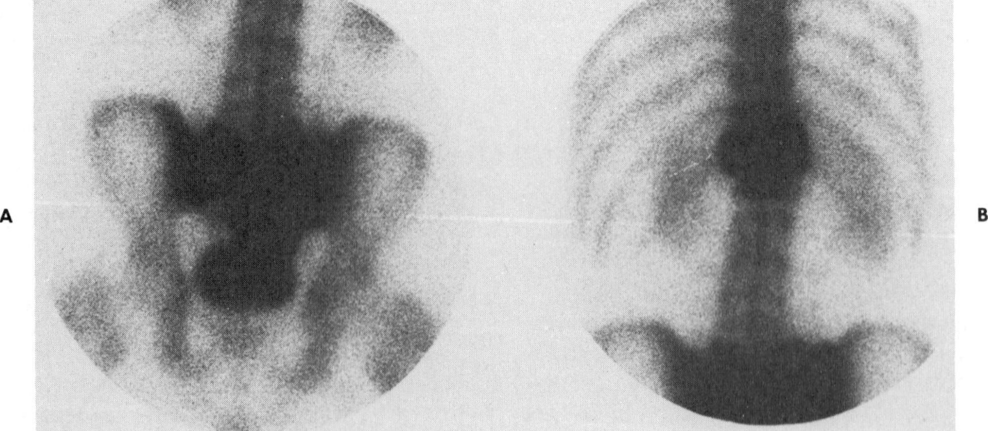

Fig. 14-32. Paget's disease. **A,** Bone images of posterior pelvis demonstrates abnormal accumulation in entire sacrum. **B,** Image of lower thoracic and lumbar spine demonstrates abnormal accumulation in entire twelfth thoracic and first lumbar vertebral bodies.

the activity decreases with time but may remain abnormal for years if the fracture is complicated and bone remodeling continues. The bone scan has been used to evaluate patients with normal radiographs suspected of having fractures. Some of these patients will have normal radiographs at the time the bone images will be abnormal.

Radionuclide bone imaging is also used in several other conditions. Paget's disease is associated with greatly abnormal radiopharmaceutical accumulation typically involving the greater part of a bone[1,41] (Fig. 14-32). The bone scan has been used to evaluate therapy of this disease.[1] The determination of the cause of pain after a total joint replacement is frequently difficult. Radionuclide imaging has been demonstrated to be a sensitive method of detecting a complication, such as loosening or infection of the prosthetic implant[19] (Figs. 14-33 and 14-34). Radionuclide imaging is also very sensitive for the detection of osteoid osteomas, a cause of skeletal pain that may be undetected for years.[30]

Joint imaging

Radionuclide imaging of the joints has been used in several institutions for the evaluation of inflammatory joint disease.[5,13,28,32-34,46,47] This imaging has been performed with either ^{99m}Tc-pertechnetate or ^{99m}Tc-phosphate compounds. The ^{99m}Tc-pertechnetate images are obtained immediately after injection of the radiopharmaceutical and abnormal accumulation is noted in

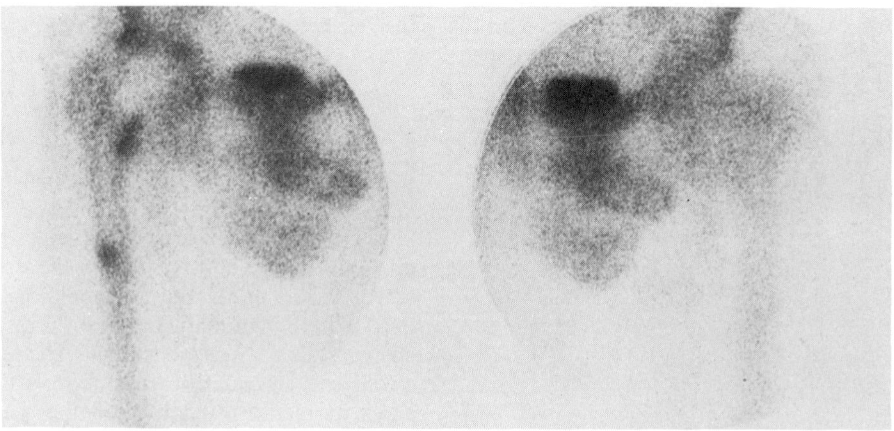

Fig. 14-33. Loosened total hip prosthesis. Focal areas of abnormal accumulation in right femur *(right)*, lesser trochanter, and tip of prosthesis are typical for loosening.

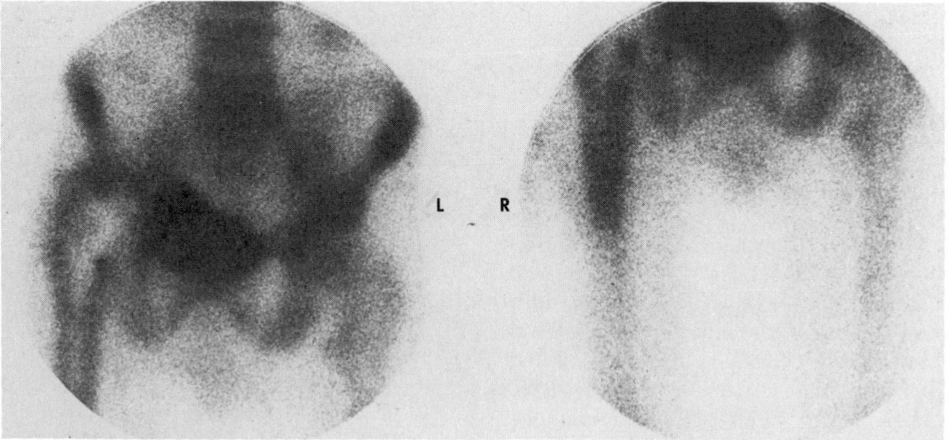

Fig. 14-34. Infected total hip prosthesis. Diffusely abnormal accumulation around entire prosthesis in right hip is characteristic of infected implant.

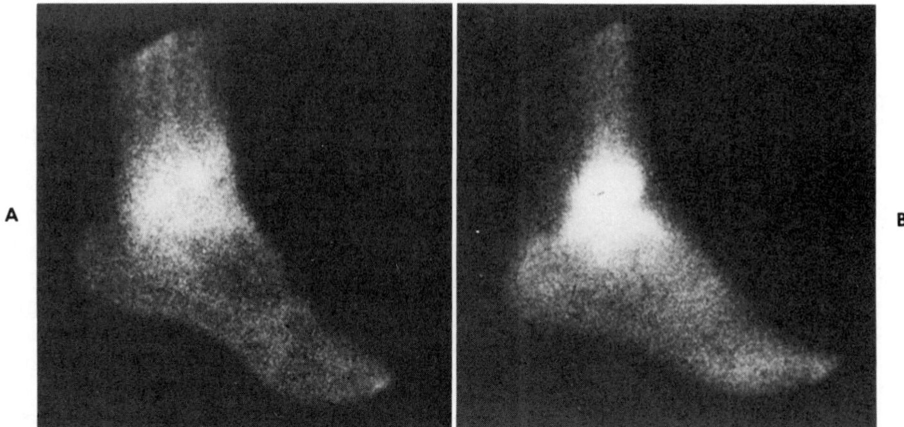

Fig. 14-35. Septic arthritis of tibiotalar joint. **A,** Blood-pool image obtained after administration of ^{99m}Tc-methylenediphosphonate (^{99m}Tc-MDP) demonstrates abnormal accumulation in ankle-joint area. **B,** Routine image obtained 2½ hours later demonstrates focal accumulation in the distal tibia and talus. Joint was aspirated, and aspirate grew pathogenic organisms. Radiographs revealed no joint abnormality.

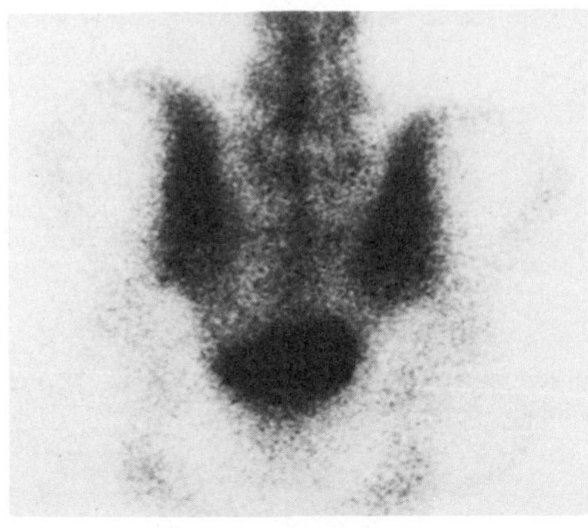

Fig. 14-36. Sacroileitis. Posterior pelvis image in patient with low back pain. Quantification revealed ratio of activity in sacroiliac area to midsacrum to be greater than 2, with normal being less than 1.5

areas of increased blood flow as found in synovitis. The ^{99m}Tc-phosphate compounds localize in areas of joint inflammation, since there is an increased turnover rate and vascularity of the adjacent bone as well as increased synovial vascularity (Fig. 14-35). Either of these radiopharmaceuticals can be used to detect early joint inflammation, often before radiographic abnormalities occur. When compared with physical examination, radiographs and arthrography, joint imaging with the ^{99m}Tc-phosphate complex is the most sensitive indicator of early degenerative disease of the knee.[47]

Several recent studies have demonstrated the utility of ^{99m}Tc-phosphate imaging in the early detection of sacroiliac inflammatory disease[13] (Fig. 14-36). Detection of the inflammatory process prior to radiographic changes has been demonstrated. The technique utilizes a computer to quantify areas of bone activity and compares the activity in the sacroiliac joint region to an area of equal size in the midsacrum.

Gallium-67 imaging in inflammatory bone and joint disease

Several studies have recently demonstrated the value of gallium-67 citrate scanning in patients with inflammatory bone and joint disease.[23,28-30] Some patients with osteomyelitis or septic arthritis may have normal ^{99m}Tc-phosphate complex images but abnormal ^{67}Ga images. Therefore, in a patient with suspected osteomyelitis or septic arthritis and a negative bone scan, a gallium scan is recommended.

REFERENCES

1. Altman, R. D., Johnston, C. C., Khairi, M. R. A., Wellman, H., Serafini, A. N. and Sanhey, R. R.: Influence of disodium etedronate on clinical and laboratory manifestations of Paget's disease of bone (osteitis deformans), N. Engl. J. Med. **28:**1379, 1973.
2. Anderson, J., Emery, E. W., McAlister, J. M., and Osborn, S. B.: The metabolism of a therapeutic dose of calcium-45 in a case of multiple myeloma, Clin. Sci. Mol. Med. **15:**567, 1956.
3. Bayer, G. C. H., and Wendeberg, B.: External counting of

Ca-47 and Sr-85 in studies of localized skeletal lesions in man, J. Bone Joint Surg. **41B:**558, 1959.

4. Belchier, J.: An account of the bones of the animals being changed to a red color by aliment only. In Bauer, G. C. H., editor: Tracer techniques for the study of bone metabolism in man, Adv. Biol. Med. Phys. **10:**228, 1965.
5. Bekerman, C., Genant, H. K., Hoffer, P. B., Kozin, F., and Ginsberg, M.: Radionuclide imaging of the bones and joints of the hand, Radiology **118:**653, 1975.
6. Bernier, D. R., and Coleman, R. E.: Impact of computed cranial tomography on radionuclide imaging and cisternography, J. Nucl. Med. Technol. **4:**180, 1976.
7. Bhansali, S. K., and Desai, P. B.: Ewing's sarcoma. Observations in 107 cases, J. Bone Joint Surg. **45A:**541, 1963.
8. Biello, D., Coleman, R. E., and Stanley, R. J.: Correlation of renal images on bone scan and intravenous pyelogram, Am. J. Roentgenol. Radium Ther. Nucl. Med. **127:**633, 1976.
9. Blau, M., Nagler, W., and Bender, M. A.: Fluorine 18: a new isotope for bone scanning, J. Nucl. Med. **3:**332, 1962.
10. Charkes, N. D., and Philips, C. M.: A new model of ^{18}F-fluoride kinetics in humans. In Medical radionuclide imaging, vol. 2, Vienna, 1977, International Atomic Energy Agency, p. 137.
11. Charkes, N. D., and Sklaroff, D. M.: Early diagnosis of metastatic bone cancer by photoscanning with strontium-85, J. Nucl. Med. **5:**168, 1964.
12. Charkes, N. D., Valentine, G., and Cravitz, B.: Interpretation of the normal ^{99m}Tc polyphosphate rectilinear bone scan, Radiology **107:**563, 1973.
13. Davis, P., Thomson, A. B. R., and Lentle, B. C.: Quantitative sacroiliac scintigraphy in patients with Crohn's disease, Arthritis Rheum. **21:**234, 1978.
14. Edelstyn, G. A., Gillespie, P. J., and Grebbel, F. S.: The radiological demonstration of osseous metastases: experimental observations, Clin. Radiol. **18:**158, 1967.
15. Frankel, R. S., Johnson, K. W., Mabry, J. J., and Johnston, G. S.: "Normal" bone radionuclide image with diffuse skeletal lymphoma, Radiology **111:**365, 1974.
16. Galasko, C. S. B.: The detection of skeletal metastases for mammary cancer by gamma camera scintigraphy, Br. J. Surg. **56:**757, 1969.
17. Galasko, C. S. B.: The mechanisms of uptake of bone-seeking isotopes by skeletal metastases. In Medical radionuclide imaging, vol. 2, Vienna, 1977, International Atomic Energy Agency, p. 125.
18. Gelfand, M. J., and Silberstein, E. B.: Radionuclide imaging. Use in diagnosis of osteomyelitis in children, J.A.M.A. **237:**245, 1977.
19. Gelman, M. I., Coleman, R. E., Stevens, P. M., and Davey, B. W.: Radiography, radionuclide imaging, and arthrography in the evaluation of total hip and knee replacement, Radiology **128:**467, 1978.
20. Gerber, F. H., Goodreau, J. J., Kirchner, P. T., and Fouty, W. J.: Efficacy of preoperative and postoperative bone scanning in the management of breast carcinoma, N. Engl. J. Med. **297:**300, 1977.
21. Gilday, D. L., Ash, J. M., and Reilly, B. J.: Radionuclide skeletal survey for pediatric neoplasms, Radiology **123:**399, 1977.
22. Goergen, T. G., Alazraki, N. P., Halpern, S. E., Heath, V., and Ashburn, W. L.: "Cold" bone lesions: a newly recognized phenomenon of bone imaging, J. Nucl. Med. **12:**1120, 1974.
23. Handmaker, H., and Giammona, S. T.: The "hot joint"—increased diagnostic accuracy using combined ^{99m}Tc phosphate and ^{67}Ca citrate imaging in pediatrics, J. Nucl. Med. **17:**554, 1976.
24. Hart, G., Hoerr, S. O., and Hughes, C. P.: Detection of bone metastases from breast cancer: an accurate, four film roentgenographic survey, Cleve. Clin. Q. **38:**1, 1971.
25. Jones, A. G., Francis, M. D., and Davis, M. A.: Bone scanning: radionuclide reaction mechanisms, Semin. Nucl. Med. **6:**1, 1976.
26. Krishnamurthy, G. T., Tubis, M., Hiss, J., and Blahd, W. H.: Distribution pattern of metastatic bone disease—a need for total body skeletal image, J.A.M.A. **237:**2504, 1977.
27. Legge, D. A., Tauxe, W. N., Pugh, D. G., and Utz, P. C.: Radioisotope scanning of metastatic lesions of bone, Mayo Clin. Proc. **45:**755, 1970.
28. Lisbona, R., and Rosenthall, L.: Radionuclide imaging of septic joints and their differentiation from periarticular osteomyelitis and cellulitis in pediatrics, Clin. Nucl. Med. **2:**337, 1977.
29. Lisbona, R., and Rosenthall, L.: Observations on the sequential use of ^{99m}Tc-phosphate complex and ^{67}Ga imaging in osteomyelitis, cellulitis and septic arthritis, Radiology **123:**123, 1977.
30. Lisbona, R., and Rosenthall, L.: Role of radionuclide imaging in osteoid osteoma, Am. J. Roentgenol. Radium Ther. Nucl. Med. **132:**77, 1979.
31. Maher, F. T.: Evaluation of renal and urinary tract abnormalities noted on scintiscans, Mayo Clin. Proc. **50:**370, 1975.
32. Merrick, M. V.: Review article—bone scanning, Br. J. Radiol. **48:**327, 1975.
33. Namey, T. C., and Rosenthall, L.: Periarticular uptake of ^{99m}technetium diphosphonate in psoriatics, Arthritis Rheum. **19:**607, 1976.
34. Park, H. M., Terman, S. A., Ridolfo, A. S., and Wellman, H. N.: A quantitative evaluation of rheumatoid arthritic activity with Tc-99m HEDP, J. Nucl. Med. **18:**973, 1977.
35. Pecher, C.: Biological investigations with radioactive calcium and strontium, Proc. Soc. Exp. Biol. Med. **46:**86, 1941.
36. Rasmussen, H.: Parathyroid hormone, calcitonin and calciferols. In Williams, R. H., editor: Textbook of endocrinology, ed. 5, Philadelphia, 1974, W. B. Saunders Co.
37. Rosenthall, L., Hill, R. O., and Chuang, S.: Observation on the use of ^{99m}Tc-phosphate imaging in peripheral bone trauma, Radiology **119:**637, 1976.
38. Schaffer, D. L., and Pendergrass, H. P.: Comparison of enzyme, clinical, radiographic and radionuclide methods of detecting bone metastases from carcinoma of the prostate, Radiology **121:**431, 1976.
39. Schall, G. L., Zeiger, L., Primack, A., and DeLellis, R.: Uptake of ^{85}Sr by an osteosarcoma metastatic to lung, J. Nucl. Med. **12:**131, 1971.
40. Shirazi, P. H., Rayudu, G. V. S., and Fordham, E. W.: ^{18}F bone scanning: review of indications and results in 1500 cases, Radiology **112:**361, 1974.
41. Shirazi, P. H., Rayudu, G. V. S., Ryan, W. G., and Fordham, E. W.: Paget's disease of bone. Bone scanning experience with 80 cases, J. Nucl. Med. **14:**450, 1973.
42. Sklaroff, D. M., and Charkes, D. N.: Diagnosis of bone metastasis by photoscanning with strontium 85, J.A.M.A. **188:**1, 1964.
43. Spencer, R., Herbert, R., Rish, M. W., and Little, W. A.: Bone scanning with ^{85}Sr and ^{18}F. Physical and radiopharmaceutical considerations and clinical experience in 50 cases, Br. J. Radiol. **40:**641, 1967.
44. Subramanian, G., and McAfee, J. F.: A new complex of ^{99m}Tc for skeletal imaging, Radiology **99:**192, 1971.
45. Subramanian, G., McAfee, J. G., Blair, R. J., and Thomas, F. D.: Radiopharmaceuticals for bone and bone-marrow imaging. In Medical radionuclide imaging, vol. 2, Vienna, 1977, International Atomic Energy Agency, p. 83.
46. Sy, W. M., Bay, R., and Camera, A.: Hand images: normal and abnormal, J. Nucl. Med. **18:**419, 1977.

47. Thomas, R. H., Resnick, D., Alazraki, N. P., Daniel, D., and Greenfield, R.: Compartmental evaluation of osteoarthritis of the knee—comparative study of available diagnostic modalities, Radiology **116:**585, 1975.
48. Thrall, J. H., Ghaed, N., Geslien, G. E., Pinsky, S. M., and Johnson, M. C.: Pitfalls in Tc^{99m} polyphosphate skeletal imaging. Am. J. Roentgenol. Radium Ther. Nucl. Med. **121:**739, 1974.
49. Wang, C. C., and Schulz, M. D.: Ewing's sarcoma—a study of 50 cases treated at the Massachusetts General Hospital, 1930-1952 inclusive, N. Engl. J. Med. **284:**571, 1953.
50. Waxman, A. D., Bryan, D., and Siemsen, J. K.: Bone scanning in the drug abuse patient: early detection of hematogenous osteomyelitis, J. Nucl. Med. **14:**647, 1973.

Chapter 15

THE HEMATOPOIETIC SYSTEM

James K. Langan and Patricia A. McIntyre

Circulating blood is an extraordinary complex mixture. Some of the representative components are listed in Table 15-1. When blood is collected with an anticoagulant (a substance that prevents normal clotting), the whole blood divides into a plasma compartment and a cellular compartment. If it is collected without an anticoagulant, the fluid that can be separated from the clot is known as serum. The clot contains most of the cellular elements as well as the proteins consumed in the coagulation process. It is important to recognize this fundamental difference between the two terms "plasma" and "serum." Many of the anticoagulants routinely used by hematologists are not applicable to nuclear hematologic studies because they prevent clotting by chelating calcium (a requirement for normal clotting) and other heavy ions such as tracer iron, which is used in some of our procedures.

The relative numbers of the basic cellular types present in circulating blood are listed in the lower portion of Table 15-1. One rarely measures the number of red blood cells in a given volume of blood to assess whether a patient has anemia unless it is included with the information routinely printed out by an automated electronic particle counter. A much simpler and far more reliable method is to prepare a hematocrit. This is done when one places a well-mixed sample of anticoagulated blood in a suitable tube and centrifuges it for an appropriate period of time and *g* force (multiples of gravity) to separate the cellular elements from the plasma phase. When hematocrits are performed on normal blood, the red cells comprise the majority of the volume of packed cells seen (Fig. 15-1, *A*). This is attributable to their relatively great number and size. The layer just above the red cells, which is slightly grayish in color, is the white cell population in that sample of blood; just above this is an even more minute layer of creamy-colored cells representing the platelets. Because of their smaller number and, in the case of platelets, their minute size, the hematocrit cannot be relied upon to measure the quantity of these cells, and they must be counted separately, preferably with an electronic particle counter. In contrast, Fig. 15-1, *B*, shows the blood of a patient who had a basic hematologic abnormality and the overwhelming majority of packed cells is made up of platelets and white cells, with the lower portion being a poorly separated mixture of white cells and red cells. If one gave only a casual glance at this hematocrit, especially if it were done as a routine in a microcapillary tube, one could easily make the serious error of overlooking the severe degree of anemia and greatly abnormal increase in white cells and platelets present.

Table 15-1. Representative components of blood (not all-inclusive)

1. Plasma compartment
   a. Water
   b. Simple solutes, such as Na^+, K^+, Cl^-, Mg^{++}, Ca^{++}, HCO_3^-, and sugar
   c. Proteins
      (1) Albumin
      (2) Immunoglobulins, such as gamma globulin (IgG) and macroglobulins (IgM)
      (3) Transport proteins, such as transferrin, transcobalamin I, and transcobalamin II
      (4) Lipoproteins (and other lipids)
      (5) Precursors and active components of the complex coagulation-fibrinolysis system
2. Cellular compartment
   a. Erythrocytes (red blood cells, RBC), about $5 \times 10^6/mm^3$
   b. Leukocytes (white blood cells, WBC), about $5 \times 10^3/mm^3$
      (1) Granulocytes
      (2) Lymphocytes
      (3) Monocytes
      (4) Plasma cells and fragments of, or whole, megakaryocytes—rarely present in routine preparations of peripheral blood for microscopic examination
   c. Platelets (thrombocytes), about 3.5×10^5 mm^3

There are two important things to remember about the interpretation of a hematocrit value: (1) It repre-

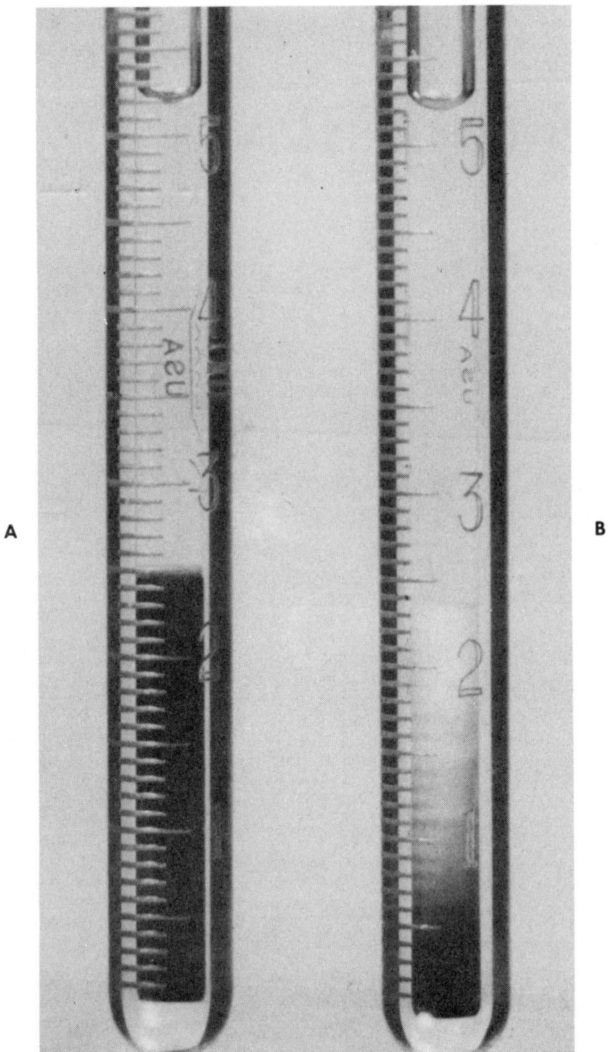

Fig. 15-1. Tube **A** contains normal blood sample and **B** a sample of blood from patient who has basic hematologic abnormality. Cellular elements have been separated from plasma by centrifugation.

sents merely a ratio between the plasma compartment and the cellular compartment of a given sample of blood. Accordingly, alterations (for example, dehydration) in the plasma compartment can make the hematocrit value seem falsely elevated. (2) A very careful examination of the hematocrit tube is necessary to make sure that one is indeed dealing with a normal red cell population in the packed cells and not a preponderance of white cells or platelets. Should the latter condition prevail and be unrecognized, tracer-labeling studies will give false and misleading results. One should use a hand-held magnifying glass or the magnifier supplied with the reading equipment when using the microhematocrit tubes.

In Table 15-2 we have summarized some of the important features of the cellular elements of the blood. Since most clinical nuclear medicine laboratories at the present time are doing only cellular labeling studies of the erythrocytes, this chapter deals solely with those tests that deal directly, or indirectly, with the mature red blood cells and factors that may influence their production.

These mature circulating red blood cells (RBC) are critical to the survival and proper function of each cell

Table 15-2. Circulating cellular elements: origin, function, approximate life-span

	Erythrocytes	Granulocytes	Monocytes	Platelets	Lymphocytes	Plasma cells
Tissue of origin in normal adults	"Red" (hematopoietically active) marrow	Same	Same; circulating through blood to become the tissue macrophages	Same	Same	Some if not all are derived from immunologically stimulated lymphocytes
Earliest recognizable precursor cell in the bone marrow	Proerythroblast	Myeloblast	Promonocyte	Megakaryocyte	Certain small marrow "lymphocytes" are morphologically indistinguishable from "pluripotential" stem cells; however, other evidence suggests that lymphocytes are not derived from same stem cell as are the erythrocytes, granulocytes, and platelets	
Function of mature cell	Oxygen transport to tissues	Phagocytosis	Phagocytosis; processing of antigens	Vital components of normal coagulation process	After release from marrow they differentiate into (1) B lymphocytes (precursors of plasma cells) with production of circulating humeral antibody, and (2) T lymphocytes (participants in cellular immunity)	Produces humeral antibody specifically directed against antigen to which they are exposed
Life-span	90 to 110 days	50% to 60% of mature granulocytes in blood are adhering to vascular endothelium, the so-called marginal pool (MGP), and are freely exchangable with those circulating (GP). Their $T_{\frac{1}{2}}$ in blood is 6 to 7 hours. They may survive up to 5 days after migration into tissues	Experimental data less firm but probably very similar to data for granulocytes in blood; once they enter and are converted to tissue, macrophages may survive months to years	8 to 10 days	B lymphocyte—unknown T lymphocyte—long lived; continue to recirculate	Highly variable; some may persist for many months

within each tissue of the body because of their oxygen-transport function. They are able to live approximately 100 days, even though with each complete transit of the circulation they are shot out of the aorta during the left ventricular contraction at speeds that come close to those of a jet airliner and at the other extreme are required to weave slowly their way through the tiny, intricate openings in the splenic sinusoids, which are much smaller than the erythrocytes themselves. In their transit through the spleen, the erythrocytes actually are required to deform themselves, with only a tiny portion initially emerging through an opening and the rest of the erythrocyte being pulled slowly after it; after this they are still able to regain their normal biconcave shape and maintain their normal functions.

Their life of approximately 100 days has a profound implication; everyday the bone marrow must replace 1% of the total circulating mass of red blood cells that have died of old age. When one considers that the mean hematocrit is of the order of magnitude of 45 volumes percent of each milliliter of circulating blood and the total blood volume is of the order of magnitude of 5 liters, one can see that the normal bone marrow performs a most efficient assembly-line function to maintain homeostasis; the same is obviously true for the production by the marrow of all the other cellular elements of the blood. Furthermore, the normal marrow contains ''reserves'' of mature cells, which can be quickly released into the circulation when needed, and with continuing stress, the normal marrow can gradually increase its daily rate of production manyfold (up to eight times normal in the case of erythrocytes).

A complete listing of all known causes and types of anemia would require several pages of this textbook; however, the following list summarizes the basic mechanisms by which anemia may be caused:

General categories of causes of anemia

1. Excessive rate of removal from circulation
   a. Blood loss
   b. Hemolysis
2. Deficient production
   a. Lack of proper ''building blocks'', that is, iron, vitamin B_{12}, folic acid, and so on
   b. Suppression of marrow activity by a wide variety of acute and chronic diseases
   c. Primary disorders of the bone marrow

Obviously anemia can result either from an excess rate of removal of erythrocytes or from deficient production. Blood loss, be it chronic or acute, remains high on the list of causes of anemia. Accelerated destruction of the red blood cell within the patient's body is a process known as hemolysis and has the same end result as blood loss, provided that either occurs at a rate that exceeds the ability of the normal bone marrow to compensate. Deficient production can result from the lack of proper building blocks, suppression of marrow activity by a wide variety of acute and chronic diseases, or, least common of all, a primary disorder of the bone marrow. Iron-deficiency anemia, a simple and rapidly curable condition, remains the most common worldwide hematologic disorder. Vitamin B_{12} and folic acid are listed, not because they represent the only other ''building blocks'' of importance but because nuclear medicine can provide useful information regarding the differential diagnosis in patients presenting with manifestations of their deficiency.

Acute, self-limited, or rapidly cured disorders, such as the common cold or acute pneumonia, will cause temporary, essentially complete, cessation of marrow erythrocyte production. Since normal erythrocytes live approximately 100 days, such a short-term illness does not result in a recognizable degree of anemia. Certain patients who have a compensated hemolytic anemia (that is, a significantly shortened life-span of their erythrocytes but a very active marrow that is maintaining a normal hematocrit by its increased rate of erythrocyte production) may very rapidly develop a severe degree of anemia because of marrow suppression from such otherwise mild illnesses. In addition, there is a wide variety of chronic diseases (for example, rheumatoid arthritis and malignant disorders) that may cause chronic suppression of marrow activity and consequent anemia.

Last are the primary disorders of the bone marrow. It is often in these complex hematologic problems that the judicious choice of nuclear medicine procedures may give unique and valuable information that could not be gathered in any other fashion.

ISOTOPIC CELLULAR ELEMENTS

All isotopic labels of the cellular elements of the blood are of two general types: cohort or pulse labels and random labels. It is important to recognize the fundamental difference between the information to be gained by the use of each of them.

Cohort or pulse label. This type of label is only available to the marrow precursors of a given cell type for a specific and limited length of time; thus it will not label cells already circulating. Incorporation of this type of label in the marrow erythroid precursors results in the appearance in the circulation of mature labeled erythrocytes of the same age. An ideal cohort label that met all these necessary criteria and had the appropriate gamma-emitting nuclide would permit study of the rate of production of erythrocytes, their kinetics, longevity, manner of death, and ultimate disposal within the body. None of the currently available radioisotopes for cohort labeling of erythrocytes satisfies all these requirements. Indeed, with the exception of the iron isotopes, none are used in routine clinical studies.

Random label. Random labels are radiopharmaceuticals that are applied to erythrocytes circulating in the peripheral blood. This process labels all cells in the sample, that is, from the youngest to the oldest circulating erythrocytes or, as classically expressed, erythrocytes of "random" age; thus these are applicable only to the study of mean cell survival, or other direct measurements of the circulating erythrocytes, as described below.

Currently many laboratories have extensive research programs to provide us with clinically useful random labels for platelets and white blood cells. These have not yet been developed to the extent necessary to justify inclusion in this text. For readers interested in the best method (and inherent limitations) for ^{51}Cr-labeled platelet studies, the International Committee for Standardization in Hematology[4] has recently published a document dealing with this subject.

ERYTHROKINETICS

Measurement of circulating red blood cell mass

The determination of red blood cell mass and plasma volume is based on the simple radioisotope dilution technique.[5] For the measurement of the red blood cell mass, ^{51}Cr-labeled erythrocytes are most often used. Whole blood is collected by use of the appropriate anticoagulant in the correct ratio to the volume of whole blood. If ACD*-NIH solution A or Strumia's ACD solution is used, the ratio is 1:5. Because of the wide variance in the composition of the many CPD† solutions, now judged to be at least as good and in some instances preferable, it is imperative to consult the manufacturer's recommendation as to the proper ratio of whole blood to CPD. Heparin and EDTA are unsatisfactory for use in this procedure. There are several satisfactory methods, both for preparing the ^{51}Cr-labeled erythrocytes and for performing the necessary measurements. We describe in detail below the one we routinely use, but readers interested in other methods should refer to a publication of the International Panel on Diagnostic Applications of Radioisotopes in Haematology.[6] Chromium 51 is not an entirely ideal label for RBC mass measurements. Only 9% of its emissions are gamma rays, and so one must inject a substantially larger amount of radioactivity to obtain statistically significant counting rates compared to an isotope having 100% gamma emission. Furthermore, the relatively long half-life of ^{51}Cr (27.8 days), coupled with its relatively slow rate (1% per day) of removal from circulating erythrocytes, means that serial red blood cell volume measurements require undesirable increases in the amount of ^{51}Cr injected for each subsequent study. For these reasons, labeling of red blood cells with ^{99m}Tc and trace amounts of stannous ion is a useful alternate method for measurement of red blood cell mass,[10,11] and the tagging method has recently been significantly improved[13a] (Scheffel, Murrell, and McIntyre: unpublished confirmatory studies). Technetium 99m has a 6-hour half-life and for practical purposes can be considered a pure gamma-ray emitter. Therefore, physically it is nearly ideal for red blood cell mass measurements. It can be used in amounts that greatly reduce the radiation dose to patients that undergo serial red cell mass measurements. Because of the more rapid loss of the ^{99m}Tc label, however, ^{51}Cr-labeled erythrocytes should be used when sampling times for a single study must extend beyond 60 minutes after injection.

Chromium 51–ascorbic acid method for labeling erythrocytes (RBC). Ten milliliters of venous blood is withdrawn from the patient into a 20 ml syringe containing 2 ml of citric acid, sodium citrate, and dextrose (ACD)—Strumia's formula—and transferred into a sterile 20 ml Vacutainer. Thirty microcuries of chromium 51 in the form of chromate ion is added to the Vacutainer with a resultant prompt transport of chromium 51 across the erythrocyte membrane. After about 10 to 15 minutes of incubation, ascorbic acid (50 mg) is added to reduce the free chromate to chromic ion, which immediately stops the tagging procedure, as the chromic ion is unable to penetrate the erythrocyte membrane. Within the erythrocyte, the chromate ion is converted to chromic.

Exactly 5 ml of the labeled blood is drawn into a syringe and the remainder is kept to make a standard. The 5 ml is injected intravenously. After adequate time to ensure complete mixing of the labeled erythrocytes within the circulation, a sample is withdrawn from a vein other than that used for the injection. In normal subjects, 10 minutes is sufficient to ensure complete mixing. However, in certain disease states, for example, splenomegaly or severe polycythemia, mixing may be greatly delayed. In this case, serial samples should be taken until there is no significant difference in their counts.

In other seriously ill patients, a less pronounced delay of mixing may occur. For this reason, our routine is to wait 30 minutes to obtain the postinjection sample (with use of a heparinized syringe).

Hematocrit (Hct) determinations are performed on the standard and blood samples. Four counting tubes are prepared to contain 1 ml volumes of the following:

Whole blood from the standard = Std WB
Plasma from the standard = Std Plas

**ACD,* Citric acid, sodium citrate, and dextrose.
†*CPD,* Citric acid, sodium citrate, sodium biphosphate, and dextrose.

Whole blood from the sample = Samp WB
Plasma from the sample = Samp Plas

The standards and samples are counted in a well counter with the spectrometer centered about the 320 keV photopeak of chromium 51 and counted for sufficient time to ensure a counting accuracy of 1% error or less. Usually there are so few counts in the postinjection plasma sample that a shorter counting time is acceptable for this tube.

$$\text{Erythrocyte volume} = \frac{[\text{Std WB} - (\text{Std Plas} \times \text{Std Plct})] \times \text{Vol Inj} \times \text{Samp Hct}}{[\text{Samp WB} - (\text{Samp Plas} \times \text{Samp Plct})]}$$

$$\text{Plct} = \text{Decimal plasmacrit} = 1 - \text{Decimal hematocrit}$$

Falsely high results are found if a faulty intravenous injection technique is used, and the entire dose is not injected into a vein. Damaged erythrocytes or excessive binding of the chromium 51 by leukocytes or platelets when these are abnormally elevated will also yield spuriously high values. Falsely low values are caused by a failure to obtain a preinjection blood sample in a patient who has had previous administration of radioactive tracers. Contamination of equipment with radioactivity will also yield spuriously low results.

For the measurement of circulating red blood cell mass, 10 μCi of chromium 51 is an adequate amount of activity and will provide enough counts so that statistically significant sample counting can be performed in a reasonable time. The specific activity of the ^{51}Cr-chromate must be such that less than 2 μg of chromium ion is present per *milliliter* of *packed erythrocytes*. This becomes particularly critical when this technique is used for erythrocyte-survival studies (see p. 409) that require larger doses of ^{51}Cr.

Plasma volume

Iodinated albumin is the conventional agent used for estimation of plasma volume. Because ^{125}I-labeled albumin provided by radiopharmaceutical manufacturers is of such high concentration, a sterile stock solution of lower concentration, on the order of 1 μCi/ml, is made with U.S.P. sterile sodium chloride as a diluent. Ten milliliters of this stock solution is drawn into a syringe and injected intravenously with care being taken that it all enters the vein. Albumin does not remain solely in the intravascular space but diffuses rapidly into extravascular compartments and produces some inaccuracies. To minimize the error that results from this, two or preferably more timed heparinized samples (for example, 10, 20, and 30 minutes) must be taken from the subject. These samples are centrifuged and 1 ml aliquots of plasma are counted.

The radioactivity in each of these samples is measured and plotted against time on semilogarithmic paper. The best straight line is drawn through these points, with only the earlier points being used if the later points deviate from the initial linear slope. The zero-time activity is estimated by extrapolation and used for the calculation of the plasma volume. A standard is prepared and counted. All counts are performed with the spectrometer adjusted to count ^{125}I (20 to 50 keV) for a time long enough to assure a 1% error or less. The plasma volume is calculated thus:

$$\text{Plasma volume (ml)} = \frac{\text{Volume injected} \times \text{Net counts per minute in standard}}{\text{Net counts per minute of plasma sample obtained by extrapolation}}$$

Having precisely measured the erythrocyte or plasma volume and knowing the venous hematocrit, one can safely calculate the volume of the other compartment and thus estimate the total blood volume, but only in normal individuals. The reason is that in normals there is a fixed relationship between the whole body hematocrit (Hct_b) and the venous hematocrit (Hct_v); the ratio of Hct_b to Hct_v on the average is 0.90. It is believed that two factors are responsible for the difference observed between the Hct_b and Hct_v; (1) the hematocrit of blood in small capillaries is lower than that found in larger vessels; (2) as discussed above, the iodinated albumin used to measure the plasma space is immediately distributed into a space larger than that of the vascular space in which the red cells are distributed.

It is important to recognize, however, that most of the patients referred to the clinical nuclear medicine service for measurement of either red blood cell volume or plasma volume are severely ill and the predictable normal relationship most likely will not be present in these individuals. For instance, in patients in whom there is moderate or gross splenomegaly, the ratio of Hct_b to Hct_v may be substantially and unpredictably increased to greater than 1; in patients with severe polycythemia, abnormalities may also be present in the plasma volume as well as in the red blood cell mass. Thus, in clinical circumstances, total blood volume can be reliably estimated only by doing simultaneous measurements of red cell mass and plasma volume.

A limitation in the interpretation of these studies is that normal values for blood volume in any given individual cannot be simply predicted from such parameters as height and weight despite the many elaborate formulas that have been proposed. In interpreting studies in adults, the simplest method of calculating the values in milliliters per kilogram is probably at

Table 15-3. Normal blood volume compartment values (ml/kg)*

	Males	Females
Total blood volume	55-80	50-75
Red blood cell volume†	25-35	20-30
Plasma volume‡	30-45	30-45

*From Rocha, A. F. G., and Harbert, J. C., editors: Textbook of nuclear medicine: clinical applications, Philadelphia, 1979, Lea & Febiger.
†95% confidence limits.
‡Because of the many variables that may influence plasma volume in normals, it is not possible to place confidence limits on these values.

least as reliable as using any of the various formulas or nomograms. The normal values published by the International Panel on Standardization in Haematology are shown in Table 15-3. Note the wide range in plasma volume observed in normal subjects; this immediately tells us that this is less than a precise test. The undesirable rapid diffusion of the radiolabeled albumin is but one factor making this procedure less than precise, even in normal subjects. Body position, recent exercise, and a number of other factors cause rapid significant changes in plasma volume. Therefore, although we can precisely measure the circulating red blood cell mass, it is best always to report the plasma volume as "estimated."

Other factors seen in patients referred for study, such as obesity, recent weight loss, and prolonged bed rest may make it impossible to estimate the red blood cell and plasma volume solely from height and weight measurements in a given patient. Since red blood cell mass is related to lean body mass, patients who are exceptionally obese or who have had recent significant weight loss should have their measured values compared to those based on "ideal" or recent body weight.

There are several specific circumstances in which blood-volume measurements have proved to be of considerable value. The use of chromium 51–labeled red blood cells to measure the red blood cell mass allows a precise determination as to whether true polycythemia is present or whether the patient has an elevated hematocrit because of a reduced plasma volume.

Hematologists see several patients each year because of a persistent elevation of the hematocrit, but the red blood cell mass is normal when this is measured by the ^{51}Cr technique. Usually these are entirely normal individuals whose red blood cell mass is near the upper limits of normal and whose plasma volume is near the lower limits of normal. The performance of this one simple, relatively inexpensive test, proving that they have a normal red blood cell mass, saves these patients an elaborate, expensive, and prolonged series of other diagnostic procedures.

It has recently been appreciated that patients with polycythemia vera and myelofibrosis may have a pronounced expansion of their plasma volume, which will be apparent only if this parameter is directly measured. Because of this combined abnormality, serial red blood cell measurements may become essential to the management of patients with polycythemia vera. It is in these circumstances that the availability of ^{99m}Tc erythrocytes becomes invaluable.

Paradoxically, in the acutely hemorrhaging patient or patient with recent severe trauma, the hematocrit may remain normal or disproportionally high for some time. In this circumstance direct measurement with ^{51}Cr-labeled erythrocytes will reveal the true red blood cell mass of the patient.

Erythrocyte survival and splenic sequestration studies

Red blood cells are labeled by use of the same technique as in the red blood cell volume determination with the exception that the dose of ^{51}Cr is adjusted to 1.5 μCi/kg of body weight. After labeling, the cells are reinjected and the first sample is obtained 24 hours later (to permit removal from the circulation of any cells accidentally damaged during the labeling procedure; during this same interval, any injected plasma radioactivity is cleared from the circulation). Samples are then obtained every other day for the next 3 weeks; a 6 ml sample of blood is withdrawn and placed into a tube containing an anticoagulant (preferably solid EDTA or concentrated heparin).

Five milliliters of whole blood is pipetted from the tubes as they are collected. (Tubes should be inverted 12 to 15 times, before samples are pipetted and hematocrits are done, to ensure thorough mixing.)

Hematocrit determinations are made on each sample on the day of collection. After this, a tiny amount of saponin powder is added to each tube and they are again gently tilted several times to ensure mixing and complete lysis of the erythrocytes. Care is taken not to allow the sample to touch the cap of the counting tube.

On the last day of the study, all the samples are counted on the gamma spectrometer with settings of 280 to 360 keV for ^{51}Cr.

The samples are counted to give a sample percent error of 1% or less (for approximately 10 minutes each).

To calculate the half-time of disappearance of the labeled red blood cells, net counts per minute of each sample are plotted on semilogarithmic paper as a function of time. The best straight line is drawn through all the points. The $T_{\frac{1}{2}}$ is obtained as follows: extrapolate the line to time zero. This is the y intercept. Divide the *y* intercept value by 2. At this value on the *y* axis, draw a straight line parallel to the *x* axis until it intersects the best straight line drawn through the observed data points. Drop a perpendicular line to the *x* axis. This is the labeled red blood cell half-time disappearance rate or survival time as measured by the ^{51}Cr technique, not corrected for elution of the isotope.

Occasionally one encounters patients whose data do not permit a satisfactory "eye fit" of a single straight line to the data points. The International Panel on Diagnostic Applications of Radioisotopes in Haematology's publication on red blood cell survival studies[7] describes alternative methods, including computer programs for handling such data. Now that most clinical nuclear medicine laboratories have one or more dedicated computers, it is suggested that the appropriate programs be added to their "software" for use as needed.

The mean half-life of normal ^{51}Cr-labeled erythrocytes is from 25 to 35 days. Normal erythrocytes are removed from the circulation when they become senescent at a rate approximating 1% per day; the true mean life-span of the normal erythrocyte therefore is between 50 and 60 days. However, this approximately 1% per day removal of senescent erythrocytes from the circulation coupled with the approximately 1% per day elution of the ^{51}Cr label from the erythrocytes combine to give the mean half-time of 25 to 35 days as measured with this technique. Tables are available for correcting for this elution, but they were derived from studies in normals and their relevance in disease states where the elution rate is known to vary is uncertain. However, the more severe the hemolytic process and thus the more rapid the rate of removal of the ^{51}Cr-labeled erythrocytes, the less significant this ^{51}Cr elution becomes.

Determination of mean erythrocyte life-span from a label randomly applied to cells of all ages is meaningful only in a patient who is in a steady state with regard to the rate of production and destruction of red cells. If either of these rates change, the mean age of the circulating red cells will be changed and will affect the ^{51}Cr results, even though the actual longevity of each individual erythrocyte has not changed. A constant hematocrit prior to and during the period of study is one index of a steady state. Obviously inaccurate results will be obtained in a patient who is being or has recently been transfused.

The study of splenic sequestration should be a routine part of any ^{51}Cr-erythrocyte survival study. Organ counting is begun 24 hours after labeled cells are reinjected and continued approximately every other day for the next 3 weeks.

The counting probe should be equipped with a flat-field collimator designed to exclude radiation from areas other than the organs of interest but still permit sampling of a large enough organ volume to give adequate count rates. The spectrometer is adjusted to count gamma rays from 280 to 360 keV.

Place the patient on the examining table in the positions as described below:

Precordium: The detector is centered over the left third intercostal interspace at the sternal border, with the patient in *supine* position.

Liver: The detector is placed over the ninth and tenth ribs on the right, in the midclavicular line with patient in the *supine* position. In elderly subjects and patients with chronic obstructive pulmonary disease, the exact location of the liver should be checked by percussion.

Spleen: The detector is placed two thirds the distance from the spinal process to the lateral edge of the body at the level of the ninth and tenth ribs, with the patient in the prone position.

The skin is marked with indelible ink, which in turn is covered by transparent nonallergenic tape to indicate the position of the external detector from one day to the next. Each area must be counted with the same geometry each time by having the detector touch the patient's skin. The areas are counted to give a sample error of 5% or less.

The results are expressed as the ratio of the count rate over the spleen to the count rate over the precordium. The count rate over the liver is also expressed relative to the count rate over the precordium. These ratios are graphed as a function of time on linear graph paper.

In normal subjects, the spleen-to-liver ratio is less than or may approximate 1:1. In patients with active splenic sequestration of cells, this ratio often rises to 2:1 or even to 4:1. The spleen-to-precordium ratio is judged to be clearly abnormal if the ratio is greater than 2:1. An initial and persistent elevation of spleen-to-precordium ratio is attributable to increased splenic blood pool. A progressive gradual increase indicates active sequestration of the labeled cells.

Sources of error

1. Inaccurate probe positioning will cause spurious results.
2. Blood loss from the gastrointestinal tract or surgical sites will cause a shortened half-time.
3. Blood transfusions during the procedure will also cause an apparent shortening of the half-time (by increasing the volume of the unlabeled cells).

Obviously, neither (2) nor (3) will affect the outcome of the splenic sequestration study and therefore do not warrant discontinuing the test, unless the hemorrhage is truly massive, leaving an insignificant amount of circulating radioactivity.

Quantitation of blood loss

Occult blood loss is difficult to demonstrate with sensitivity and specificity. Over the years, many methods of stool collection, homogenation, and counting have been devised by a great number of technologists in order to make this procedure more esthetic. Our current procedure has been demonstrated to be sensitive, specific, and acceptable to the technical staff! Erythrocytes are labeled as in the erythrocyte survival and sequestration study and returned to the patient intravenously. The patient is instructed to collect all stools for 4 days in clean paint cans and to avoid contaminating the collection with urine. Five milliliters of concentrated phenol in water is added to the stool collections as they arrive in the lab. The total weight of the can containing the fecal specimen and phenol is then brought to 2 kg by the addition of tap water and the lid is tightly shut on the can. The stool is homogenized in the can by shaking the can on a commercial paint shaker for about 10 minutes. Blood samples are drawn on the first and third days and counted with identical geometry and compared to the counts of the homogenized stool samples for determination of blood loss.

$$\frac{\text{Total net cpm in 24-hour stool}}{\text{Net cpm in 1 ml of WB}} = \text{Blood loss (ml)}$$

Normal values are 1.2 ± 0.5 ml with a range of 0.3 to 2.8 ml per 24 hours. Any blood in the stools in excess of this amount suggests enteric blood loss.

In vivo cross matching

There are rare instances when blood banks are unable to identify a satisfactory donor for a patient requiring transfusion.[7] In these unusual circumstances, the use of chromium-labeled *donor* red cells to do an in vivo cross match may provide an invaluable lifesaving service.

The general principle is that one infuses into the patient no more than 1 ml of donor cells after they have been labeled with chromium 51. Carefully timed serial blood samples are then taken from the recipient at 3, 10, and 60 minutes, and both whole blood and plasma radioactivity are measured in the samples. The technique is as follows:

Using sterile technique, add 50 μCi of sodium ^{51}Cr-chromate to 5 ml of the donor blood in a sterile test tube. Invert this mixture gently several times to ensure proper mixing and allow to incubate for 15 minutes at room temperature with occasional inverting. Centrifuge the tube and aseptically withdraw the supernatant plasma using an 18-gauge spinal needle. Fill the tube with sterile isotonic saline and centrifuge as before after having gently inverted the tube several times. Repeat the washing procedure, and then resuspend the cells in isotonic saline to the initial volume. Draw 1 ml of the chromium 51–tagged cells into a 3 ml syringe, and keep the remaining labeled cells to make a standard.

Technique and sample preparation. Do a hematocrit on the 3-minute sample and pipette 1 ml of whole blood from each of the blood samples into tubes and label. Centrifuge the remaining whole blood from the 10- and 60-minute samples and pipette 1 ml of the plasma into tubes and label. Pipette 2 ml of labeled whole blood from the dose tube into a 100 ml volumetric flask containing 50 to 60 ml of distilled water. The volume in the flask is then filled to the mark with water and mixed. Pipette a 1 ml sample from the flask into counting tubes and label. All samples are then counted in a well counter with spectrometer settings for chromium 51 (280 to 360 keV) and count for a sufficient time to give a counting accuracy of 1% error or less.

Interpretation. Estimated red blood cell mass is obtained from tables based on the sex, body weight, and venous hematocrit of the recipient. The predicted red blood cell mass is compared to the calculated value by use of the 3-minute sample.

$$\text{Calculated red blood cell mass} = \frac{\text{Volume injected ([cpm RBC Std/1 ml][Dilution factor])}}{\text{cpm 3 min whole blood/1 ml}} \times \text{Decimal hematocrit}$$

If there has not been immediate removal of a significant portion of the donor red blood cells from the circulation, the estimated and the calculated red blood cell masses should be the same order of magnitude.

When compatible red blood cells have been injected, about 99% of the radioactivity in the 3-minute whole-blood sample will be found in the 60-minute sample (range: 94% to 104%) and no radioactivity is seen in any of the plasma samples. In cases of urgency or when there is great difficulty in finding completely compatible red blood cells, donor red blood cells may be transfused with minimal hazard when 70% of the radioactivity in the 3-minute sample is found in the 60-minute sample and the amount of radioactivity in the 10- and 60-minute plasma samples is less than 5% of the radioactivity injected.

Ferrokinetics

The administration of radioactive iron permits one to obtain clinically relevant data on net red cell production. A tracer amount of high specific activity ^{59}Fe citrate in isotonic saline is preincubated with plasma prior to injection. The other isotopes of iron are unsuitable, because of their physical characteristics.

It is important to note that the iron nuclide must be bound initially to transferrin (the normal iron-transport protein) by prior incubation with plasma. If non–transferrin bound iron is injected into a patient whose iron-binding capacity is saturated, the iron will be rapidly cleared as a foreign substance by the reticuloendothelial system instead of being available for tracing iron metabolism. Patients with significant reduction of their unsaturated iron-binding capacity are frequently encountered among subjects referred for ferrokinetic studies, that is, patients with hemolytic or aplastic anemia and patients who have recently been treated with iron or transfusions. The determination of the serum iron (SI) and the unsaturated iron-binding capacity (UIBC) is an obligatory first step in the planning of a ferrokinetic study. Note that with the usual tests one rarely if ever gets a zero value for UIBC, even in patients dying from iron overload. The reason is that once transferrin is saturated, a significant amount of added iron will bind loosely to other plasma proteins.

The sample for these determinations should be drawn at the same time of day the study is to begin in the laboratory (for example 9 AM or 2 PM). If the UIBC is greater than 100 μg/dl, then one may continue the procedure. If, however, these tests indicate a significant reduction in the UIBC (that is, unsaturated transferrin), the following must be done: a sample of the patient's blood is sent to the blood bank requesting that a professional ABO-compatible donor be identified who is known to be hepatitis B antigen negative and asked to donate 30 ml of blood for the study. One ideally should use only professional donors whose blood has been used for transfusions by the blood bank for a substantial period of time without incidences of hepatitis occurring in the recipients.

This sample must be collected using heparin; other anticoagulants will chelate the iron and thus negate the study. This blood is centrifuged for 10 minutes; using sterile techniques, 2 ml of plasma is pipetted into a vial and incubated for 30 minutes with 12 μCi of ^{59}Fe citrate. If the patient's UIBC is normal, the ^{59}Fe citrate is added to 12 ml of sterile sodium chloride. Five milliliters of the solution is drawn into a 10 ml syringe and the remainder is kept to make the standard. The injection is made very slowly.

Plasma iron clearance. To determine the initial clearance rate of iron from plasma, serial heparinized 6 ml blood samples are drawn at 10, 30, 60, and 90 minutes after the injection of ^{59}Fe from a vein other than the one used for the injection. Even in patients with greatly accelerated erythrocytosis, no ^{59}Fe will be present in the erythrocytes during this initial phase. Therefore whole-blood samples may be counted.

The 5 ml samples are counted in a well counter with the gamma spectrometer set to accept 1 to 1.4 meV ^{59}Fe events. Net counts per minute for the 10-, 30-, 60-, and 90-minute samples are plotted on semilogarithmic paper as a function of time. A straight line is usually obtained (at least from the earlier points) and the $T_{\frac{1}{2}}$ of initial rate of plasma iron clearance can be determined from the graph. If the tracer iron has been preincubated with plasma and therefore bound to transferrin, one may extrapolate the initial straight line portion of this curve to time zero and thereby use this transferrin-bound ^{59}Fe and the standard to calculate the volume of distribution (that is, plasma volume).

It should be emphasized that this initial rapid single exponential removal of iron from the plasma does not accurately reflect the overall turnover of iron in the plasma. If the clearance rate is followed for longer periods of time, there is slowing of the clearance of the remaining iron with two or more exponential components to the curve, even in normal subjects. However, this simply obtained $T_{\frac{1}{2}}$ of initial plasma clearance does vary considerably in a wide number of disease states, but of and by itself is never diagnostic. The normal range of the $T_{\frac{1}{2}}$ of plasma clearance by this method is 60 to 120 minutes. This clearance rate can change in disease states because of alterations in the rate of erythropoiesis and of the activity of the macrophages of the reticuloendothelial system, where iron is normally retained as storage iron. An increased rate of clearance is seen in such diseases as iron-deficiency anemia, pernicious anemia, recent blood loss, hemolytic anemia, polycythemia vera, and paradoxically, myelofibrosis with ineffective erythropoiesis. The clearance rate is generally greatly slowed in patients with aplastic anemia.

This portion of the test should not be deleted because it serves as an invaluable quality control; if the ^{59}Fe is inadvertently not bound to transferrin, there will be essentially no counts in the first specimen, where no matter how rapid the clearance is in disease states, sufficient radioactivity will remain to allow accurate measurement of this initial rapid exponential phase of plasma iron clearance.

Incorporation of iron into erythrocytes. Determining the rate of incorporation of the radioactive iron into the circulating erythrocytes provides some insight into the effectiveness of erythropoiesis. Twenty-four hours after the injection of the iron-59 citrate a 6 ml sample of blood is withdrawn and additional samples of heparinized whole blood are then obtained every other day for at least 10 and preferably 14 days. Pipette 5 ml of whole blood from the samples as they are collected. Hematocrit determinations are made on each sample on the day of collection. On the last day of the study, all the samples are counted with settings of 1 to 1.4 meV on a scintillation spectrometer. The following formula is used to calculate the percentage of red blood cell iron-59 incorporation.

$$\% \text{ RBC incorporation of } {}^{59}\text{Fe for any day} = \frac{\text{cpm of each day's whole blood} \times \text{RBC volume} \times 100}{\text{cpm of the standard} \times \text{Dilution factor} \times \text{Decimal Hct (for each day)}}$$

A measurement of the red blood cell mass must be made just prior to the beginning of the ferrokinetic studies. This data is necessary to calculate the iron incorporation into red blood cells. The percentage of red blood cell iron-59 incorporation is plotted on linear paper against time in days.

In normal subjects from 60% to 80% of the administered dose will be incorporated into the circulating erythrocytes by 7 to 10 days and the radioactivity will remain at that same level for the period of observation. In some patients with hemolytic anemia, there may be immediate accelerated incorporation of iron into the circulating erythrocytes, but by the seventh to tenth day many of these labeled erythrocytes may already have been removed from the circulation; a single sample obtained at this time would indicate that the net incorporation of iron was subnormal. In patients with ineffective erythropoiesis one may see a very slow increase in red blood cell iron-59 counts, because iron continues to flow back into the plasma and once again through the marrow. These are but two examples where obtaining frequent samples over the 2-week period and applying "pattern recognition" techniques to the interpretation will provide accurate and clinically important data (Fig. 15-2).

If one wishes to calculate the variety of parameters listed in many texts with precision in such complicated cases as just mentioned, it is necessary to have (1) daily or every other day samples for erythrocyte and plasma radioactivity (because the latter is so low after the first day, this may require dialysis to remove traces of contaminating hemoglobin and does require prolonged counting times), (2) multiple samples for serum iron determinations, drawn at the same time as (1), (3) ideally, serial red blood cell mass measurements, and (4) profound patience or a computer program to handle these data properly.

This is clearly beyond the scope of the ordinary nuclear medicine laboratory. In our opinion, the simple "pattern recognition" approach described above usually provides the answers to the basic clinical question being asked.

Surface counting to determine the organ localization of iron 59 often gives additional clinically useful information. The technique and probe positioning are similar to those described for external counting for organ localization of ^{51}Cr-labeled erythrocytes. In this case, however, appropriate areas to be counted include the sacrum as well as the precordium, the spleen, and the liver. In normal individuals, one sees a relatively rapid increase in iron-59 counts over the sacrum during the first few hours of the study and then a gradual decline as erythrocytes bearing their iron-59 label are released from the marrow. Little radioactivity normally accumulates in the spleen and liver; the counts noted over these areas in normal subjects undoubtedly represent iron-59 accumulation in adjacent areas of active marrow. Abnormal patterns of surface counting may be seen in patients with ineffective hematopoiesis or in patients with significant extramedullary hematopoiesis.

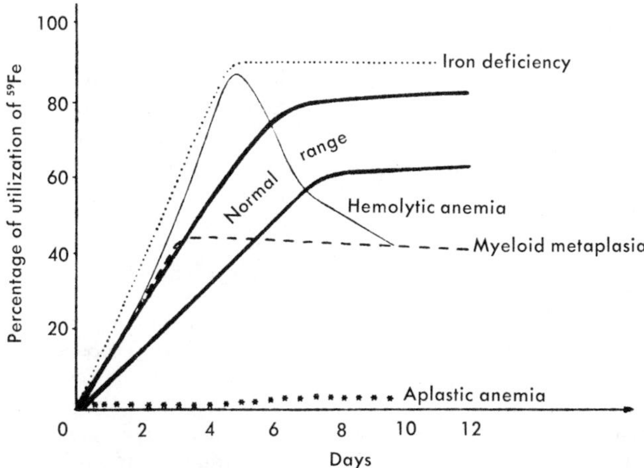

Fig. 15-2. Curves compare normal red blood cell utilization of radioiron with that in various disease states. (By permission from Wagner, H. N., Jr., editor: Nuclear medicine, New York, 1974, Hospital Practice Publishing Co., Inc.)

MEASUREMENT OF ABSORPTION AND SERUM LEVELS OF ESSENTIAL NUTRIENTS

Vitamin-B_{12} (cyanocobalamin) absorption

Nuclear medicne has furnished important diagnostic tools for the diagnosis of vitamin-B_{12} deficiency. The consequences of untreated vitamin-B_{12} deficiency include anemia, thrombocytopenia, leukopenia, crippling spinal cord degeneration, and death.

The importance of measuring vitamin-B_{12} absorption in patients with unexplained anemia deserves emphasis, since the principle that anemia is not a disease per se but only a symptom of some underlying disorder is not always reflected in practice. The onset of clinical symptoms from vitamin-B_{12} deficiency is notoriously insidious and the initial complaints of the patients are often vague; in the early stages the classic erythrocyte changes are not present.

Table 15-4 summarizes the causes of vitamin-B_{12} deficiency. Table 15-5 summarizes factors important in vitamin-B_{12} nutrition and absorption in man. Isolated "pure" (apart from several prolonged protein deprivations) dietary deficiency is very rare. Therefore, the overwhelming number of cases of vitamin-B_{12} deficiency are caused by some underlying disorder attributable to malabsorption. The most common cause of vitamin-B_{12} malabsorption is a deficiency in intrinsic factor, a protein secreted by the parietal cells of the stomach, which is an obligatory requirement for normal vitamin-B_{12} absorption by the terminal ileum.

Thus the availability of radioactive vitamin B_{12} for specific testing of a patient's ability to absorb physiologic amounts of this essential nutrient has been of great clinical value. Vitamin B_{12} is a complex corrinoid compound, the central ligand of which is cobalt; several radioactive isotopes of cobalt are available. The earliest in use was ^{60}Co, but ^{57}Co and ^{58}Co are now preferred for routine clinical studies because of their shorter half-lives and smaller radiation dose (Table 15-6). The Schilling test of urinary excretion is generally accepted as the standard method of measuring absorption of radioactive vitamin B_{12}. This test requires (1) the oral administration and retention of a tracer dose of vitamin B_{12} (it is important that this oral dose be in the range of 0.25 to 2 μg, a quantity similar to one that might be present in a normal meal, because quantities above this level may be absorbed by mechanisms not dependent on intrinsic factor) and (2) a transient saturation of normal binding sites in the plasma that is achieved by injection of a "flushing" dose of 1 mg of nonradioactive vitamin B_{12}.

Patients may drink water before and after the test; however, they should have nothing to eat after midnight before the day of the test and remain fasting for 2 hours after the oral dose of ^{57}Co-vitamin B_{12}. The patient's doctor should be instructed not to give any enemas or laxatives, or schedule the patient for barium enema or intravenous pylogram for the duration of this study. The patient should be questioned before the dose is given regarding these medications, which may interfere with the results: vitamin-B_{12} injections, colchicine corticosteroids, and ACTH. Because of hepatobiliary recirculation, it is theoretically possible

Table 15-4. Causes of vitamin-B_{12} deficiency*

1. Inadequate intake
2. Malabsorption
   a. Caused by gastric abnormalities
      (1) Absence of intrinsic factor
         (a) Congenital
         (b) Addisonian pernicious anemia
         (c) Total gastrectomy
         (d) Subtotal gastrectomy
      (2) Excessive excretion of hydrochloric acid: Zollinger-Ellison syndrome
   b. Caused by intestinal malabsorption
      (1) Destruction, removal, or functional incompetence of ileal mucosal absorptive sites
      (2) Competition with host for available dietary vitamin B_{12}
         (a) *Diphyllobothrium latum* (fish tapeworm)
         (b) Small-bowel lesions associated with stagnation and bacterial overgrowth (jejunal diverticula, strictures, blind loops, and so on)
      (3) Pancreatic insufficiency
      (4) Drug therapy†
         (a) Para-aminosalicylic acid (PAS)
         (b) Neomycin
         (c) Colchicine
         (d) Calcium-chelating agents
   c. Caused by genetic abnormality in the transport protein transcobalamin II

*From Rocha, A. F. G., and Harbert, J. C., editors: Textbook of nuclear medicine: clinical applications, Philadelphia, 1979, Lea & Febiger.

†Although any of these agents may produce abnormalities in vitamin-B_{12} absorption, only patients on long-term PAS therapy have been reported to develop clinical evidence of vitamin-B_{12} deficiency.

Table 15-5. Absorption of dietary vitamin B_{12} in man*

1. Available for human nutrition only in animal food sources.
2. Vitamin B_{12} is bound to intrinsic factor by gastric mucosa.
3. Normal ileal mucosal absorptive sites depend on presence of ionic Ca^{++} and on pH of ileal contents of more than 6.
4. Normal "transport" protein (transcobalamin II) conveys vitamin B_{12} from ileal absorptive sites to areas of active utilization and storage.

*The same factors apply to absorption of tracer amounts of radioactive vitamin B_{12} used in absorption studies.

to block all the absorptive sites (in the terminal ileum) if large (1 mg or greater) daily doses of vitamin B_{12} are being administered. If the patient has normal renal function, however, all excess vitamin B_{12} is promptly excreted in the urine and the test only needs to be delayed for 24 to 48 hours after discontinuing the vitamin-B_{12} injections.

If the patient has previously been given radioactive materials, a 24-hour urine collection is obtained for background. The dose of 0.5 μCi of ^{57}Co-vitamin B_{12} is administered orally and 2 hours later 1 mg of stable vitamin B_{12} is given intramuscularly. Two 24-hour urine collections are obtained, one for each 24-hour period. The patient is instructed to collect all urine during this period and avoid losing any urine during defecation.

The total volume and specific gravity of each 24-hour collection is measured. The urine samples and a standard are counted in a well counter with the spectrometer set to count gamma rays from 105 to 145 keV.

$$\% \text{ of } ^{57}\text{Co-vitamin B}_{12} \text{ in 24-hour urine} = \frac{\text{cpm in urine sample} \times \dfrac{\text{Urine volume}}{\text{Sample volume}}}{\text{cpm in Std} \times \text{Dilution factor}}$$

Malabsorption of vitamin B_{12} can be documented by the appearance of less than 9% of the administered dose in the first 24-hour urine collection.

The major problem with this test is its dependence on a complete 24-hour urine collection. The loss of just one urine specimen may cause falsely low results. The 24-hour test also requires that urinary function be intact. Erroneously low values will result from abnormal urinary retention, as in men with benign prostatic hypertrophy, or in patients with renal disease. In such patients the amount excreted in the first 24-hours will be reduced, but significant radioactivity will continue to be excreted for the next 24 to 48 hours; total excretion will eventually be within normal limits. For this reason and because it often helps tell when the first 24-hour collection was incomplete, our routine is to have the patient collect two separate 24-hour urines, after the single flushing dose. We measure volume, specific gravity and the percent of the administered dose of radioactivity separately in each 24-hour specimen. Table 15-7 gives some typical patient results and illustrates the value of this minor modification of the Schilling test. If less than 6% of the dose is excreted in 24 hours, the test should be repeated with the manufacturer's recommended dose of intrinsic factor (IF)* given with the dose of ^{57}Co-vitamin B_{12}. Three to 7 days must elapse before the repeat test. A normal urinary excretion value after the administration of intrinsic factor occurs in pernicious anemia.

Serum vitamin-B_{12} assays

Conventional microbiologic assays have recently been replaced by tracer techniques for the measurement of serum vitamin-B_{12} levels. The principles underlying the use of radioactive vitamin B_{12} for such measurements are essentially the same as those for any other competitive binding assay; competition between radioactive and nonradioactive vitamin B_{12} for the binding sites on a protein, and separation of the protein-bound vitamin B_{12} from the free vitamin. The theoretical danger present in this type of competitive protein-binding assay is that the binder will "recognize" a chemically similar, but biologically inactive substance. This has been shown to be the case with

*Unfortunately these products vary greatly from time to time and at times are totally ineffective. For that reason alone the products where radiolabeled vitamin B_{12} is prebound to normal human gastric juice are more reliable. Furthermore, there are occasional patients who have antibody to hog intrinsic factor and who will therefore not respond to even potent preparations; such patients do respond normally to this human source of intrinsic factor.

Table 15-6. Characteristics of selected radioisotopes of cobalt*†

Isotope	Physical half-life	Effective half-life in liver‡	Radiation	Principal photon energies (meV)	Relative dose to liver
^{57}Co	270 days	161 days	Electron capture	0.122 (87%)	1§
^{58}Co	72 days	60 days	Electron capture, β^+, γ	0.810 (99%) 0.511 (30%)	2
^{60}Co	5.2 years	331 days	β^-, γ	1.17 (100%) 1.33 (100%)	29

*From Rocha, A. F. G., Harbert, J. C., editors: Textbook of nuclear medicine: clinical applications, Philadelphia, 1979, Lea & Febiger.
†Adapted from Rosenblum, C.: In Heinrich, H. C., editor: Vitamin B-12 und Intrinsic Factor. 2. Europäisches Symposium über Vitamin B-12 und Intrinsic Factor, Hamburg, 1961, Stuttgart, 1961, Ferdinand Encke Verlag, p. 306.
‡Assuming a biologic half-life of 400 days after administration as radioactive cobalt-labeled vitamin B_{12}.
§Approximately 0.051 rads per 0.5 μCi of ^{57}Co-labeled vitamin when parenteral dose of 1 mg of vitamin B_{12} is given, resulting in renal excretion of approximately 30% of the absorbed dose of radioactive vitamin B_{12}.

Table 15-7. Representative results of Schilling test using two 24-hour urine collections (single nuclide without intrinsic factor)*

	First 24-hour urine			Second 24-hour urine		
	Volume	Specific gravity	% of dose excreted	Volume	Specific gravity	% of dose excreted
A	640	1.010	3.0	1230	1.010	0.8
B	1210	1.012	3.0	1120	1.012	0.8
C	1200	1.010	3.0	1150	1.010	4.0
D (normal)	1210	1.012	14.0	1200	1.012	0.3

Patient A had an incomplete first 24-hour urine collection because of inadvertent loss of urine during cleansing enemas, which had been ordered to prepare her for gastrointestinal x-ray examinations.
Patient B subsequently had normal excretion when the test was repeated with the addition of a potent intrinsic factor. Other studies confirmed the diagnosis of addisonian pernicious anemia.
Patient C was recognized on reexamination to have benign prostatic hypertrophy with significant bladder retention. The delayed pattern of excretion of the radioactive vitamin B_{12} was the first clinical indication of this condition.
Patient D was a cooperative normal volunteer.

*From Rocha, A. F. G., and Harbert, J. C., editors: Textbook of nuclear medicine: clinical applications, Philadelphia, 1979, Lea & Febiger.

these vitamin-B_{12} assays. Some patients with pernicious anemia in relapse were observed to have normal test results using these competitive protein-binding assays.[8] The future of these tests is uncertain: intrinsic factor (IF) will bind only vitamin B_{12}, and in gastric juice there is another binder that can provide false-normal results. Separation of pure, nondenatured intrinsic factor is a rather delicate and time-consuming procedure.

Furthermore, a single injection of vitamin B_{12} results in a normal serum value that may persist for many weeks, despite the patient's inability to absorb any dietary vitamin B_{12}. Accordingly, normal results obtained even with the most accurate microbiologic assay in patients who otherwise have clinical evidence suggestive of vitamin-B_{12} deficiency should be confirmed by radioactive vitamin B_{12}–absorption studies.

Radioactive vitamin B_{12} can also be utilized in vitro to test gastric juice for intrinsic factor content. It is especially useful in following some of the childhood endocrinopathies and pre–pernicious anemia states because it does not expose the children to any radiation. This assay is based on the fact that free vitamin B_{12} will be absorbed by charcoal-coated protein whereas intrinsic factor–bound vitamin B_{12} will not. The patient's gastric juice is titrated with tracer vitamin B_{12} with and without charcoal, and the binding that occurs is compared with that in a similar titration to which antibody to intrinsic factor has been added. The amount of binding inhibited by the antibody reflects the intrinsic factor level present. With a pool of normal human gastric juice, this method can be used to detect and measure antibody to intrinsic factor.

Serum folate assays

As with vitamin-B_{12} assays, it was hoped that the tedious microbiologic methods could be discarded. A competitive protein-binding (CPB) assay of serum folate, with use of a folate-binding protein (β-lactoglobulin) present in cow's milk, has been adopted by a number of laboratories and forms the basis for several commercially available kits. This method has, however, inherent limitations:

1. It is difficult to standardize and tedious to perform within acceptable limits of quality control.
2. At present the only folate available in high enough specific activity for use in such an assay is the simple folic acid. The folate compound normally present in serum is 5-methyl-tetrahydrofolate (5-MTHF), a reduced and substituted form of folic acid. It has been noted that patients on drugs that inhibit the normal "reducing" enzyme for absorbed folates (dihydrofolate reductase) may have normal serum levels as measured by this method while suffering from severe clinical folate deficiency.
3. Serum folate levels are very sensitive to relatively brief periods of dietary deprivation. Erythrocyte folate levels more accurately reflect the clinical status of the patient. The erythrocyte folates include reduced and polyglutamate forms, and their assay is even more difficult to standardize with this binder than the serum folate measurement is.

A recent evaluation of the commercially available kits using this binder for the radioassay of serum folate showed that all failed one or more standard quality

Table 15-8. Physical characteristics of radiopharmaceuticals that have been used for bone-marrow scanning*

Class of agent	Dose†	Physical half-life	Photon energy (meV)	Liver dose (rads)	Bone-marrow dose (rads)	Kidney (rads)
Transferrin-bound metals						
^{59}Fe	40 μCi	45 days	1.1 1.3	—	2	—
^{52}Fe‡	100 μCi	8.2 hours	0.165 0.511	—	2.5	—
^{111}In	2 to 5 mCi	2.8 days	0.173 0.247	6.4 to 16	1.3 to 3.3	13.2 to 33
Radiocolloids						
Gold-198 colloid	1 to 2.5 mCi	2.7 days	0.411	50 to 100	4 to 10	—
Technetium-99m–sulfur colloid	6 mCi	6 hours	0.140	1.8	0.2	—

*From Rocha, A. F. G., and Harbert, J. C., editors: Textbook of nuclear medicine: clinical applications, Philadelphia, 1979, Lea & Febiger.
†Average dose administered to an adult patient for a marrow scan.
‡This dose adequate for imaging only with positron camera; 500 μCi required if properly equipped rectilinear scanner is to be used (see text).

control tests.[15] Other binders, more recently described, have not yet been adequately tested, but no matter how good they prove to be, the stable radiolabeled folate compound will remain the same; so there seems little hope of developing a reproducible, stable, sensitive, and specific assay for folates in biologic materials by the CPB assay approach.

Serum ferritin assay

In contrast, the recent development of an immunoradiometric assay for human ferritin has made quantitative measurement of this substance in the serum possible for the first time and has already been proved to be clinically useful. This test is at present of greatest clinical use in the differential diagnosis of patients with low serum iron concentrations; those with iron deficiency have a greatly reduced serum ferritin level, whereas patients with low serum iron associated with the anemia of chronic disease have a normal or high level of circulating ferritin. These assays are far more reliable in this regard than the older measurements of iron-binding capacity, and often will save the patient the need for a bone marrow aspiration solely for the purpose of visually assessing body-iron stores.

Commercial kits are available for this assay, but ongoing thorough quality control by each laboratory introducing this test is necessary to ensure valid test results.

IMAGING THE HEMATOPOIETICALLY ACTIVE BONE MARROW IN MAN

Bone marrow aspiration and biopsy are useful clinical tools, but they suffer from the limitations that they sample only a small portion of that organ. A method that evaluated the functional integrity of the total blood-forming organ would serve to provide much more useful information, particularly if radiopharmaceuticals were available to delineate the functional status of each cell line (erythrocytes, leukocytes, and so on). Marrow scanning offers one such approach[9,16] and is useful in selected patients, but is limited to date by the nature of the radiopharmaceuticals available. To date only two physiologic processes of the functional bone marrow can be studied by scanning of that organ: (1) tracer doses of transferrin-bound radioactive iron are rapidly cleared from the circulation and deposited in areas of the marrow with active erythropoiesis; these agents permit scanning of the erythroid marrow, or "erythron." (2) Phagocytic cells in the marrow accumulate radiocolloids; although a smaller percent of an injected radiocolloid accumulates in the marrow than in the liver and spleen, use of the permissible larger doses of colloids made of short-lived gamma ray–emitting nuclides allows scanning of the functional reticuloendothelial marrow. Table 15-8 summarizes the physical properties of these radiopharmaceuticals.

Iron 59 (^{59}Fe) is not suitable for imaging the active erythrocyte-producing ("erythron") areas of the marrow with satisfactory spatial resolution because of its high gamma energy. Iron 52 (^{52}Fe), a short-lived positron emitter, provides excellent images with a positron camera[1] or, after a substantially larger patient dose of ^{52}Fe, with rectilinear scanners equipped with special high-energy collimators. Several investigators[14,18,19] have shown it to be highly satisfactory as an erythron label both in the presence of disease and under nor-

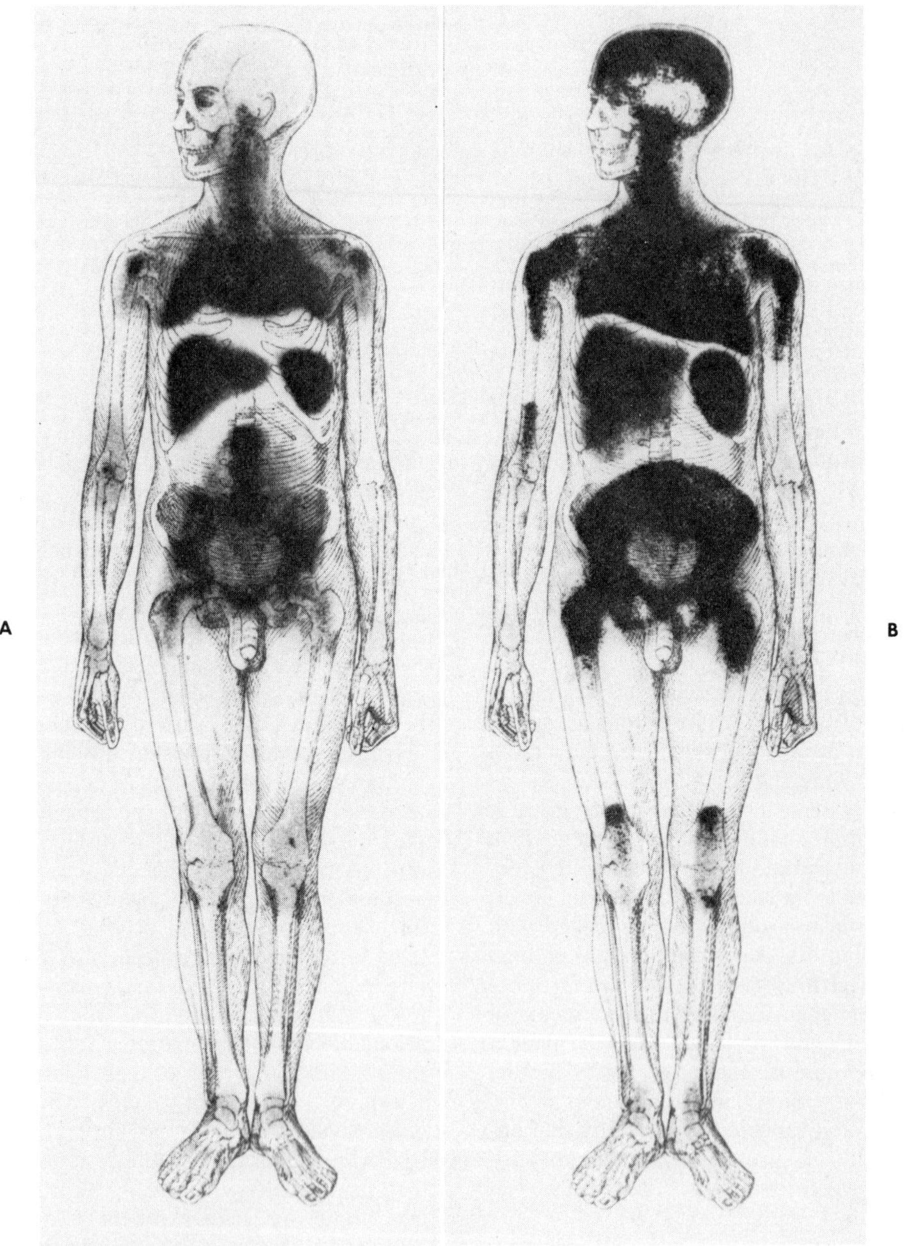

Fig. 15-3. A, Normal patient showing reticuloendothelial-system marrow activity only in axial bones and proximal parts of humeri and femora. **B,** In polycythemia vera, hyperplasia of central and peripheral expansion of RES marrow are seen. (By permission from Wagner, H. N., Jr., editor: Nuclear medicine, New York, 1974, Hospital Practice Publishing Co., Inc.)

mal conditions. Because of its short half-life and because it is cyclotron produced, it is not widely available.

There was transitory hope that indium-111 chloride might provide a substitute for ^{52}Fe for marrow scans in man. The basis for this expectation was the fact that ionic indium at low pH binds, like iron, to unsaturated transferrin.[13] However, studies have demonstrated that the biologic behavior of indium-bound transferrin is significantly different from that of iron bound to transferrin.[2,3,12,17,20]

Regardless of the type of radiopharmaceutical agent used, the pattern of marrow-activity distribution in normal humans is identical; in adults, the active marrow is confined to the axial skeleton and the proximal one third of both humeri and femora; in young children, some degree of peripheral marrow activity, especially in the long bones of the leg, is a normal variant. Abnormalities in the scan of the marrow may include one or more of the following: (1) There is a decrease or increase in activity in the central (axial) portion of the marrow. (2) There is a reduction or increase of activity in the proximal portions of the long bones, or varying degrees of extension of marrow activity farther down the long bones (in extreme instances of marrow hyperplasia, such as seen in some patients with chronic, severe hemolytic anemias, active marrow may be visualized in other osseous structures, that is, the maxillae and mandible). In these other conditions active erythroid marrow may be seen in nonosseous structures; that is known as extramedullary hematopoiesis. (3) There are focal defects, which may be single or multiple in areas of normal marrow activity. These most often are clearly distinguished in pelvic views by a camera.

Direct comparison of ^{52}Fe and ^{99m}Tc-sulfur colloid scans done in subjects with a wide variety of hematologic disorders have shown them to be nearly identical. One clear exception occurs in patients with pure erythrocyte aplasia wherein no ^{52}Fe is present in the marrow, whereas the reticuloendothelial-system marrow scan shows both hypertrophy and expansion of those phagocytic cells of the marrow. Since there are no erythrocyte precursors in the marrow of patients with this disorder, this discrepancy could have been predicted, but here is an excellent example of the fact that the marrow scan pattern alone is rarely diagnostic. It should always be interpreted in light of other clinical and hematologic features of the patient.

The dose of ^{99m}Tc-sulfur colloid is calculated to body surface area with use of a ratio of 12 mCi for an average 70 kg adult area of 1.7 meters. Anterior and posterior whole body scans or camera images of specific areas are routine. The camera views include the lateral skull, both shoulders, anterior pelvis, lumbar spine, posterior pelvis, both hips, and both knees. All the camera images are done for the same preset time. Thus, with a standardized dose, and careful attention to scan and camera-image factors, one can make a visual semiquantitative assessment of the overall and regional reticuloendothelial-system function (Fig. 15-3).

Liver and spleen scans should be obtained after appropriate adjustments in the instrument settings. This additional information is often of importance in patients with hematologic or malignant disorders.

REFERENCES

1. Anger, H. O., and Van Dyke, D.: Human bone marrow distribution shown in vivo by ^{52}Fe and the positron scintillation camera, Science **144:**1587-1589, 1964.
2. Beamish, M. R., and Brown, E. B.: The metabolism of transferrin-bound ^{111}In and ^{59}Fe in the rat, Blood **43:**693-702, 1974.
3. Beamish, M. R., and Brown, E. B.: A comparison of the behavior of ^{111}In and ^{59}Fe-labeled transferrin on incubation with human and rat reticulocytes, Blood **43:**703, 1974.
4. Belcher, E. H., Berlin, N. I., Eernisse, J. G., et al.: Recommended methods for radioisotope platelet survival studies by the panel, Blood **50:**1137-1144, 1977.
5. Belcher, E. H., Berlin, N. I., Eernisse, J. G., et al.: Standard techniques for the measurement of red cell and plasma volume, Br. J. Haematol. **25:**801-814, 1973.
6. Belcher, E. H., Berlin, N. I., Dudley, R. A., et al.: Recommended methods for measurement of red cell and plasma volume, J. Nucl. Med. **21:**793-800, 1980.
7. Belcher, E. H., Berlin, N. I., Eernisse, J. G., et al.: Recommended methods for radioisotope red-cell survival studies, Br. J. Haematol. **21:**241-250, 1971.
8. Cooper, B. A., and Whitehead, V. M.: Evidence that some patients with pernicious anemia are not recognized by radiodilution assay for cobalamin in serum, N. Engl. J. Med. **299:**816-818, 1978.
9. Dibos, P. E., Judisch, J. M., Spaulding, M. B., Wagner, H. N., Jr., and McIntyre, P. A.: Scanning the reticuloendothelial system (RES) in hematologic diseases, Johns Hopkins Med. J. **130:**68-81, 1972.
10. Ducassou, D., Arnaud, D., Bardy, A., Beydon, J., Hégésippe, M., and Baquey, C.: A new stannous agent list for labeling red blood cells with ^{99m}Tc and its clinical application, Br. J. Radiol. **49:**344-347, 1979.
11. Eckelman, W., Richards, P., Hausen, W., and Atkins, H.: Technetium-labeled red blood cells, J. Nucl. Med. **12:**22-24, 1971.
12. Graber, S. E., Hurley, P. J., Heyssel, R. M., and McIntyre, P. A.: Behavior of iron, indium and iodine labeled transferrin in the pregnant rat, Proc. Soc. Exp. Biol. Med. **133:**1093, 1970.
13. Hosain, F., McIntyre, P. A., Poulose, K. P., Stern, H. S., and Wagner, H. N., Jr.: Binding of trace amounts of ionic indium to plasma transferrin, Clin. Chim. Acta **24:**69-75, 1969.

13a. Jones, J., and Mollison, P. L.: A simple and efficient method of labelling red cells with ^{99m}Tc for determination of red cell volume, Br. J. Haematol. **38:**141, 1978.

14. Knosde, W. H., Rayudu, G. V. S., Cardello, M., Friedman, A. M., and Fordham, E.: Bone marrow scanning with ^{52}Fe. Regeneration and extension of marrow after ablative doses of radiotherapy, Cancer **37:**1432-1442, 1976.
15. Kubasik, N. P., Volosin, M. T., and Sine, H. E.: Comparison of commercial kits for radioimmunoassay. III. Radioassay of serum folate, Clin. Chem. **21:**1922-1926, 1975.

16. McIntyre, P. A.: Agents for bone marrow imaging: an evaluation. In Subramanian, G., Rhodes, B., Cooper, J., and Sodd, V., editors: Radiopharmaceuticals, New York, 1975, The Society of Nuclear Medicine, Inc.
17. McIntyre, P. A., Larson, S. M., Eikman, E. A., Colman, M., Scheffel, U., and Hodkinson, B. A.: Comparison of the metabolism of iron labeled transferrin (Fe-TF) and indium labeled transferrin (IN-TF) by the erythropoietic marrow, J. Nucl. Med. **15**:856-862, 1974.
18. Van Dyke, D., Anger, H. O., and Pollycove, M.: The effect of erythropoietic stimulation on marrow distribution in man, rabbit and rat as shown by ^{59}Fe and ^{52}Fe, Blood **24**:356-371, 1964.
19. Van Dyke, D., Shkurkin, C., Price, D., Yano, Y., and Anger, H. O.: Differences in distribution of erythropoietic and reticuloendothelial marrow in hematologic disease, Blood **30**:364-374, 1967.
20. Wochner, R. D., Adatepe, M., Van Amburg, A., and Potchen, E. J.: A new method for estimation of plasma volume with the use of the distribution space of indium-113m-transferrin, J. Lab. Clin. Med. **75**:711-720, 1970.

Chapter 16

INFLAMMATORY PROCESS AND TUMOR IMAGING

Sara Jane Davis and David F. Preston

Carrier-free gallium-67 citrate is the most frequently used radiopharmaceutical for the detection and staging of cancer. In the last 6 years, it has also been used for inflammation and abscess detection. The physiologic, anatomic, radiopharmaceutical, historic, and technical basis of gallium imaging is summarized.

PHYSIOLOGY AND ANATOMY

Cancer

Cancer is an uncontrolled overgrowth of cells often associated with the development of tumor nodules at sites remote from the original tumor usually leading to the death of the patient. In the last 15 years remarkable improvement in life expectancy has occurred in several types of cancer. Early stages of Hodgkin's disease and choriocarcinoma are now considered curable. The concept of cancer as a systemic process, involving the entire body, perhaps through altered immune mechanisms, has been popularized only in the last several years. The increasing success of chemotherapy, radiation therapy, and surgery is to a great extent dependent on early diagnosis of cancer. Staging, defining the extent of the disease at the time of diagnosis, has permitted appropriate therapy to be instituted. The stage of the disease and its response to treatment are parts of a data base with which results of new innovations in therapy may be measured against the established therapeutic modalities. It is in this area of staging that ^{67}Ga imaging had its initial use.

No one is sure when a cancer begins. There are situations where a sequence of cellular change, whose final outcome is frank cancer, can be identified under the microscope. An incomplete list of organs where premalignant lesions have been identified includes the skin, lung, cervix, and colon. The pathologist identifies the premalignant lesions by unusual changes in the nuclei of the cells, by changes in the cytoplasm, and by loss of the usual orientation of cells. If the atypical cells have invaded the surrounding tissue or blood vessels, a malignancy is considered to exist.

For cancer to continue to grow, new blood vessels must develop. When a cancer reaches a certain size, capillaries from surrounding tissue grow toward the cancer and provide it with an adequate blood supply. Cancer implants in the anterior chamber of rabbit eyes appear to release a substance that causes local capillary proliferation. The increased blood supply permits increased nutriments, leukocytes, and antibodies to be exposed to the cancer. Many cancers are associated with large accumulations of serum proteins.[1]

There are many occasions when the center of a cancer will become necrotic because the central blood flow is insufficient to maintain cellular life. Often these are fast-growing cancers whose rapid growth at the periphery usurps the blood needed centrally. The anoxic center has implications for radiation therapy. Decreased oxygenation is associated with decreased radiation responsiveness; therefore the implication for nuclear medicine is obvious: the radiopharmaceutical is not delivered to the central portion of the cancer and these tumors are imaged as having intense activity peripherally with decreased activity centrally.

The surface of a tumor cell contains antigens that are characteristic of the tumor. Antibodies to these antigens have been labeled with gamma ray–emitting radionuclides. In experimental situations, tumor localization by external imaging has been demonstrated when the antibody specific for the tumor has been labeled.[2]

Abscess

Pyogenic abscesses may be found in any part of the body. Typically an abscess will begin with a small nidus of inflammation, increased capillary permeability, capillary leakage of serum proteins and increasing concentrations of white cells. The increased permeability of the surrounding capillaries is caused by release of histamine and the capability of some bacteria to release toxins.

The neutrophil is the white cell that is most involved in the defense against pyogenic bacteria. If the blood supply does not bring adequate neutrophils to the nidus of infection, the bacteria will increase in number. The process of inflammation causes release of certain substances, called "leukotaxines," that cause leukocytes to migrate to the area of inflammation. Some bacteria such as staphylococci release a toxin, a coagulase, that causes deposition of fibrin, thereby walling off the bacteria from neutrophils and antibiotics. Streptococci produce hemolysins, which cause destruction of erythrocytes. A large cluster of vigorously growing bacteria may produce toxins that destroy neutrophils. As local blood flow brings more neutrophils to the scene, the neutrophils attempt to engulf the bacteria and digest them with packets of enzymes called "lysosomes." The mixture of dead bacteria, dead granulocytes, and fluid is commonly known as pus. If the pus accumulates faster than the local circulation can remove it, the inflammatory volume expands and its center becomes a small volume of pus with viable bacteria. This is an abscess. At the periphery of the abscess new neutrophils arrive, fibrinogen and other serum proteins accumulate, fibrin is deposited, and the abscess becomes walled off. This wall is called the "pyogenic membrane."

The pyogenic membrane helps to isolate the abscess and limit its spread. Unrecognized abscesses are a common cause of death in seriously ill hospitalized patients.

There are five major areas of localized infection in which gallium-67 imaging may play a major role. Bacterial endocarditis is a serious medical emergency where bacteria colonize a heart valve, usually the aortic or mitral valve. If not detected in time, the valve may be destroyed or scarred to the point of deformity and incompetence. Additionally, small particles of fibrin and bacteria may break off from the valve and be carried by the bloodstream to embolize any area. Embolization of the brain, eyes, and kidneys is most common. The diagnosis of bacterial endocarditis is difficult, especially in a patient with previous unsuccessful antibiotic therapy. Recent dental extractions, intravenous drug abuse, and infections from other areas of the body may precede and cause bacterial endocarditis.

Lung abscesses may occur from certain types of pneumonia or as a result of chronic lung disease or infection anywhere in the body. Lung cancer obstructing a bronchus may cause a localized pneumonia and eventually an abscess behind the obstruction.

A pelvic abscess may occur from pelvic inflammatory disease, a ruptured diverticulum of the colon, appendicitis, regional ileitis, or prior surgery. Subdiaphragmatic and intra-abdominal abscesses may be associated with perforated duodenal ulcers. Even in the antibiotic era, an abscess usually requires surgical drainage. Successful antibiotic treatment of a well-organized abscess may be impossible and may result in organisms resistant to antibiotics; therefore precise localization is imperative.

HISTORICAL PERSPECTIVES OF GALLIUM

The element gallium was discovered in 1875 by the French chemist Lecoq de Boisbaudran. Gallium is a metal with a low melting point of about 30° Celsius. It has been used in industrial high-temperature thermometers, has been investigated as a reactor coolant, and more recently has found use in light-emitting diode displays. Gallium is similar to aluminum in many of its chemical properties.

CHEMICAL TOXICITY

Gallium toxicity[3] is characterized by symptoms of vomiting, skin rash, proteinuria, anemia, and leukopenia when given to humans in doses of up to 71 mg/kg. Gallium toxicity is variable depending on the experimenal animal.[4] Six millicuries of ^{67}Ga contain only 10 ng[5] of elemental gallium, providing a substantial chemical-toxicity safety factor. In present-day clinical studies, carrier-free gallium citrate is the radiopharmaceutical used. In early preparations, excess citrate became bound to calcium and caused hypocalcemia.[6] This has not been a problem with the amounts of citrate currently used (2 mg of sodium citrate per 2 mCi of ^{67}Ga).

Gallium has 14 known isotopes ranging in mass number from 63 to 78. Because of an inappropriate half-life, type of emission, and production problems, only ^{67}Ga, ^{68}Ga, and ^{72}Ga seem likely to be useful in clinical nuclear medicine. Between 1949 and 1951, ^{72}Ga was first investigated by Dudley[7-9] as a diagnostic and therapeutic agent for osteogenic sarcoma and metastases to bone. ^{72}Ga was not especially valuable in these situations, but the bone-seeking property of gallium was demonstrated. In the early 1960s Brookhaven National Laboratories developed a germanium-68/gallium-68 generator. ^{68}Ge has a long half-life, 280 days, and decays to ^{68}Ga, a positron emitter with a half-life of 68 minutes. The long-lived germanium parent and the short-lived gallium daughter looked like a promising combination for clinical use. ^{68}Ga as ethylenediaminetetraacetic acid (EDTA) was used with some success as a brain-imaging agent.[10,11] The citrate was investigated as a bone-imaging agent; however neither radiopharmaceutical was widely used. By 1965 the technetium generator was commercially available, and pertechnetate quickly became the agent of choice for brain imaging. The scintillation camera with its ½-inch-thick crystal was rather inefficient in stopping the 511 keV annihilation photon of ^{68}Ga. A 360 keV collimator was the standard high-energy collimator provided, and resolution was greatly impaired by septal penetration. In 1967 a prototype two-detector positron camera was available but was not mass produced. With the advent of newer positron imaging devices the germanium-68/gallium-68 generator may return to nuclear medicine.

In 1965 there was no technetium-labeled phosphate for bone imaging. That year Hayes[12] from the Medical Division, Oak Ridge Institute of Nuclear studies, reconfirmed earlier work[13] showing ^{67}Ga administered with carrier gallium to localize in bones within hours, with carrier-free ^{67}Ga being concentrated in bones much later. After 2 to 3 days there was enough bone-to-background difference with carrier-free ^{67}Ga that an investigation of the usefulness of this product as a bone-imaging agent was begun. In 1968, while performing bone scans with carrier-free ^{67}Ga citrate on patients with a known malignancy and suspected bone lesions, Edwards and Hayes noted intense uptake in tumor.[14] In this initial report, they found that carrier-free ^{67}Ga citrate concentrated in soft-tissue tumors, especially in those without prior radiation therapy or chemotherapy. They also found that false negatives did occur, and they found tumor sites not previously detected by other modalities. With this evidence of tumor detection, Oak Ridge Associated Universities (ORAU) in a cooperative study with 16 universities performed nearly 3000 scans between 1970 and 1974, firmly establishing the utility of carrier-free ^{67}Ga citrate in staging and detecting cancer. Over the last 6 years there have been numerous reports of the utility of gallium tumor-and-abscess imaging, in addition to the ORAU Cooperative Group publications.[15-17]

PRODUCTION OF GALLIUM 67

Carrier-free ^{67}Ga is cyclotron produced by the proton bombardment of a zinc oxide target. The reactions are as follows:

$$^{67}Zn(p,n)^{67}Ga$$
$$^{68}Zn(p,2n)^{67}Ga$$

^{67}Zn and ^{68}Zn occur with a natural abundance of 4% and 18%, respectively.

How "free" is "carrier free"? If natural zinc targets are used, as much as 4 μg of stable gallium may contaminate each milliliter of the final "carrier-free" gallium[18] depending on the amount of stable gallium in the target. Ten millicuries of ^{67}Ga contain 15×10^{13} atoms of ^{67}Ga. The 40 μg of stable gallium in 10 ml contains 36×10^{16} atoms, about 2400 stable gallium atoms for each radioactive atom when the target is from natural zinc. Carrier-free gallium made from a natural zinc target is not really carrier free. Recently improvements have been made in enriching the target so that it is 99% ^{68}Zn. ^{67}Ga made from such a target will contain no stable gallium in the final injectate.

Additional production methods such as alpha-particle bombardment of a zinc target, deuteron bombardment of a zinc target, and alpha-particle bombardment of a copper target are available.

BIODISTRIBUTION DIFFERENCES BETWEEN CARRIER-FREE AND CARRIER-ADDED GALLIUM CITRATE

When nanograms of ^{67}Ga per kilogram of body weight are injected into humans, the percent activity per organ is far different from the percent activity per organ when the same amount of ^{67}Ga is accompanied with milligram per kilogram body-weight quantities of stable gallium.[12] In the carrier-free state ^{67}Ga concentrates first in the liver, soft tissues, abscesses, and some cancers. After 2 to 3 days, it will concentrate slightly in bone. With carrier gallium added, ^{67}Ga will initially concentrate more heavily in bone. Differences in the citrate concentration between manufacturers has been found and may account for diagnostic differences reported in the literature.[19]

DISTRIBUTION OF CARRIER-FREE GALLIUM CITRATE

After the intravenous injection of carrier-free ^{67}Ga citrate there is binding to serum proteins probably transferrin[20,21] and alpha and beta globulins with little activity in albumin and gamma globulins.[22] Blood clearance is fairly rapid initially, with only 25% of the injected dose remaining in the blood at 3 hours. Only 7% remains at 24 hours, 5% remains at 40 hours, and only 2% remains in the intravascular space at 5 days. Once gallium has entered a tissue, it will remain there. Ten to 15% of the injected dose is excreted in the urine in the first 24 hours, whereas approximately 10% of the injected dose will be excreted in the stool. Accounting for decay, 65% remains in the body.[23] Twenty percent of the dose is eliminated with an effective half-life of 69.5 hours[24] (Fig. 16-1).

There have been attempts in the past to increase the target-to-background ratio of gallium images. The first involved the administration of stable scandium, an element with properties similar to gallium. Administered to animals, scandium caused a definite decrease in background gallium. When scandium administration was tried with humans, a hemolytic anemia was caused. In animals there has been success with the administration of iron-dextran complex (Imferon) to decrease the blood background and significantly enhance the target-to-background ratio.[25,26]

From autopsy studies the five organs with the greatest mean percent injected dose per kilogram are the spleen (4%), the renal cortex (3.8%), bone marrow (3.6%), liver (2.8%), and bone (1.4%).[23] From patient to patient there was a tenfold range of activity

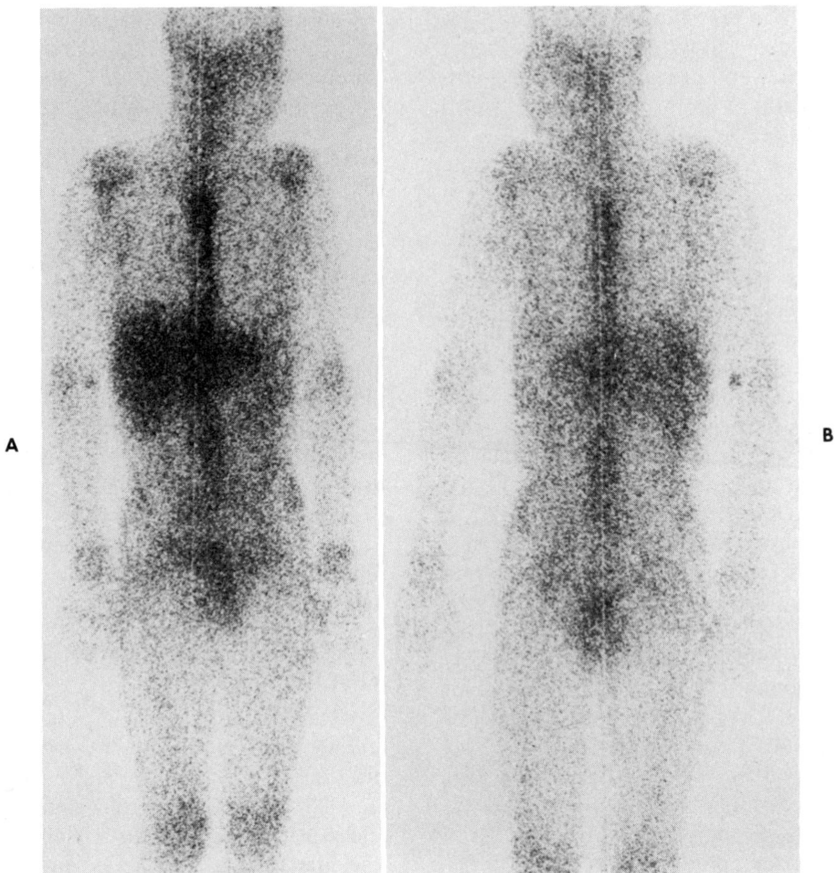

Fig. 16-1. Scintigrams demonstrating normal distribution of carrier-free gallium citrate. **A,** Anterior. **B,** Posterior.

for each organ. Brain and muscle contained one seventh to one fortieth the activity of the five most active organs.

The mechanism of gallium concentration in tumor tissue remains unknown. Several proposed mechanisms of gallium uptake in tumors include increased tumor vascularity, increased pore size of tumor cell membranes, increased localization in rapidly growing tumors, binding of gallium to tumor proteins after dissociation caused by a drop in pH, and intracellular exchange of gallium for calcium. The most probable and most important mechanism involves a tumor's increased avidity for serum proteins. The engulfing of serum proteins by tumor cells is called "pinocytosis" and may be responsible for the ^{67}Ga-protein complex entering the cells. Careful fragmentation of the tumor into its various intracellular components showed gallium to reside in the lysosomal fraction of the tumor cell.[27,28] Lysosomes are intracellular structures that contain enzymes and lysozymes useful in digesting bacteria and intracellular debris.

Great variations in tumor uptake are seen from one tumor to another within the same patient. In general, tumors with a significant fibrotic or necrotic component will accumulate less than usual amounts of gallium. Tumors with less than 5% of injected dose per kilogram are very difficult to visualize, as well as those tumors under 2 cm in diameter.

Does gallium concentration by a tumor and the rate of DNA synthesis have an association? This question was examined in experimental animals with tumors. In small tumors, Harding-Passey melanomas, there was decreased gallium uptake with increased DNA synthesis, but in larger tumors there was increased gallium uptake associated with increased DNA synthesis. Chemotherapy of some experimental tumors caused a sharp reduction in DNA synthesis but no change in gallium uptake.[29]

TECHNICAL CONSIDERATIONS

Imaging protocols usually consist in establishing guidelines for dosages, optimal time after injection

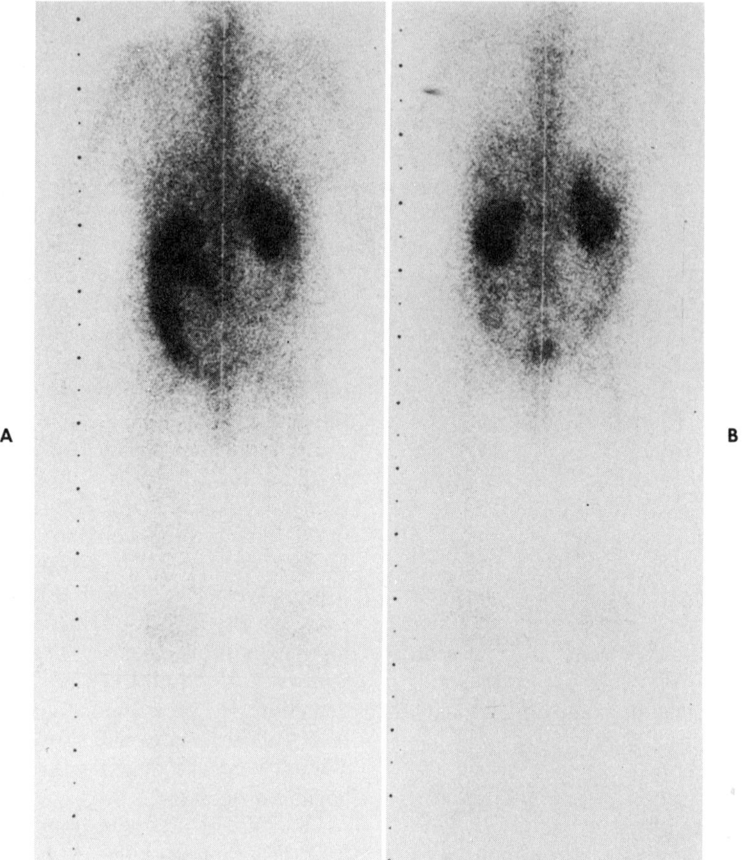

Fig. 16-2. Scintigram demonstrating accumulation of gallium-containing feces in colon before, **A,** and after, **B,** cleansing enema. Note excessive renal uptake.

for imaging, photopeak settings, information density, collimation, and positioning. Certain data such as decay mode and dosimetry must be presented as a rationale for these guidelines. Variations of the guidelines will occur depending on the instrumentation available.

Preparation prior to scanning with ^{67}Ga citrate must be twofold: physical and emotional.

The physical preparation is primarily concerned with the elimination of gallium containing feces from the colon (Fig. 16-2). Nine to 15% of the gallium is excreted through the bowel, especially in the first 24 hours. At that time gallium that accumulates in the bowel is seen as areas of increased activity that may be mistaken for cancer, abscess, or inflammation. In the first 24 hours gallium may attach itself to newly forming colon mucosal cells, which over the course of several days may be shed into the lumen of the colon. During the time when the gallium is in the mucosa, bowel cleansing will not be successful in removing activity from the abdomen.

The more commonly used bowel preparations are a combination of bisacodyl tablets and magnesium citrate, or cleansing enemas. Little research has been done on the efficacy of this type of preparation. Zeman and Ryerson[30] reported that patients given bisacodyl tablets and magnesium citrate showed no greater bowel clearance than did patients without preparation. Other reports claim bowel preparation to be necessary.[31] The patient's diet is another variable. It is likely, but as yet unproved, that patients on a normal diet will have a greater clearance of gallium from the bowel than will patients on a low-bulk, or liquid, diet. If possible, a regular diet should be continued. If the patient has diarrhea, bowel preparation is unnecessary and may aggravate dehydration and electrolyte loss. Accumulation of gallium in the abdomen in patients with diarrhea is almost always indicative of a pathologic condition.

The emotional aspect of gallium scanning is important and often unappreciated. Adequate emotional preparation can yield many benefits: decreased motion, decreased imaging time, fewer repeat views, and less time spent explaining the examination after the fact. Credibility is greater when the explanation is initiated by the person performing the test. Ethically and practically, a technologist should never inform a patient of anything related to the patient's specific condition nor supply a patient with any records that his physician has not cleared; however the patient should be informed of the duration of the overall gallium study. Depending on the type of equipment and on the dose, this will range from 40 minutes to 3 hours. A longer examination than expected may be a threatening experience that can be prevented by the patient's prior knowledge of the duration of the test. The patient should also know that he needs to be still during the procedure and various views may be required.

Using a camera with a scanning table or its equivalent, the patient should be placed comfortably supine and imaged posteriorly from below the table and then anteriorly from above to include all the body from the top of the head to approximately midthigh. If a prone position is used, the head, neck, and perhaps shoulder will be rotated in an undesirable semioblique position that requires a static image of the neck so that both right and left cervical areas may be compared. In addition, the prone position is usually painful if there has been recent abdominal surgery.

Doses for intravenous injection of carrier-free ^{67}Ga citrate range from 2 to 5 mCi for a 70 kg adult. Several institutions use 10 mCi doses for larger adults with known cancer. The injection site should be chosen to avoid a potential site of clinical interest. The technologist should always record the date, time, and site of injection.

RADIATION CHARACTERISTICS OF GALLIUM

Gallium 67 has a 78-hour (3.25-day) half-life and decays by electron capture. It has four principal gamma-ray energies, shown in Table 16-1. The radiation-absorbed dose from 5 mCi of ^{67}Ga citrate is recorded in Table 16-2.[32]

Table 16-1. Gallium-67 radionuclide characteristics*

Nuclide	Production	Half-life	Principal radiations MeV	%
Gallium 67	^{67}Zn(p,n)^{67}Ga	78 hours	0.093	40
	^{68}Zn(p,2n)^{67}Ga		0.184	24
			0.296	22
			0.388	7

*From Radiological health handbook, Washington, D.C., 1970, Bureau of Radiological Health, U.S. Department of Health, Education, and Welfare.

IMAGING TIME AFTER INJECTION

Imaging of a patient injected with ^{67}Ga citrate may range from 6 hours to 1 week after injection. Gallium will remain in tissue once it is deposited, and the target-to-background ratio will increase with the passage of time as blood clearance progresses. Considerations other than target-to-background ratios, such as the urgency of possible surgery for an abscess, the cost of hospitalization, the fact that imaging time increases with physical decay, and the necessity of delaying other studies that might interfere, may dictate earlier rather than later imaging.

Hopkins and Mende have evaluated ^{67}Ga citrate imaging for subphrenic abscess 6 hours after injection.[33] They found no additional positive sites at 24 or 72 hours when compared with the 6-hour scans. In another study,[34] it was noted that gallium citrate was not yet in the bowel at 6 hours, and in that study focal activity in the abdomen was indicative of a pathologic condition. Beihn[35] used combined technetium 99m–sulfur colloid liver and ^{67}Ga imaging for abscess detection. He subtracted technetium counts in the liver from gallium counts and showed that increased gallium counts were associated with early detection of intrahepatic abscesses.

Our own results with imaging at 12 to 24 hours has been less than optimal. Although it is true that many abscesses have been demonstrated at this time, we have found that more than half were equivocally detected and reimaging at 48 and even 72 hours was required.

Table 16-2. Radiation dosimetry for ^{67}Ga citrate*

Organ	^{67}Ga citrate (rads/5 mCi)
Whole body	1.3
Skeleton	2.2
Liver	2.3
Bone marrow	2.9
Spleen	2.65
Kidney	2.05 (calyx)
Ovary	1.4
Testes	1.2
Stomach	1.1
Small intestine	1.8
Upper colon	2.8
Lower colon	4.5
Thyroid	

*From Medical internal radiation dose (MIRD): dose estimate report no. 2, J. Nucl. Med. **14**:755, 1973.

INSTRUMENTATION AND TECHNIQUE VARIATIONS

There is a variety of equipment that may be used for gallium imaging. Initially rectilinear scanners, especially those with whole-body and minification capabilities, were used. In recent years, the evolution of the scintillation camera with its increase in field size and the introduction of multiple pulse-height analyzers has supplanted the rectilinear scanner. Scintillation cameras with whole body–imaging capabilities have also contributed to the demise of the rectilinear scanners.

Today there is a tomographic scanner (Pho-Con) that combines the focusing collimation of the rectilinear scanner with the multiple photomultiplier-tube electronics of the scintillation camera. This scanner uses a stationary table and moving detector heads and has proved to be a very satisfactory and perhaps superior instrument for gallium imaging (Figs. 16-3 and 16-4).

The use of medium-energy collimators (rated at 300 keV at least) is necessary because of the physical characteristics of gallium photon emission. If a low-energy collimator is used and the pulse-height analyzer is set at the 93 keV peak, scatter and septal penetration from the high-energy photons will destroy meaningful

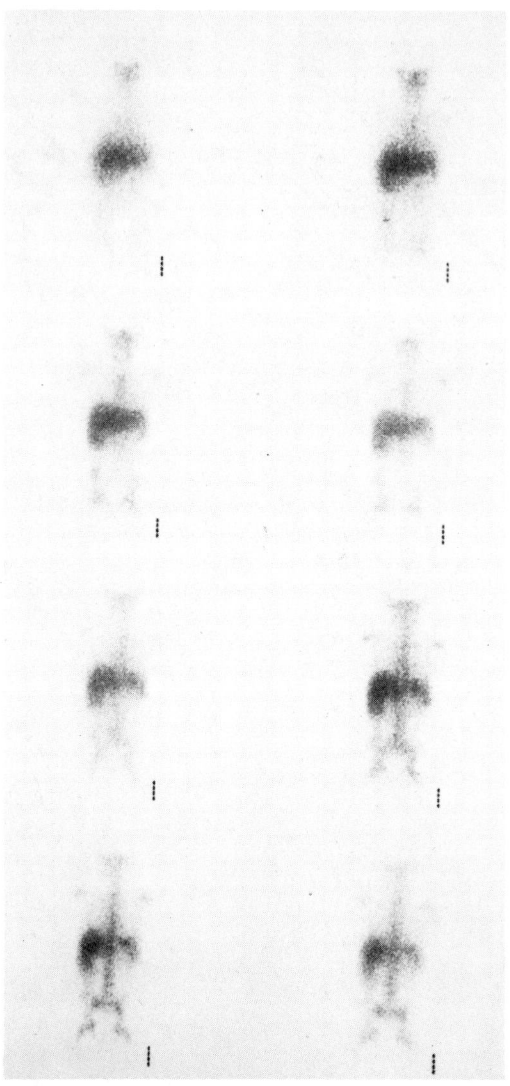

Fig. 16-3. Normal gallium scan using tomographic scanning camera (Pho/Con). (Courtesy Dr. Donald R. Germann, St. Luke's Hospital, Kansas City, Missouri.)

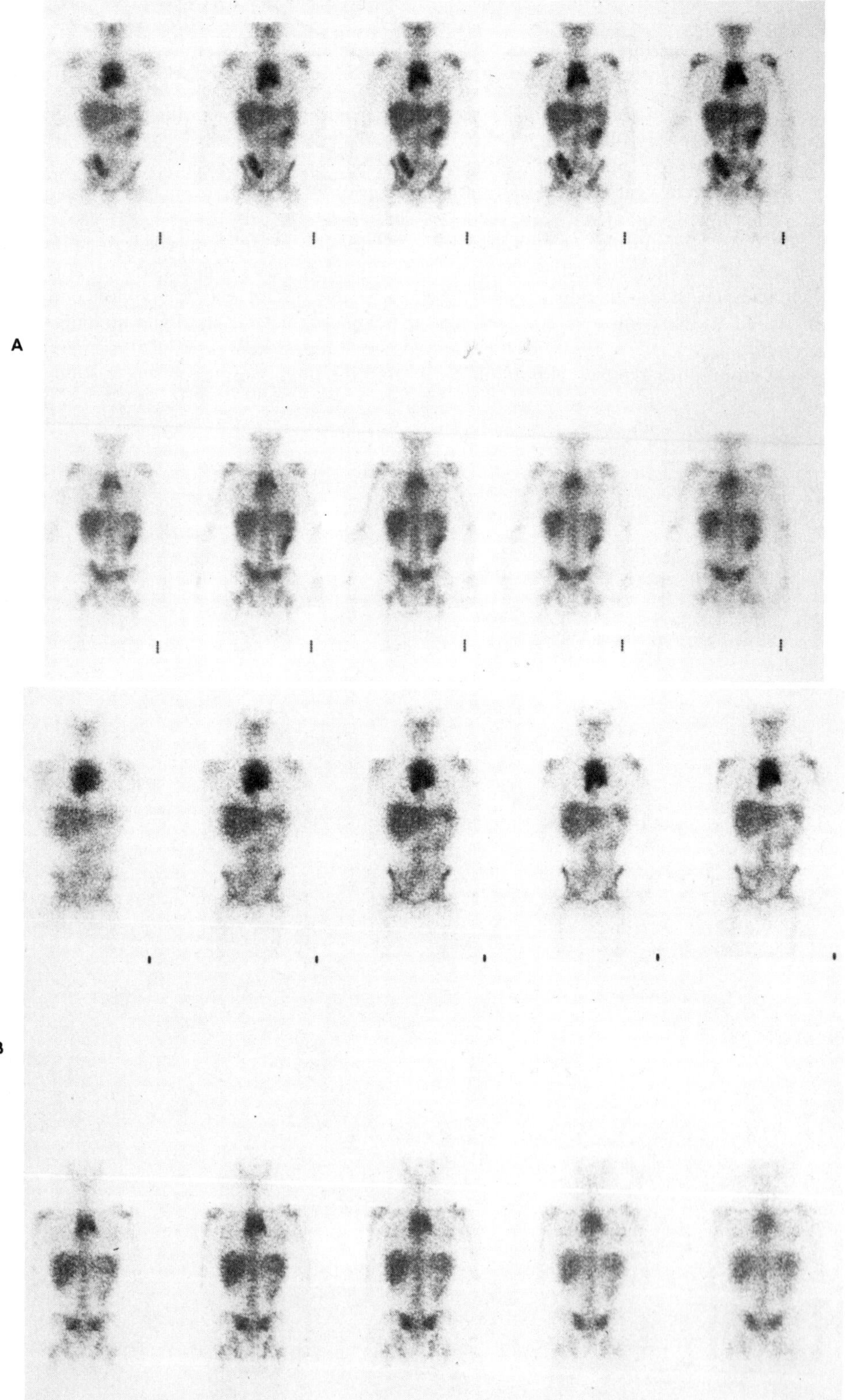

Fig. 16-4. A, Sixteen-year-old male with lymphoma is imaged at 24 hours. Bilateral mediastinal activity is abnormal. Right lower quadrant abdominal activity is probably in cecum. Left upper abdominal activity could be in spleen but probably is in colon. **B,** Scanned at 48 hours. Mediastianal activity is still present. Cecal activity has disappeared and left upper quadrant activity has decreased dramatically as would be expected with colon activity. (Courtesy Dr. Donald R. Germann, St. Luke's Hospital, Kansas City, Missouri.)

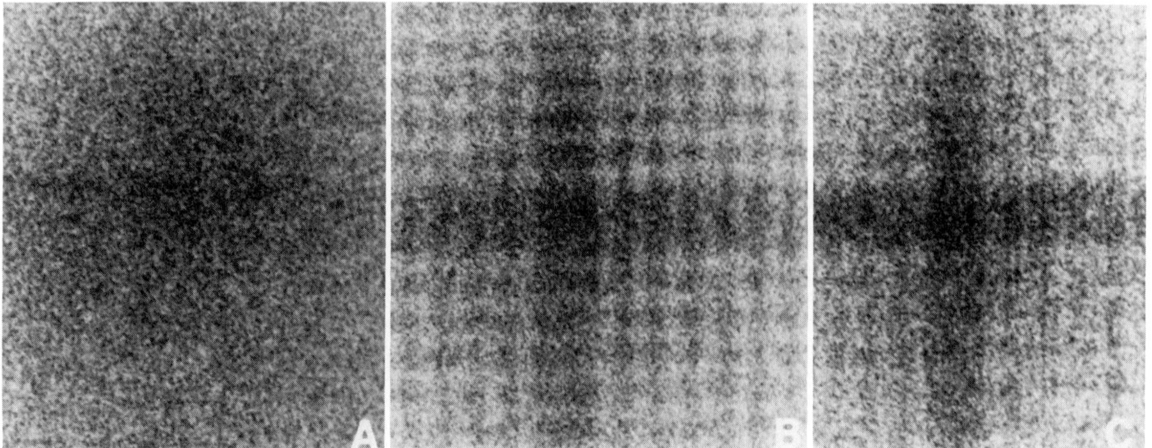

Fig. 16-5. Scintiphoto of a line phantom of gallium 67. Center cross has 1 cm line spacing, remainder has 2 cm line spacing. Scintiphoto was taken through 10 cm of scattering material with three photopeaks of gallium 67 being used: 93, 184, and 296 keV. All images are 2×10^6 counts. Collimator rated to, **A,** 140 keV; **B,** 280 keV; **C,** 400 keV.

resolution (Fig. 16-5). If a single photopeak is used, a medium-energy collimator and a 93 keV peak will usually be best. If two photopeaks can be summed, the 93 and the 184 keV peaks are chosen. Optimally the 93, 184, and 296 keV peaks with a medium-energy collimator are utilized. When three peaks can be used, the imaging time is halved with a constant information density when compared to the 94 keV peak alone. With all peaks we use a 20% window centered on each photopeak. This is critical when one uses the 93 keV peak because small amounts of 40-degree scatter will be detected even at 88 keV. Acceptance of excessive scatter will degrade spatial resolution.

Technically suboptimal images are the major cause of difficulty in the confident, accurate interpretation of gallium-67 studies. There must be adequate counts, and the intensity of those counts must be distributed over the dynamic range of the film. In whole-body scanning the sternal activity is made to correspond to a midpoint in the dynamic range of the film. Areas of increased or decreased activity will usually remain within the dynamic range of the film. If equivocal areas are noted, additional static images of 300,000 counts for a standard-field-of-view camera and 500,000 counts for a large-field-of-view camera are adequate. Repeating selected views, especially of the abdomen, at 48 hours and occasionally more delayed views at 72 and 96 hours are important to accurate clinical results.

SUMMARY

At this time, there is no radiopharmaceutical that is specific for cancer. Carrier-free ^{67}Ga citrate has had the greatest clinical experience. Even so, some nuclear medicine departments find it difficult to produce results that are helpful to clinicians. The nuclear medicine physician must develop confidence in the accuracy of his interpretation. If he lacks confidence in the ability of gallium imaging to detect abscesses and tumors, his report will be equivocal and nondiagnostic.

The future of nuclear medicine lies in the development of new radiopharmaceuticals that demonstrate altered biochemistry and physiology prior to the occurrence of an anatomic defect. To some degree, nuclear medicine has this capability now with carrier-free ^{67}Ga citrate. New radiopharmaceuticals, perhaps labeled antibodies, may dramatically improve the specificity of tumor imaging in the future. At present, carrier-free ^{67}Ga citrate used by informed technologists and physicians is the most satisfactory agent for tumor and abscess imaging. A nuclear physician must have an optimum image based on standard technical factors. Without a stable technique the physicians' report may become an expensive ''weather report'' which points in all directions and does little to aid the clinician.

REFERENCES

1. Ghose, T., Nairn, R. C., and Fothergill, J. E.: Uptake of proteins by malignant cells, Nature **196:**1108-1109, 1962.
2. Goldenberg, D. M., Preston, D. F., Primus, F. J., and Hanson, J. J.: Photoscan localization of GW-39 tumors in hamsters using radiolabeled anticarcinoembryonic antigen immunoglobulin G Cancer Res. **37:**1-9, 1974.
3. Dudley, H. C., and Levine, M. D.: Studies of the toxic action of gallium, Pharmacol. Exp. Ther. **95:**487-493, 1949.
4. Burner, H. D., Cooper, B. M., and Rehback, D. J.: A study of gallium. Part IV. Toxicity of gallium citrate in dogs and rats, Radiology **61:**550-555, 1953.

5. Quimby, E. H., and Feitelberg, S.: Physics and instrumentation, ed. 3, Philadelphia, 1970, Lea & Febiger, pp. 25-27.
6. Porter, J., Kawana, M., Krizek, H., Lathrop, K. A., and Harper, P. V.: ^{67}Ga production with a compact cyclotron, J. Nucl. Med. **10:**352, 1970. (Abstract)
7. Dudley, H. C., Maddox, G. E., and LaRue, H. C.: Studies of the metabolism of gallium, J. Pharmacol. Exp. Ther. **96:**135-138, 1949.
8. Dudley, H. C., Imirie, G. W., Jr., and Istoek, J. T.: Deposition of radiogallium (Ga^{72}) in proliferating tissues, Radiology **55:**571-578, 1950.
9. Mulry, W. C., and Dudley, H. C.: Studies of radiogallium as a diagnostic agent in bone tumors, J. Lab. Clin. Med. **37:**239-252, 1951.
10. Anger, H. O., and Gottschalk, A.: Localization of brain tumors with the positron scintillation camera, J. Nucl. Med. **4:**326-330, 1963.
11. Shealy, C. N., Aronow, S., and Brownell, G. L.: Gallium-68 as a scanning agent for intracranial lesion, J. Nucl. Med. **5:**161-167, 1964.
12. Andrews, G. A., Knisely, R. M., and Wagner, H. N.: Radioactive pharmaceuticals, AEC Symposium Series 6, Washington, D.C., April 1966, U.S. Atomic Energy Commission/Division of Technical Information, pp. 603-617.
13. Bruner, H. D., Hayes, R. L., and Perkinson, J. D.: Preliminary data on gallium-67, Radiology **61:**602-612, 1953.
14. Edwards, C. L., and Hayes, R. L.: Tumor scanning with ^{67}Ga citrate, J. Nucl. Med. **10:**103-108, 1969.
15. Johnston, G., Benua, R. S., Teates, C. D., et al.: ^{67}Ga-citrate imaging in untreated Hodgkin's disease: preliminary report of the cooperative group, J. Nucl. Med. **15:**399-403, 1974.
16. Greenlaw, R. H., Weinstein, M. B., Brill, A. B., et al.: ^{67}Ga-citrate imaging in untreated malignant lymphoma: preliminary report of the cooperative group, J. Nucl. Med. **15:**404-407, 1974.
17. DeLand, F. H., Sauerbrunn, B. J. L., Boyd, C., et al.: ^{67}Ga-citrate imaging in untreated primary lung cancer: preliminary report of the cooperative group, J. Nucl. Med. **15:**408-411, 1974.
18. Hirsch, J. I., Fratkin, J. M., and Sharpe, A. R., Jr.: Gallium-67 citrate, Drug Intell. Clin. Pharm. **7:**519-523, 1973.
19. Waxman, A. D., Kawada, T., Wolf, W., and Siemsen, J. K.: Are all gallium citrate preparations the same? Radiology **117:** 647-648, 1975.
20. Clausen, J., Edeling, C. J., and Fogh, J.: ^{67}Ga binding to human serum proteins and tumor components, Cancer Res. **34:** 1931-1937, 1974.
21. Gunasekera, S. W., King, L. J., and Lavender, P. H.: The behavior of tracer gallium-67 towards serum proteins, Clin. Chim. Acta **39:**401-406, 1972.
22. Hartman, R. F., and Hayes, R. L.: Gallium binding by blood serum, Fed. Proc. **26:**780, March 1967. (Abstract)
23. Nelson, B., Hayes, R. L., Edwards, C. L., Knisely, R. M., and Andrews, G. A.: The distribution of gallium in human tissues after intravenous administration, J. Nucl. Med. **13:**92-100, 1972.
24. Goswitz, F. A., Andrews, G. A., and Viamonte, M.: Clinical uses of radionuclides, AEC Symposium Series 27, Washington, D.C., Dec. 1972, U.S. AEC Office of Information Services.
25. Hill, J. H., Merz, T., and Wagner, H. N., Jr.: Iron-induced enhancement of ^{67}Ga uptake in a model human leukocyte culture system, J. Nucl. Med. **16:**1183-1186, 1975.
26. Oster, Z. H., Larson, S. M., and Wagner, H. N., Jr.: Possible enhancement of ^{67}Ga-citrate imaging by iron dextran, J. Nucl. Med. **17:**356-358, 1976.
27. Hayes, R. C., Nelson, B., Swartzendruber, D. C., Carlton, J. E., and Byrd, B. L.: Gallium-67 localization in rat and mouse tumors, Science **167:**289-290, 1970.
28. Swartzendruber, D. C., Nelson, B., and Hayes, R. L.: Gallium-67 localization in lysosomal-like granules of leukemic and nonleukemic murine tissues, J. Natl. Cancer Inst. **46:**941-952, 1971.
29. Subramanian, G., Rhodes, B. A., Cooper, J. F., and Sodd, V. S., editors: Radiopharmaceuticals, New York, 1975, The Society of Nuclear Medicine, Inc., pp. 447-451.
30. Zeman, R. K., and Ryerson, T. W.: Bowel preparation in ^{67}Ga-citrate scanning, J. Nucl. Med. **18:**886-889, 1977.
31. Bakshi, S. J., and Parthasarathy, K. L.: Combination of laxatives for cleansing of ^{67}Ga-citrate activity in the bowel, J. Nucl. Med. **15:**470, 1974.
32. Medical internal radiation dose (MIRD): dose estimate report no. 2: J. Nucl. Med. **14:**755-756, 1973.
33. Hopkins, G. B., and Mende, C. W.: Gallium-67 and subphrenic abscesses—Is delayed scintigraphy necessary? J. Nucl. Med. **16:**609-611, 1975.
34. Hopkins, G. B., Kan, M., and Mende, C. W.: Early Ga^{67} scintigraphy for the localization of abdominal abscesses, J. Nucl. Med. **16:**990-992, 1975.
35. Beihn, R. M., Damron, J. R., and Hafner, T.: Subtraction technique for the detection of subphrenic abscess using ^{67}Ga and ^{99m}Tc, J. Nucl. Med. **15:**371-373, 1974.

Chapter 17

PEDIATRIC IMAGING

Paul Cole and Philip O. Alderson

The principles of nuclear medicine apply equally well to adults and children. Nevertheless there are important differences that must be considered from both the clinical and technical standpoint.

TECHNICAL CONSIDERATIONS

The scintillation camera is the instrument of choice for pediatric nuclear imaging procedures. Its ability to produce high-resolution images in a short period of time has made the rectilinear scanner obsolete in pediatric work.

The use of magnification to improve resolution is applied when neonates and infants are studied. The use of either a pinhole or converging collimator will give magnification when small objects are imaged at short distances. The resultant improvement in resolution is a decided diagnostic advantage. A detailed description of these collimators will be found in Chapter 3.

Data-storage devices are also useful in pediatric studies, since they ensure that the study will not have to be repeated because of improper photographic techniques.

Dose considerations

Exposure to ionizing radiation is an important consideration in children undergoing nuclear medicine procedures. The radiopharmaceutical dose chosen must produce a statistically valid image within a reasonable amount of time. The imaging time should be kept to 5 minutes or less. Longer exposure times are not acceptable because patient motion is likely to interfere with image quality.

There are several methods for calculating the administered dose in pediatric nuclear medicine, which include the body weight of the patient, body surface area, or estimated organ volume.

Body weight. The body-weight method is the most commonly used procedure for calculating radiopharmaceutical doses for pediatric patients.[1] The Talbot nomogram (Fig. 17-1) is used to determine the percentage of the adult dose the child should receive based on either the child's weight or body-surface area. A child weighing 140 pounds (63 kg) and having a body surface area of 1.7 square meters would receive a full adult dose employing the nomogram.

EXAMPLE: A child weighing 40 pounds (18 kg) will have a body surface area of approximately 0.72 square meters and should receive 42% of the adult dose.

Body-surface area. Body-surface area can also be used for dose calculations in children.[1] The West nomogram (Fig. 17-2) gives a close approximation of body surface area based on the height and weight of the child. The Talbot nomogram (Fig. 17-1) should then be used to determine the percentage of an adult dose the patient will receive.

Organ volume (estimated). Another dose-calculation method was developed by Webster.[2] Using this method, one strives to obtain a constant activity per unit volume of organ in children of various ages. The dose is calculated when one reduces the adult dose by the fraction

$$\frac{\text{Age in years} + 1}{\text{Age in years} + 7}$$

EXAMPLE: A 5-year-old child is scheduled for a liver study. The adult liver imaging dose is 3 mCi of ^{99m}Tc-sulfur colloid. With Webster's method

$$\frac{5 + 1}{5 + 7} = \frac{6}{12}$$

the radiopharmaceutical dose will be 50% of 3 mCi, or 1.5 mCi.

Minimum dose. Although we want to keep the radiation exposure to the patient as low as possible, we must administer a dose that will allow a satisfactory study to be obtained. The dose schedules discussed above may yield doses for neonates that are too low to produce a quality image in a reasonable amount of time. Therefore a "minimum-dose" schedule has been developed[3] (Table 17-1).

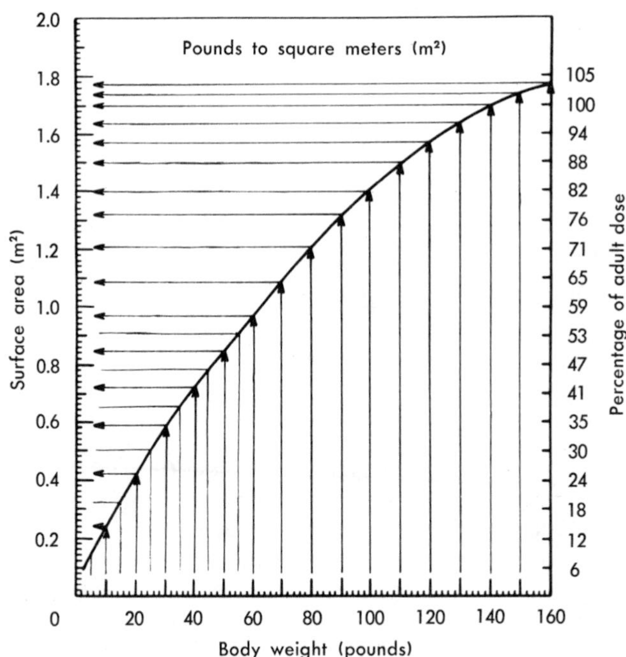

Fig. 17-1. Talbot nomogram can be used to calculate percentage of adult dose with pediatric patient's body weight or surface area in square meters being used.

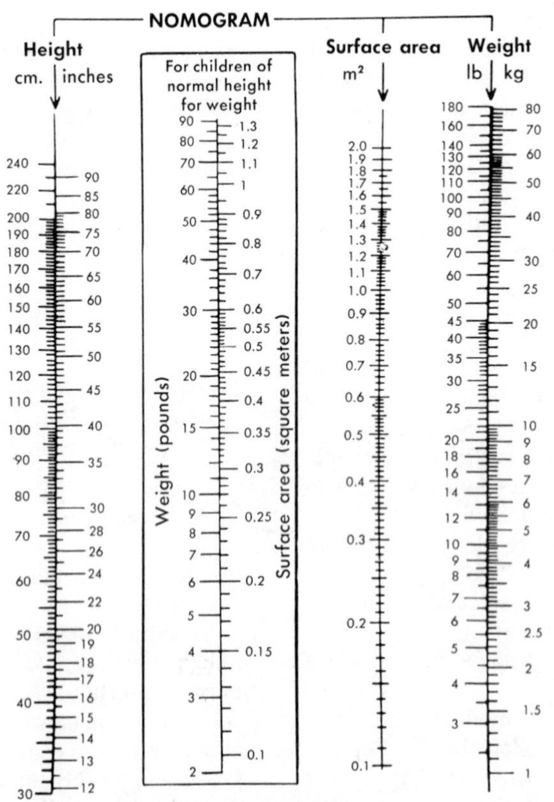

Fig. 17-2. West nomogram is used to calculate body surface area. Straight line drawn across surface area column connecting patient's height and weight will give approximate body surface area in square meters. Surface area can also be determined with weight being used if child is of normal height (enclosed column).

Table 17-1. Minimum pediatric doses*

Examination	Radiopharmaceutical	Dose
Brain scan	$^{99m}TcO_4^-$	2 mCi
Meckel scan	$^{99m}TcO_4^-$	2 mCi
Angiocardiogram	$^{99m}TcO_4^-$	2 mCi
Thyroid scan	$^{99m}TcO_4^-$	1 mCi
Bone scan	^{99m}Tc-phosphate	2 mCi
Lung scan	^{99m}Tc-HAM or ^{99m}Tc-MAA	500 μCi
Liver scan	^{99m}Tc-sulfur colloid	750 μCi
Renal scan	^{99m}Tc-DTPA or ^{99m}Tc-DMSA	500 μCi
Tumor scan	^{67}Ga citrate	500 μCi
Cisternogram	^{111}In-DTPA	25 μCi

*From Alderson, P. O., Gilday, D. L., and Wagner, H. N., Jr.: Atlas of pediatric nuclear medicine, St. Louis, 1978, The C. V. Mosby Co.

Injection technique

The administration of intravenous radiopharmaceuticals is often a problem when one is working with pediatric patients. Suitable injection sites for infants are frequently different from those used for older children and adults. As a rule, the largest convenient vein just distal to a venous junction should be used.

Injection sites. Veins on the dorsum of the hands or feet are recommended because of their superficial location and accessibility.[3,4] One can easily immobilize the hand of an infant by placing the patient's wrist between the index and third fingers and pressing the fingers down with the thumb (Fig. 17-3). A similar procedure can be used for the foot. Flexing the infant's wrist will make the vein less mobile and increase the likelihood of a successful venipuncture.

Antecubital veins are a second choice for venipuncture, but they are usually deeper in infants, are more difficult to immobilize, and have often been traumatized by blood sampling. However, these veins are often large, even in neonates, and should be considered when one is searching for the best injection

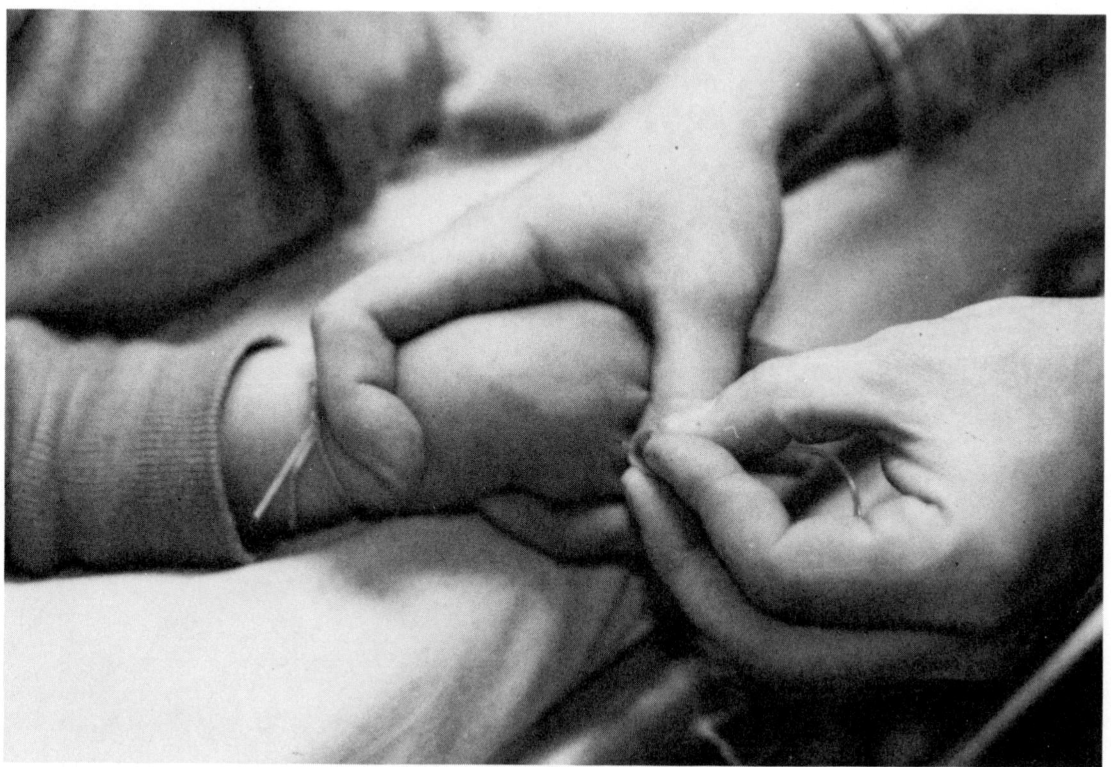

Fig. 17-3. Placing patient's wrist between your index and third fingers and pressing fingers down with your thumb will immobilize hand and vein.

site. The arm can be best immobilized when it is secured to an armboard (Fig. 17-4).

External jugular veins are considered a safe site for venipuncture, provided that careful technique is used. The patient should be placed in the supine position with the neck extended and the head rotated to the side. If the patient is crying, these veins are usually more prominent (Fig. 17-5). Jugular vein puncture may be a frightening experience for the child and should be performed only when the veins on the dorsum of the hands and feet or the antecubital veins are unacceptable as injection sites. This injection should only be performed by a physician, because nerves and vessels in the neck and the apex of the lung are near the vein and must be avoided during venipuncture.

Scalp veins are prominent in some infants but have a low priority on the list of acceptable injection sites. They should never be used if the patient is having a brain scan because residual activity at the injection site is likely to interfere with image interpretation. Scalp-vein injection can also be a frightening experience for the patient because the head is held securely, the injection site is shaved (usually not necessary for neonates), and a tourniquet is placed around the scalp to make the veins more prominent. If the child is crying, the scalp vein usually becomes prominent and the tourniquet can be eliminated.

Femoral veins should be used only as a last resort because of the high incidence of complications occurring after venipuncture at that site. Septic arthritis of the hip is a potential complication as well as venous thrombosis of the lower extremity.[5] These veins are usually difficult to locate because they are not palpable. The vein is located approximately 0.5 cm medially to the femoral artery. This injection should be performed only by a physician.

Injection of radiopharmaceutical. A special injection set is recommended for use with pediatric patients[3] (Fig. 17-6). It consists of a scalp-vein infusion needle (usually 23G or 25G), a three-way stopcock, a 10 ml syringe filled with saline, a syringe containing the radiopharmaceutical dose, a syringe shield,

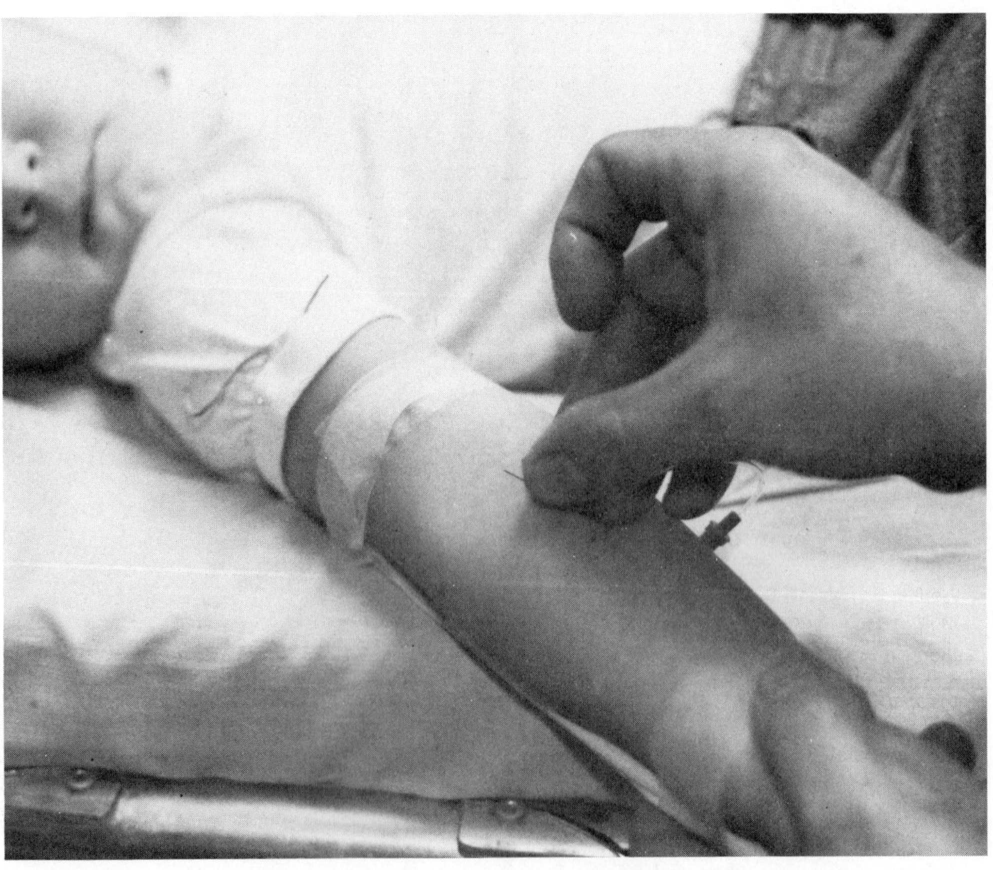

Fig. 17-4. Arm should be secured to board for antecubital injections.

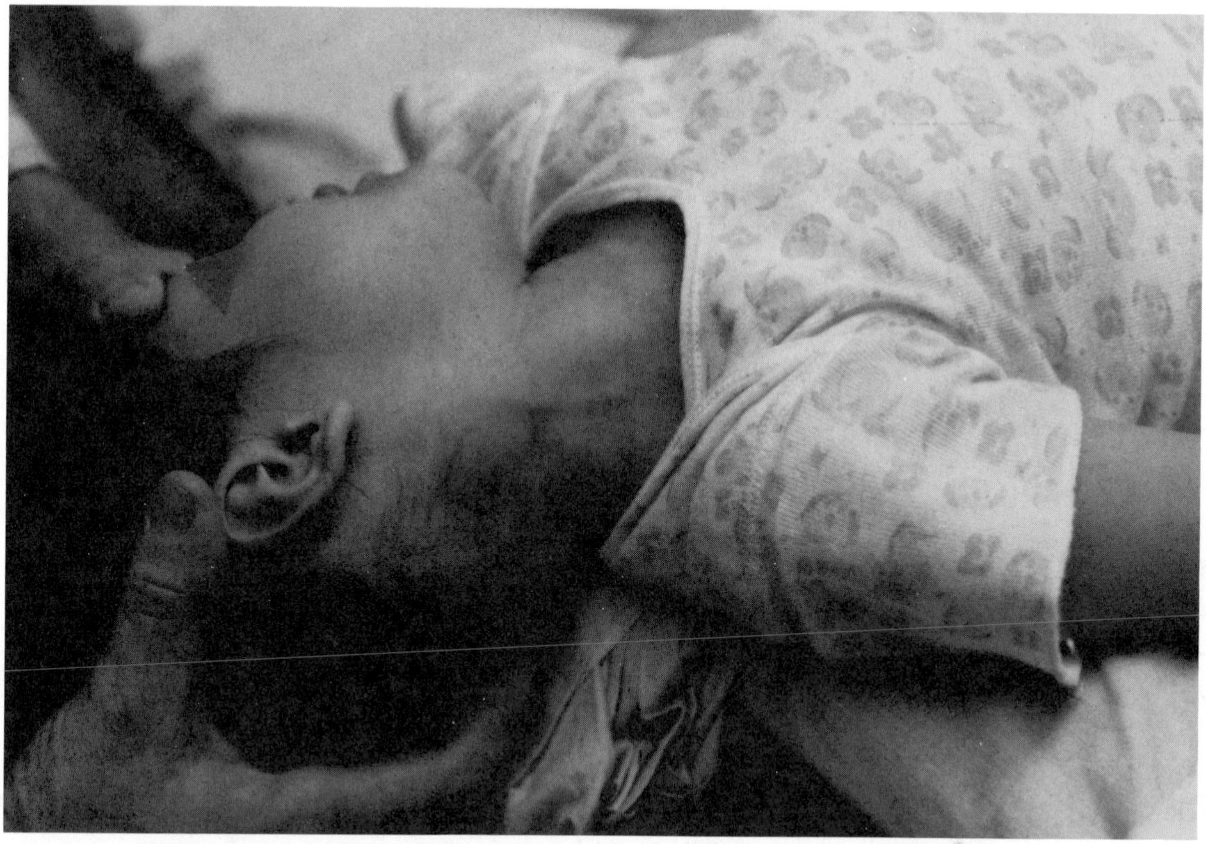

Fig. 17-5. External jugular vein can be made accessible when patient is placed supine with neck extended and head rotated to side with patient crying.

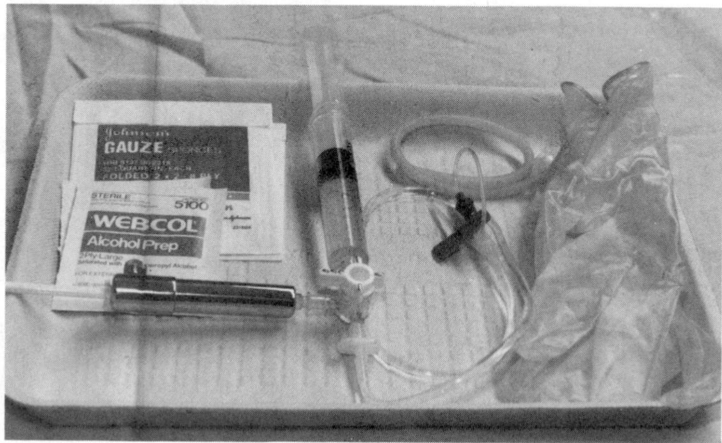

Fig. 17-6. Injection set should include everything needed for venipuncture and administration of radiopharmaceutical.

a tourniquet, alcohol sponges, and dry sterile sponges.

The injection apparatus should be assembled prior to the venipuncture. The lead-shielded syringe containing the radiopharmaceutical is connected to the three-way stopcock along with the syringe containing the saline flush. A small amount of saline is injected into the stopcock to avoid injection of an air bubble into the patient.

After the injection site has been determined, the area is immobilized and swabbed with an alcohol sponge and a tourniquet is applied. The vein is cannulated with the bevel of the needle facing down, which decreases the possibility of the needle penetrating the posterior lumen (Fig. 17-7). When the vein is successfully entered, blood will flow back into the tubing. The tourniquet is removed. No attempt should be made to "thread" the needle into the vein, since this will only increase the chances of dislodging it. As soon as the tubing has filled with blood, it is connected to the stopcock and a small volume of saline solution is injected to check for swelling around the needle. Absence of swelling is an indication that a successful venipuncture has been accomplished. The radiopharmaceutical can then be injected. After the radiopharmaceutical is injected, the syringe that contained the dose is flushed with saline solution several times to ensure that all the dose has been injected.

If a bolus is desired, a 12-inch extension tube with a volume of 1.5 ml should be connected between the infusion set and the stopcock. The radiopharmaceutical is injected through the stopcock into the extension tube, and a rapid injection of saline then propels the dose into the vein. The radiopharmaceutical syringe should be flushed with saline to ensure that all of the dose has been delivered.

Handling techniques

Most scintigraphic procedures require a patient to remain completely motionless for 3 to 5 minutes. This task is often difficult to accomplish when dealing with children. Every effort should be made to create a comfortable environment for the patient. Starting the procedure with the detector behind the patient is less frightening (Fig. 17-8) and will give the child a chance to become more confident with the technologist. The child will be less frightened if the detector must later be positioned above him.

The psychologic relationship between the technologist and the child is extremely important. Often a frightened child can be reassured by gently talking to him. Such interactions with children are simple and yet surprisingly are often overlooked. Their importance cannot be overemphasized. The child should be informed about each step in the procedure before it occurs. Many pediatric patients can be better dealt with if a parent is in the room to reassure them. However, a parent who is upset or overprotective may upset the child and should be discouraged from staying in the room.

Physical immobilization is not the most effective way to handle a child over 6 months of age. This is a frightening experience and will cause the child to become even more apprehensive. This method should be used only after the communicative approach has failed and the patient's condition precludes the use of sedation. Several methods can be used to immobilize the pediatric patient. Forcibly holding the child is most commonly used. Alternatively, the child may be wrapped in a sheet or strapped to a board. These techniques are not recommended unless other attempts at immobilization fail.

Sedation will help to ensure that a good study can

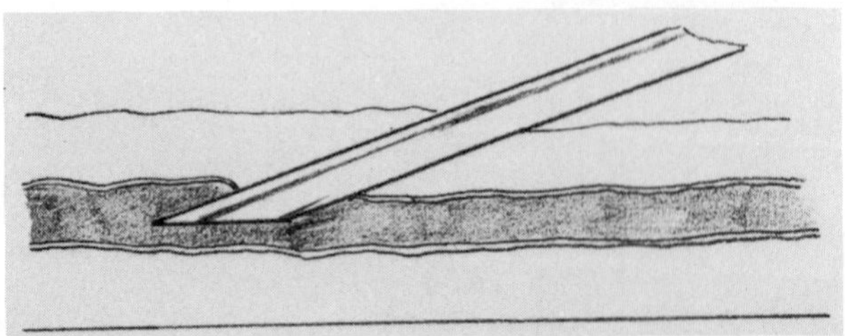

Fig. 17-7. Bevel of needle should face down when small vein is cannulated.

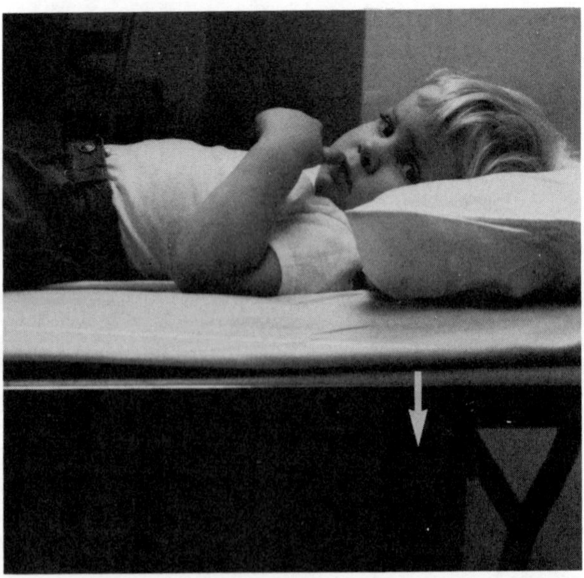

Fig. 17-8. Patient is usually less frightened if detector *(arrow)* is placed behind him.

be performed. It is most often used on patients between 6 months and 5 years of age. The sedative should be given on the hospital floor about 20 to 30 minutes before the study is begun. The most commonly used sedatives are pentobarbital sodium (Nembutal), diazepam (Valium), chloral hydrate, and DTP (Demerol, Thorazine, Phenergan). In our experience, an intramuscular injection of Nembutal (5 mg/kg of body weight) has proved to be the most effective sedative. Sedatives are always administered by authorized personnel after consultation with the nuclear medicine and pediatric physicians.

CLINICAL APPLICATIONS

In this section selected clinical topics and techniques are reviewed.

Central nervous system

Static brain imaging has proved to be a reliable diagnostic examination in children.[6,7] The radionuclide angiogram improves the accuracy of the study by revealing abnormalities in a small portion of children (about 11%) presenting with focal neurologic signs and who have normal static images.[8] Studies of the regional circulation aid the diagnosis of subdural hematomas, cerebral vascular abnormalities, and cerebral cysts. The flow study is unable to detect mild or moderate degrees of hydrocephalus. When both the flow study and static images are obtained, the yield of true-positive brain scans in children with a proved subdural pathologic condition increases to well over 90% with a false-positive rate of less than 5%.[8] Brain scans may be especially useful in children with possible encephalitis or cerebritis, as these diseases may be detected earlier by brain scans than by cranial computerized axial tomography.

Cisternography is useful in demonstrating obstructive hydrocephalus and for studying the patency of cerebrospinal fluid diversionary shunts in children with treated hydrocephalus.[3,9] Ventriculoperitoneal (VP) and ventriculoatrial (VA) shunts are assessed in identical fashion, except that the distal end of the shunt is imaged in the thorax (VA shunt) or abdomen (VP shunt). In this study, the scintillation camera records the passage of the radioactive tracer through the shunt from the reservoir to its distal end. A small dose (100 μCi of ^{111}In-DTPA or ^{99m}Tc-DTPA) is injected into the shunt reservoir under sterile conditions. Reflux into the ventricles may occur but is often not seen with modern high-pressure valve systems. In patients with two ventricular catheters, it is advisable to inject both reservoirs and determine the flow from each; often only one will be functioning. Images of the reservoir and shunt tubing are taken immediately and every 5 minutes for 30 minutes after injection. If necessary, additional images are obtained at 45, 60, and 120 minutes after having the child sit up to increase the pressure gradient down the shunt tubing. It may be helpful to quantify the clearance-rate constant describing the disappearance of the tracer from the reservoir. If the volume of the reservoir is known, the flow rate can be calculated in milliliters per minute.

In the normal functioning VP or VA shunt, the radiopharmaceutical injected into the reservoir passes through the tubing to disperse in the peritoneal cavity or right atrium within 15 to 30 minutes. The rate of clearance depends on the release pressure of the valve. Sequential images of the head reveal a rapid decrease in the amount of radiopharmaceutical within the reservoir as the flow of cerebrospinal fluid through the tubing carries the radiopharmaceutical to the peritoneum or atrium. Depending on the type of shunt malfunction, characteristic abnormal patterns may be seen. When radioactivity flows in only one direction into the ventricle and a flap-valve type of obstruction prevents its exit, there is no decrease in the amount of radioactivity within the ventricle during the course of the study, even for as long as 24 hours. When the distal end of the VP or VA shunt is totally obstructed, there is no tracer flow through the distal shunt tubing. In cases of partial distal obstruction, the radiopharmaceutical may pass slowly to the distal end of the shunt tubing. Another pattern results when the radioactivity passes into the peritoneal cavity but, because of peritoneal adhesions, remains in focal collections.

Lung

Radioactive-tracer studies have proved to be a valuable diagnostic aid in a variety of pediatric lung diseases.[3,10,11] They can be performed in children of any age, but the margin of safety in perfusion studies is reduced in neonates, as both the number of precapillary arterioles and the internal diameter of these vessels are reduced (perhaps as much as a factor of 3).[12] The statement that roughly 1 in 1000 pulmonary arterioles are blocked by a dose of 500,000 to 600,000 particles is a good approximation in an adult,[13] but not in a neonate. No more than 100,000 labeled particles should be injected when one is performing perfusion lung studies in neonates and young infants.

Xenon-133 studies have been used to assess ventilation in children.[10,14] Children age 4 or older can be examined by use of a standard plastic mouthpiece to administer the radioactive gas. Younger children are less likely to cooperate, in which case the ^{133}Xe gas may be delivered by use of a tight-fitting pediatric anesthesia mask. The mask is placed over the infant's face and the ^{133}Xe gas is administered during tidal respiration. The exhaled ^{133}Xe is cleared from the laboratory by a venting system or into a trap. One may also administer ^{133}Xe to uncooperative children by introducing it directly through nasal prongs or a nasal cannula. Alternatively, a saline solution of gas can be injected intravenously to obtain perfusion images, and a rebreathing system used during the ventilation phase of the study. Because of its short physical half-life (13 seconds), low radiation dose (less than 100 mrad/exam), and ease of administration, krypton 81m may become widely used for pediatric ventilation studies.[15]

Both ventilation and perfusion imaging have been useful in the study of children with congenital heart disease. For example, in infundibular pulmonic stenosis, perfusion of the right lung is usually much greater than that of the left.[16,17] Asymmetric pulmonary perfusion may also be seen in tetralogy of Fallot,[17,18] isolated pulmonic stenosis,[16] transposition of the great vessels,[19] and other anomalies of the right side of the heart.

Ventilation-perfusion studies with radionuclides can provide quantitative, regional lung-function analysis. Young (less than 5-year-old) children with obstructive lung disease often cannot cooperate to the degree necessary for performance of standard quantitative pulmonary function tests; thus ventilation or perfusion studies have been used to assess regional lung disease in children with obstructive airway diseases including cystic fibrosis, asthma, congenital lobar emphysema, or central airway obstruction (such as foreign-body aspiration). Severe bilateral perfusion abnormalities are found in most patients with advanced cystic fibrosis.[14,20,21] Bilateral segmental and nonsegmental perfusion defects are common, with the most severe defects often being located in the upper lung fields.

Probably the most common indication for pulmonary-tracer studies in adults is suspected pulmonary embolism. This is not the case in children, as this disease is relatively rare. There are certain conditions, such as sickle-cell disease[22,23] or the presence of a ventriculoatrial shunt or hyperalimentation catheter in the superior vena cava,[24] that predispose children to pulmonary emboli.

Heart

Radionuclide studies of the heart in children are commonly used to detect and quantitate left to right (L-R) cardiac shunts. A tracer (such as ^{99m}Tc-pertechnetate, ^{99m}Tc-albumin, or ^{99m}Tc–red blood cells) is injected intravenously as a compact bolus by use of the techniques described on p. 436. Its transit through the cardiopulmonary circuit is monitored when several 0.4- to 1-second images are obtained while the patient lies supine beneath a scintillation camera. The injected activity appears initially in the superior vena cava and right side of the heart, then in the lungs, then in the left ventricle, and finally in the aorta. Shortly after the appearance of aortic activity, lung activity disappears. Characteristic abnormalities in this sequence of radionuclide transit make possible the diagnosis of certain cardiac abnormalities by visual inspection of serial images alone.[25,26] The major advantage of radionuclide angiocardiography is that it permits quantitation of the size of the shunt. The technique for this procedure is described below.

Left-to-right shunt quantitation. When an infant or child is found to have a heart murmur, the possibility of a cardiac shunt exists. If the child is not cyanotic, the murmur is usually caused by valvular heart disease or a left-to-right (L-R) shunt through an atrial or ventricular septal defect, or a patent ductus arteriosus. Simple radionuclide studies can be used to differentiate children with L-R shunts from those with murmurs of other causes.

Folse and Braunwald[27] first showed that monitoring the pulmonary time-activity curve after intravenous injection of radioactive tracers could be used to diagnose L-R shunts. They used a simple count ratio (C_2/C_1) to indicate the presence of L-R shunt. More accurate results can be obtained from mathematical fitting techniques that analyze the areas under the pulmonary transit curve.[28] Maltz and Treves[29] proposed a gamma-function curve-fitting method for analyzing the pulmonary time-activity curve, and this method has been widely used. The gamma-variate function is used to fit the first-transit curve and to extrapolate this fitted function as if the pulmonary circulation were normal. The fitted curve is then subtracted from the real data. If no shunt is present, there is little or no difference between the two curves and the pulmonary-to-systemic flow ratio (Q_P/Q_S ratio) is calculated as 1. If a difference does exist, the "difference curve" is also fitted by use of the gamma variate and the ratio of the areas of the first-transit curve and the abnormal recirculation area is used to calculate the Q_P/Q_S ratio. Using this method, Askenazi et al.[30] evaluated over 100 children and found precise quantitation of L-R shunts with pulmonary-to-systemic ratios of 1.2 to 3. The correlation between shunt size determined by the radionuclide method and by oximetry was excellent (r = 0.94).

In addition to its use in evaluating children with murmurs of undetermined etiology, quantitative radionuclide angiocardiography is useful in serial studies of children who have small L-R shunts, which often close spontaneously. It can also be used to determine whether an infant in respiratory distress has a cardiac shunt or lung disease or to document the success of surgical closure of shunts. The major advantages of the technique include its noninvasive nature, its rapidity (less than 1 minute between injection and completion of the study), and its low radiation dose compared to the alternative procedures, such as cardiac catheterization and contrast angiography.

Right-to-left cardiac shunts. The cyanotic child with congenital heart disease usually has a right-to-left (R-L) cardiac shunt. Surgery is often required for correction or palliation. Preoperative cardiac catheterization is the most common diagnostic procedure, and oxygen saturation measurements are used to quantitate the magnitude of shunting. Radionuclide studies are used to screen patients for catheterization and to monitor their clinical course, especially after palliative surgery. Although radionuclide angiocardiography with ^{99m}Tc-pertechnetate can be used to quantitate R-L shunts,[31] they are usually quantified by use of lung-scanning microspheres. After these particles are injected intravenously, the partition of activity between the systemic circulation and the lungs is determined. If no R-L shunt is present, more than 95% of the injected activity will be trapped in the pulmonary vascular bed. If a R-L shunt is present, some of the labeled particles will pass through the shunt to be distributed throughout the systemic circulation, including the kidneys, brain, and other organs. If activity is seen in the kidneys, the shunt is usually greater than 15%.[32]

The exact magnitude of the R-L shunt can be determined when the whole body distribution of activity is quantified with the pulmonary net counts:

$$\%\text{R-L shunt} = \frac{\text{Total body count} - \text{Total lung count}}{\text{Total body count}}$$

Although these studies have been performed in many children without complications, caution is in order because the technique results in embolization of systemic end arteries. When one uses this technique, we recommend that the total number of injected particles be restricted to a 70,000 to 100,000 maximum.

Ventricular dysfunction. Gated blood-pool imaging and myocardial imaging have been used more widely in adults than in children, and these techniques are described in detail in Chapter 11. Ejection fraction studies have been used to determine ventricular function and regional wall motion in children with cardiomyopathy or cystic fibrosis and to follow cardiac effects of the drug doxorubicin HCl (Adriamycin). Myocardial imaging with ^{201}Tl has been used to evaluate neonates with transient myocardial ischemia, children with cardiomyopathy, and rare problems like anomalous origin of the left coronary artery.[3] Further applications of these techniques in children will undoubtedly be made.

Abdomen

Meckel's diverticulum. Nuclear medicine techniques are used to investigate the possibility that abdominal pain or gastrointestinal bleeding in children is caused by Meckel's diverticulum. Nearly 20% of these diverticula contain heterotopic gastric mucosa, which at times ulcerates the adjacent normal bowel and results in abdominal pain or lower gastrointestinal bleeding. Since radiographic detection of Meckel's diverticula is difficult, radionuclide studies have been used.[3,33] A Meckel's diverticulum containing functional gastric mucosa is visualized after an intravenous injection of 5 mCi of ^{99m}Tc-pertechnetate (Fig. 17-9). The child should be fasting prior to the study and not receive intestinal irritants such as barium, laxatives, or aspirin for at least 3 days prior to the study. Images should be obtained from several projections, including supine, posterior, and right lateral views, to better localize the site of increased activity. Accumulation of activity in Meckel's diverticulum parallels that of the stomach, being seen best about 10 to 15 minutes after injection. It is not necessary to continue imaging beyond 60 minutes after injection.

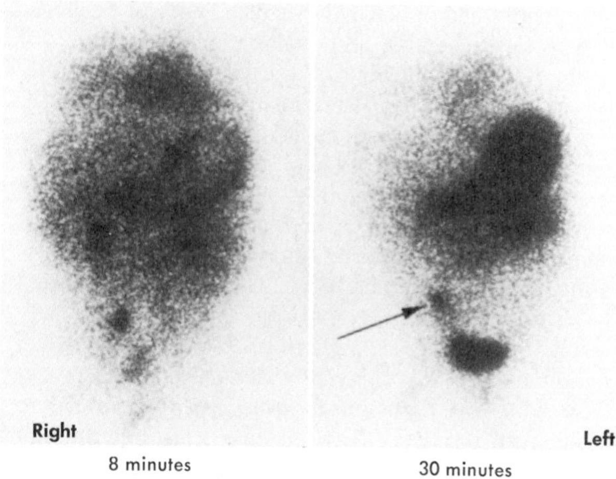

Fig. 17-9. Meckel's diverticulum is represented by area of increased activity in right lower quadrant, *arrow*. (From Alderson, P. O., Gilday, D. L., and Wagner, H. N., Jr.: Atlas of pediatric nuclear medicine, St. Louis, 1978, The C. V. Mosby Co.)

Not all Meckel's diverticula are located in the right lower quadrant of the abdomen. They are occasionally found in the right upper quadrant or midabdomen. Failure to image these areas may be a source of false-negative examinations. Other causes for a false-negative study include absence of gastric mucosa in the diverticulum, insufficient gastric mucosa to be resolved by imaging, or necrosis of the mucosa because of a decreased vascular supply. False-negative studies can be minimized if careful techniques are used. Because of the low prevalence of a Meckel's diverticulum (1% to 3% of the population) most studies in children with nonspecific abdominal pain or bleeding will be negative. A false-negative study will be found in about 25% of the patients with Meckel's diverticulum. The study has its greatest value when positive.

Urinary tract infections. A problem of great importance in pediatrics is urinary tract infection. In children, recurrent urinary infections are often secondary to vesicoureteral reflux, which promotes urinary stasis and may lead to the development of chronic pyelonephritis. Vesicoureteral reflux can be accurately detected by radiographic cystography, but this procedure may result in gonad doses as high as 300 mrads.[34] Direct radionuclide cystography provides an alternate procedure with less radiation exposure. In this procedure 0.5 to 1 mCi of ^{99m}Tc-pertechnetate is instilled through a catheter into the bladder.[35] A 500 ml bottle of sterile saline is attached to the catheter and allowed to fill the bladder for about 10 minutes. The catheter is then clamped and images are obtained while the child strains to urinate with the catheter still clamped and then again after its release. Reflux is indicated by ascent of activity from the bladder into the ureters or the upper collecting system of the involved kidneys. Conway[34] has shown that this procedure is nearly as sensitive in the detection of reflux as radiographic urethrocystography. The radiation dose to the gonads is about 1% of that received during a radiographic cystogram. Approximately 30 mrads are delivered to the bladder mucosa during a 30-minute radionuclide study performed with 1 mCi of pertechnetate.

Indirect voiding cystography using *intravenously* administered ^{99m}Tc-DTPA may provide information as helpful as that obtained at direct radionuclide cystography, while the hazards of infection associated with bladder catheterization are avoided.[36] In this procedure ^{99m}Tc-DTPA (250 μCi/kg) is injected intravenously and the patient is instructed not to void. After a waiting period of about 2 hours, most of the injected activity will have been excreted into the bladder. At this point the patient is placed in front of a scintillation camera interfaced to a digital computer, and the patient is instructed to void. Increasing activity over the ureters or kidneys during voiding is evidence of reflux. A disadvantage of the indirect method is the requirement for patient cooperation. Reflux is a problem in young (ages 1 to 3), as well as in older children. Detection of reflux at the earliest possible age is needed to prevent chronic pyelonephritis. Unfortunately, many of these young children are not able to cooperate to the degree needed for indirect cystography.

Testicular imaging. Scrotal imaging after intravenous injection of ^{99m}Tc-pertechnetate or human serum albumin (^{99m}Tc-HSA) is useful in distinguishing testicular torsion from acute intrascrotal inflammation in a child with a swollen, painful testis. This procedure was first used in adult patients but has subsequently proved useful in children.[3,37] In inflammatory lesions there is increased activity in the painful testis, but a testis that has undergone torsion has decreased activity (Fig. 17-10). Torsion of the appendix testis is not so common as torsion of the vascular pedicle but may be present in similar fashion. It is usually associated with normal images for the first 12 hours after onset of pain, mild hyperemia for 12 to 48 hours, and pronounced hyperemia for 7 to 10 days thereafter. Scrotal imaging should precede surgical exploration in children if the clinical diagnosis is in doubt. It is important to obtain a high-quality radionuclide angiogram of the testes to evaluate arterial perfusion. During static imaging a lead shield should be placed beneath the scrotum to block activity from the thighs.

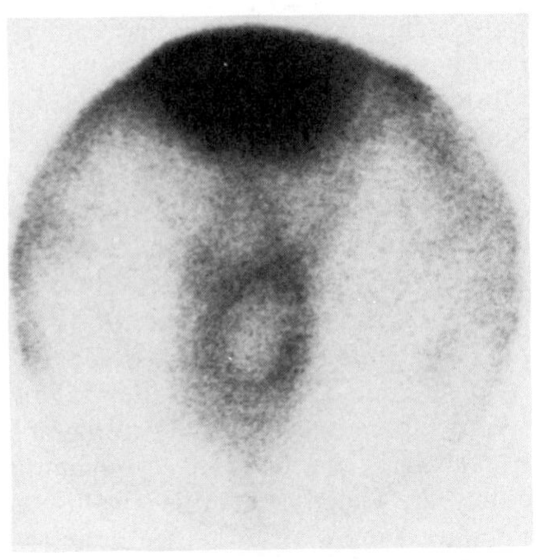

Fig. 17-10. Decreased activity in testis is indication of torsion.

Bone imaging

Bone scanning in children is often performed in three phases: (1) a radionuclide angiogram (1 film per 3 seconds) over the involved site, (2) a blood-pool image (400,000 counts) immediately after the angiogram, and (3) delayed static images (after 2 to 3 hours). The utility of these three-phase studies is determined by the specific clinical problem being investigated. Bone scanning has been shown to be a sensitive indicator of metastatic skeletal disease in children (such as neuroblastoma, osteosarcoma, or Ewing's sarcoma)[38] but is used even more frequently to diagnose nonmalignant disease. For example, the cause of bone pain in pediatrics is often obscure, particularly if radiographs are normal. The ^{99m}Tc-phosphate bone scan has provided a useful tool for solving this diagnostic problem.

Osteomyelitis or cellulitis. The clinical diagnosis of osteomyelitis is based on the occurrence of a focal, well-defined area of bone tenderness in a patient with

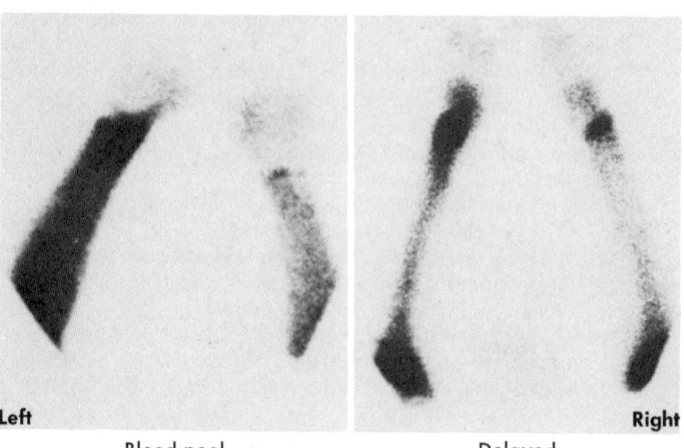

Fig. 17-11. Osteomyelitis appears as well-defined area of increased activity in left distal forearm on delayed bone images. (From Alderson, P. O., Gilday, D. L., and Wagner, H. N., Jr.: Atlas of pediatric nuclear medicine, St. Louis, 1978, The C. V. Mosby Co.)

clinical signs of infection. Radiologic examination is difficult because both cellulitis and osteomyelitis cause swelling of the soft tissues and loss of fat planes. Infections are often present for 7 to 14 days before bone is demineralized to the extent that changes become apparent radiographically. Bone scans have been found to be a sensitive test for diagnosing pediatric osteomyelitis during its early stages.[39-41] They usually become abnormal about 48 hours after the onset of symptoms. The typical appearance of osteomyelitis is a well-defined area of increased activity on delayed bone images (after 3 hours) (Fig. 17-11), often associated with an area of hyperemia in the blood-flow phase of the study. Cellulitis also has a distinctive appearance consisting of a diffuse increase in radioactivity throughout the soft tissues and bone in the blood-pool image. In the delayed bone scan there is *no* well-defined focal area of increased activity seen within the bone. The ratio of radioactivity in the bone compared to soft tissues is similar to that of the opposite side, but the overall activity of the affected side is increased. This is attributable to the hyperemia that is associated with cellulitis. Bone scanning can reliably differentiate between osteomyelitis and cellulitis in most patients[39,42] and is most valuable in assessing patients whose skeletal radiographs are normal.

Hip pain. The differential diagnosis of a child with hip pain is difficult and includes the possibility of transient synovitis, Legg-Perthes disease, and septic arthritis. Bone imaging can help in this differential diagnosis. Adequate imaging of the affected hip requires magnification, accomplished by use of pinhole or converging collimation of the hip and pelvis. Magnification provides anatomic detail sufficient to make the diagnosis in cases such as avascular necrosis or Legg Perthes disease, in which the abnormality may only be poorly seen in conventional scintillation-camera images. Paul[43] employs a 2.3 mm pinhole inserted in a pinhole collimator. Counts of 30,000 to 50,000 are collected over the normal hip, and an image of the affected hip is taken for the same time as that required for the normal hip. The femoral head is seen best when the hip is in maximum internal rotation.

Synovitis of the hip is usually characterized by a diffuse increase in radioactivity involving the acetabulum, the hip, and the neck of the femur. In contrast, patients with Legg-Perthes disease have a definite area of decreased activity, usually in the lateral portion of the femoral head. Hip pain may also be attributable to septic arthritis. This condition is characterized by a pronounced generalized increase in radioactivity in bones adjacent to the joint space, with no focal area of increased activity. Generalized increased activity in adjacent bony surfaces is apparent in both blood-pool and delayed bone images. Images of the hip with ^{67}Ga citrate are also positive in septic arthritis and may aid in making this diagnosis during the early phase of the disease.[44]

CONCLUSION

Children present a variety of unique and challenging problems to the nuclear medicine technologist. High-quality studies can be obtained if careful attention is paid to imaging techniques and patient handling. Nuclear medicine procedures provide a great deal of useful information to pediatricians. In addition, they are noninvasive and expose children to only small amounts of radiation. Thus every effort should be made to design these studies especially for children so that the maximum yield of diagnostic information can be extracted.

REFERENCES

1. Shirkey, H. C.: Pediatric therapy, St. Louis, 1972, The C. V. Mosby Co., pp. 39-46.
2. Webster, E.: Comparison of radiation dosage in pediatric nuclear medicine and diagnostic radiographic procedures. In James, A. E., Wagner, H. N., and Cooke, R. E., editors: Pediatric nuclear medicine, Philadelphia, 1974, W. B. Saunders Co., pp. 36-38.
3. Alderson, P. O., Gilday, D. L., Wagner, H. N., et al.: Atlas of pediatric nuclear medicine, St. Louis, 1978, The C. V. Mosby Co.
4. Conway, J. J.: Sedation, injection and handling techniques in pediatric nuclear medicine. In James, A. E., Wagner, H. N., and Cooke, R. E., editors: Pediatric nuclear medicine, Philadelphia, 1974, W. B. Saunders Co., pp. 97-98.
5. McKay, R. J., Jr.: Diagnosis and treatment: risks of obtaining samples of venous blood in infants, Pediatrics **38:**906-908, 1968.
6. Conway, J. J.: Radionuclide imaging of the central nervous system in children, Radiol. Clin. N. Am. **10:**291-312, 1972.

7. Hurley, P. J., and Wagner, H. N.: Diagnostic value of brain scanning in children, J.A.M.A. **221**:877-881, 1972.
8. Alderson, P. O., Gilday, D. L., Mikhad, M., et al.: The value of routine cerebral radionuclide angiography in pediatric brain imaging, J. Nucl. Med. **17**:780-785, 1976.
9. Gilday, D. L.: Paediatric neuronuclear medicine. In Harwood-Nash, D. C., and Fitz, C. R., editors: Neuroradiology in infants and children, St. Louis, 1976, The C. V. Mosby Co., pp. 572-607.
10. Treves, S., Ahnberg, D. S., Laguarda, R., and Strieder, D. J.: Radionuclide evaluation of regional lung function in children, J. Nucl. Med. **15**:582-587, 1974.
11. Alderson, P. O.: Radionuclide studies in pediatric lung disease. In Bibliography of pediatric nuclear medicine literature, Des Plaines, Ill., 1976, Searle Radiographics, Inc.
12. Davies, G., and Reid, L.: Growth of the alveoli and pulmonary arteries in childhood, Thorax **25**:679-681, 1970.
13. Harding, L. K., Horsfield, K., Singhal, S. S., and Cumming, G.: The proportion of lung vessels blocked by albumin microspheres, J. Nucl. Med. **14**:579-581, 1973.
14. Alderson, P. O., Secker-Walker, R. H., Strominger, D. B., McAlister, W. H., Hill, R. L., and Markham, J.: Quantitative assessment of regional ventilation and perfusion in children with cystic fibrosis, Radiology **111**:151-155, 1974.
15. Li, D. K., Treves, S., Heyman, S., et al.: Krypton 81m: a better radiopharmaceutical for assessment of regional lung function in children, Radiology **130**:741-747, 1979.
16. Chen, J. T. T., Robinson, A. E., Goodrich, J. K., and Lester, R. G.: Uneven distribution of pulmonary blood flow between left and right lungs in isolated valvular pulmonary stenosis, Am. J. Roentgenol. Radium Ther. Nucl. Med. **107**:343-351, 1969.
17. Lin, C. Y.: Lung scan in cardiopulmonary disease. I. Tetralogy of Fallot, J. Thor. Cardiovasc. Surg. **61**:370-379, 1971.
18. Puyau, F. A., and Meckstroth, G. R.: Evaluation of pulmonary perfusion patterns in children with tetralogy of Fallot, Am. J. Roentgenol. Radium Ther. Nucl. Med. **122**:119-124, 1974.
19. Muster, A. J., Paul, M. H., von Grondelle, A., and Conway, J. J.: Asymmetric distribution of the pulmonary blood flow between the right and left lungs in transposition of the great arteries, Am. J. Cardiol. **38**:352-361, 1976.
20. Samanek, M., Houstek, J., Varona, V., Ruth, C., and Snobl, O.: Distribution of pulmonary blood flow in children with cystic fibrosis, Acta Pediatr. Scand. **60**:149-157, 1971.
21. Piepsz, A., Decostre, P., and Baran, D.: Scintigraphic study of pulmonary blood flow distribution in cystic fibrosis, J. Nucl. Med. **14**:326-330, 1973.
22. Barrett-Connor, E.: Acute pulmonary disease and sickle cell anemia, Am. Rev. Resp. Dis. **104**:159-165, 1971.
23. Barrett-Connor, E.: Pneumonia and pulmonary infarction in sickle cell anemia, J.A.M.A. **224**:997-1000, 1973.
24. Emery, J. L., and Hilton, H. B.: Lung and heart complications of treatment of hydrocephalus by ventriculoauriculostomy, Surgery **50**:309-314, 1961.
25. Kriss, J. P., Freedman, G. S., Enright, L. P., et al.: Radioisotopic angiocardiography: findings in congenital heart disease, J. Nucl. Med. **13**:31-40, 1972.
26. Stocker, F. P., Kinser, J., Weber, J. W., and Rosler, H.: Pediatric radiocardioangiography: shunt diagnosis, Circulation **47**: 819-826, 1973.
27. Folse, R., and Braunwald, E.: Pulmonary vascular dilution curves recorded by external detection in the diagnosis of left-to-right shunts, Br. Heart J. **24**:166-172, 1962.
28. Alderson, P. O., Jost, R. G., Strauss, A. W., Boonvisut, S., and Markham, J.: Radionuclide angiocardiography: improved diagnosis and quantitation of left-to-right shunts using area ratio techniques in children, Circulation **51**:1136-1143, 1975.
29. Maltz, D. L., and Treves, S.: Quantitative radionuclide angiocardiography: determination of $Q_P:Q_S$ in children, Circulation **47**:1049-1056, 1973.
30. Askenazi, J., Ahnberg, D., Korngold, E., La Farge, C., Maltz, D. L., and Treves, S.: Quantitative radionuclide angiocardiography: detection and quantitation of left-to-right shunts, Am. J. Cardiol. **37**:382-393, 1976.
31. Hurley, P. J., Strauss, H. W., and Wagner, H. N.: Radionuclide angiocardiography in cyanotic congenital heart disease, Johns Hopkins Med. J. **127**:46-54, 1970.
32. Gates, G. F., Orme, H. W., and Dore, E. K.: Cardiac shunt assessment in children with macroaggregated albumin technetium 99m, Radiology **112**:649-653, 1974.
33. Conway, J. J.: The sensitivity, specificity and accuracy of radionuclide imaging of Meckel's diverticulum, J. Nucl. Med. **17**:553, 1976.
34. Conway, J. J., King, L. R., Belman, A. B., et al.: Detection of vesicoureteral reflux with radionuclide cystography, Am. J. Roentgenol. Radium Ther. Nucl. Med. **115**:720-727, 1972.
35. Weiss, S., and Conway, J. J.: The technique of direct radionuclide cystography, Appl. Radiol. **4**:133-137, 1975.
36. Handmaker, H., McRae, J., and Buck, E. G.: Intravenous radionuclide voiding cystography (IRVC). An atraumatic method of demonstrating vesicoureteral reflux, Radiology **108**:703-705, 1973.
37. Gilday, D. L., Hitch, D., Shandling, B., et al.: Testicular imaging for testicular torsion in pediatric surgery, J. Nucl. Med. **17**:553, 1976.
38. Gilday, D. L., Ash, J. M., and Reilly, B. J.: Radionuclide skeletal survey for pediatric neoplasms, Radiology **123**:399-406, 1977.
39. Gilday, D. L., and Paul, D. J.: The differentiation of osteomyelitis and cellulitis in children using a combined blood pool and bone scan, J. Nucl. Med. **15**:494, 1974.
40. Duszynski, D. O., Kuhn, J. P., Afshani, E., and Riddlesberger, M. M.: Early radionuclide diagnosis of acute osteomyelitis, Radiology **117**:337-340, 1975.
41. Treves, S., Khettry, J., Broker, F. H., Wilkinson, R. H., and Watts, H.: Osteomyelitis: early scintigraphic detection in children, Pediatrics **57**:173-186, 1976.
42. Majd, M., and Frankel, R. S.: Bone scanning in osteomyelitis, cellulitis and bone infarct in children, J. Nucl. Med. **16**:547, 1975.
43. Paul, D. J., Gilday, D. L., Gurd, A., and Bobechko, W.: A better method of imaging the abnormal hips, Radiology **113**: 466-467, 1974.
44. Handmaker, H., and Leonards, R.: The bone scan in inflammatory osseous disease, Semin. Nucl. Med. **6**:95-105, 1976.

Chapter 18

RADIOIMMUNOASSAY

Thomas J. Persoon

The technique of radioimmunoassay, like so many other scientific discoveries, was developed as a result of some serendipitous events and careful observation on the part of two investigators. In the mid-1950s Solomon Berson and Rosalyn Yalow, working at the Veterans Administration Hospital in Bronx, New York, were studying the role of insulin in diabetics when they noted that treated diabetics carried antibodies to the peptide hormone. They discovered that these antibodies could bind radioactively labeled insulin[1,26] and the science of radioimmunoassay was born. For her contribution of this important analytical technique to medical science, Rosalyn Yalow shared the 1977 Nobel Prize in Medicine and Physiology. (Solomon Berson died in 1975.)

It was not long before other investigators discovered that radioimmunoassay could be used to measure other molecules besides peptide hormones. Assays for the thyroid hormones, drugs, and many more compounds were devised. Their effectiveness in readily measuring substances that previously could be measured only by long and laborious bioassays or indirect chemical methods led radioimmunoassay to become accepted first by the medical research community and then by the nuclear medicine laboratory as a standard technique. Despite forecasts that it reached its peak in the early 1970s, the field of radioimmunoassay has continued to grow. The list of substances measurable by radioassay has grown to well over 100, and new assays are added yearly. Although not all of these are of clinical usefulness, the core of clinically useful assays has also grown and spawned a new health care–product industry to supply the needed reagents and supplies. The purpose of this chapter is to provide the nuclear medicine technologist with a basic understanding of how radioimmunoassay works, what type of substances radioimmunoassay can be used to measure, and the techniques necessary to make it a viable part of the nuclear medicine laboratory.

THEORY OF COMPETITIVE-BINDING RADIOASSAYS

Radioimmunoassay is an elegant yet simple analytical technique. There are four elements needed for a radioimmunoassay. The material that is to be measured, usually referred to as the *ligand,* must be available in a pure form to be used as a standard. A *radiolabeled analog* of the ligand must also be available. Perhaps the most important element of the system is the *specific reactor substance,* a molecule that will selectively react with the ligand and its radiolabeled analog. Finally, some *method of separating* the reacted ligand from the nonreacted ligand must be available. The basic chemical reaction in a radioimmunoassay is competition between the chemically identical ligand species for binding sites on the specific reactor substance, which is present in limited quantity, followed by separation of the bound and unbound substances.

The important chemical law of mass action governs the behavior of the reacting molecules. The law of mass action states that when two *chemically identical* molecules, L and L*, participate in a reaction with a third molecule, S, the ratio of LS to L*S, the final products, will be the same as the ratio of L to L* in the initial reactant mixture. Since the presence of a radioactive atom in a molecule does not alter its chemical properties, a ligand L and its radiolabeled analog L* obey the laws of mass action. The fact that the law of mass action is obeyed does not in itself permit the reaction of L and S to be used in a chemical system that measures L. Equally important is the fact that reagent S must be the limiting reagent; that is, there must be fewer molecules of S present than the sum of radiolabeled and nonradiolabeled L molecules. Only when this is true can the radiolabeled and nonradiolabeled L *compete* for the limited number of S molecules. Once the reaction of L and S has gone to completion we know that (1) there is no unreacted S left and (2) the ratio of LS to L*S is the same as the ratio of L to L*

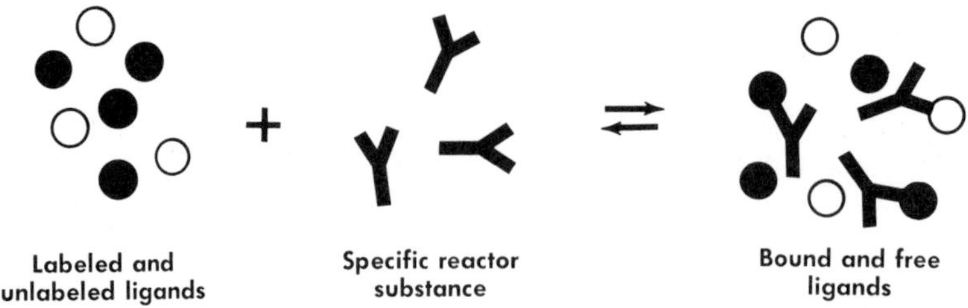

Fig. 18-1. Radioimmunoassay involves competition between labeled and unlabeled ligands for limited number of binding sites on specific reactor molecules.

before the reaction occurred, as predicted by the law of mass action.

If the amount of radioactive ligand in the system is held constant, an increase in the amount of L in the reaction mixture reduces the number of L* molecules that finally react with S, since the L/L* ratio has been changed. By separating the reacted L and L* from the nonreacted material and counting the radioactivity in either fraction, a relative measure of the amount of L added is obtained. Unknown amounts of L may be determined by comparison with a series of samples where L is known. Fig. 18-1 depicts this "assay" system, which is known as competitive-binding radioassay. The term "saturation analysis" is also used because the binding sites of S are saturated with L.

CHEMICAL EQUILIBRIUM

The competitive-binding radioassay is designed to be used with biologic molecules, and the reactions are thus biochemical reactions. Few, if any, biochemical reactions are as simple or as complete as implied by the one-line equations written to describe them. In fact, the net position of many biochemical reactions lies somewhere between the totally unreacted mixture implied on the left side of the chemical equation and the completely reacted products written on the right side. Furthermore, many of the reactions are reversible; that is, the "products" normally written on the right side of the reaction arrow become "reactants" for the reverse reaction. In this situation chemists write a double-reaction arrow ($\rightleftharpoons$) one pointing in each direction, and the system is said to obey the laws of chemical equilibrium. If a reaction is partially reversible, the upper arrow is shorter ($\leftrightarrows$). Although I cannot present a detailed discussion of chemical equilibrium and its thermodynamics in this chapter, it is important to remember that the biochemical reactions to be studied generally are equilibriums.

There are three key properties of equilibriums. First, chemical equilibrium is a dynamic state, and the system expressed by the chemical equation represents only the net state of the entire system at equilibrium, not the state of any individual molecule at some particular point in time. The classic experiment demonstrating dynamic equilbrium is shown in Fig. 18-2. A slightly soluble ionic salt (solid) is in equilibrium with its ions in solution. If some of the solution is removed and replaced with an equal amount of solution containing a radioactive nuclide of the same element, and equilibrium is allowed to be reached, radioactivity will be present in the solid phase, an indication that there has been a constant dissolution of individual salt molecules accompanied by an equal number of precipitation events. The net concentrations remain the same as expressed in the chemical equation, but the reaction between solid and solution is continuous.

The second property of equilibriums is the existence of the equilibrium constant, written K_{eq}. The numerical value for K_{eq} is defined in equation (1).

$$K_{eq} = \frac{[\text{Products}]}{[\text{Reactants}]} \tag{1}$$

where "[products]" indicates the mathematical product of the concentrations of the chemical products and "[reactants]" indicates the mathematical product of the concentration of the chemical reactants. For the chemical system

$$A + B \rightleftharpoons C + D \tag{2}$$

the equilibrium is

$$K_{eq} = \frac{[C][D]}{[A][B]} \tag{3}$$

where the brackets indicate concentrations of the respective species. Since an equilibrium constant is a true constant under defined physical conditions, the "position" of an equilibrium system will change if either concentration of products or reactants is changed. If more A is added to the system in (2), more A and B molecules will react to form C and D until the concentrations of all components are such that (3) is true. Similarly, if some D is removed from the system, A and B will react to form more C and D until the concentrations of all components are such that (3) is again

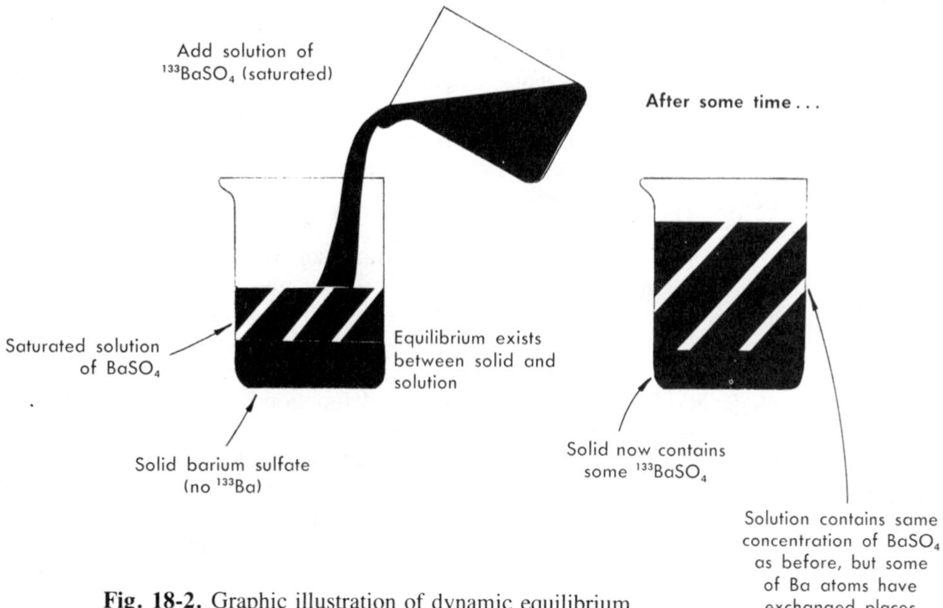
Add solution of
$^{133}BaSO_4$ (saturated)
After some time...
Saturated solution
of $BaSO_4$
Equilibrium exists
between solid and
solution
Solid barium sulfate
(no ^{133}Ba)
Solid now contains
some $^{133}BaSO_4$
Solution contains same
concentration of $BaSO_4$
as before, but some
of Ba atoms have
exchanged places

Fig. 18-2. Graphic illustration of dynamic equilibrium.

true. This ability of a chemical system to maintain equilibrium despite perturbations is known as Le Châtelier's principle. Le Châtelier's principle also applies to perturbations of the physical conditions (the environment) of an equilibrium system, though the mechanism responsible is different. If the temperature of a system at equilibrium is changed, the system is perturbed, because the value of K_{eq} is temperature dependent. With a new value for K_{eq}, the molecules in equation (2) react until equilibrium as defined in equation (3) is again achieved. Le Châtelier's principle is the third property of equilibriums, which is important.

A number of physical and chemical properties affect the value of K_{eq} and the position of the equilibrium. Among them are pH, ionic strength, and especially temperature. The former two chemical properties affect equilibrium because they affect the reactivity of the biologic molecules involved. The latter physical property affects the value of K_{eq} because of thermodynamic principles too complex to address here. In future discussions of the individual components of competitive-binding radioassays those physical and chemical properties that may affect the behavior of individual components will be considered.

With this discussion of chemical equilibrium in mind, an equation describing the reaction between L, L*, and S can be written

$$\begin{matrix} L \\ L^* \end{matrix} + S \rightleftharpoons \begin{matrix} LS \\ L^*S \end{matrix} \qquad (4)$$

An equilibrium constant K_{eq} for this system exists. For the system to be used as the basis for a competitive-binding radioassay, K_{eq} must be very large, on the order of 10^{-8} liter-mol^{-1}. Few biologic equilibriums meet this criterion, but those that do make excellent choices for competitive-binding radioassays.

SPECIFIC REACTOR SUBSTANCES

The properties of the specific reactor substance determine the utility of a competitive-binding radioassay. For an analysis scheme to be of maximum value it must measure only one substance; in other words it must be specific. In competitive-binding radioassay the specificity is determined by the material for which the rabiolabeled and nonlabeled ligand compete—S in equation (4)—hence the name *specific reactor substance*. In addition to the property of specificity (also called selectivity, since the substance must *select* to react with only one of the thousands of molecules present in a biologic fluid), the analysis should also be sensitive—able to detect the selected molecule in very small concentrations. The sensitivity of a competitive-binding radioassay is partially determined by two related properties of the specific reactor substance (SRS). The first of these properties, *affinity,* refers to the ability of the SRS to seek out the ligand of interest from among the thousands present in the biologic fluid and react with it spontaneously and as completely as possible. Since the biochemical reaction between ligand and SRS is likely to be an equilibrium (remember, few biochemical reactions are not in equilibrium), it is desirable to have the equilibrium go as far toward the products as possible, with little dissociation of the product complex (the reverse reaction). The reluctance of the reverse reaction in the equilibrium to occur is known as *avidity,* and a specific reactor substance that binds its ligands tightly is known as an avid SRS. Avidity is the second property of a specific reactor substance that contributes to sensitivity. In the situation where both the affinity and avidity are large, the equilibrium constant is also large. The larger the equilibrium constant, the smaller the concentration of ligand needed to saturate the SRS-binding sites, and the more sensitive the system is to small amounts of L. Therefore in a search for a specific reactor substance it is important to seek one with a large K_{eq}.

Fortunately, two classifications of biologic molecules meet the criteria of specificity, affinity, and avidity needed to make them good specific reactor substances. The first of these are carrier proteins. Dozens of these proteins exist in the body; their purpose is to transport important regulatory molecules throughout the tissues, releasing their cargo of hormone or vitamin to individual cells as needed. Generally, the hormone or vitamin bound to a carrier protein is inactive, whereas the released or ''free'' molecule is biochemically active. Some of the carrier proteins, such as albumin, are very nonspecific and will transport many different molecules. Other such as thyroid-binding globulin (TBG) and transferrin are very specific, carrying only one kind of molecule. Obviously it is the latter than can serve as specific reactor substances.

One of the advantages of using a carrier protein is the ease with which many of these materials can be obtained. In the original competitive-binding assay for thyroxine, Murphy and Pattee used serums from pregnant women, diluted with a buffer, as their source of TBG.[18] De la Pena and Goldzieher used a simple dilution of human plasma to obtain a suitable concentration of cortisol-binding globulin (CBG) for their cortisol assay.[5] β-Lactoglobulin, the so-called folate milk binder, can be obtained by dialysis of ordinary nonfat dry milk obtained at the grocery store. Other competitive-binding proteins such as intrinsic factor (isolated from hog intestinal mucosa for use as the SRS in the assay for vitamin B_{12}) and fish vitamin B_{12}–binding protein[15] are not quite so easily obtained but are still useful.

Unfortunately, some carrier proteins are not perfect specific reactor substances. The lack of complete specificity has been the downfall of these carrier proteins. The discovery in 1976[21] that serum-free fatty acids bind to TBG caused an almost total abandonment of TBG as an SRS. Similar interferences have been found for CBG. Other SRS materials with larger equilibrium constants have also led to the abandonment of carrier proteins.

The second and most common type of biologic molecule used as a specific reactor substance is the antibody. The study of antibodies, their formation, and their chemical reactions is called ''immunology.'' A review of the basic principles of this complex subject is in order.

BASIC IMMUNOLOGY

Mammalian bodies are complex and delicately tuned chemical systems. The process of evolution has resulted in each species' biochemical mechanisms developing an ability to recognize its own molecules from those of other species, even though the molecules have identical functions in the other species. For instance, treatment of diabetes mellitus in man with porcine insulin results in the diabetic regaining his ability to metabolize carbohydrates, but at the same time his immune system recognizes the procine insulin molecules as not coming from *Homo sapiens* and prepares to rid the body of them. Similarly, invasion of the human body by viruses is recognized by the body's immune system as a threat to its well-being, and it fights the invader by attempting to capture and destroy it.

A class of important molecules called ''immunoglobulins'' or ''antibodies'' is responsible for this defense mechanism. The immunoglobulin molecule's basic structure is shown in Fig. 18-3. Two heavy chains (of amino acids) and two light chains are bound together by disulfide (sulfur-to-sulfur) bonds. These molecules are synthesized by plasma cells, a type of lymphocyte that has its origins in the bone marrow and that has the unique ability to recognize ''foreign'' molecules. Recognition is achieved when the charge distribution and shape of a molecule are matched

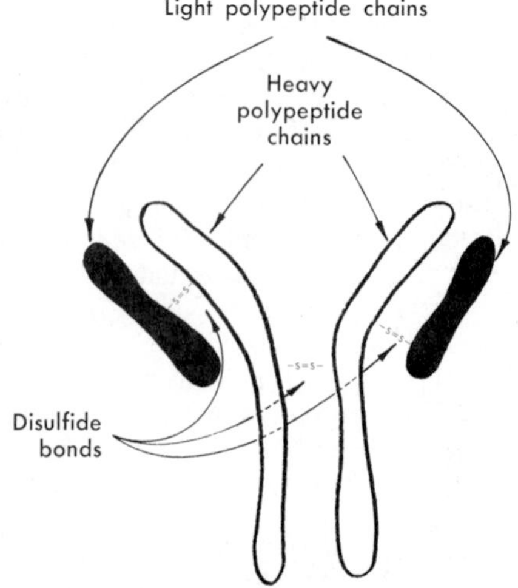

Fig. 18-3. Basic structure of immunoglobulins.

with some as yet undefined cellular ''knowledge'' about the species' own molecules. For instance, the amino acid sequence of porcine insulin differs from that of human insulin. The human immune system recognizes the difference and responds by producing immunoglobulins to porcine insulin. The immunoglobulin molecules react with the porcine insulin by binding it tightly. The recognition is stereochemical in nature; that is, the immunoglobulin recognizes the shape as being foreign. It is similar to the way in which a lock ''recognizes'' the key designed to open it. Once binding has occurred, the complex is destroyed either by a phagocyte or, in the case of whole-cell antigens, by the complement system.[25]

It is important to remember that antibodies to molecules of other species are not inherent in an organism, but rather are produced in response to a stimulus. It is this discovery that made Edward Jenner famous and founded the science of immunology. In 1796 Jenner noted that milkmaids who had been exposed to cowpox by coming into contact with the sores of animals who had the disease were immune to smallpox, the virulent plague of that time. In the famous experiment, Jenner inoculated a young boy with pus from a cowpox sore and then later exposed him to smallpox. The boy remained free of the disease—he was immune to it. We now know that the viruses that cause smallpox and cowpox are similar. Inoculation of the young boy with the pus that contained cowpox viruses caused his immune system to produce antibodies to the viruses. Later, when he was exposed to smallpox virus, these same antibodies bound to the viruses and permitted them to be destroyed before they could invade cells and cause the disease. Jenner called his cowpox pus preparation ''vaccine,'' and the process ''vaccination.''

There are five classes of immunoglobulin molecules. They differ in their molecular weight, valence (number of bonds that may be formed), their lifetime, and their rate of production. Table 18-1 lists these molecules and some of their properties. Despite the wide range of molecular weights, all except IgM have the same basic configuration shown in Fig. 18-3. IgM is a pentamer containing five such structures.

Like most biochemical reactions, the reaction between immunoglobulin and its intended target (known as an antigen) is an equilibrium with a K_{eq} on the order of 10^{10} liters per mole. A K_{eq} that large means that it is very difficult to separate immunoglobulin from antigen once they have reacted. Immunoglobulins are thus very avid molecules. They also undergo a unique polymerization reaction known as the ''precipitin reaction.'' Each immunoglobulin molecule has two or more identical binding sites. In a solution where the concentration of immunoglobulin is greater than that of the antigen, each molecule will bind only one antigen molecule, with some immunoglobulins having no antigen bound. In a solution whose antigen concentration is much greater than the immunoglobulin concentration, each immunoglobulin will bind two or more antigens, with some antigen being left over. In the zone of equivalence, the antibody/antigen ratio is such that a chain or polymer of antibody-antigen-antibody is formed. Eventually this chain grows to such a length that it can no longer remain in solution, and it precipitates out. This is the precipitin reaction. Detection of the precipitin reaction is important in an analytic method called ''radial immunodiffusion.'' It is also important in certain separation methods (to be discussed later).

Immunoglobulins make excellent specific reactor substances in competitive-binding radioassays. The specificity of the antibody-antigen reaction and the large K_{eq} (hence high affinity and avidity) of immunoglobulins give them the ideal properties needed. A competitive-binding radioassay where an immunoglobulin is used as the specific reactor substance is called a ''radioimmunoassay,'' or RIA. The ease with which the word and its abbreviation roll off the tongue have led to its being used to describe all competitive-binding radioassays, whether they involve an immunoglobulin or not. This text will follow that practice.

Preparation of antiserums

Since the ability to produce immunoglobulins is possessed by all mammals, the use of experimental animals to prepare antiserums (serums containing antibodies) is the obvious route to follow. Large molecules such as insulin are natural antigens, and injection of insulin from one species into another results in antibody formation. The tendency to form antibodies and the potency of those antibodies is dependent in part on the separation of the species in the phylogenetic chain. The more unrelated the species, the greater the production of potent antibodies. To induce antiserum production, the antigen is mixed with a material known

Table 18-1. Types of immunoglobulins*

Type	Molecular weight	Mean serum concentration (mg/ml)	Half-life (days)
IgG	150,000	11.4	23
IgA	170,000-500,000†	1.8	5.8
IgM	900,000‡	1	5.1
IgD	180,000	0.03	2.8
IgE	200,000	0.0003	2.3

*Modified from Kyle, R. A., and Greipp, P. R.: Mayo Clin. Proc. **53**:719-739, 1978.

†Tends to form polymers of the monomer.

‡Forms a pentamer.

as Freund's adjuvant, which is a suspension of killed bacteria, waxes, and emulsifiers in mineral oil. The components of this mixture serve to ''sensitize' or stimulate the immune system while preventing resorption of the adjuvant. Only small amounts (0.2 to 2 mg) of the potential antigen are necessary. One injects the adjuvant-antigen solution into the animal and then waits for antibody formation. Booster or secondary immunizations may be given at biweekly intervals to enhance antibody production, though the specificity of the antibody is determined by the primary immunization. After a suitable period, usually 2 to 3 months, a sample of the animal's blood is removed and tested for specificity and titer in the manner described below. The animal is not killed, for it will continue to produce antibodies as long as booster injections are given. A high-titer, high-specificity antiserum can be of real monetary value to the person who prepares it, and there have been some ''million-dollar'' rabbits that produced exceptionally good antiserums. Rabbits and goats, and to a lesser extent guinea pigs, have been commonly used for antiserum production because they are easy to care for and cooperative, yielding good antiserums.

The immunoglobulins produced under these conditions are usually of the IgG type. The determining factor is the time required for production, and IgG is usually the first immunoglobulin produced. Occasionally, immunoglobulins used in RIA are of the IgM class.

In some cases, the molecules toward which an antiserum is desired cannot be used directly as an antigen. This situation occurs when the molecule is not species-specific and hence not antigenic (as in the case of thyroxine), or when the molecule is too small to produce an immune response. (The immune response is, as you recall, a defense mechanism designed to rid the body of foreign ''invaders.'' It is primarily useful against larger molecules [molecular weight 5000 or greater]. Smaller molecules are eliminated by renal excretion or detoxified by conjugation in the liver.) When an antibody to a small molecule is desired, it must be conjugated (chemically attached) to a larger molecule that is antigenic. In that instance the small molecule is known as a ''hapten.'' A number of conjugation schemes have been utilized, the most common being the carbodiimide condensation. The basic principle behind any conjugation scheme is to (1) put a reactive group on the molecule of interest and (2) react this combination with a true antigen, which then serves as a carrier. This is schematically shown in Fig. 18-4. The animal immunized with this conjugate will (one hopes) produce antibodies to the carrier and the hapten. This brings out an important point about antibodies. Although an antibody, once produced, is specific for the stereochemical entity that served as the antigen, a large molecule has many antigenic sites and thus a family of antibodies is produced. It becomes a goal of the immunochemist to separate the antibodies of value in a radioimmunoassay from those produced to other than the desired hapten. The term ''antiserum'' usually indicates that a relatively unpurified solution of antibodies is being used.

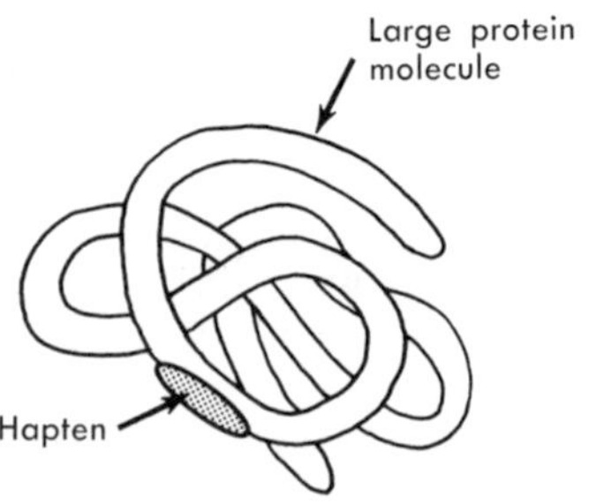

Fig. 18-4. Immunogen is produced when a hapten is bound to a larger carrier molecule. The binding process is called ''conjugation.''

Purification and characterization of antiserums

In order for an antiserum to be of maximum utility in a radioimmunoassay, it is desirable to know both the specificity and the titer, which is an indirect way of expressing the affinity, avidity, and K_{eq}. Before determining these properties, the immunochemist often purifies the immunoglobulins by a variety of techniques. Gel permeation chromatography may be used first to separate out molecules by molecular weight. The fraction containing the immunoglobulin molecules is then subjected to affinity chromatography. In this technique, the antigen is chemically bound to a solid carbohydrate support, which is then packed in a column. The immunoglobulin solution is passed through the column, and the antibodies of interest bind to the immobilized antigen. The column is washed, and the antibodies of interest are eluted from the solid support with a buffer that acts by changing the environment from one that allowed the antibody-antigen reaction to occur to one that favors release of the antigen. This is an example of the equilibrium nature and reversibility of the antigen-antibody reaction. If the antibody were perfectly avid, it would not be possible to isolate and purify it by this technique.

Another purification step is used to reduce the population of cross-reacting antibodies. Large molecules, especially polypeptide and steroid hormones, contain many regions that are stereochemically identical and that therefore may react with antibodies directed toward another member of that class of materials. This phenomena is called ''cross-reactivity'' and is a major problem in radioimmunoassay, since it reduces the

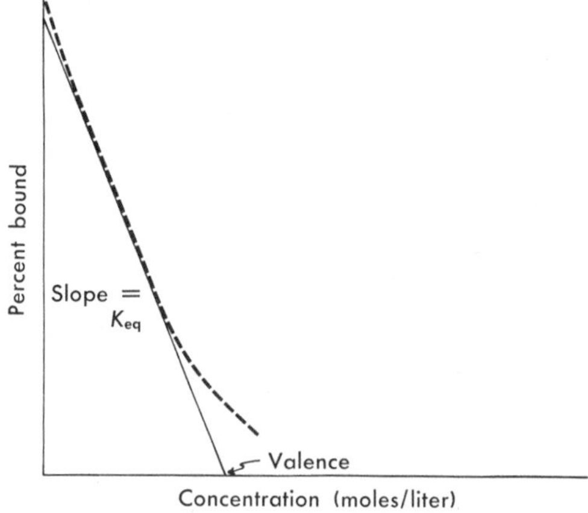

Fig. 18-5. Scatchard plot. Slope of line is equal to equilibrium constant. The *x* intercept is valence, or number of ligands that may be bound.

specificity of the assay. The affinity-chromatography purification process outlined above does not separate out cross-reacting antibodies. However, by attaching the cross-reacting *antigens* in a similar manner and passing the antiserum through a column packed with these, the antibodies that cross-react are retained in the column while those that do not react pass through the column. In this case the retained antibodies are discarded, and the antibody solution that passes through is used in further characterization steps.

Usual characterization steps include determination of K_{eq} by the method of Scatchard[20] and final determination of cross-reacting species. In the Scatchard analysis aliquots of the antibody at a suitable dilution are mixed with a constant amount of radiolabeled ligand and varying amounts of nonradiolabeled ligand. The unbound ligand is separated from the bound ligand and the ratio of bound to unbound radiolabeled ligand is plotted versus the bound concentration, which can be expressed as counts per minute (cpm). The graph that results is shown in Fig. 18-5, and the line is described by the equation

$$R = K(q - B) \qquad (5)$$

where R is the ratio of bound to unbound radiolabeled ligand, K is the equilibrium constant K_{eq}, q is the molar concentration of free antibody at equilibrium, and B is the radiolabeled ligand bound. The student of mathematics will recognize this equation as a form of the equation for a straight line

$$y = mx + b$$

where $y = R$, $m = K$, $x = (q - B)$, and $b = 0$. R and B are determined experimentally, and a plot of R versus B yields a straight line with slope k and a y intercept of 0 (since, when $R = 0$, $q - B$ must equal 0.) From this graph, K_{eq} and q, the maximum number of binding sites, may be determined. These values can be expressed as the molar quantities if the specific activity of the radiolabeled ligand is known and cpm is converted to moles per liter bound. Remember that K_{eq} is a measure of the affinity and avidity of a specific reactor substance.

Cross-reactivity is usually expressed as a percentage and is determined in the following way. Varying amounts of the cross-reacting substance are added to a mixture of the specific reactor substance and the labeled ligand toward which it is directed. A plot of percent radiolabeled ligand bound versus log concentration of cross-reacting material is made. Fig. 18-6 is an example of such a graph. The cross-reactivity is defined as the amount of cross-reacting material required to displace 50% of the radiolabeled ligand, divided by the amount of the substance of interest (cold ligand) required to displace 50% of the radiolabeled ligand. Cross-reactivity is often expressed as a percentage, the value from above being multiplied by 100. The degree of cross-reactivity tolerable in an RIA varies with the expected physiologic concentration of the cross-reacting species. One percent is a suitable cross-reactivity for the other aminoglycosides in the gentamicin radioimmunoassay, since the cross-reacting species is unlikely to be found in greater concentrations than gentamicin and 1% is better than the precision of the assay. On the other hand, the cross-reactivity of thyroxine (tetraiodothyronine, T_4) in the RIA for triiodothyronine (T_3) must be less than 0.01%, since T_4 is present in serum at a concentration of around 100 ng/ml and T_3 has a normal concentration of 0.1 ng/ml in serum.

The *titer* of a specific reactor substance is the dilu-

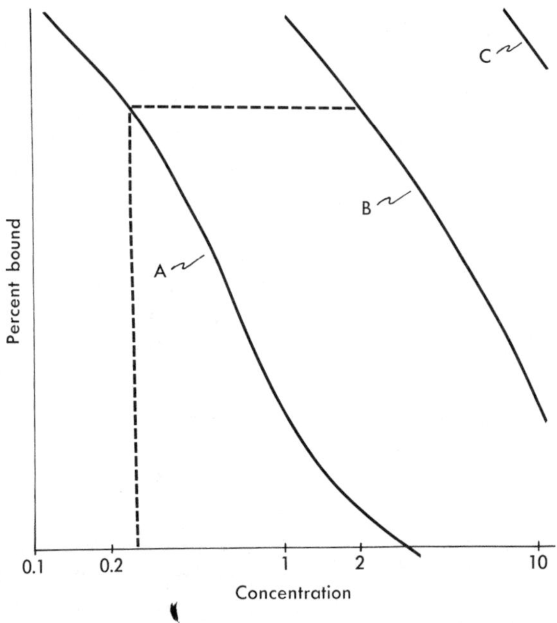

Fig. 18-6. In this typical cross-reactivity graph, substance *A* is being measured. Substance *B* cross-reacts about 10%, and substance *C* less than 2%.

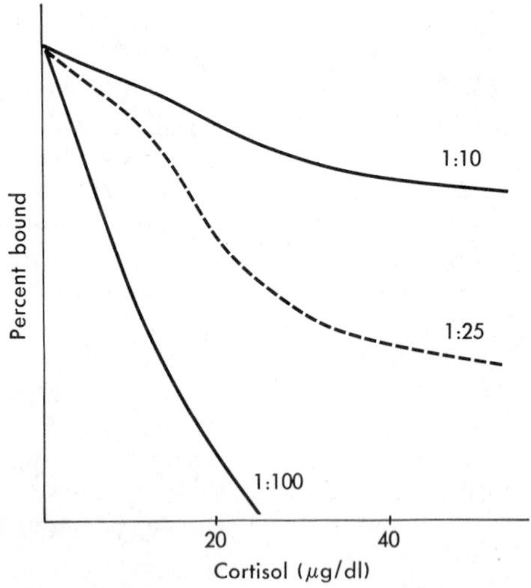

Fig. 18-7. Measuring percentage of ligand bound to specific reactor substance at various dilutions gives titer of specific reactor substance. In this example, 1:10 dilution does not give a very sensitive response and thus is not desirable. The 1:100 dilution gives a sensitive response, but it does not cover entire range of interest. The 1:25 dilution gives adequately sensitive response over concentration range of interest.

tion of the antibody required to give a solution of desired and useful concentration. Titers are determined by successive dilutions of the straight antiserums. The desired dilution is one in which 50% of the added radiolabeled ligand is bound. Fig. 18-7 shows the way in which the appropriate titer is determined.

The properties of specificity (expressed as cross-reactivity) and titer, as well as K_{eq}, are not unique to immunoglobulins, but also apply to carrier proteins and are determined in the same way. For all but a few special instances, notably vitamin B_{12} and folic acid, antibodies have replaced carrier proteins as the specific

Table 18-2. Properties of immunoglobulins and binding proteins of specific reactor substances

	Immunoglobulins	**Binding proteins**
Source	Immunized animals	Native human or animal serums or tissues
Typical K_{eq}	10^{10} liters/mol	10^{8} liters/mol
Specificity	High	Moderate
Avidity	High	Moderate
Preparation	Time-consuming immunization and purification	Simple dilution
Relative cost	Moderate	Low

reactor substance of choice, Table 18-2 compares the properties of these two classes of specific reactor substances.

RADIOLABELED LIGAND

The key to the sensitivity of a radioimmunoassay lies in the ability to prepare a radiolabeled ligand of high specific activity that is easily counted. The high degree of specificity obtainable with an antibody requires that the radiolabeling of the ligand be carried out in such a way as to leave the immunoreactive end of it intact. The radiochemist is challenged to prepare a radioligand that is immunoreactive and at the same time easily and efficiently counted.

Since biochemicals are primarily organic molecules, all contain hydrogen and carbon, and substitution of tritium (^{3}H) or ^{14}C is the first way of labeling that might be tried. Such simple substitution has the advantage of ensuring immunoreactivity of the product, since ^{3}H and ^{1}H are chemically identical. However, these beta particle–emitting nuclides present two other problems that make them less than ideal as labeling agents. First, their relatively long half-lives (12.3 years for ^{3}H, 5730 years for ^{14}C) mean that high specific activity is not easily achieved, even if more than one atom is substituted. Long counting times are therefore necessary to achieve precise determination of the radioactivity bound. Second, as beta-particle emitters these nuclides must be counted in a liquid scintillation counter, involving expensive and somewhat messy scintillation cocktails. Furthermore, serum, the biologic matrix that serves as the unknown sample in most radioimmunoassays, may contain bilirubin and hemoglobin, both excellent blue-light absorbers and consequently excellent quenching agents in liquid scintillation counting. Although some radioimmunoassays are still performed by use of ^{3}H-labeled ligands, the majority of labeled ligands are now of the gamma ray–emitting type.

Many early radioimmunoassays utilized the gamma-ray emitter iodine 131 as the radiolabeling agent. ^{131}I-labeled materials had been used in nuclear medicine for a long time. Furthermore, it was well known that the thyroid hormones could easily be labeled with radioactive ^{131}I, a substitution that allowed introduction of RIA into studies of thyroid function. Unfortunately, the relatively short half-life of ^{131}I and the difficulty in obtaining it in a pure form for use as a labeling reagent limited its use. It was not until ^{125}I became widely available in the early 1960s did iodination become the optimal way of preparing radiolabeled ligands.

For those molecules such as thyroxine, which already contained iodine, simple substitution of ^{125}I for the normal ^{127}I yielded a reagent of high specific activity. Unfortunately, the thyroid hormones are the exception; few of the biochemicals for which radioimmunoassays have been developed have iodine as a native atom. In these instances it becomes necessary to alter the molecule to attach the radiolabel. In the early 1960s it was discovered that iodine could be easily added to the aromatic ring of the amino acid tyrosine by reduction of the iodide ion with the oxidizing agent chloramine-T* in an aqueous medium. Now any protein containing a tyrosine or histidine residue could be easily iodinated by use of the so-called Hunter-Greenwood technique.[9] This led to development of radioimmunoassays for a number of important protein hormones, among them TSH and FSH. However, development of radioimmunoassays for smaller or nonprotein hormones and drugs was still limited by the necessity to use ^{3}H- or ^{14}C-labeled ligands. When chemists discovered techniques to attach tyrosine to a variety of nonprotein molecules, the field began to expand, since these tyrosines could be iodinated in the same way as proteinaceous tyrosine. One of the first small molecules to which this technique was applied is the cardioactive drug digoxin, shown in Fig. 18-8. The digitose sugars were removed and replaced by a succinyl tyrosine ester, which could be easily iodinated. Later, a tyrosine methyl ester of digoxin, which could be iodinated, was also prepared and is now the common labeled ligand used in the digoxin RIA. An essential feature of these radioligands is that they continue to react with the antidigoxin antibody identically to pure digoxin. In the preparation of any labeled derivative for use in RIA, the location of the derivatizing group must be chosen so that the immunoreactivity of the molecule remains unchanged. This requirement has been cleverly met for a number of molecules, so that iodinated derivatives of many drugs and steroid hor-

*Chloramine-T is a trivial name for *N*-chloro-4-methylbenzenesulfonamide sodium salt.

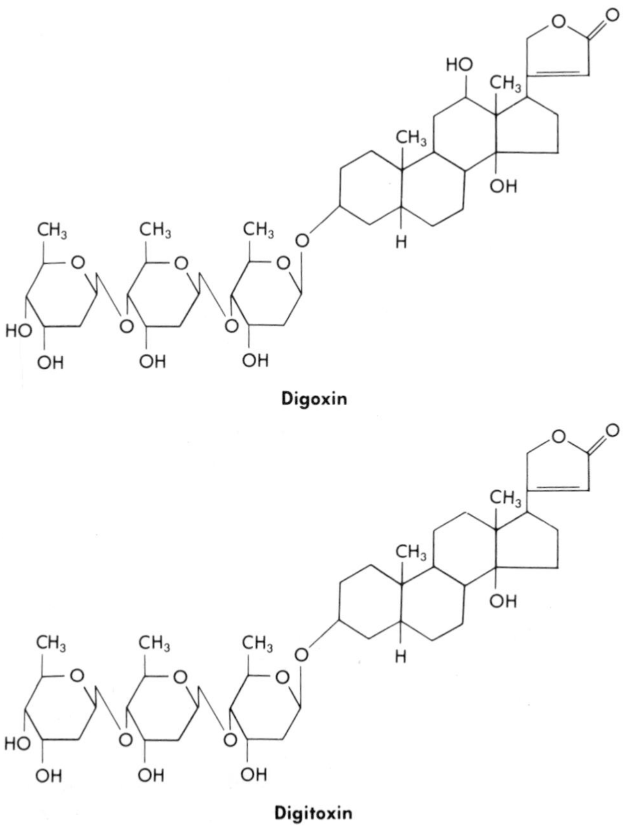

Fig. 18-8. Digoxin and digitoxin. Note difference of hydroxyl group, —OH, on third ring from right.

mones are available for use in radioimmunoassays today.

Iodine 125 is now the standard nuclide used in radioimmunoassays. It is a low-energy gamma-ray emitter that is safe to handle, easy to count, and has a reasonable half-life and therefore shelf-life. It can be obtained in essentially pure form as NaI, so that labeled ligands of extremely high specific activity are obtainable. (The specific activity of some ligands is so high that some kit manufacturers deliberately add unlabeled ligand to their labeled reagent to keep count rates at a reasonable level.) Because ^{125}I is a "pure" gamma-ray emitter, compounds labeled with it do not undergo the radiation damage that may result from use of ^{131}I, which decays to give a beta particle as well as gamma radiation. However, it is still difficult to label some peptide materials even with ^{125}I, by the chloramine-T technique, since chloramine-T can cause some structural damage to the molecule. In 1973 Bolton and Hunter[2] devised a modified chloramine-T method that spared the protein from exposure to the oxidizing agent. In the Bolton-Hunter technique, the activated ester *N*-succinimidyl-3(4-hydroxyphenyl)propionate is first iodinated by the chloramine-T method; then the protein is reacted with the purified iodinated ester to form a derivative that contains the iodine. This technique is of considerable importance in preparing labeled analogs of peptides that are difficult and expensive to obtain.

Although ^{125}I is the standard nuclide for use in radioimmunoassays, there are a number of instances where other nuclides are more advantageous. It is still not possible to prepare good iodinated derivatives of some steroid hormones, and so ^{3}H must be used to label these. In at least one case, a better gamma-ray emitter is available—that case being vitamin B_{12}, whose corrin shell surrounds an atom of cobalt. ^{57}Co has been successfully placed in the corrin shell to provide a labeled compound of such high specific activity that picogram amounts of the vitamin can be detected in serum. Selenium 75 has also been used to label some molecules for RIA.

SEPARATION METHODS

The chemistry of specific reactor substances and radiolabeled molecules lend specificity and sensitivity

Table 18-3. Separation methods

Method	Advantages	Disadvantages	Restrictions
Adsorbents	Rapid		
Dextran-charcoal	Cheap	Stripping	Control temperature and contact time
Silicates	Convenient	Nonspecific	
Ion-exchange resin	Cheap Rapid Convenient		Free ligand must be ionic
Molecular sieving	Cheap	Slow	Works best for small molecules
Protein denaturation $(NH_4)_2SO_4$ Polyethylene glycol Alcohols	Cheap	Trapping	Restricted to small molecules
Double antibody	Specific	Expensive Time consuming	
Solid-phase antibody	Convenient	Expensive Variable	Limited to small molecules

to radioimmunoassays, but the benefit of these two parameters cannot be realized unless separation of the bound and free ligands are achieved. A good separation is thus important to a useful radioimmunoassay.

Early investigators separated bound from unbound ligands by electrophoresis, a technique for separating proteins based on their charge. However, electrophoresis is a time-consuming process not easily adapted to large numbers of samples, and so it is seldom used in modern radioimmunoassays. Its place has been taken by a number of other separation techniques, listed in Table 18-3. As each of these is reviewed, remember that none of them is the "perfect" technique. Each has its advantages, and the separation method must therefore be tailored to meet the individual radioimmunoassay.

Adsorption of the unbound ligand was the separation method that became popular when the large volumes of samples being assayed precluded the use of electrophoresis. Separation by adsorption depends on the fact that certain materials have the property of forming weak, Van der Waals bonds with almost any polar molecules. (A van der Waals bond is an attraction between the charged portions of two molecules, known as dipoles.) These materials have been put to use as separating agents in RIA. Among them are activated charcoal and certain silicate minerals.

The process of adsorption is a surface phenomenon. A small molecule containing a weak dipole (slight excess or deficit of electron concentration around a nucleus) can form a van der Waals bond between itself and the adsorbent. Molecules that are nonpolar, or whose dipoles are hidden by nonpolar parts of the molecule, are less easily adsorbed. Furthermore, the particles of adsorbents contain many millions of interstices, through which smaller molecules pass with ease but which larger molecules may not enter because of their size. These properties of adsorbents make them potential separating agents for RIA, since most ligands are small whereas antibody-antigen complexes are large. Another advantage in using surface adsorption as a separation method in RIA is that tremendous surface area is available for adsorption on the particles. A gram of charcoal may have many square meters of available surface area. Thus even a small amount of charcoal is sufficient to adsorb all polar molecules rapidly. Fast adsorption is desirable for two reasons. First, as free ligand is removed from solution, Le Châtelier's principle dictates that the immunoglobulin-ligand complex dissociate to form free ligand again and attempt to reestablish an equilibrium between free and bound ligand. Unless a high-avidity immunoglobulin is used, such dissociation can be enough to destroy the sensitivity of the assay. A more practical reason for desiring fast adsorption is that it reduces total assay time and thus increases the productivity of the individual performing the assay.

Adsorption is not without its disadvantages, and thus its popularity as a separation method is decreasing. The greatest disadvantage is that adsorbents, especially activated charcoal, have a tendency to strip the ligands off of antibodies of low avidity. The time during which the adsorbent is allowed to be in contact with the solution containing the full ligand must be carefully controlled to minimize stripping. The time of contact for all tubes in the assay must be kept constant to maintain reproducibility. The need for exact timing, then, is the most serious disadvantage is using adsorbents. Another disadvantage is the nonselectivity of adsorbents, which results in the removal of some ligand-antibody complex. This problem can be overcome, however, by use of a coated adsorbent, dextran-coated charcoal being the most common. Dextran is a polymeric carbohydrate that, if magnified large enough so that individual molecules may be seen, would look like a net or sieve. Coating charcoal particles with dextran further reduces the surface area available to adsorb large molecules, since only smaller molecules (free ligands) can pass through the "holes" in the dextran sieve. Coating charcoal thus increases the selectivity of this separating medium.

In practice, separation by adsorption of free ligand is achieved by the addition of a constant aliquot of adsorbent suspension to each tube in the assay, followed by centrifugation of the tubes for a period of time, usually 10 minutes. With a good centrifuge, the adsorbent is usually concentrated in the bottom of the tube in the first half-minute of centrifugation, effectively completing the separation. The remainder of the time is necessary to pack the adsorbent into a hard pellet so that the supernate solution can be poured off. Theoretically either the bound (supernate) or free (pellet) fraction can be counted, but in practice the bound is usually transferred to another tube and counted. A refrigerated centrifuge is often used, since the lower temperature increases the avidity of the antibody.

A somewhat related method of separating bound and free ligands on the basis of molecular size is known as "gel permeation chromatography," or "gel filtration." Certain polymeric materials, of which cross-linked dextran (Sephadex) is the most common, are in fact porous particles that can be compared to sponges. Each particle has thousands of interstices that small molecules can migrate into but that are too narrow for large molecules to pass through. When this material is packed into a column and the mixture of free and bound ligand added, the free ligands migrate into the particles and get trapped in the myriad of interstices. Meanwhile, the larger, antibody-ligand complexes pass around the particles and exit from the column first. Control of the size of particles and their interstices can yield a very effective separation. However, because of the need for a separate column for each tube and the expense of collecting fractions, separation by gel permeation is usually reserved for those radioimmunoassays where other methods prove ineffective.

A separation technique that has proved particularly useful in the radioimmunoassay of thyroid hormones is ion exchange. By changing the pH of the media it is dissolved in, one can make thyroxine (see Fig. 18-15) anionic. There is a class of materials known as ion-exchange resins in which a plastic (polystyrene) bead is chemically modified to add a side chain to its structure. The side chain contains a functional group that is ionic. Under the proper conditions of pH and ionic strength, the thyroxine ion will exchange with the counter-ion of the ionic side chain, becoming bound to the bead. Only free thyroxine can react in this manner; antibody-bound thyroxine is either nonionic or the ionic site is shielded and unable to react. Physical removal of the resin beads from the solution completes the separation. A number of gimmicks have been used to facilitate the removal, including immobilization of the resin beads in a polyurethane sponge or on a plastic strip, use of a fine sieve to retain the beads while the solution is being poured off, and reduction of the size of the beads to the point where they pack upon centrifugation. The obvious disadvantage of ion exchange is that it works only for those small molecules that can be made ionic, and its use has been limited chiefly to radioimmunoassays for thyroxine. Fig. 18-9 illustrates ion exchange.

All the above separation methods have made use of the physical properties of the free ligand to achieve separation. The next three separation methods take advantage of properties of the antibody to separate bound from free.

Precipitation of the immunoglobulin complex by protein denaturation is an old biochemical technique that has been successfully applied in radioimmunoassays. Modern analytic techniques such as x-ray diffraction have demonstrated that a protein's activity and solubility depend on its three "structures." The primary structure is the order in which the amino acids are arranged; the secondary structure is the coiling of the molecule into spirals and loops; and the tertiary structure is the folding of the coils and loops on top of one another. Disruption of the secondary and tertiary structures results in denaturation of the protein, making it insoluble.

A number of chemicals will cause this denaturation. Saturated ammonium sulfate and alcohols including polyethylene glycol are the most commonly used substances. Addition of either of these to a solution of immunoglobulins will cause the immunoglobulins to precipitate, though the antigen still remains bound to

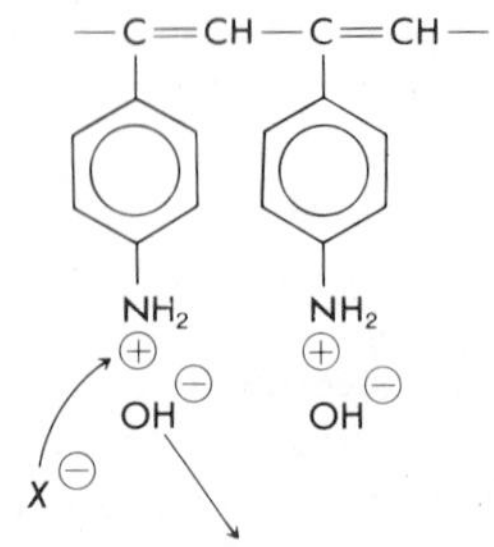

Fig. 18-9. In ion exchange, negatively charged ion (anion, X^-) replaces ion of like charge (in this case hydroxide ion, OH^-) from its binding site on polystyrene resin.

the immunoglobulin. If the antigen is not a protein itself, this technique can be used to separate bound from free, with centrifugation removing the precipitate from the solution. Since the amount of active immunoglobulin in one tube of an RIA is quite small, some neutral protein such as albumin is usually added to increase the bulk of the precipitate. Aside from its restriction to use with nonprotein antigens, the chief disadvantage of this technique is the tendency of some unbound radiolabeled ligand to become either physically trapped in the precipitate pellet or adsorbed to it, making the separation inconsistent or incomplete.

Immunoglobulins are proteins that themselves become antigens when introduced into another species, and this leads to a separation technique known as the double-antibody precipitation. First described almost simultaneously by Morgan and Lazarow[17] in 1962, and Hales and Randle[6] in 1963, the technique requires two antibodies—one raised to the ligand of interest, the other raised toward immunoglobulins from the species producing the first antibody. In double-antibody separation, the original antigen-antibody reaction is allowed to reach equilibrium, and the second antibody is added to the solution in a quantity that will give a final antibody concentration in the zone of equivalence. The precipitin reaction occurs and the precipitated antibody complex, still containing the original radiolabeled antigen, is centrifuged to achieve physical separation. The resulting supernate is poured off or aspirated and discarded, and the bound radioactivity present in the centrifuged pellet is counted. One of the advantages of the double-antibody precipitation is that it can be used with any size of antigen. It was originally used mainly for hormones, but its use has expanded to include all ligands. Nearly 25% of all commercially available RIA kits use the double-antibody separation. A disadvantage of the double-antibody technique is that the precipitating reaction may be slow, requiring a lengthy incubation after addition of the second antibody. This problem has been overcome by use of the pre-precipitated double antibody. One carries out the reaction between the first and second antibodies in bulk prior to performing the actual RIA. When the RIA is performed, aliquots of the suspension containing the double-antibody precipitin are added to each tube. If the second antibody was correctly prepared, the active site of the first antibody is still available for reaction with the ligands. When that reaction is complete, centrifugation completes the separation process. A difficulty that can be encountered with use of the double antibody is the tendency of the precipitin pellet to begin floating once centrifugation has ceased. To prevent this occurrence, it is important to remove the supernate by pouring or suction immediately after centrifugation is complete.

The final method for the separation of bound and free ligands is to attach the antibody to a solid supporting medium, which can be physically removed from the solution once the reaction is complete. Attachment of the antibody may be through a covalent bond, or a form of adsorption to a surface may be used. More recently, microencapsulation of the antibody in a membrane that is permeable to the antigen has been described.* Solid phases that have been used include polypropylene tube walls, glass beads both large and small, and cross-linked dextran (Sephadex) particles. Binding of the antibody to a tube wall results in the easiest radioimmunoassay to perform, since a pipetting step (antibody addition) is eliminated, as is centrifugation. However, this type of solid-phase antibody is not without its disadvantages. It is difficult to achieve a uniform lot-to-lot coating of the tube walls, which may lead to lot-to-lot variations in the results. Because the antibody is immobilized, the rate of reaction between antibody and antigen is controlled by the rate at which antigen-containing solution can be brought into contact with the tube walls. For undisturbed solutions, this rate is the rate of diffusion of the ligands in that medium, which is slow. Periodic mixing increases the rate, but it still does not approach that of a soluble antibody. For this reason, relatively long incubation times are required for some coated-tube assays. This is not true of those solid-phase RIAs where the antibody is bound to small particles such as Sephadex or glass microbeads. These systems behave similarly to a pre-precipitated double antibody with physical separation achieved by centrifugation. Large glass beads coated with antibody behave similarly to coated tubes.

Another innovation in solid-phase separation is the use of magnetic microparticles. Both antibodies bound covalently to magnetic particles[8,19] and microparticles encapsulated by sorption reagents or binding proteins[10] have been described. Separation is achieved when a magnet is placed next to the tube and the solution is poured off while the magnetic particles are retained.

Table 18-3 lists the separation methods and their advantages and disadvantages.

MANIPULATION OF RADIOIMMUNOASSAY DATA

The performance of a radioimmunoassay involves the mixing of hot and cold ligands with an antibody, a suitable incubation period, separation of bound and free ligands, and counting of the radioactivity in one of these fractions. The resulting data, in the form of accumulated counts, must be analyzed in some way to

*Patent applied for by the Damon Corporation, Needham Heights, Massachusetts.

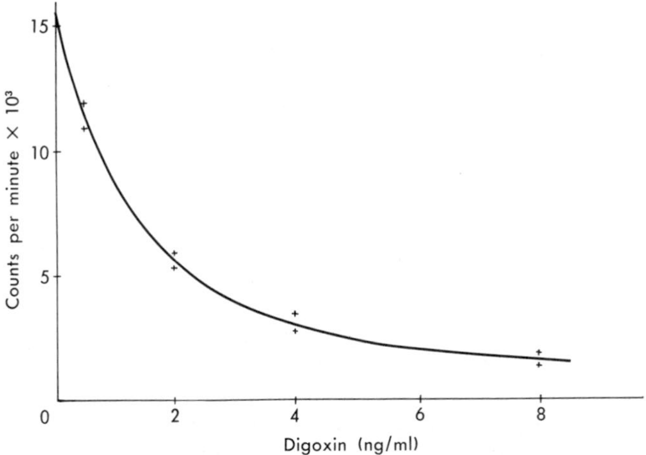

Fig. 18-10. Plot of counts per minute bound versus concentration is simplest way to plot radioimmunoassay data. Curve that results is hyperbolic in shape.

yield information about the concentration of the substance of interest in the unknown specimens. This data analysis must take into account not only the amounts of radioactively labeled ligand bound for the various standards, but also the amount of radioligand bound in the absence of any cold ligand (the zero standard) and the amount of radioactivity nonspecifically bound to tube walls, precipitating antiserums, etc. (the nonspecific binding, or NSB). Evaluation of these two parameters is conducted by use of zero standard tube (contains labeled ligand and antibody but no unlabeled ligand) and an NSB tube (contains labeled ligand but no unlabeled ligand or antibody) in each assay.

Since the nonspecific binding of radiolabeled ligand is not related to the concentration of unlabeled ligand, counts accumulated for NSB tubes are always subtracted from all other tubes before further data analysis is begun. It is desirable for the NSB counts to be at a minimum, and certainly no more than 10% of the counts for the zero standard. When NSB counts are subtracted, the background is also automatically subtracted, since it is assumed that the background is part of the NSB. A separate subtraction step is therefore not necessary. The exception to this is in assays where separation is achieved by solid-phase antibodies. A true NSB cannot be obtained in a solid-phase system, and so this tube is left out. Subtraction of counter background is thus necessary for a solid-phase RIA.

Having completed the first step of data analysis, NSB/background subtraction, the next step is to plot the accumulated counts (or some quantity related to counts) versus the concentration of the standards employed in the assay. The simplest method is to plot counts bound versus concentration on rectilinear graph paper (Fig. 18-10). For most radioimmunoassays this will result in a hyperbolic curve. Note the following features of this plot: (1) The sensitivity of the curve varies, that is, the number of counts required to achieve the same change in concentration is fewer on the right end of the curve than it is on the left (upper) end. (2) The plot is not linear, and some degree of skill is required to draw the best smooth line through all points on the curve. A linear relationship is therefore more desirable than a curve. Notice that the points do not all fall directly on the line. A "roller-coaster" curve connecting all points does not truly reflect the relationship between counts-per-minute bound and concentration because it can be mathematically shown that the relationship is a smooth curve. The variation between a point's actual y coordinate and the position of the curve (estimated y coordinate) for the same x coordinate is subject to experimental error, discussed in the section on quality control.

The two features mentioned above represent drawbacks to this type of plot of RIA data. It would be much better if a method of plotting that yielded a linear relationship were available. Fig. 18-11 shows another method of plotting data that yields a better (but still not perfect) approximation of a straight line. In this instance, the fraction or percent of the total radioactive ligand bound is plotted against the logarithm of the concentration. To simplify this, semilogarithmic graph paper is used. (One may determine the total radioactive ligand present by either including a special "total count" tube in the run [this tube need only contain an aliquot of the labeled ligand] or by counting any one of the assay tubes before the separation step.) A sigmoid curve results, with the center portion approaching linearity. However, this method of displaying the

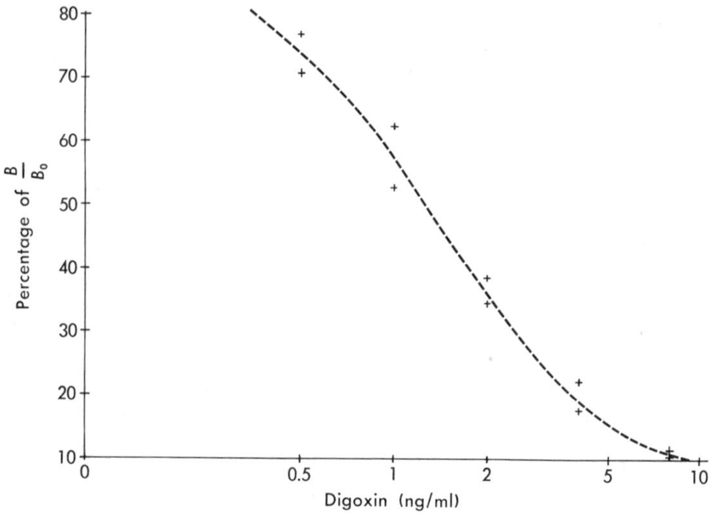

Fig. 18-11. Same data shown in Fig. 18-10 has been plotted here in form of percentage of B/B_0 versus log concentration. Curve approaches linearity in central region but is noticeably nonlinear near extremes.

data requires the subjective drawing of the curve at the extreme ends of the data set, thus not satisfying our goal of a linear relationship.

Fortunately, there is a simple mathematical transformation known as the logit, which permits the plotting of RIA data in a linear fashion. The logit of y is defined as

$$\ln\left(\frac{y}{1-y}\right)$$

If we choose y as the fraction of the radiolabeled ligand bound relative to the fraction bound for the zero standard (commonly written B/B_0), then

$$\text{logit } B/B_0 = \ln\left(\frac{B/B_0}{1 - B/B_0}\right)$$

If B/B_0 is expressed as a percent, then

$$\text{logit } B/B_0 = \ln\left(\frac{B/B_0}{100 - B/B_0}\right)$$

A plot of logit B/B_0 versus the log of the concentration will yield a straight line if the system were allowed to come to equilibrium. (It will not be linear for nonequilibrium or sequential saturation analyses). Such a plot is shown in Fig. 18-12. Although the actual sensitivity of the assay remains the same as it was with the first plotting method, the apparent sensitivity changes when this method is used. The reason is that the distance separating 1% bound is much greater on the ends of the line than in the middle, as illustrated by the percentage-bound scale on the right side of the graph paper. However, the main advantage of using the logit-log plot for RIA data is that it gives a straight line and is less subject to interpretation and drawing errors than either of the two methods discussed above. The logit has become the generally accepted method of plotting RIA data.

Logit plots have some disadvantages. One disadvantage is that no zero point exists on a logit graph, and in fact the relationship between zero and the smallest standard concentration is not defined on the graph. It is therefore not justified to read or report an unknown value less than the lowest nonzero standard—only a "less than" report should be issued. Another disadvantage is that the logit transformation results in a pronounced nonuniformity of the variance at the extreme ends of the curve. This property is known as "heteroskedasticity."[19a] The effects of heteroskedasticity will be reviewed when computer analysis of data is discussed.

These two disadvantages are more than compensated for by the advantage of using the logit transformation. In addition to the ease of preparing the correct standard curve, the logit transformation makes it easy to check parallelism, a desirable property of all RIAs. An RIA is said to exhibit parallelism if the line produced by a series of standards is parallel to one produced when one dilutes out a high unknown sample and plots the result of each dilution. If the plot of logit B/B_0 versus log standard concentration is not parallel to the line of logit B/B_0 versus log concentration of a diluted patient sample, the RIA is not correctly measuring the substance of interest at both ends of the concentration range. The usual cause of nonparallelism is

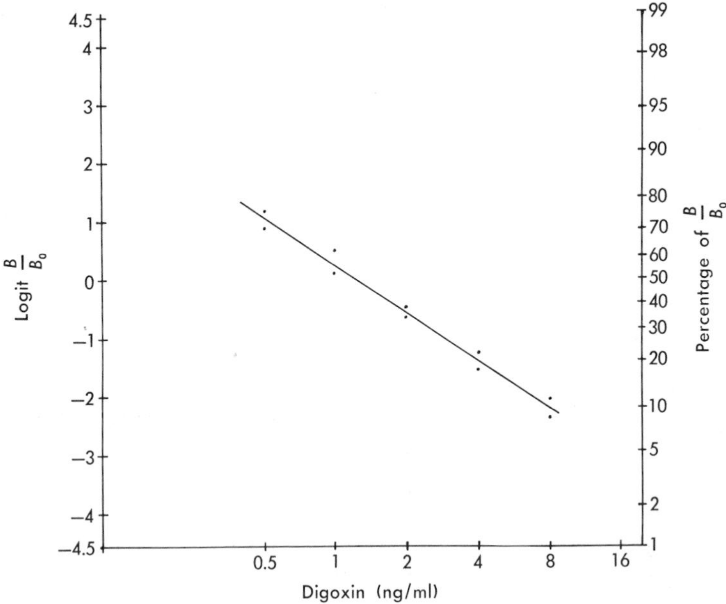

Fig. 18-12. Data from Fig. 18-10 plotted as logit percentage bound versus log concentration. Notice linearity of line over two orders of magnitude. Some radioassays have linear logit plots over three orders of magnitude.

cross-reactivity at the high end, since the cross-reacting substance is diluted out more quickly than the true ligand. The presence of an autoantibody to the ligand, a phenomenon observed in insulin-treated diabetes, for example, would also be evident in an evaluation for parallelism.

The logit transformation also permits confirmation that true equilibrium conditions exist in the RIA, that the antibody is saturated (all binding sites occupied), that the NSB is sufficiently low, and that the B_0 counts are correct.[22] If these conditions do not exist, the logit plot becomes curved, a situation that the technologist can quickly discern when plotting the data. Nonequilibrium can occur because of destruction of the labeled ligand, an insufficient incubation time, or a variation in temperature during the run or between tubes within a run.

Another simple method of graphing RIA data which results in a curve approaching linearity is to plot some reciprocal function of counts bound vs. concentration on a linear scale. The reciprocal function may be $1/B$, T/B, F/B, or B_0/B, where B, T, F, and B_0 are counts bound, total counts, counts "free," and zero standard counts bound respectively. Recognize that all these expressions except F/B are essentially equivalent, differing only by a constant. A plot of $1/B$ versus concentration is shown in Fig. 18-13 for the same set of data plotted in the other examples. Note that the points become curved as the line approaches zero. The accuracy of this type of graph is thus limited in regions of low concentration. An additional disadvantage is the fact that the highest concentration point exerts a greater influence on the line than do the other points. This is a more severe problem when computer analysis of the data is used. The reciprocal method of plotting does have the advantage of giving a nonlinear graph when certain assay conditions are not met.[7]

Electronic processing of radioimmunoassay data

The proliferation of pocket and desktop programmable calculators during the same period of time that RIA was growing in popularity led to a great amount of interest in electronic evaluation of RIA data. All the methods of data plotting discussed previously can be adapted to a programmable calculator or minicomputer. The limiting factors to such electronic data processing are the user's knowledge of the properties of the equations that represent the data and the cleverness of the programmer.

Most electronic data processing programs for determining standard curves are based on a variation of the least-squares concept. Briefly, the least-squares concept states that the best line through a group of data $(x_1, y_1, x_2, y_2, \ldots x_n, y_n)$ representing a relationship is the line where the sum of $(y_{\text{actual}} - y_{\text{calculated}})^2$ for all values of y is the smallest. This concept can be applied to both linear and nonlinear relationships. It is easily programmed on a computer or calculator

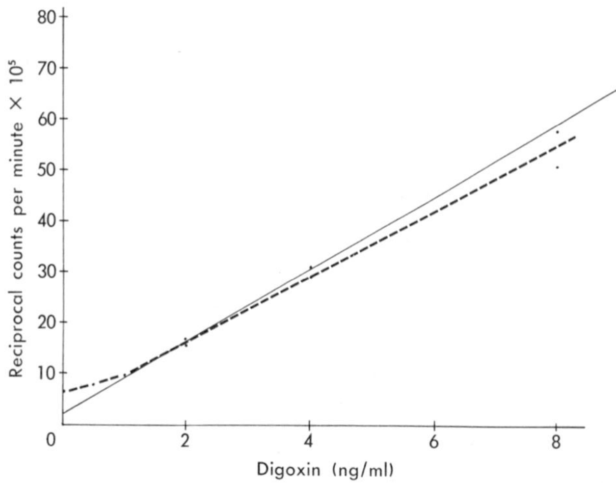

Fig. 18-13. Plot of reciprocal counts per minute versus concentration yields line that approaches linearity at high concentrations but is noticeably nonlinear at low concentrations. *Dashed line,* Actual data; *solid line,* computer-calculated best-fit straight line.

(some pocket calculators have a built-in capability for calculating the least-squares line for linear data sets).

The use of the least-squares technique for analyzing data in the counts-per-minute versus concentration and B/T versus log concentrations forms is limited because of the difficulty in defining the nonlinear equations that represent these curves. If several terms are required to define the curve, more calculation steps are necessary and more computer time and memory space is used. The equations for handling the nonlinear relationships frequently exceed the storage capacity of desktop calculators, negating their use. The logit equation, on the other hand, has only one x and one y term and thus is well-suited to analysis by desktop calculators. However, use of the logit data directly in a linear least-squares program can lead to erroneous results because of heteroskedasticity: the points on the ends have more influence on the slope of the line than do the ones in between. This can be remedied by use of a weighted least-squares program. Here, the line is determined by the sum of $\frac{1}{x} \cdot (y_{\text{actual}} - y_{\text{calculated}})^2$, with $\frac{1}{x}$ being the weighting factor. When such a program is used, the linear least squares becomes a powerful tool, for it not only defines the best line for the standard curve but also gives the user a slope and intercept with which he can calculate his unknown results instead of reading them from a graph. In a correctly written program, the user need only enter the raw data and the calculator will respond with an answer in concentration units.

The reciprocally weighted least-squares program may also be adapted to handling standard curves plotted by one of the reciprocal equations. However, the nonlinearity of these equations in the low concentration ranges will result in a positive bias on the calculated line, which may be significant. The degree of such bias for this plot and any least-squares plot can be determined by graphing $(y_{\text{actual}} - y_{\text{calculated}})$ versus y. If the equation to which the data was fitted is appropriate, the points will be scattered above and below zero over the entire range of y. If a bias exists, there will be a definite trend for all points to be above or below zero. This type of graph is known as a residuals plot and may be made without the benefit of a computer.

Since most radioimmunoassays are done in duplicate, the question of how to handle the duplicate sets of data for each concentration often arises. Each duplicate tube should be handled separately, since this minimizes the shift caused by one outlier in a pair of data points. Similarly, averaging of data on unknowns should be done with the final result, not the raw data.

QUALITY CONTROL IN RADIOIMMUNOASSAYS

An important part of any laboratory system performing routine analyses is the maintenance of a quality control program. Analysts are concerned with performing their work with accuracy and precision. Accuracy refers to the agreement of the measured value with the actual value of the parameter of interest. Precision refers to the degree of reproducibility one can obtain in measuring the same sample repeatedly. Quality control is the way of defining both the precision and the accuracy of analytical methods.

The accuracy of a method is dependent on the chemical and physical characteristics of the substance being measured and on the methodology used. Some methods are much more accurate than others. Part of the analyst's job is to know where both inaccuracy and imprecision exist in his methodology.

The type of error described by consistent inaccuracy in measurements is known as a systematic error. Random error is the term used to describe the fact that man and his inventions are not perfect, so that when he measures a parameter many times some variation in the result will occur just because of his imperfections. The attempt to define how close man can come to perfection in his measurement is the premise for statistical quality control. Statistical quality control is based on the phenomenon known as normal distribution. Normal distributions occur widely in nature. For instance, if one were to measure the height of 1000 men selected at random from across the United States, one would find that the average height of all 1000 men is about 5 feet 10 inches; furthermore, more men would be 5 feet 10 inches tall than any other height. There would be a few men only 5 feet tall and a few almost 7 feet tall, with the number of men of a certain height increasing as the height approaches 5 feet 10 inches. A graph of height versus the number of men having that height gives the familiar bell-shaped curve we call a normal, or gaussian, distribution.

The same type of distribution exists for many other body parameters, such as the concentration of various substances in the blood of healthy people. Most importantly, the measurement of a single sample for one of these substances, done repeatedly, also follows a normal distribution. It is the mathematical nature of this distribution that is defined with statistical quality control.

A mathematic equation for the normal distribution has been described, and from this equation the most important statistical parameter, the standard deviation, was derived. The formula for the standard deviation, SD, is

$$SD = \sqrt{\frac{\sum(x - \bar{x})^2}{n - 1}} \qquad (6)$$

where x is an individual measurement, $\bar{x}$ is the average of all measurements, and n is the number of measurements. A close look at the formula reveals that it is a function of the differences between an individual measurement and the average of all measurements. Either the symbol s, or the symbol σ, is sometimes used to denote standard deviation.

It can be shown that for a normal distribution, 68.3% of the values measured lie within ±1 SD of the mean, and 95.5% lie within ±2 SD of the mean. The normal distribution curve, with these limits indicated, is shown in Fig. 18-14.

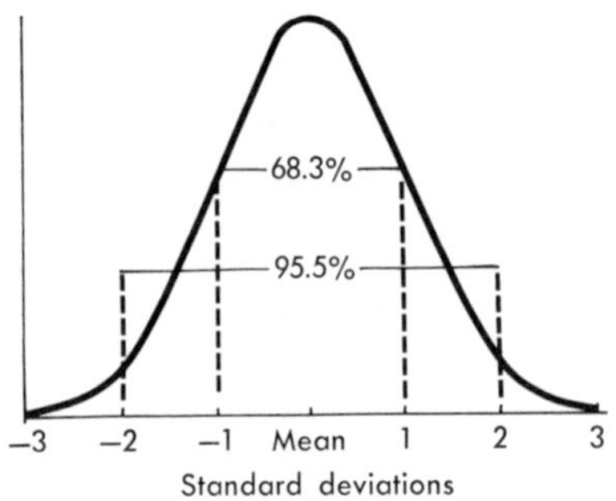

Fig. 18-14. In gaussian relationship 68.3% of values lie within 1 standard deviation of mean and 95.5% lie within 2 SD of mean.

As is evident from the figure, the standard deviation is an indicator of how widely a population varies. In the previous example, the population consisted of 1000 men and the measured parameter was height. Deviation from the mean exists because nature does not make all men the same. What if the measured parameter is the concentration of component z in a serum sample? There can be only one absolute concentration of z in that serum sample. However, if that concentration is measured many times, the measurements comprise a normal distribution, because z cannot be measured perfectly every time. The smaller the standard deviation, the more precise the measurement of z is. If the procedure is accurate (measures true z exactly), then the standard deviation is an indicator of how well z can be measured.

It is easy to see the value of statistical quality control. If a sample is assayed each and every time a particular procedure is done, in a short period of time enough values are accumulated for the sample to determine the standard deviation for measurement of that sample and, by implication, for all other samples measured at the same time. The standard deviation thus allows one to set limits on the precision of measurement of any one sample. Such a sample is a quality control sample, often called simply a "control." If the control value lies within the 95.5% range, the value for any other sample from the same run is precise and accurate to the same degree of confidence. Furthermore, a control value outside of the 95.5% range is a flag to tell us that there may be a problem with that particular run. Some laboratories use the ±2 SD range as a cutoff, with control values falling outside the limits being an indication that the run should be repeated. Other laboratories use the ±2 SD limits as "warning limits" to draw attention to a particular procedure, and ±3 SD as "action limits" to necessitate repeating the run (±3 SD represents 99% of all values in the distribution). To facilitate visualization of the 2 and 3 SD limits, the individual values from various runs are plotted on a graph known as a Shewhart chart.

The standard deviation is not a static number that is calculated once and then used continuously. Rather, standard deviations should be recalculated periodically to redefine the confidence limits of the procedure. A good rule to use is that standard deviation should be calculated once a month or whenever 20 values have been determined. There is often confusion over the inclusion of elimination of the value that falls outside of the ± 3 SD range in the next calculation of the standard deviation. A general rule to use is that if the run is turned out, the control value is included; if the run is not turned out, the control value is discarded in the next recalculation of the mean and standard deviation.

Quality control samples

The ideal quality control sample is identical in all ways to the samples being analyzed. The control for the RIA of thyroxine in human serum should also be human serum. Unfortunately, it is not always possible to obtain controls whose matrix is identical to the patient samples. Two sources of control serums are generally available: commercially available lyophilized controls and locally prepared controls. Ideally, the controls should be not only an indication of precision but also of accuracy. The latter can be achieved only if the constituent of interest has been determined independently by a known accurate method. This is best illustrated by examples. Suppose a control for serum digoxin is desired. (Digoxin is a cardioactive drug. See section on radioimmunoassay for drugs.) The first step would be to acquire a quantity of human serum that has no digoxin in it. One could do this by collecting specimens from people known to have no digoxin intake, and pooling these specimens. As a double check, a sample of this pool should be sent to a reputable reference laboratory for digoxin assay. Once the pool is assured to be digoxin-free, a known amount of pure digoxin can be carefully weighed out and added to it. If this is done, the control prepared can serve as an accuracy check as well as a precision check, since the digoxin concentration was determined by an independent absolute method (weighing out pure digoxin). Of course, one must be certain that all digoxin is dissolved, decomposition has not occurred, and so forth. The sample should again be sent to a reputable reference laboratory as a double check. Finally, the control serums should be parceled out into appropriate aliquots and frozen in tightly closed containers. It is important when one uses both commercial and locally prepared controls to purchase or make enough material to last a long time, preferably a year. Switching control lots frequently is not conducive to maintaining good statistical quality control data.

Another commonly used method of locally prepared controls is the simple pool. This may be used when it is impossible to purchase or prepare a control serum containing the component desired. One prepares the control by pooling a number of samples, mixing well, and then aliquoting the pool and freezing or lyophilizing for future use. This type of control is not useful as an accuracy check, since the concentration of the constituent of interest is not independently determined. Whenever serum is pooled, two safety checks should be made on the pool. Samples should be screened for the presence of interfering substances, and the pool should be checked for the presence of pathogenic organisms and hepatitis-associated antigen before it is aliquoted. Fortunately, the demand for good quality control samples is such that a large number of them are commercially available. They have generally been prepared in the way described above and checked for accuracy.

An important consideration in choosing a control is the approximate level of constituent present. Although there is no ideal level, some rules should be followed. If only one control is used, it should have a constituent level in the normal range. Consideration should be given to using a second control with an abnormal level in such circumstances. In most cases it is desirable to have a control whose value falls near some threshold level. A good example of this is digoxin, which has a toxicity threshold near 2 ng/ml. A control having this digoxin concentration serves the additional function of a marker separating the toxic and nontoxic ranges.

A good quality control program includes accurate and functional record keeping. The values obtained for all control samples should be recorded, both with the data from the respective runs and graphically on the Shewhart chart. As mentioned previously, one should calculate new statistical parameters periodically by using the previous period's data. Graphic displays should also be observed for the occurrence of trends that are indicative of changing standards, controls, or analysis conditions. Although the systematic error that results in trending occurs much less often with radiobioassays than with automated chemical analyses, any trend away from a random distribution of the control values should prompt an investigation of the assay, with special attention paid to possible decomposition of reagents.

Refer to the excellent references listed at the end of this chapter for a more comprehensive review of quality control.

PRACTICAL RADIOIMMUNOASSAY

The establishment of a radioimmunoassay laboratory requires not only an understanding of the theory of radioimmunoassay, but also a firm grasp of the technology and techniques that make it possible. In this section these practical considerations will be reviewed.

Should my department do radioimmunoassay?

The decision by a nuclear medicine department to establish an RIA laboratory should be made on the basis of the demand for the services the lab could offer and on the ability of the lab to provide these services with high quality. There is no point in doing an RIA unless it is done well; and RIA cannot be done well unless it is done frequently enough to maintain technologist skills and good statistical quality control. Expected volume of tests should play a major part in determining if an RIA lab is established, and the same criteria should be used by an existing lab to justify establishment of a new RIA test.

The physical location of an RIA laboratory must be chosen to optimize the quality of the results produced. A room separated from the rest of the nuclear medicine department is almost mandatory, since the amount of radioactivity used in RIA is so small in comparison to in vivo nuclear medicine techniques that a significant contamination hazard exists when these two operations are combined. Design of the actual physical space is very dependent on personal preference and no attempt will be made to suggest designs of laboratory areas. Most often the newly created laboratory must move into existing space with no remodeling. In those instances where a new physical facility is being constructed, an architect familiar with laboratory design should be consulted.

Equipment

In order to operate, an RIA lab needs four basic pieces of equipment: a well type of scintillation counter, a centrifuge, pipetting devices, and a refrigerator. An existing scintillation counter may be used if it is kept clean and located in a place where the background is low (50 to 100 cpm). If a new scintillation counter is to be purchased, thought must be given to an automated versus manual counter. If there is sufficient volume to warrant establishing an RIA lab, then there is sufficient volume to choose an automated counter. It will more than pay for itself in reduced labor costs and increased capability. Sample capacities from 50 to 1200 tubes are available, and a size should be chosen to reflect projected RIA volume 3 years from now. Either manual or preset windows are available on most models. An ^{125}I window is standard on all models, and a preset ^{57}Co is usually standard also. Many counters now come with time-saving data reduction microprocessors to perform at least part of the RIA calculation (NSB subtract and percent bound). These devices also generally pay for themselves in reduction of errors and technologist time saved.

A centrifuge is necessary in an RIA lab for both processing blood specimens and separation of bound and free ligands with certain separation methods. One of the larger benchtop centrifuges is adequate for most RIA labs. The centrifuge should have a swinging bucket (not fixed-angle head) rotor with a capacity of at least 50 tubes. Models that meet these specifications can achieve speeds of around 3000 rpm, providing the 1000 g necessary to achieve good separations. For most RIAs a refrigerated centrifuge is not necessary, but individual kits or methods should be checked for this requirement. Laboratories having larger run sizes should consider larger, floor-mounted centrifuges with larger tube capacities.

Pipetting devices are the most critical pieces of equipment in an RIA laboratory, because pipetting is the single largest cause of error in RIA. For a typical RIA, pipetting is required to dissolve or dilute reagents, mix samples and reagents together, and add a separating agent. Dissolving or diluting reagents, which may come as a lyophilized material or a concentrate, require glass volumetric pipets. Only pipets that meet the National Bureau of Standards specifications for class A pipets should be purchased. They are available in sizes from 0.5 to 50 ml. It is unsafe to draw solutions into any pipet by mouth, and mouth pipetting should be absolutely forbidden. A number of bulbs and mechanical devices are available to safely draw solutions into glass pipets.

The pipetting of reagents and samples into reaction tubes involves smaller volumes and larger number of pipets. It is impractical to use glass volumetric pipets for these steps. The alternatives are to use manually operated pipettor/samplers (MOPS) or an automated pipetting device. The latter is discussed in the section on automation. MOPS are hand-held devices that use a piston/cylinder arrangement to draw liquid up into a disposable plastic tip. The liquid is dispensed when the piston is compressed and the liquid is expelled into a vessel. The process requires only one motion of the finger or thumb for each fill and each expel cycle, and thus it can be repeated with rapidity. The same plastic tip may be used if one solution is being transferred. A new tip should be used for different samples or reagents. The MOPS themselves are made of aluminum or plastic and come in sizes ranging from 10 to 1000 μl. Before one of these devices is put into use, it must be calibrated to ensure that it delivers the proper volume reproducibly. Calibration instructions are provided with the MOPS. The most common calibration method is to transfer 10 aliquots of pure water into separate vessels that have been tared on an analytical balance. Since water weighs 0.997 g/ml of 25° C, weighing the water transferred is in effect measuring the volume. The mean and standard deviation of the 10 transfers gives the accuracy and precision of the pipettor. An accuracy of ±2% and a precision of ±1% are the minimum tolerances that should be used.

A refrigerator is necessary for the RIA laboratory, primarily for storage of specimens and reagents. Household refrigerators are quite adequate for this purpose if no flammables are stored in them. (Food or beverages should *never* be stored in the same refrigerator with reagents and specimens.) A minor inconvenience with household refrigerators is the presence of egg trays, butter boxes, and so on, which often cannot be used and are thus wasted space. An advantage to the household refrigerator is the freezer compartment, necessary for storage of some radioassay samples. Since these refrigerators are available in many sizes, one appropriate to the laboratory can be chosen.

Some smaller pieces of laboratory equipment are also desirable for the RIA lab. A vortex type of mixer for mixing tubes is important. Some procedures may require incubation in a water bath. A double-trap vacuum apparatus for suctioning off supernatants is valuable for some radioimmunoassays.

The vessels in which an RIA is performed are usually disposable test tubes, which come in several sizes and materials. The 12 × 75 mm tube has become almost the standard of the industry. Glass, polystyrene, and polypropylene are the commonly available materials. The use of glass is not recommended, since glass absorbs about 10% of the gamma radiation from ^{125}I and presents a hazard if breakage should occur. It has also been shown to adsorb some antigens.[14] Polystyrene is the least expensive and most commonly used material. It is a clear material and tubes are available in several thicknesses. The thin wall (0.3 mm) type is not recommended for RIA, since it can be cracked by application of pressure with the fingers and it has been known to disintegrate during high-speed (3000 rpm) centrifugation. The thick wall (1 mm) type does not suffer from these problems and is an excellent choice for RIA use. Polypropylene tubes are somewhat more expensive but give the added feature of heat stability necessary for some assay such as vitamin B_{12}. Certain substances have been shown to adsorb to polystyrene, and polypropylene tubes must be substituted in RIAs for these materials. Polypropylene's nonadsorptive properties, as well as its unbreakable nature, make it ideal for specimen storage.

An important quality control parameter in any RIA is sample preparation, for an analysis can be only as good as the sample on which it is performed. Most RIAs are performed on serum, though plasma is acceptable for some of them. Serum is the straw-colored liquid that remains after blood is allowed to clot and the clot removed. Plasma, on the other hand, is a similar-looking liquid that results when the clotting process is inhibited and the cells are removed by centrifugation. Since the clotting process results in the use of some biochemicals present in the plasma and release of others from platelets, the two liquids cannot be considered identical. Table 18-4 lists the preferred specimen for the commonly performed RIAs as well as information regarding alternate specimens and storage conditions.

Table 18-4. Specimens and storage conditions for common radioimmunoassays

Substance	Specimen	Minimum storage temperature (°C)
Cortisol	Plasma	−20
Digoxin	Serum	4
	Plasma	4
Other drugs	Serum	4
Folate	Serum	−20 in dark
	Erythrocytes	−20 in dark
Insulin	Serum	−4
	Plasma	−4
Renin	Plasma	−20
Steroid hormones	Plasma	−20
Thyrotropin	Serum	−4
Thyroxine	Serum	4
Triiodothyronine	Serum	−4
Vitamin B_{12}	Serum	−20

Preparation of serum for RIAs may begin after the blood has been withdrawn from the patient and allowed to clot—usually about 20 minutes. If the blood has been drawn into an evacuated blood-collection tube, the cap of the collection tube should be removed to release the vacuum and loosen any clot that may be stuck to the cap. When removing the cap, hold the tube away from the face, since an aerosol, which may contain hepatitis viruses,* is often produced. The tube should then be recapped and centrifuged at a minimum of 2000 rpm for 5 minutes in a swinging-bucket centrifuge. When centrifugation is complete, the serum is transferred to another vessel for storage. Transfer may be by pouring or by use of a pasteur pipet. With either method, be careful not to transfer any cells into the storage vessel.

*Viral hepatitis is a serious occupational hazard for all health care workers, but particularly laboratory personnel. Since one never knows which patient samples are potential hepatitis transmitters, all specimens should be treated as capable of transmitting the virus. The safety rules for avoiding exposure to the disease include the following: (1) no eating, drinking, or smoking in the laboratory; (2) wash hands with disinfectant soap before leaving the laboratory; (3) never put anything, including pipets, pens, and fingers, into your mouth while in the laboratory; (4) avoid direct skin contact with biologic specimens.

RIA KITS

For most laboratories, radioimmunoassay is performed with commercially available kits. These kits contain all the reagents needed to perform the RIA. The reagents and standards are generally shipped in lyophilized form and must be reconstituted before use. An RIA kit should always be used exactly according to the manufacturer's directions.

The number and variety of kits in the marketplace make choosing a radioimmunoassay kit a difficult task. Before a kit is chosen, the potential user should list the qualities of the kit desired. What is the maximum sample size acceptable? What separation methods work best for the compound the lab wishes to measure? Does the lab want to automate the assay, and can this be done? What type of precision and accuracy is acceptable (The College of American Pathologists provides information about kit precision to laboratories on a subscription basis.) What do colleagues and other laboratories recommend? When these questions have been answered, the technologist can narrow the choice down to less than a half-dozen kits. Evaluation kits can then be requested and tried. The choice of an RIA kit should never be based on one trial. Those kits passing the first trial should be subjected to additional rigorous analysis. If possible, comparison should be made with an existing method or another laboratory known to provide reliable results. (Upon written request, some laboratories will provide leftover samples that have been analyzed, especially to another lab in the same region.)

Potential cross-reacting materials or abnormal samples should be run to determine how well the kit can handle them. Precision both within and between runs should be checked. Finally, when the choice has been made, a normal range should be confirmed with specimens from healthy people in your own locale. Once a kit is chosen and put into use, it should not be changed again for at least a year. Frequent methodology changes wreak havoc with quality control and make establishment of a stable laboratory difficult.

AUTOMATION IN RADIOIMMUNOASSAY

One of the most valuable assets of radioimmunoassay is the rapidity with which it can be done, especially when compared to a bioassay. However, the growth of radioimmunoassay has meant a sharp increase in the number of repetitive steps, chiefly volume transfers (pipetting), which must be performed for each run. In an attempt to improve the precision of the pipetting steps and at the same time reduce labor (and labor costs), the radioimmunoassay industry has turned, as Americans always do, to automation. This discussion of automation in RIA is divided into two parts—automated pipetting devices and total automated RIA systems.

Automated pipetting devices are designed to accurately and precisely perform the repetitive pipetting steps of a radioimmunoassay. Although the details of design vary from manufacturer to manufacturer, all the automated pipetting devices operate on the piston and cylinder, or syringe, principle. An electric motor drives a mechanical mechanism or gear train, which moves the plunger (piston) in the syringe barrel (cylinder) in two cycles. In most of these machines, two pistons operate simultaneously, one drawing up solution through a sampling probe while a second larger piston fills a cylinder-reservoir with a diluent or reagent. In the second cycle, the action of the pistons is reversed, with a valve routing the diluent out through the first cyclinder so that the sample is flushed into a waiting receptacle. Triggering of the cycle is accomplished by either a foot pedal or hand switch. Usually each cycle is triggered separately, though sòme dilutions can be set so that both cycles are performed after one trigger step. This requires an operator with fast hands, since he must remove the sample container from under the sampling probe and quickly replace it with the receptable for the sample plus diluent. Some pipettors have infinitely variable delivery volumes within the range of the syringes; others can deliver sample and diluent at only a few fixed volumes or ratios.

A calibrated, well-maintained automatic pipettor can achieve an accuracy of ±1% of the assigned delivery value, with a precision of less than 1%. This is better than the best technologist can do with a manually operated pipettor-sampler (MOPS). In addition to the improved precision and accuracy, the technologist operating an automatic pipettor can generally pipet twice as fast as his fellow with a MOPS (because he is performing two liquid transfers with one step). However, this gain in time is somewhat offset by the time required to prime the system before and wash out the system after the pipetting. The priming-rinsing process also wastes some reagents, the major disadvantage of automatic pipettors.

A variation of the automatic pipettor-dilutor combines it with a transfer table to create an automatic pipetting station. Two sets of tubes are placed on the transfer table—one containing the samples or standards to be assayed, the other a set of empties. The motion of the table is designed such that a probe picks up a sample from one of the sample tubes and then dispenses it and a reagent into one of the empty tubes. This process is repeated without operator intervention until all the samples loaded on the table have been so treated. Another variation of the automatic pipettor is the reagent dispenser, which is essentially a mechanically powered syringe that precisely dispenses an aliquot of a single reagent when triggered. The reagent dispenser does not transfer a sample, but because the reagent may be stored in the cylinder, it eliminates the problem of waste because of priming and rinsing.

Completely automated radioimmunoassay systems made their debut in the mid-1970s, as manufacturers attempted to sell automated devices designed to reduce the most expensive part of RIA, the labor. Five automated machines, each operating on a different principle, have been marketed. The first of these, Micromedic Systems' Concept 4,* is an extension of that firm's automatic pipetting stations. The sequence involved in Concept 4 is identical to a manually performed RIA. Sample and reagents are pipetted into antibody-coated tubes in a movable rack. The rack is then mechanically cycled for a defined period of time to achieve equilibrium before the supernatant liquid is aspirated from the tube. The tubes containing the bound ligands are then passed to an analyzer module where they are counted. Finally, a microprocessor calculates the best standard curve and patient-sample results. Concept 4 uses conventional separation technology and is the most "robotlike" of the automated RIA devices. Because it can process batches of up to 300 tubes, it is somewhat faster (per sample) than the continuous-flow type of RIA systems. Its major disadvantage is that it operates only with 8 × 50 mm antibody-coated tubes, limiting the user to those assay kits supplied with these instead of the conventional 12 × 75 mm tubes.

Union Carbide's Centria† RIA system applies that firm's experience with centrifugal chemical analyzers to radioimmunoassay. Although Centria is not completely automated (some operator manipulation is required), it still qualifies as an automated system. The heart of the system is a rotor disk containing two sets of wells arranged radially. Sample and labeled ligand are pipetted automatically into the outermost set of wells. Antibody is pipetted into the other set. The operator then places the rotor in the instrument where it is spun. Centrifugal force causes each aliquot of antibody to flow into the corresponding well containing sample and label. After an appropriate incubation time, the rotor is spun again at a higher speed, forcing the antibody-ligand solution from each set of wells through individual columns containing cross-linked dextran (Sephadex). Separation of bound and free labeled ligand occurs by molecular sieving. The free ligand is retained by the Sephadex, while the bound ligand passes through the column and is collected in a series of tubes. When the separation is complete, counting of the bound fractions is accomplished by three separate counting wells arranged at 120-degree angles to each other. A microprocessor again compiles the data and calculates the standard curves, controls, and patient samples. Centria can handle 36 samples at one time, requiring between 1 and 2 hours for completion of the analyses.

The other three automated radioimmunoassay systems are based on continuous flow technology rather than the batch processes of Concept 4 and Centria. The ARIA II,* now sold by Becton-Dickinson Diagnostics, is based on a rechargeable antibody chamber. A syringe dilutor system introduces a mixture of labeled and unlabeled ligand into the chamber, which contains a solid-phase antibody. As the mixture of ligands passes through the chamber, binding to the solid-phase antibody occurs in proportion to the ratio of labeled to unlabeled ligand. When the free ligand has cleared the chamber, an eluting solution is passed through it, eluting the previously bound ligand into a counting well where it is counted. Alternatively, the eluted bound ligand may be mixed with a liquid scintillation cocktail if a beta particle–emitting nuclide is used to label the ligand. (The instrument comes equipped for counting both gamma-ray and beta-particle emitters.) While the bound ligand is being eluted from the chamber, the instrument is setting up to analyze the next sample. The key to the ARIA is obviously the antibody chamber, and the means by which the antibody is regenerated is proprietary information. Antibody cartridges for a number of hormones and drugs are available. The recycle time for each sample is from 2 to 5 minutes, for analysis rates of 12 to 30 samples per hour. The antibody chambers are reported to last for up to 3000 samples. As with the other instruments, a microprocessor controls the operations and processes the data.

The Technicon Instruments Corporation, long a leader in the area of continuous flow analysis systems, has used their knowledge of flow technology to develop a continuous flow automated radioimmunoassay system called STAR.† The system is based on a peristaltic pump that separates the reagents and samples into a segmented stream, with the segments being evenly separated by air bubbles. Samples are picked up by a probe and mixed with labeled ligand and a solid-phase antibody when the segmented streams are combined. The solid phase for the antibody is fine particles of ferric oxide, which can be attracted to a magnetic field. The mixed, segmented stream is passed through a coil whose length determines the incubation period for the assay. Finally, the stream passes between the poles of an electromagnet. The magnet is first turned on to hold the magnetic particles containing bound

*Micromedic Systems, Horsham, Pennsylvania 19044.
†Union Carbide Corp., Rye, New York, 10580.

*Becton-Dickinson Diagnostics, Orangeburg, New York 10962.
†Technicon Instruments Corporation, Tarrytown, New York 10591.

antigen, allowing the free antigen to pass by and into a waste container. Then the magnet is turned off and a following wash segment carries the particles on to a counting chamber. This sequence is continued for each sample-containing segment. Pneumatic valves control sampling and reagent additions and route the sample and waste segments to the proper containers. A separate minicomputer gathers the data from the scintillation counter and calculates the standard curve and patient results.

An automated system somewhat similar in design to the Technicon system was developed by Brooker and his associates at the University of Virginia.[4] Called "Gammaflow," it also uses a peristaltic pump to pull reagents and samples through tubing. It differs from the Technicon system in that reagents are discretely introduced into the sample segment rather than flowing continuously. It also uses a preset timing sequence and miniature solenoid values to control the routing of the segments through various parts of the instrument. A stopped-flow technique is used for counting the bound ligand, which was separated from free by a column containing either a mixed-bed ion exchange resin, charcoal, or both. As usual, a minicomputer processes the data. Gammaflow is being marketed by E. R. Squibb Co., Princeton, New Jersey.

In the early stages of development of the automated RIA systems, it was hoped that they would improve the precision of radioimmunoassays. However, none of the systems discussed have been able to significantly improve on the precision obtained by a good technologist using properly calibrated pipetting and counting equipment. Data presented for all of the automated systems indicates that the precision obtainable is on the order of 4% to 7%. This may be the best precision obtainable with the current state of the radioimmunoassay art.

The obvious major advantage to using an automated RIA system is the reduction in the cost of labor and expendable supplies. These savings are offset by the high initial cost of the system and the per tube cost, which may run higher than for a nonautomated RIA. The decision to purchase an automated system must be made carefully, based on calculation of projected test volume and savings attributable to decreased labor costs.

RADIOIMMUNOASSAY OF THYROID HORMONES

Radioimmunoassay has made its greatest impact on endocrinology, particularly thyroid endocrinology. Measurement of thyroxine, the principal thyroid hormone, has become a commmonplace laboratory measurement, partly because of the ease with which it can be done by RIA.

Thyroid physiology

The thyroid gland produces hormones that control the utilization of energy by the cell. There are two principle hormones, thyroxine (T_4) and triiodothyronine (T_3) (Fig. 18-15). These hormones circulate in the blood on their way to tissues. Thyroxine, the more abundant hormone, is present in a concentration of 4.5 to 11.5 μg/dl* in euthyroid individuals' serum. Of the thyroxine, 99.95% is bound to serum proteins, with thyroxine-binding globulin, TBG, carrying 68% of the thyroxine, thyroxine-binding prealbumin (TBPA) binding another 15%, and albumin the remainder. Endocrinologists now know that the 0.05% not bound to these proteins (the "free" thyroxine) is the physiologically important fraction, since it is readily available to cells. The remainder, or bound fraction, can be considered to be in transit or storage, though it can be made available as free T_4 quickly by dissociation of the binding protein thyroxine complex.

The amount of total (free and bound) thyroxine in circulation is regulated by a complex mechanism of hormones, the thyroid feedback mechanism. A decrease in circulating thyroxine triggers the hypothalamus to release the tripeptide thyrotropin-releasing hormone, TRH. TRH in turn stimulates the pituitary to release thyrotropin, also called thyroid-stimulating hormone (TSH). It is the TSH that ultimately stimulates the thyroid gland to produce its hormones. Fig. 18-16 illustrates the thyroid feedback mechanism. This mechanism by itself is not completely responsible for maintaining adequate thyroid hormone in circulation. Remember that it was the free thyroxine concentration that regulated TRH. Free thyroxine is also regulated by the concentration of the binding proteins, with which it is in equilibrium. An increase in binding protein concentrations results in more of the circulating free T_4 being bound, in accordance with Le Châtelier's principle. The drop in free T_4 stimulates the feedback mechanism, and more thyroxine is produced. A percentage of this is bound, and the system continues to react until the free thyroxine is at an acceptable level. If the binding protein concentration increases, an increase in the total thyroxine is expected and observed. The free thyroxine, however, should remain relatively constant.

Ideally, measurement of free thyroxine is the best way to determine a person's thyroid status. However, free thyroxine can only be measured by the time-consuming and difficult technique of equilibrium dialysis. Total T_4, however, is easily measured by RIA, and binding protein status can be indirectly estimated. These two measurements can be combined to give an indication of free thyroxine.

*This "reference range" may vary slightly depending on method of analysis and geographic location.

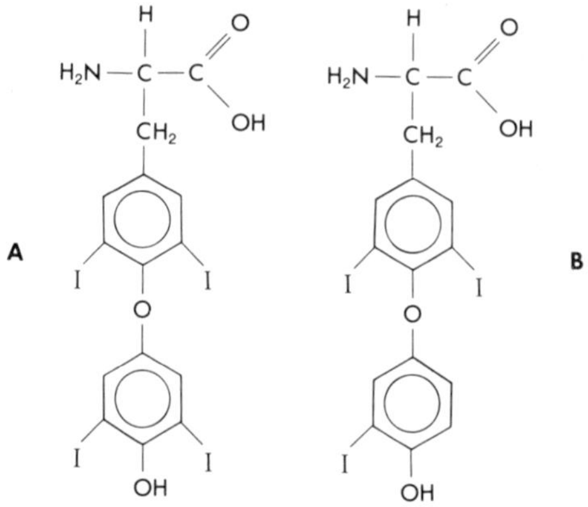

Fig. 18-15. A, Thyroxine. Note fourth iodine. **B,** Triiodothyronine.

The second major thyroid hormone is triiodothyronine. T_3 has been shown to have 4 to 5 times the calorigenic effect that T_4 has, and most endocrinologists believe it to be the true active thyroid hormone. The gland produces some of the T_3 utilized by the tissues; the rest is believed to arise from peripheral deiodination of free T_4. The circulating concentration of triiodothyronine is only around 100 ng/dl, roughly 100 times less than T_4. Both of the major thyroid hormones as well as TSH are measurable by RIA.

Radioassays for thyroid hormones

The earliest radioassays for thyroxine were based on the pioneering work of Murphy and Pattee at the Queen Mary Veterans Hospital in Montreal.[18] The Murphy-Pattee assay for thyroxine is not an immunoassay but instead uses the native protein thyroxine-binding globulin (TBG) as the specific reactor substance. Thyroxine, T_4, is extracted from serum by the addition of an alcohol, usually ethanol, that denatures the proteins binding T_4 in serum and frees the T_4. An aliquot of this alcoholic extract is used as the sample, being mixed with the labeled T_4 and TBG obtained from human serums. Separation of bound from free was usually carried out with an ion-exchange resin at pH 8.6, where T_4 is anionic. A number of commercial kits using this same methodology were available, the main distinction between them being the mechanics of adding and removing the ion-exchange resin. Although the Murphy-Pattee thyroxine assay was a great advantage over the previously used T_4 by column and protein-bound iodine (PBI) assays, it suffered from two disadvantages. A relatively large amount (0.5 ml) of serum was required for each assay, and a number of drugs including salicylates (aspirin) and phenytoin (diphenylhydantoin, Dilantin) interfered with the analysis because they cross-reacted with TBG. Despite

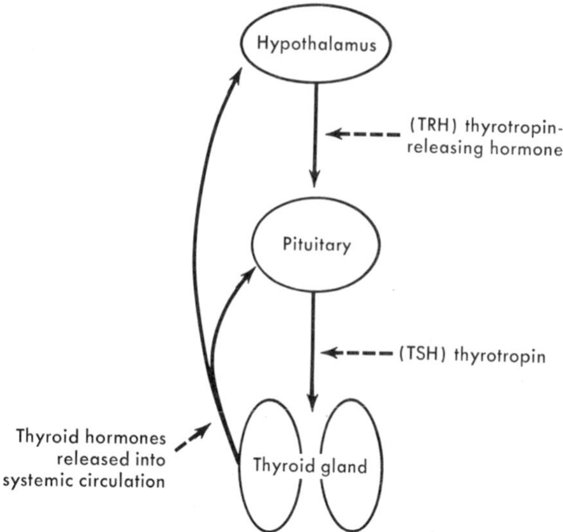

Fig. 18-16. Thyroid feedback mechanism. Circulating thyroid hormone stimulates or represses release of more hormone through control of hypothalamic and pituitary hormone secretions.

these limitations, the TBG-based assay for T_4 was widely used until the mid-1970s. In 1976, Shaw, Hubert, and Spierto of the Center for Disease Control reported that the naturally occurring fatty acids in serum could severely affect the TBG-based radioassay for T_4 by competing as if they were T_4.[21] After these reports, the TBG-based kits were largely abandoned in favor of true radioimmunoassays for the hormone. Radioimmunoassays have the advantages of requiring no alcohol extraction, a small (10 to 50 μl) sample, and freedom from interference by drugs and fatty acids. Because serum protein denaturation is not usually performed prior to radioimmunoassay, the TBG and other binding proteins present in the serum pose a potential problem, since their binding constants may approach that of the antibody. This problem has been solved by the addition of 8-anilino-1-naphthalene sulfonic acid (ANS) and salicylate to the reaction solution. ANS blocks the specific T_4 binding sites on TBG; salicylate blocks the nonspecific sites on serum albumin. Nearly every separation technique has been successfully applied to RIAs for T_4. The number of T_4 radioimmunoassay kits available approaches 40, giving the consumer a wide choice of separation techniques, sample size, and ease of performance.

The reference range for thyroxine is derived from studies done on euthyroid individuals, who have normal binding proteins. The binding protein concentration, however, does not always remain normal. Natural occurrences such as pregnancy and disease states such as cancer cause alteration of the binding protein concentrations. The situation that occurs in pregnancy is the most common and will serve to illustrate the operation of the regulatory mechanisms. In pregnancy, an overall increase in binding protein concentration occurs. To maintain chemical equilibrium, more of the free T_4 becomes bound to the proteins. Were there no physiologic mechanism, the decrease in free T_4 would result in hypothyroidism. However, the thyroid feedback mechanism detects the drop in free T_4 and responds with an increase in thyroxine output, until both physiologic (free) and chemical (total) equilibrium concentrations of T_4 are achieved. The net result is an increased total T_4, though the individual remains clinically euthyroid. Correct assessment of the thyroid status during pregnancy is not possible with the T_4 alone; evaluation of the binding protein saturation, and thus the free T_4, must also be performed.

The companion test to the T_4 RIA, which measures binding protein saturation, is the T_3 uptake test, or T_3U. The T_3U is not a radioimmunoassay but uses radiolabeled T_3 as a quantitative marker. An aliquot of the patient's serum is mixed with an amount of radiolabeled T_3. T_3 will bind to TBG, TBPA, and albumin, though not so strongly as T_4. Another medium that has an affinity for T_3 is added and allowed to react, picking up the T_3 not bound by the proteins. This "uptake" of radiolabeled T_3 is measured after the medium is separated from the serum and the former is counted. The more T_3 taken up by the medium, the fewer the binding sites available. Although no absolute standards exist, the uptake is relative to available binding sites on a reference serum. The medium used to take up the T_3 can be either an ion-exchange resin, an antibody, or a solid adsorbing material. The uptake is usually expressed as a percentage of the total radioactivity added.

The T_3 uptake cannot be used by itself to diagnose thyroid disease, since it does not measure a true thyroid-dependent parameter. However, it is invaluable to the evaluation of T_4 results. Such evaluation is usually done with a calculation known as the free thyroxine index (FTI). The FTI is defined as

$$\frac{T_4 \times T_3U}{100} \qquad (7)$$

The FTI is a way of expressing the T_4 concentration, corrected for binding protein status. It correlates very well with actual measurements of free thyroxine. The reference range is dependent, of course, on the particular methods used for the T_4 and T_3U.

One disadvantage to the FTI is that it requires two separate laboratory measurements. Because of this, there have been devised a number of modified radioassays for T_4 that, by the addition of one step, eliminate the need for a T_3U. Although the details of the various procedures differ, the principle in each is basically the same. A T_4 radioassay using TBG as the specific reactor substance is used; after the alcoholic extract of the serum is added, a smaller amount of unextracted serum is also added; the assay is then completed as usual. The small aliquot of serum contains TBG and proportionally increases or decreases the number of TBG molecules available for binding T_4 and labeled T_4. In the case of hyperthyroidism or hypothyroidism, the additional TBG added does not offset the increased or decreased thyroxine, and the test result appears abnormal. In the case of euthyroidism accompanied by binding protein increase (such as is found in pregnancy) the TBG from the patient serum significantly adds to the total TBG present and thus compensates for the increased T_4; the result appears normal. The result may be expressed as a thyroxine concentration, or it may be expressed as a ratio to a euthyroid reference serum, in which case it is known as an effective thyroxine ratio, or ETR[16] (Mallinckrodt Chemical Works, St. Louis, Missouri).

Radioimmunoassays for triiodothyronine (T_3) are similar to those for T_4 but are less commonly used because they are useful only in the documentation of cases of hyperthyroidism. The assay buffer contains blocking agents similar to those used in T_4 RIAs. The most critical factor in the T_3 RIA is the antibody—it must have a cross reactivity with T_4 of less than 0.1% (1 part in 1000), since there is approximately 100 times more T_4 in a milliliter of serum than there is T_3.

In addition to measuring the hormones of thyroid origin, radioimmunoassay is the common technique utilized for measuring thyrotropin (TSH). Thyrotropin is a glycoprotein with a molecular weight of 13,000; it has two peptide chains designated α and β, and β is believed to be the active portion. Both equilibrium radioimmunoassays and sequential saturation have been developed. Because of its size, TSH does not lend itself well to separation by adsorbents or ion exchange. Its size also limits it use in solid-phase RIAs that are diffusion controlled. The double-antibody technique is therefore most commonly used for separation of free from bound antibody in TSH radioimmunoassays. The TSH RIA may be used directly to establish whether hypothyroidism is primary (a failure of the thyroid gland—TSH will be greatly elevated above normal) or secondary (a pituitary insufficiency—TSH is low or normal). A challenge test known as the TRH stimulation also utilizes the TSH radioassay. In this test, the patient is given a dose of TRH and serial TSH levels are drawn. Fig. 18-17 illustrates the TSH response to the TRH stimulation in euthyroid individuals and in various disease states.

Table 18-5 illustrates the patterns seen in the various

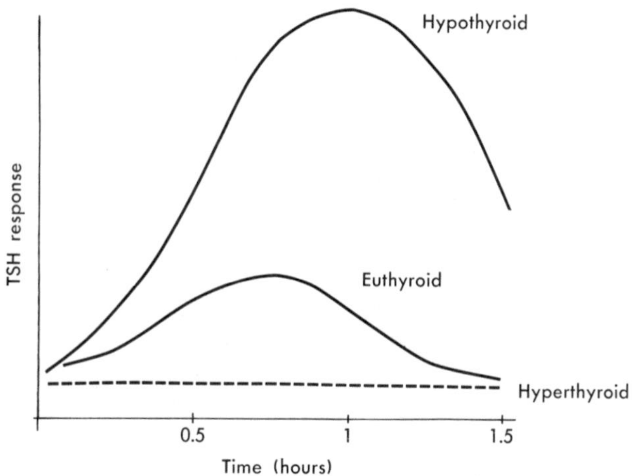

Fig. 18-17. TSH response to stimulating dose of thyrotropin-releasing hormone in euthyroid, hyperthyroid, and primary hypothyroid individuals.

Table 18-5. Pattern of thyroid tests

Disease state	T_4	T_3U	T_3	TSH	Thyroid index
Euthyroidism	N	N	N	N	N
Hypothyroidism					
Primary	↓	↓	N	↑	↓
Secondary	↓	↓	N	N	↓
Hyperthyroidism	↑	↑	↑	N	↑
T_3 thyrotoxicosis	N	N	↑	N	N
Euthyroid pregnancy	↑	↓	N	N	N
Hyperthyroid pregnancy	↑	N	↑	N	↑

thyroid hormone radioassays because of various thyroid conditions.

RADIOIMMUNOASSAY FOR THERAPEUTICALLY MONITORED DRUGS

The application of radioimmunoassay to the measurement of circulatory digoxin concentration marked the beginning of modern therapeutic drug monitoring. To grasp the importance of RIA drug measurements, one needs to understand some basic pharmacology, and although a comprehensive study of that subject will not be pursued here, a review of a few principles is in order.

Basic pharmacology

Pharmacology uses mathematical models to explain the behavior of drugs introduced into the body. The simplest of these models, the one-compartment model, views the body essentially as a tank, with the drug entering and leaving by simple pathways much as water would. As is true with many simple models, the one-compartment model has limited applicability, since it implies that all tissues and the blood are instantly homogeneous with respect to drug concentration, a fact known to be erroneous. A more reasonable pharmacologic model is the two-compartment model, which can be viewed as a semipermeable chamber within a tank. Drug is introduced into the outer tank or compartment directly and is excreted from this compartment in an equally direct fashion. However, the drug's site of action is the inner chamber or compartment, and it reaches that compartment by being transported, either actively or passively, through the semipermeable wall. In the body, if the bloodstream represents the outer compartment, the organs or tissues are the inner compartment. Obviously, the mathematical models used to describe the two-compartment model are much more complex than for the one-compartment model. Equally obvious is the difficulty of measuring drug concentration in the inner compartment of the two-compartment model. Drug concentration measurements in the outer compartment are valid only if the relationship between inner and outer compartments are well established for the particular drug.

Drugs can be introduced into the body in one of three ways—intravenously (IV), intramuscularly (IM), or orally. Intravenous administration results in a peak (or highest) drug concentration in the circulation being reached almost immediately. With an intramuscular injection, the drug must be absorbed from the IM site, and so the effect is not so immediate as with IV and the peak concentration is reached somewhat slower. Oral administration of the drug results in absorption of the drug over an even longer period of time, with the time required to reach the peak concentration depending on, among other things, the speed in which the drug dissolves in gastric juices before being transported across the mucosa. The so-called time release drug formulations control this dissolution process so that drug absorption takes place over a long period of time.

The process of removal of the drug from the circulation begins almost immediately even while drug absorption is taking place. There are two major routes of elimination—renal excretion and hepatic detoxification. In the latter case the hepatic enzymes act on the drug to destroy its chemical functions; it may then be excreted by the renal route. For many, but certainly not all, drugs, excretion follows the same first-order kinetics as radioactive decay. Consequently, the term "half-life" is used to describe the time it takes to reduce the concentration of drug in the circulation by half after a single dose of the drug. Drug half-lives vary from a few minutes to as long as 5 days. Knowledge of a drug's half-life permits a physician to choose a correct dose and dosing interval.

Another characteristic of some drugs is the existence of a *therapeutic window,* a range of concentration where the desired effect is achieved without occurrence of toxic symptoms. For drugs that have such a window, subtherapeutic concentrations result in no effect, whereas concentrations above the window result in toxicity. When a person is on long-term drug therapy, it is desirable to establish a dosing regimen that always maintains the circulatory concentration within the therapeutic range. This implies that each dose contains only enough drug to replace that percentage of the previous dose lost by excretion. When this situation exists, the person is said to be in steady state with respect to that drug, and the dose that keeps him there is called a "maintenance dose." Steady-state concentration is reached after approximately five half-lives if the same same dose is administered at the end of one half-life and then after each subsequent half-life. Since this may be too long a period to wait for efficacy, a loading dose, usually three or four times the maintenance dose, is often given to attain therapeutic concentration before the maintenance dose schedule is begun.

In order for monitoring of serum drug concentrations to be useful, the following must apply to the drug to be monitored: (1) The circulating drug concentration must be directly related to the desired effect of the drug; (2) significant danger to the patient must exist if the therapeutic window concentration is not achieved or is exceeded; and (3) other means of verifying drug efficacy and toxicity (that is, physical signs and symptoms) must be less reliable than the drug measurements. All the drugs to be discussed in the remainder of this section meet these requirements for effective therapeutic monitoring. For a more detailed discussion of pharmacology, consult the references by Gibaldi and Levy listed at the end of this chapter.

Digitalis glycosides

The digitalis glycosides are drugs with excellent ability to control cardiac arrhythmias. There are several members of this family, all isolated from species of the plant genus *Digitalis.* The most widely used of these is digoxin (Fig. 18-8), which is isolated from *Digitalis lanata.* It is available as the pure crystalline compound. The drug is administered either intravenously (for a loading dose) or orally for maintenance doses. It is eliminated through renal excretion, and its half-life in the bloodstream is around 36 hours for a person with normal renal function. A patient on maintenance digoxin therapy usually takes his digoxin only once a day. The therapeutic range of concentrations for digoxin is from 1 to 2.1 ng/ml in adults, with toxic symptoms likely above 2.1 ng/ml. However, there is some overlap between the therapeutic and toxic ranges. In pediatric patients, greater concentrations may be tolerated without toxicity.[12,24] Sampling time plays an important part in determining digoxin toxicity. The therapeutic and toxic ranges above are based on blood samples drawn 8 hours after the last digoxin dose was taken. This is now considered the standard time when blood for digoxin concentration measurements should be drawn.

The first RIAs for digoxin were developed in the late 1960s using antibodies prepared in goats and ^{3}H-labeled drug as the hot ligand. Subsequently iodinated derivatives were introduced as labeled ligands. Nearly every separation technique has been successfully applied to digoxin RIA. At one time, serum digoxin concentrations were believed to be influenced by albumin concentration in the patient's serum, but later studies indicate that the so-called albumin effect may instead be a function of the labeled derivative used, with the digoxigenin succinyl tyrosine methyl ester derivative in particular causing the problems.[13,23] Most manufacturers of digoxin kits now use the digoxin-tyrosine-methyl ester derivative. Both serum and plasma may be used as samples in the digoxin RIA.

Digitoxin (Fig. 18-8) is another digitalis glycoside, isolated from *Digitalis purpurea* (foxglove). Despite its structural similarity to digoxin (it differs by only the absence of a hydroxyl group in the 12 positions on the steroid ring), it has vastly different properties. Instead of being excreted directly by the kidneys, it is first conjugated in the liver. It has a mean half-life of 172 hours (7.1 days) and a therapeutic concentration range of from 10 to 26 ng/ml. Toxicity occurs above 26 ng/ml, but like digoxin there is a considerable overlap between therapeutic and toxic ranges. Because its long half-life means long times are necessary for dosage adjustment, digitoxin is less frequently used than digoxin.

The radioimmunoassay for digitoxin is identical to that for digoxin. Occasionally, a patient may have both drugs in his serum as he is being switched from one to another. In this case, the cross-reactivity of the antibody plays an important role in determining how accurate the measurement is. In measuring digitoxin, the cross-reactivity of digoxin with the antibody can be large, since the amount of digoxin required to make a significant difference in the measured digitoxin concentration would be fatal to the patient. In the opposite instance, a 10% cross-reactivity of digitoxin with the digoxin antibody can make a therapeutic digoxin concentration appear toxic. Fortunately, digoxin antibodies can be prepared with a digitoxin cross-reactivity of 3% or less. Other potential cross-reacting compounds include spironolactone and some of the gonadal hormones. Occasionally, digitalis leaf is prescribed for a patient instead of the pure crystalline compound. Since digitalis leaf is usually the purpurea species, digitoxin should be measured. Gitalin, another related drug, cannot be monitored with serum levels because it is an amorphous mixture of several digitalis compounds.

Aminoglycoside antibiotics

Use of radioimmunoassay to measure the circulating concentration of aminoglycoside antibiotics represents a case where monitoring of the drug both significantly improves chances of successful therapy and diminishes the occurrence of toxicity. The aminoglycoside antibiotics are widely used for the treatment of gram-negative sepsis, especially burns. These drugs must be used with caution, because serum concentrations above about 10 to 12 μg/ml may result in serious ototoxicity and permanent hearing loss, as well as nephrotoxicity. On the other hand, concentrations below the minimum inhibitory concentration (MIC, the minimum drug concentration that will inhibit bacterial growth) for the infecting organism not only presents the probability of a therapeutic failure but also may lead to the development of organism resistance to the antibiotic. Careful monitoring of serum concentrations to keep the drug at bactericidal levels but below the ototoxic range ensures that the infecting organisms are combated without the treatment harming the patient.

Monitoring of aminoglycoside therapy is not a new technique. The introduction of radioimmunoassays for these drugs made such monitoring feasible, however. Previous aminoglycoside assays were bioassays, involving many dilutions of the patient specimen, followed by inoculation of organism-containing broths and a long wait to see which dilution resulted in inhibition of growth. Obviously, an RIA that required only one dilution of the sample followed by a few minutes' incubation with reagents and another few minutes counting time considerably reduced total assay time. Cost, too, is a factor in favor of RIA, as is specificity in this day of multiple drug therapy.

The nuclear medicine laboratory wishing to provide aminoglycoside monitoring does not need to have RIAs for all aminoglycosides available. In any one hospital it is likely that only one or two of the aminoglycosides will be available for use. Communication with the pharmacy will aid the laboratory in determining which aminoglycoside RIAs should be provided.

The assays themselves are straightforward, with most using the double-antibody separation method. Because RIA is three orders of magnitude more sensitive than therapeutic concentrations of the drugs, a 1:100 dilution of patient serum samples, standards, and controls is made first with a buffer being used as diluent. Sample storage, dilution, and analysis should be performed in polystyrene or polypropylene tubes, since the aminoglycosides have a tendency to bind to glass. While individual antibiotic concentrations are of some usefulness, half-life determinations are more valuable. Some physicians prefer to draw a "peak" sample at about 1 hour after dose, and a "trough" level just before the next dose. However, determining a half-life based on only two points is risky, since anyone can draw a straight line between two points. A more valid half-life is obtained with three points separated by at least an hour. In most cases the antibodies are specific enough to permit measurement of one aminoglycoside in the presence of the others; however, the literature supplied with the antibody should be checked for possible cross-reacting substances.

Radioimmunoassays for other drugs

The bronchodilator theophylline is another drug whose use has been revolutionized by therapeutic monitoring. Theophylline is a small molecule, chemically related to caffeine. The importance of therapeutic monitoring of this drug was brought out by the report of grand mal seizures and death from overdose in several patients in Denver in 1 year.[27] Radioimmunoassays for the drug were not developed until several years later, and they had to compete with other established monitoring methods. However, RIA offers a batch capability that none of the other techniques have, making it most useful to the laboratory that has a high volume of requests for theophylline determinations. The antiepileptic drugs, particularly phenytoin, have also been monitored by RIA. Because antiepileptic drugs are often administered in combination, an assay that is specific is important.

RADIOIMMUNOASSAY FOR NONTHYROID HORMONES

Radioimmunoassay for the nonthyroid hormones presents a greater challenge to the radioimmunoassayist than does that for the thyroid hormones. The nonthyroid hormones can be divided into the polypeptide hormones and the steroid hormones. A third class of compounds, the prostaglandins, though not strictly hormones, are also considered in this discussion.

Polypeptide hormones

Although the first hormone to be measured by radioimmunoassay was insulin, the clinical usefulness of insulin measurements has declined. The major clinical use of this RIA is in the detection of an insulinoma, a malignant tumor of the pancreas that causes increased insulin production. Occasionally, serum insulin as well as glucose may be measured during a glucose tolerance test (GTT) to determine the physiology of an abnormal response to glucose stimulation, but insulin levels are not necessary to establish a diagnosis of diabetes, which is a common disease caused by a lack of insulin production.

There are several other polypeptide hormones that are measured by RIA, but these analyses are usually performed only at specialized diagnostic centers because of the infrequency of requests and the complexity of the assays. These include adrenocorticotropin (ACTH), follicle-stimulating hormone (FSH), luteinizing hormone (LH), and the human chorionic gonadotropin (HCG). The first three are produced by the pituitary, the last by the ovaries. FSH, LH, and HCG are active in the maintenance of the normal menstrual cycle. HCG levels are related to the implantation and maturation of the egg in the uterus. Sensitive RIAs for HCG that can detect pregnancy as soon as 9 days after conception, even before the first missed menstrual period, have been developed. However this is of limited clinical usefulness and primary pregnancy testing will continue to be done by nonradioisotopic methods, which are much simpler and less expensive.

Steroid hormones

The steroid hormones are a large group of related compounds that influence a variety of body functions. Fig. 18-18 shows the basic steroid nucleus, from which the hormones are derived. The first hormone in the synthesis pathway, pregnenolone, is synthesized from cholesterol, and a multitude of pathways exist for interconverting hormones to various antecedents. As you might suspect, the similarity of these compounds makes preparation of specific antiserums difficult. Preparation of iodinated derivatives is also difficult and may in fact result in a loss of specificity for the assay. For this reason many of the steroid hormone RIAs are conducted with ^{3}H-labeled derivatives.

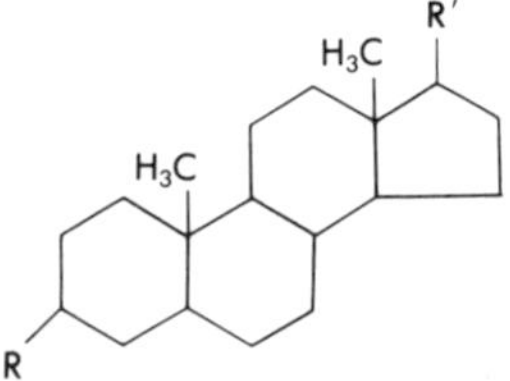

Fig. 18-18. All steroid hormones are derived from this basic structure. *R* may be either a hydroxyl (—OH) or oxo (=O) group. *R'* may have three or four carbons and contain hydroxyl, aldehyde, or carboxylic acid functional groups.

The measurement of the steroid hormones can tell the endocrinologist about many different disorders. Assessment of the sex steroids (testosterone and its derivatives; progesterone and its derivatives) can differentiate several diseases of the gonads as well as of the adrenal cortex. However, these diseases are all relatively uncommon and the RIAs for the sex-related steroids are generally done only at the specialized diagnostic centers, or large commercial laboratories. Another of the steroid hormones, aldosterone, is associated with the control of the mechanism that causes the kidney to retain or excrete salts. Aldosterone is controlled in part by the renin-angiotensin system. Renin is an enzyme that converts angiotensinogen to angiotensin. Both renin and angiotensin can be measured by RIA—angiotensin directly, and renin by measurement of the amount of angiotensin produced by an aliquot of renin-containing plasma. The instability of these materials necessitates measurement within a few hours of sampling. Some smaller laboratories are therefore involved in the measurement of renin and angiotensin. Aldosterone presents a different problem. It cannot be measured directly in plasma or urine but first must be extracted with a nonpolar organic solvent such as dichloromethane. Chromatography on lipophilic cross-linked dextran (Sephadex) is also used to achieve separation. A recovery sample of labeled aldosterone is usually carried through the procedure since complete recovery is not always achieved. Because of these complexities, aldosterone is another compound whose measurement is usually done only in larger laboratories.

By far the most commonly measured steroid hormone is cortisol. It is the primary adrenal cortex hormone, and knowledge of its concentration in plasma can aid in the diagnosis of a number of disorders, including adrenal insufficiency and adrenocortical overactivity (Cushing's syndrome). Cortisol is analogous in many ways to thyroxine in that it circulates as both the free hormone and a bound fraction, with the free hormone being physiologically active. The bound fraction is carried by cortisol binding globulin (CBG), analogous to TBG. The first radioassays for cortisol

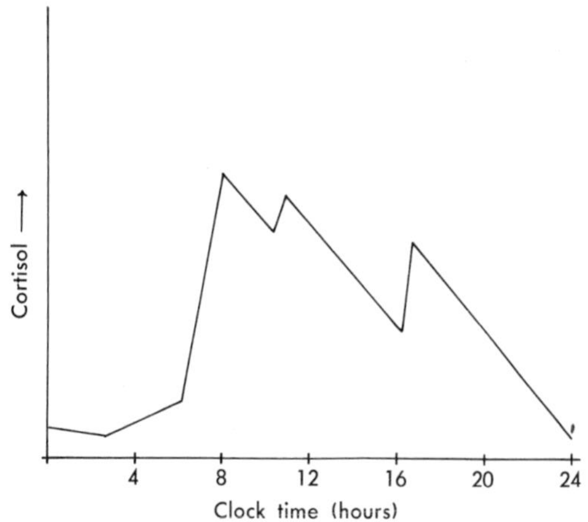

Fig. 18-19. Circulating cortisol concentration varies with time of day. In most individuals, there is a peak in hours around sunrise, a dip late in afternoon, and another peak early in evening. Levels are lowest between midnight and 4 A.M.

used CBG as the specific reactor substance,[5] though antibodies have been developed and are now in general use. Similarly, only tritiated cortisol was originally available as a labeled ligand, but now both iodine 125 and selenium 75 (a gamma-ray emitter) derivatives are used in RIA kits for cortisol. All the common separation techniques have been used in cortisol radioassays.

The largest problem associated with the measurement of the corticosteroid hormones (and some of the polypeptide hormones as well) is the necessity for careful sampling. Most of the hormones exhibit a time-dependent variation in concentration. For the female sex hormones, this variation occurs over a month's time, corresponding to the menstrual period. For cortisol, the variation is diurnal (varies within the course of a day). Fig. 18-19 shows a typical blood cortisol cycle. Obviously, the time of day in which the blood sample is drawn will affect the cortisol concentration measured. It is common practice, in measuring cortisol levels, to sample at 8:00 A.M., when most individuals have a cortisol peak. The physician may designate other sampling times.

A common technique used in endocrine diagnosis is challenge or stimulation testing. The presence of normal physiologic and biochemical mechanisms controlling hormones may be tested by administration of a drug that either stimulates or blocks a hormonal action. For example, adrenal insufficiency can be screened for by the ACTH-stimulation test. In this test, a blood sample for cortisol is obtained prior to stimulation. An aliquot of synthetic human ACTH is then administered to the patient intramuscularly, and another

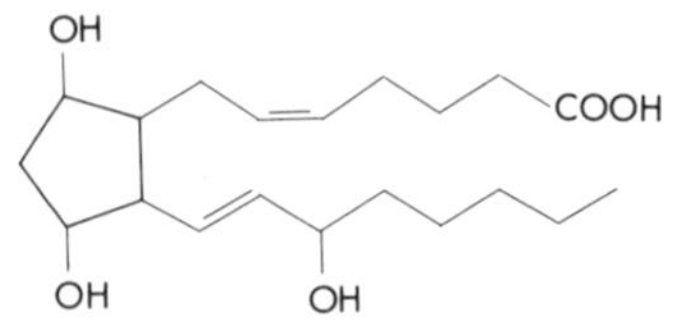

Fig. 18-20. Prostaglandin F-2, typical member of this class of compounds.

blood sample for cortisol drawn 1 hour later. In a normal individual, the serum cortisol will increase at least 10 μg/dl over the base line (prestimulation) in 1 hour. Adrenal insufficiency will result in a lesser response, and this diagnosis must be confirmed by subsequent more complete testing. A variety of stimulation tests of this nature exist and all require careful timing of the sampling. The laboratory that engages in measurement of any of these hormones must therefore be prepared to ascertain that correct blood-drawing procedures have been followed and to reject those specimens that were obtained at incorrect times.

Prostaglandins

Prostaglandins are a series of small molecules whose presence and functions were discovered in the early 1970s. They differ from most biologic molecules in that they are neither aromatic nor polar. A typical prostaglandin is shown in Fig. 18-20. The exact roles of these molecules has not been fully explained, but they are known to be related to gonadal function and fertility. Many have been measured by radioimmunoassay, and although the clinical usefulness for these assays has not been defined, the situation may change as their true role is discovered.

RADIOASSAYS FOR VITAMIN B_{12} AND FOLATES

Folic acid and its congeners are vitamins, that is, compounds necessary for life that cannot be synthesized by the organism. The active form of folate, *N*-5-methyltetrahydrofolic acid, is necessary for the transfer of one-carbon moieties in the metabolic cycle that produces purines. This cycle is shown in Fig. 18-21. Cell replication requires the purines thymidine and cytosine, which are incorporated in DNA. Production of these nucleic acids is dependent on the cycle, which in turn requires vitamin B_{12} to catalyze the conversion of homocysteine to methionine. Lack of vitamin B_{12} halts the tetrahydrofolate cycle and production of purines. The cell perceives that its nucleus is incomplete, and it continues to grow forming a megaloblast. This effect is most dramatically seen in those cells that are growing and dividing rapidly, such as erythrocytes. A vitamin B_{12} or folate deficiency thus results in the formation of megaloblasts (large cells)

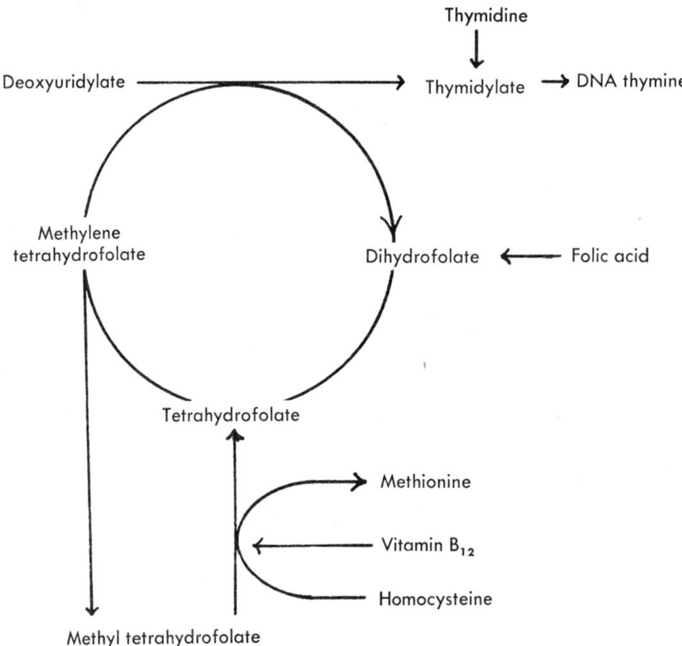

Fig. 18-21. Contribution of vitamin B_{12} and folates to synthesis of nucleotides is illustrated in cycle shown here.

and leads to a megaloblastic anemia. Megaloblastic anemia is seen only in cases where there is a long-term deficiency.

Vitamin B_{12} is synthesized by microorganisms in the rumen of grazing animals. Red meat is thus the source of the vitamin for man. The vitamin is absorbed through the ileal mucosa with the aid of intrinsic factor (IF), a glycoprotein (molecular weight 50,000). Intrinsic factor binds vitamin B_{12} and attaches to ileal cell walls, facilitating transport through the cell. From there, the vitamin is transferred to transcobalamin I, a beta globulin that transports the vitamin to the liver and marrow, where it is immediately absorbed. The vitamin B_{12} is also bound by transcobalamin II, an alpha globulin that serves to store the vitamin. Greater than 90% of the circulating vitamin is bound to these two proteins, and normal circulating levels are 130 to 700 picograms/ml.

Man requires about 100 ng of vitamin B_{12} per day. However, lack of vitamin intake does not become immediately apparent, since the body stores 2 to 3 μg (200 to 3000 ng) and has some capability to reuse vitamin B_{12}. Long-term vitamin B_{12} deficiency usually manifests itself first as a megaloblastic anemia. Today, dietary vitamin B_{12} deficiencies are usually seen in chronic alcoholics (who generally drink their meals) and occasionally in vegetarians. If discovered early, this megaloblastic anemia is treatable with oral vitamin therapy and improved diet. However, long-term deficiency results in more serious and irreversible problems, chiefly neuropathy caused by degradation of the lipoprotein myelin sheath. A form of vitamin B_{12}, coenzyme B_{12}, is required to maintain this important tissue.

A relatively rare though often-mentioned disease involving vitamin B_{12} is pernicious anemia, a megaloblastic anemia resulting from a deficiency of intrinsic factor. In the absence of this glycoprotein, dietary vitamin B_{12} cannot be absorbed and the megaloblastic anemia occurs by the mechanism mentioned above. Pernicious anemia is diagnosed by low serum vitamin B_{12} levels and by the Schilling test, which involves oral administration of radioactive (^{57}Co) vitamin B_{12} followed by measurement of ^{57}Co in the urine. Pernicious anemia is treated with biweekly or monthly intramuscular injections of the vitamin.

Folate deficiencies are caused by poor dietary habits. Leafy green vegetables are the main natural source of folates. However, many processed breakfast foods (dry cereals) now contain added amounts of folate. Inclusion of these foods in one's diet can cause phenomenal rises in serum folate levels. There is no known pathologic effect of increased serum folates.

Measurement of serum vitamin B_{12} and folate

Prior to the 1970s, serum vitamin B_{12} levels were measured by a microbial assay. The microbial assay is time consuming and cannot be done if the patient is on antibiotics. For these reasons a competitive binding radioassay has supplanted the microbial assay. Intrinsic factor, isolated from hog ileal mucosa, is one specific reactor substance that is commonly used. Certain proteins isolated from a variety of fish species have also been described as good specific reactor substances.[15] No attempts have been made to use vitamin B_{12} antibodies. The labeled ligand for vitamin B_{12} radioassay is ^{57}Co-labeled vitamin B_{12}, a natural choice since B_{12} contains cobalt in its structure. Separation of bound and free ligand is usually achieved by dextran-coated charcoal. Before analysis, the vitamin must be hydrolyzed from its binding proteins. This can be accomplished by either acid or base hydrolysis, the acid being somewhat more effective.

Although the correlation between the microbial assay and the competitive binding radioassay for vitamin B_{12} is generally good, many clinicians have observed patients with apparent pernicious anemia who did not exhibit low vitamin B_{12} levels. This anomalous situation was explained in 1978 when Kolhouse and his co-workers[11] demonstrated that a substance known as R-protein was present as a contaminant in the intrinsic factor most laboratories used for their vitamin B_{12} radioassays, and that R-protein bound biologically inactive vitamin B_{12} analogs, leading to falsely elevated vitamin B_{12} levels. Most manufacturers of vitamin B_{12} kits responded to this discovery by either adding cobinamide to their kits to block the effect of the R-proteins, or by changing to highly purified intrinsic factor as the specific reactor substance.

Folate levels were classically measured by microbiologic assays, but these have been replaced by competitive binding radioassays. In the radioassay, all folate congeners in the serum are converted to pteroylglutamic acid (folic acid, PGA). The PGA then competes with radiolabeled PGA for binding sites on the specific folate binder, beta lactoglobulin, which is obtained from cow's milk. Either ^{125}I or ^{3}H can be used to label the PGA, but the need for a liquid scintillation counter and the problems of quenching have all but doomed ^{3}H-folate radioassays. The bound and free PGA are separated by dextran-coated charcoal.

Some hematologists prefer to measure red blood cell folate, since it may more correctly reflect the true hematologic picture. The same radioassay kits that are used to measure serum folate may also be used for red blood cell folate. A hemolysate of the cells is made and then diluted 1 to 50 or 1 to 100 before being assayed.

All folates are chemically unstable and sensitive to photochemical oxidation. For this reason, samples for folate analysis should be protected from heat and light. Common practice is to remove the serum from the clot as soon as possible and freeze at $-20°$ C. Some investigators recommend the addition of ascorbic acid to samples prior to storage, to prevent oxidation.

In the late 1970s several simultaneous vitamin B_{12}/folate radioassays were developed. The simultaneous assays are possible because two different gamma nuclides are used, the separation method is suitable for both compounds, there is no cross-reactivity and all reagents are compatible. Simultaneous vitamin B_{12}/folate assays represent a significant time-saver for the laboratory. The critical quality control parameter in performing a simultaneous assay is the counter windows. They must be set so that there is less than 3% spillover from the other isotope.

IMMUNORADIOMETRIC ASSAYS

Classic radioimmunoassay, as described in the previous pages, uses radiolabeled antigen as the marker for analysis. There are several techniques where antibodies rather than antigens are radioactively labeled. These are sometimes called immunoradiometric assays (IRMA) to distinguish them from true RIAs. The most commonly used of these assays is for hepatitis B surface antigen, HB_sAg. This material is present in the serum of individuals who have active viral hepatitis or are carriers of the disease even though they may be free from symptoms. The IRMA for HB_sAg is performed by the addition of an aliquot of the patient's serum to a tube or well containing anti-HB_sAg bound to a solid support. After a suitable incubation during which the antigen, if present, binds to the solid-phase antibody, anti-HB_sAg labeled with ^{125}I is added. Since HB_sAg is divalent, a second binding site is available to the labeled antibody. An antibody sandwich, consisting of solid phase Ab-HB_sAg-Ab-^{125}I forms. The remaining labeled antibody is then washed away. The solid support is counted and compared to known negative and positive controls, before being reported out as either positive or negative for HB_sAg. The largest use of the IRMA for hepatitis antigen is in blood banking, since every unit of blood transfused must be screened for hepatitis antigen.

Another form of IRMA is the radioallergosorbent test, or RAST.* The RAST is used by allergists to determine which allergens a patient may react to. Since allergies are immune reactions, the RAST is in essence a test to determine the presence of antibodies of the IgE type, which are responsible for the allergic response. In the RAST, the patient's serum is incubated with paper disks each having a specific allergen coupled to it. If the person has an IgE to that allergen, it binds to the disk. The nonspecific IgE is then washed away and a radiolabeled antibody to IgE is added. The labeled anti-IgE binds to any IgE present and again the excess is washed away. The disks are counted, and those to which the patient has an allergy are compared to reference samples to yield a classification of the re-

*Pharmacia, Inc., Uppsala, Sweden.

sponses. A standard radioimmunoassay for IgE is also available in kit form to aid in the diagnosis of latent or rare allergies.

GLOSSARY OF RADIOIMMUNOASSAY TERMS

affinity The attraction of a specific reactor substance for a ligand.

antibody See *immunoglobulin*.

antigen A molecule or particle capable of eliciting an immune response.

antiserum Serum containing antibodies. In RIA the term often indicates an antibody solution that has not been subjected to purification steps.

avidity The tendency of a specific reactor substance to hold its ligands.

binder See *specific reactor substance*.

binding constant The equilibrium constant for a reaction between an antibody or binding protein and its antigen or ligand.

buffer A solution of a weak acid and one of its salts that resists change in pH; a buffer is usually used to maintain a constant pH for a reaction in solution.

competitive protein binding A type of competitive-binding radioassay in which the specific reactor substance is a native nonimmunologic protein.

control See *quality control serum*.

cross-reactivity The reaction of a molecule with an immunoglobulin directed toward another substance.

dose-response curve The graphic relationship between counts bound and amount of standard added in a radioimmunoassay; a standard curve.

equilibrium constant A true constant that relates the concentration of products and reactants in a reversible chemical system when no further net change is occurring in those concentrations.

hapten A molecule that cannot elicit immunoglobulin response by itself but can when bound to a larger carrier molecule.

immunoglobulin A type of protein, isolated from the globulin fraction of serum, having a characteristic structure and the ability to bind to molecules that are not endogenous to the species producing the immunoglobulin.

ligand In the general chemical sense, a molecule that binds reversibility to another. In radioimmunoassay, ligand usually means an antigen or small molecule that binds to a native carrier protein.

logit The mathematical relationship defined as

$$\ln \frac{y}{1-y}$$

nonspecific binding The binding of the radiolabeled ligand to substances or surfaces other than the specific reactor substance.

percent trace binding The amount of radioactivity bound by a specific reactor substance in a solution containing the substance of interest, divided by the amount of radioactivity bound by the same amount of specific reactor substance in a solution where the substance of interest in undetectable, times 100. Mathematically:

$$100 \times \frac{\text{Counts bound}}{\text{Counts bound in absence of substance}}$$

Often written as $\% B/B_0$

pH The negative logarithm of the hydrogen-ion concentration.

quality control serum A serum sample that is analyzed many times to yield data about the statistical reproducibility of a radioassay.

saturation analysis A type of competitive-binding assay where the specific reactor substance–binding sites are all occupied (saturated) with ligand. RIA is a type of saturation analysis.

solid-phase antibody An antibody chemically linked to a solid surface.

specific reactor substance A material capable of specifically and reversibly reacting with another molecule.

specificity The ability of a substance to recognize and bind to only one other molecule.

standard A solution of a pure substance of known concentration to which unknown substances may be compared.

total count tube A tube in an RIA to which an aliquot of radiolabeled ligand only has been added to serve as a check on the delivery of that material.

REFERENCES

1. Berson, S. A., and Yalow, R. S.: Immunoassay of endogenous plasma insulin in man, J. Clin. Invest. **39:**1157, 1960.
2. Bolton, A. E., and Hunter, W. M.: A new method for labeling protein hormones with radioiodine for use in radioimmunoassay, J. Endocrinol. **55:**xxx, (1972).
3. Bowker, A. H., and Lieberman, G. H.: Engineering statistics, Englewood Cliffs, N.J., 1972, Prentice-Hall, Inc., p. 492.
4. Brooker, G., Terasaki, W. L., and Price, M. G.: Gammaflow: a completely automated radioimmunoassay system, Science **194:**270, 1976.
5. de la Pena, A., and Goldzieher, J. W.: Practical determination of total plasma cortisol by use of competitive protein binding, Clin. Chem. **20:**1376, 1974.
6. Hales, C. N., and Randle, P. J.: Immunoassay of insulin with insulin-antibody precipitate, Biochem. J. **88:**137, 1963.
7. Hatch, K. F., Coles, E., Busey, H., and Goldman, S. C.: End-point parameter adjustment on a small desk-top programmable calculator for logit-log analysis of radioimmunoassay data, Clin. Chem. **22:**1383, 1976.
8. Hersh, L. S., and Yaverbaum, S.: Magnetic solid phase radioimmunoassay, Clin. Chim. Acta **63:**69, 1975.
9. Hunter, W. M., and Greenwood, F. C.: Preparation of iodine-131 labeled human growth hormone of high specific activity, Nature **194:**495, 1962.
10. Ithakissios, D. S., and Kubiatowicz, D. O.: Use of protein-containing magnetic microparticles in radioassays, Clin. Chem. **23:**2072, 1977.
11. Kolhouse, J. F., Kondo, H., Allen, N. C., Podell, E., and Allen, R. H.: Cobalamin analogs are present in human plasma and can mask cobalamin deficiency because current radioisotope dilution assays are not specific for true cobalamin, N. Engl. J. Med. **299:**785, 1978.
12. Krasula, R., Yanagi, R., Hastreiter, A. R., Levitsky, S., and Soyka, L. F.: Digoxin intoxication in infants and children: correlation with serum levels, J. Pediatr. **84:**265, 1974.
13. Kroening, B., and Weintraub, M.: Reduced variation of tracer binding in digoxin radioimmunoassay by use of ^{125}I-labeled tyrosine–methyl ester derivative; relation of thyroxine concentration to binding, Clin. Chem. **22:**1732, 1976.

14. Kubasik, N. P., Hall, J. L., and Sine, H. E.: Selection of assay tubes for radioassay procedures, Clin. Chem. **22:**1745, 1976.
15. Kubiatowicz, D. O., Ithakissios, D. S., and Windorski, D. C.: Vitamin B_{12} radioassay with oyster toadfish *(Opsanus tau)* serum as binder, Clin. Chem. **23:**1037, 1977.
16. Mincey, E. K., Thorson, S. C., and Brown, J. L.: A new in-vitro blood test for determining thyroid status—the effective thyroxine ratio, Clin. Biochem. **4:**216, 1971.
17. Morgan, C. R., and Lazarow, A.: Immunoassay of insulin using a two-antibody system, Proc. Soc. Exp. Biol. Med. **110:**29, 1962.
18. Murphy, B. E. P., and Pattee, C. J.: Determination of thyroxine utilizing the property of protein binding, J. Clin. Endocrinol. Metab. **24:**187, 1964.
19. Nye, L., Forrest, G. C., Greenwood, H., et al.: Solid phase magnetic particle radioimmunoassay, Clin. Chim. Acta **69:**387, 1976.
19a. Rodbard, D.: Statistical quality control and routine data processing for radioimmunoassays and immunoradiometric assays, Clin. Chem. **20:**1255-1270, 1974.
20. Scatchard, G.: The attractions of proteins for small molecules and ions, Ann. N.Y. Acad. Sci. **51:**660, 1949.
21. Shaw, W., Hubert, I. L., and Spierto, F. W.: Interference of fatty acids in the competitive protein binding assay for serum thyroxine, Clin. Chem. **22:**673, 1976.
22. Shaw, W., Smith, J., Spierto, F. W., and Agnese, S. T.: Linearization of data for saturation-type competitive binding assay and radioimmunoassay, Clin. Chim. Acta **76:**15, 1977.
23. Soto, A. R., Brotherton, M., Castellanos, M. E., and Chambliss, K. W.: Causes of variability of assay values in radioimmunoassay of digoxin, Clin. Chem. **22:**1183, 1976.
24. Wettrell, G., and Andersson, K. E.: Clinical pharmacokinetics of digoxin in children, Clin. Pharmacokinetics **2:**17, 1977.
25. Whicher, J. T.: The value of complement assays in clinical chemistry, Clin. Chem. **24:**7, 1978.
26. Yalow, R. S., and Berson, S. A.: Quantitative aspects of the reaction between insulin and insulin binding antibody, J. Clin. Invest. **38:**1996, 1959.
27. Zwillich, C. W., Sutton, F. D., Neff, T. A., Cohn, W. M., Matthey, R. A., and Weinberger, M. M.: Theophylline-induced seizures in adults, Ann. Intern. Med. **82:**784, 1975.

ADDITIONAL READINGS

Besch, P. K., editor: Clinical radioassay procedures: a compendium, Washington, D.C., 1975, The American Association for Clinical Chemistry.

Brown, J., Chopra, I. J., Cornell, J. S., Hershman, J. M., Solomon, D. H., Uller, R. P., and Van Henle, A. J.: Thyroid physiology in health and disease, Ann Intern. Med. **81:**68, 1974.

Dvorchik, B. H., and Vesell, E. S.: Pharmacokinetic interpretation of data gathered during therapeutic drug monitoring, Clin. Chem. **22:**868, 1976.

Evered, D.: Diseases of the thyroid gland, Clin. Endocrinol. Metab. **3:**3, 1974.

Freeman, L. M., and Blaufox, M. D., editors: Radioimmunoassay I, Semin. Nucl. Med., vol. V, no. 2, April 1975.

Freeman, L. M., and Blaufox, M. D., editors: Radioimmunoassay II, Semin. Nucl. Med., vol. V, no. 3, July 1975.

Gibaldi, M., and Levy, G.: Pharmacokinetics in clinical practice: concepts, J.A.M.A. **235:**1864, 1976.

Gibaldi, M., and Levy, G.: Pharmacokinetics in clinical practice: applications, J.A.M.A. **235:**1987, 1976.

Parker, C. W.: Radioimmunoassay of biologically active compounds, Englewood Cliffs, N.J., 1976, Prentice-Hall, Inc.

Prince, J. R., and Schmidt, L. D.: Statistics and mathematics in the nuclear medicine laboratory, Chicago, 1976, The American Society of Clinical Pathologists.

Ransom, J. P.: Practical competitive binding assay methods, St. Louis, 1976, The C. V. Mosby Co.

Rothfeld, B.: Nuclear medicine in vitro, Philadelphia, 1974, J. B. Lippincott Co.

Shaw, W., Smith, J., Spierto, F. W., and Agnese, S. T.: Linearization of data for saturation-type competitive binding assay and radioimmunoassay, Clin. Chim. Acta **76:**15, 1977.

Chapter 19

PATIENT CARE

Carolyn Weisberg and L. David Wells

As we look at the medical care complex, with its many departments and specialty areas, one single component of the operation is clearly predominant in all areas. This single component is the patient. Without the patient we would have little need for health care institutions.

NUCLEAR MEDICINE TECHNOLOGIST AS A MEMBER OF THE HEALTH CARE TEAM

Health is defined by the World Health Organization as "A state of complete physical, mental and social well-being, and not merely the absence of disease or infirmity. The enjoyment of the highest attainable standard of health care is one of the fundamental rights of every human being without distinction of race, religion, political belief, economic or social condition. The health of all people is fundamental to the attainment of peace and security and is dependent upon the fullest cooperation of individuals and states."

The health team consists of everyone concerned with the operation of the hospital. This includes physicians, technologists, technicians, nurses, social workers, and others. In order for the operation to be effective, the responsibilities of good teamwork must be applied. Each member must be aware of the responsibilities of the other members. It is of great advantage to the nuclear medicine technologist to communicate with and possibly observe other departments so that each member's role may be perspectively placed in the total picture of health care services. A good exercise in observing the health care team would be to select a particular patient and follow him from admission to discharge. You will be surprised at how many people are directly and indirectly involved with his plan of care.

Realization of your role as a nuclear medicine technologist will help you deal with patients and other team members. The studies you produce will directly affect the physician's plan of care. The performance of such a service makes you a vital part of the health care team.

Observing the patient

When a patient arrives in the nuclear medicine department, the technologist must formulate a plan to efficiently complete the study. The first step in this plan is the initial observation of the patient. In what condition is the patient? Is he in pain? Will he be able to hold still for the necessary imaging time? Will he be able to lie flat? These are only a few questions that, depending on the answer, will directly affect how well your study will turn out and how well the patient will tolerate the procedure.

Signs and symptoms may be either subjective or objective. Objective symptoms also may be called physical signs. They are symptoms that may be discovered by the technologist, physician, nurse, or anyone monitoring the patient. Examples of objective symptoms are changes in vital signs, bleeding, and changes in level of consciousness. These signs, if noticed by the technologist, must be reported to the patient's physician immediately.

Subjective symptoms are the signs that the patient feels. Examples of these are pain, nausea, apprehension, and fear. If a patient informs you of any such symptom, it, like the objective symptoms, must be reported. Depending on the problem, certain steps must be taken to alleviate or reverse the problem. In some cases, for example, medication may be given to relieve pain or nausea.

Relief of the discomfort will allow the technologist and the patient to procede with the study.

Fear and apprehension are frequently observed subjective symptoms. These feelings take many forms and may or may not interfere with the study. The patient who refuses his study may seem angry and hostile when, in truth, he is afraid. Perhaps he is afraid of the study, or of his illness, or of the outcome of his many tests. Another patient may just become silent, almost mechanical. He follows instruction without question. Although the latter may seem like an ideal situation, it is neither ideal or beneficial.

In either situation, gaining the patient's confidence must be placed high on the technologist's priority list. How do you gain the patient's confidence? In most cases the easiest way is to tell the patient what you are going to do to him before you do it. So often, members of the health care team, in the rush of completing technical tasks, forget that patients are people. Place yourself in the patient's shoes. Let him know that you know what you are doing and that you do it well.

Body mechanics and patient safety

Body mechanics are techniques that provide safety to you and to the patient. When used properly, they will make your work easier and your patient more comfortable. Always employ correct body mechanics when moving a patient. Some general rules of body mechanics are the following:

- Good posture and positioning the feet slightly apart with one foot forward will provide a base of support.
- Always bend your knees when lifting. Back strain or injury may occur if you bend only at the hips.
- Stand as close as possible to the object you are lifting.
- When you work at a stretcher or bed, be sure that the height is at a comfortable level for you.

In addition to using body mechanics to make your task safer for you, there are some rules that provide safety for the patient. Patient safety is extremely important, and it is your responsibility while the patient is in your care.

- Never place a patient on a stretcher without using side rails or stretcher straps.
- Never leave a disoriented, senile, unconscious, sedated, psychiatric, geriatric, or pediatric patient alone.
- Never restrain a patient without an order from his physician.
- Never restrain a patient's arms without elevating his head, especially if he is lethargic or unconscious.

These are only some of the rules of patient safety. Using common sense and protecting your patient from what might happen to him should always be foremost in your mind.

Transporting the patient

Wheelchairs. Wheelchairs are generally used for patients who are alert, coherent, and physically able to sit in a chair. Several things should be considered when one uses a wheelchair to transport a patient. Look at the patient's total physical picture. He may be alert and coherent but have a paralyzed extremity. If this extremity is not properly and safely positioned by you, it could become caught in the wheels of the chair and cause serious injury. Patients should not be placed in wheelchairs if they cannot stand or walk. It would be very difficult to move them from chair to stretcher for their study. Consideration should also be given to tubes, intravenous fluids and indwelling catheters to be sure that they are safely away from the wheels.

Stretchers. Stretchers are used for patients who cannot safely or comfortably sit in a chair. Perhaps they have had a test requiring them to lie flat, such as a lumbar puncture. You as a nuclear medicine technologist must be familiar with the reason your patient is traveling on a stretcher.

Whether your patient travels by wheelchair or stretcher, safety rules must be considered. These rules are of such great importance that they are worth mentioning over and over gain. In addition to safety, remember:

- Do not push the patient backwards.
- If you are going over a rough spot, warn him ahead of time.
- Take the shortest route to your destination.
- Check the patient's identification band.
- Tell the patient where you are taking him.

Vital signs

"Vital sign" is a term used to denote one or more of the measurements of pulse, body temperature, respirations, and blood pressure. Each of these measurements is a direct indication of certain physiologic functions. Any deviation from the normal range or the previous measurements means that a change is taking place in the patient's condition.

Although you will not be expected, in most cases, to routinely take vital signs, it is wise to learn how to do it correctly. If a change occurs in the patient while you are doing his study, his physician may ask you to give one or more of the measurements. In order to know whether the measurement has changed, you must know the previous measurement. You will find this information in the patient's chart.

Pulse. To obtain the pulse, place two fingers over the radial, carotid, or femoral artery and count the beats for one full minute. The radial pulse is the most commonly used site, but if this is difficult to feel, you may use the other sites mentioned. Note the character of the beat. The normal range is from 70 to 80 beats per minute.

Temperature. The temperature may be taken orally, rectally, or at the axilla. Be sure the reading is below 96° F or (36° C) before you insert the thermometer. Allow it to remain in place at least two full minutes. Before choosing the route, refer to the physician's orders. Patients who are on seizure precautions, for example, or are unconscious should not have oral temperatures taken. On the other hand, patients who have cardiac problems should not have rectal temperatures taken. Check the patient's chart. Normal body temperature is 98.6° F (37° C).

Respirations. If the patient is conscious, count his respirations for one full minute. If he is unconscious, place your hand on his chest and count for one full minute. Like the pulse, the character and regularity should also be noted. Respirations normally occur 16 to 20 times per minute.

Blood pressure. Place the cuff around the upper arm (unless contraindicated) and close it comfortably. Place the diaphragm of the stethoscope over the brachial artery. Pump the cuff until it reaches approximately 170 mm Hg. Slowly release the cuff and record the first and last sound you hear. The first sound will be the systolic reading and the last will be the diastolic. Never leave an inflated cuff around a patient's arm longer than necessary. Besides being extremely uncomfortable, it will act as a tourniquet and may cause injury. Normal blood pressure is 120 mm/80 mm Hg.

Asepsis and sterile technique

Another aspect of safety for both you and the patient is preventing the spread of infection. "Medical asepsis" is a term used to describe techniques to prevent the transmission of infection. This ranges from simple handwashing to complex isolation procedures.

"Surgical asepsis" is a term to describe the techniques used to protect the patient against infection or contamination, for example, sterilizing the skin prior to injection of a radioisotope and using sterile equipment is a method of surgical asepsis. Washing your hands between patients is a method of medical asepsis. Many times these techniques overlap in their use.

Much of the equipment in health care institutions today comes prepackaged and sterile. Before using these materials, however, we must double-check their sterility. Most equipment will have a date of expiration. Do not use expired equipment. Check the package to be sure it is not damaged or open. Microorganisms need only a tiny portal of entry. If the package has watermarks or is wet, it must be considered contaminated. If you are at all suspicious, discard the item.

In your role as a nuclear medicine technologist you will deal with patients that require isolation. When you receive a patient who is on isolation, your first step is to find out what type of isolation you are to use. Each institution has its own policy for isolation procedures. It is up to you to learn the policies of your particular institution.

Some types of isolation require gowns, masks, gloves, and complete disinfection of the room when the study is complete. Other types require only mask or gloves and simple washing of used equipment.

Terminal disinfection refers to the care of equipment when an isolated patient leaves the area. Again, different institutions use different procedures, but some of the rules are nearly universal. The disinfectant used must be effective against the particular organism, and the strength of the solution must be sufficient to destroy the organism.

After disinfection it is extremely important to rinse and dry articles so that residual chemicals are not absorbed or ingested by another patient.

Special patient care

Surgical patients. Many of your patients will have had recent surgery. It will be your responsibility to find out what procedure has been performed so that you may perform your study with maximum efficiency and comfort to the patient. Orthopedic surgery with traction, for example, requires direct communication with the patient's physician before you move or turn the patient. You will also need to be aware of special dressings and drains so that any drainage can be reported should it change in character or become profuse.

Psychiatric patients. Occasionally you may have a patient who has a psychiatric illness. Perhaps his physician is ruling out medical etiology or perhaps he has a medical problem unrelated to his psychiatric disorder. In either case there are several things you will need to recall in dealing with this particular patient.

You must first employ your usual practice of gaining his confidence and explaining the procedure. Perhaps you will need to provide this explanation more than once or in segments as you procede through the study. Never leave a psychiatric patient alone. Always maintain reality and your professionalism. Do not indulge in the patient's fantasy or delusions, should he present them to you.

Pediatric patients. Children are people. You must gain their confidence and explain the procedure according to their level of comprehension. Never lie to a child. If he is being extremely difficult to handle, you may discover that it is because he has been lied to about a previous procedure. Sometimes it is possible to successfully complete a study if someone whom the child knows and trusts is allowed to remain with him. Upon occasion, especially with younger children, it may be necessary to request that he be sedated. If this is the case, be sure you know what the child has been given and that you have been made aware of possible adverse reactions. Never leave a child of any age alone. Keep dangerous objects out of his reach.

Physically handicapped patients. Physically handicapped patients require little special attention. They should be treated as any other patient. If a part of the patient's body has been injured so that he has no feeling in that particular area, it is your responsibility to see that no additional injury occurs. Be sure that it is safely protected from wheels or from getting caught between the stretcher and the wall. Allow these patients to do as much for themselves as possible and assist only as needed. If your patient is blind, do not attempt to lead him by taking his arm. Let him hold your arm and follow you. If your patient cannot talk or is deaf, be sure to provide him with a paper and pencil.

Elderly patients. Older people are often unique in that they are more or less set in their ways. It becomes, once again, important for you to gain their confidence and explain procedures. Frequently older people have much to say to us, and it is worthwhile for us to stop and listen. Like physically handicapped patients, older people need to be protected from injury. Geriatric skin is especially susceptible to injury. Be particularly cautious about placing adhesive tape on the skin of older people.

Special equipment

Parenteral fluids. Mismanagement or neglect of intravenous tubing, flow rate, or needle site by ancillary departments is the most common cause of conflict with nursing unit personnel. A patient receives intravenous fluids for various reasons, all of them extremely important. He may be getting fluid replacement or medications, or an intravenous line may have been established to maintain an avenue for emergency drugs. Frequently the veins of ill people are not easy to find and the need to preserve the site is great.

When the patient comes to the nuclear medicine department, it is your responsibility as a technologist to protect and preserve his intravenous line. Protect the needle site and monitor the flow rate. The correct rate may be found on the bottle label or in the patient's chart. Watch the fluid level in the bottle to be sure it does not empty. If the line is not running properly or you suspect a malfunction, notify the patient's physician or appropriate nursing personnel.

Remember that an intravenous line is a direct entry into the bloodstream. It must remain a closed, sterile system and must be protected from air bubbles and contamination.

Gastric suction. Occasionally you may have a patient with a gastric-suction or nasogastric tube. This is a tube inserted through the mouth or nose for the administration of fluids and medication or connected to suction to drain the stomach contents. You will need to observe the patient for discomfort and preserve the placement of the tube. Do not use the tube for the administration of fluids such as potassium perchlorate unless you have permission from the patient's physician and you are sure that the tube is in the stomach and not in the lung.

Chest suction. Patients have chest tubes to maintain respiratory function in the event of lung collapse, injury, or surgery. These tubes serve to assure the necessary pressure. Working with patients who have chest tubes in place requires a great deal of caution. You must be sure that the chest tubes do not become disconnected. Most chest suction sets will have a clamp attached to them. In the event that a tube becomes disconnected or suction is broken, the tube must be clamped immediately and the physician notified.

T-tubes. T-tubes are special drains placed in an incision at the time of surgery. They need only be kept intact. An unusually large amount of drainage or change in character of drainage should be reported.

Urinary retention catheters. Urinary retention catheters are tubes that are placed in the bladder to allow continuous drainage of urine. Because the chance of infection is great with such a device, you must maintain its closed sterile system. If a patient complains of severe discomfort from an indwelling catheter, notify his physician.

Surgical dressings. As mentioned earlier, surgical patients usually have dressings over their incisions. The technologist must be aware of these dressings. Excess drainage or change in character of drainage must be reported. Do not remove a dressing but reinforce it if necessary.

Cardiac monitors. Patients whose heart beats must be monitored on an oscilloscope may occasionally come to your department. These patients should be accompanied by someone trained in reading the monitor and capable to treating possible complications should they arise.

Central venous pressure lines. Commonly called "CVP lines," these lines are generally used to measure circulating blood volume. They are treated in much the same way that you would treat intravenous fluids. The main difference is that this catheter is directly inserted into a large vessel near the heart and lungs. Extreme caution must be taken to preserve sterility and maintain a patent line. Generally you should not inject anything into a central line. If using the central line is a last resort for injection, it should be done by a physician.

Colostomy care. At some time you may be asked to perform a study on a patient with a colostomy. A colostomy is merely an opening in the abdomen through which fecal material is excreted. A colostomy is performed for the removal of sections of diseased bowel. If the patient has had his colostomy for some time, he will generally care for it himself. If it is new, he is probably learning to care for it and acquire some sequence and regularity. If it is new, he may need supportive care from you. It may be necessary to provide him with equipment such as a new bag or dressing reinforcements until he can complete his study and return to his room.

Oxygen administration. Responsibility for oxygen administration varies somewhat between institutions. One institution may use piped oxygen directly from a wall outlet, whereas another may use oxygen cylinders. You should be familiar with the procedure to be followed in your particular institution.

Oxygen is administered to a patient to treat anoxia. The amount to be given and the method of administration is determined by the physician. If you are performing a study on a patient who is receiving oxygen, you have several responsibilities.

1. Maintain the correct flow as prescribed.
2. Do not remove oxygen from the patient unless you have permission from the physician.
3. Even where wall oxygen is used, you must provide a cylinder for the patient while he is in transit to his floor.
4. Be sure the cylinder is secure. A poorly supported cylinder is extremely dangerous.
5. Smoking must not be permitted in areas where oxygen is in use. Appropriate signs should be posted.
6. Do not permit oil or grease to come into contact with any part of an oxygen cylinder.

Emergency care

Emergency care refers to the care given to patients with immediate and possibly life-threatening needs. Because you are dealing with patients who have known medical problems, the chance of having to provide emergency care would seem to be greater. Emergencies vary in their type and severity. Convulsions, hemorrhage, syncope, and respiratory and cardiac arrest are among those you may encounter in the health care setting.

Seizures. Seizures are a symptom of an underlying illness and not a disease in itself. They vary in etiology and type. A seizure may involve one part of the body or the entire body. Loss of consciousness may range from only momentary to several minutes. Frequently patients with a history of seizure disorders will be placed on special precautions. When such a patient is scheduled for your department, these precautions should be made known to you. Usually such precautions include padded side rails on the bed, and a padded tongue blade and airway accompany the patient at all times.

If you observe a patient during a seizure, you must protect the patient from injury without restraining him. You must maintain a patent airway at all times. Immediate notification of the patient's physician is essential. Description of the seizure and its exact length of time is extremely useful information for the physician.

Hemorrhage. Hemorrhage is a term used to describe a large amount of blood lost within a short period of time. You must attempt to stop the bleeding and prevent shock. Immediate notification of the physician is imperative. Do not leave the patient. Send someone for help.

Syncope. Syncope and fainting may occur for many reasons. Sometimes it is a manifestation of heart disease or depleted oxygen in the circulation. Employment of safety precautions frequently will prevent serious injury in susceptible patients. If a patient should faint, you should measure his vital signs and report the incident to his physician as soon as possible.

Cardiopulmonary resuscitation. Respiratory and cardiac arrests are emergency situations that require immediate treatment. Because every second counts in such a situation, it should be stressed that everyone be completely skilled in the technique and application of cardiopulmonary resuscitation (CPR). The American Heart Association and the American National Red Cross continuously provide courses in CPR. Health care institutions frequently include these courses as part of their orientation or make them available through inservice education.

Application of basic CPR may be necessary anywhere and at anytime.

The technique of CPR must be applied correctly to be effective. You cannot learn it completely by reading a book or watching a movie. A complete training program must include manikin practice and must meet the standards of the American Heart Association.

SUMMARY

As a member of the health care team you are a provider of essential information leading to the treatment of illness and the maintenance of health. You must be concerned with the many aspects of care, including observation of the patient and the application of certain techniques.

You must become efficient in handling patients, providing for their safety as well as your own.

You must act responsibly and professionally in all facets of your role.

REFERENCE

Matheney, R. V., Nolan, B. T., Hogan, A. E., and Griffin, G. J.: Fundamentals of patient-centered nursing, ed. 3, St. Louis, 1972, The C. V. Mosby Co.

GLOSSARY

A **number** See *atomic mass.*
ablation (1) Separation or detachment; (2) destruction, that is, by radiation.
abscess Localized collection of pus within tissue.
absorption (μ) coefficient Constant representing the fraction of ionizing radiation absorbed per centimeter thickness of absorbing material.
accelerator Device imparting high kinetic energy to a charged particle causing it to undergo nuclear or particle reaction.
access time The time required to locate and retrieve information from a specified location. In the case of memory, this is related to the electronic speed of the address register and read/write circuits. In the case of disks, the access time is the sum of the time taken for the read/write head to locate a particular track plus the time required for information to rotate into the read/write position.
accumulator Register or data buffer used for temporary storage of data.
acid Any chemical compound that can either donate a proton or accept a pair of electrons in a chemical reaction.
acidophilic (1) Stains easily with acid dyes; (2) grows best on acid media.
acinus Smallest lobule of a gland; secretes the product of the gland.
acquisition Intake of data to the computer.
activation analysis Analytical procedure detecting and measuring trace quantities of elements after exposure to a flux of neutrons.
ADC See *analog-digital converters.*
A/D converter See *analog-digital converters.*
address Label, name, or number that designates a location where information is stored.
adenohypophysis Anterior lobe of the pituitary.
adenoma Epithelial tumor composed of glandular tissue.
adenylate cyclase Enzyme found in the liver and muscle cell membranes.
adrenal cortex Outer portion of the adrenal gland; it produces cortisone.
adrenal medulla Central portion of the adrenal gland; it produces adrenalin.
adrenocorticotropin Compound isolated from the anterior pituitary having a stimulating effect on the adrenal cortex.
afferent Carrying or conveying toward a center.
affinity Attraction of a specific reactor substance for a ligand.
affinity chromatography Separation of compounds based on differences in their affinities for a given species.
akinesia Abnormal reduction of muscle movement.
ALARA NRC operating philosophy for maintaining occupational radiation exposures "as low as is reasonably achievable."
albumin Class of simple proteins, found in most tissues.
alcohol Organic molecule containing the functional —OH group.
aldehyde Organic molecule containing the $-\overset{\displaystyle O}{\overset{\|}{C}}-H$ group.
aldosterone Sodium-retaining hormone of the adrenal cortex.
ALGOL (ALGOrithmic Language) High-level compiler language particularly well suited to arithmetic and string manipulations.
algorithm Prescribed set of well-defined rules or processes for the solution of a problem in a finite number of steps.
aliquot Specific measured amount of liquid.
alimentary canal Food tract starting with the mouth and ending with the rectum and anus.
alkane Hydrocarbon with a general formula of C_nH_{2n+2}.
alkene Hydrocarbon that has one double bond and a general formula of C_nH_{2n}.
alkyl Alkane with one hydrogen atom removed.
alkyne Hydrocarbon that contains a triple bond and a general formula of C_2H_{2n-2}.
alpha cells Cells in pancreatic islands containing large granules.
alpha particle Nucleus of a helium atom emitted by certain radioisotopes upon disintegration.
ALU See *arithmetic unit.*
alveoli Terminal air pockets in the lungs.
amelioration Improvement of a disease.
amide Organic molecule with the functional group $-\overset{\displaystyle O}{\overset{\|}{C}}-NH_2$.
amine Organic molecule containing the functional group $-NH_2$.
amino acid Organic acid containing an NH_2 and a COOH group; thus having both basic and acidic properties.
AMP Adenosine monophosphate; nucleotide containing adenine, a pentose sugar, and one phosphoric acid; product of metabolism.
ampulla of vater Dilation of ducts from the liver and pancreas where they enter the small intestine.
AMU See *atomic mass unit.*
analog (1) Representation of a parameter by a signal the magnitude of which voltage, current, or length is proportional to the parameter; (2) structure with a similar function.
analog computer Computer that parameterizes data in terms of the magnitude of the incoming signals.

analog-digital converters (ADC) Electronic module used to convert an analog signal such as a pulse height into digital information recognizable by a computer.
anastomose To unite an end to another end; to bridge two vessels with a section of a vessel.
androgenic hormone Hormone stimulating male characteristics.
anemia Deficiency of red blood cells.
aneurysm Dilation of part of the wall of an artery.
Anger camera Type of gamma-ray scintillation camera, named for its inventor Hal O. Anger.
angiography X-ray photography of the blood vessels with use of a radiopaque substance.
angiotensin Vasoconstrictor substance present in blood.
anion Negatively charged ion.
annihilation Reaction between a pair of particles resulting in their disintegration and the production of an equivalent amount of energy in the form of photons.
anode Positive electrode.
anoxia Deficiency of oxygen.
antecubital Area in front of the elbow.
antibiotics Drugs used to destroy bacteria, extracted from living organisms.
antibody Substance capable of producing specific immunity to a bacterium or virus, found in the blood.
anticholinergic Drug blocking passage of impulses through the autonomic nerves.
antigen Molecule or particle capable of eliciting an immune response.
antineutrino Neutral nuclear particle emitted in either positron decay or electron capture.
antiserum Serum containing antibodies.
aorta Large artery stemming from the left ventricle.
apatite Crystalline phosphate of lime.
aplasia Failure of an organ to develop.
aplastic anemia Anemia characterized by absence of red blood cell regeneration.
application program Program that performs a task specific to a particular user's needs.
aqueous Referring to anything dissolved in water.
arachnoid Membrane covering the brain and spinal cord.
arene Hydrocarbon compound that contains an aromatic portion.
arithmetic and logical unit (ALU) See *arithmetic unit*.
arithmetic unit Unit within the computer architecture that performs all mathematical and logical operations. Sometimes called "arithmetic and logic unit (ALU)."
aromatic compound Chemical compound containing a ring system that has $(4n + 2)\pi$ electrons.
Arrhenius concept Concept stating that an acid is a compound that acts as a proton donor.
arrhythmia Variation of the heartbeat.
arterial thrombus Blood clot formed in an artery.
arthrography Radiography after the introduction of opaque contrast material into a joint.
ASCII Abbreviation for American Standard Code for Information Interchange, consisting of 128 seven-bit binary codes for upper- and lower-case letters, numbers, punctuation, and special communication control characters.
ascorbic acid Vitamin C.
asepsis Sterile state.
assembler Programs that assemble symbolic programs into binary form.
assembly language Commands for the minicomputer system written in symbolic or mnemonic form. Typically, three-letter abbreviations, called mnemonics, are used to represent each instruction, and each mnemonic can usually be equaled to one machine-code or binary instruction. An assembly language program is translated to binary code by an assembler.
astrocytoma Central nervous system tumor composed of star-shaped cells.
asynchronous Mode of operation in which an operation is started by a signal that the operation on which it depends is completed. When referring to hardware devices, it is the method in which each character is sent with its own synchronizing information. The hardware operations are scheduled by "ready" and "done" signals rather than by time intervals. In addition, it implies that a second operation can begin before the first operation is complete.
asynchronous transfer Sequential computer-operational signal that starts an operation when a necessary previous operation is completed.
ataxia Disorder of the neuromuscular system; lacking muscle coordination.
atherosclerosis Arterial hardening.
atom Smallest unit of an element that can exist and still maintain the properties of the element.
atomic mass Mass of a neutral atom usually expressed in atomic mass units.
atomic mass unit Exactly one twelfth the mass of carbon 12; 1.661×10^{-24} gram.
atomic number Number of protons in an atom, the symbol of which is Z.
atomic weight Average weight of the neutral atoms of an element.
atrium Cavity of the heart receiving blood.
attenuation Any condition that results in a decrease of radiation intensity.
Auger electrons Electrons that participate in the production of x rays; pronounce "Auger" as "o-zháy."
Avogadro's number Number of atoms in the gram atomic weight of a given element or the number of molecules in the gram molecular weight of a given substance: 6.022×10^{23} per gram mole.
avidity Tendency of a specific reactor substance to hold its ligands.
background Detected disintegration events not emanating from the sample.
backscattering Scattering of particulate radiation by more than 90 degrees.
barn Area unit expressing the area of nuclear cross section; 1 barn = 10^{-24} cm^2.
base Any compound that either acts as a proton acceptor or an electron pair donor in a chemical process.
base line Normal evaluation; evaluation before administration of a substance.
BASIC (beginner's all-purpose symbolic instruction code) High-level interactive, interpreter language for mathematical and string-variable manipulations.
batch mode Automatic computer mode that does not require specific programming instruction.

batch operation Computer operation that runs consecutively without operator intervention.
beta cells Pancreatic cells in the islets of Langerhans.
beta (β^-) particle Electron whose point of origin is the nucleus; electron originating in the nucleus by way of decay or a neutron into a proton and electron (beta particle).
biconcave Having two concave surfaces.
bifunctional chelates Complexing agent with two sites for complexation.
bifunctional drug Drug with ability to attack two types of symptoms or diseases.
biliary system System including the liver serving both a digestive and an excretory function.
binary Pertaining to the number system with a radix of two.
binary digit One of the symbols 1 or 0; called a "bit."
binding energy Energy released when a chemical bond is formed; amount of stabilization energy holding a nucleon in the nucleus.
binding sites Sites on a protein where they bind to radionuclides.
bioassay Determination of chemical strength by tests of living tissues.
biochemical Referring to the chemistry of living organisms.
biochemical analogs Chemicals of the living system that resemble one another in function but not in structure.
bioeffects Effects on the biologic system.
biologic distribution Normal distribution of a substance within the living system.
biologic matrix Basic materials of living systems.
biopsy Examination of tissue taken from the living body usually without entirely removing the organ.
biosynthesis Formation of a compound from other compounds by living organisms.
bisacodyl tablets Drugs used as a laxative.
bit An individual binary digit, either 1 or 0; acronym for *bi*nary digi*t*.
bleomycin An antibiotic substance having antineoplastic properties.
blood pool Vascular cavity.
bolus Rounded mass or lump quantity; a concentrated radiopharmaceutical given intravenously.
bombardment Exposure of a target to any ionizing radiation.
bootstrap loader Routine whose first instructions are sufficient to load the remainder of itself into memory from an input device and normally start a complex system of programs.
Bowman's capsule Sac at the end of uriniferous tubules in the kidneys.
Bragg curve Curve showing specific ionization as a function of distance or energy.
bremsstrahlung x rays Photonic emissions caused by the slowing down of beta particles in matter.
briggsian logarithmic system System of logarithms based on the decimal system, using the base 10.
bromination Chemical addition of bromine to a compound.
bronchiectasis Dilation of the small bronchial tubes.
bronchioles Small bronchial tubes leading to air cells.
bronchus Large passage carrying air within the lungs.
Brönsted-Lowry concept Concept stating that an acid is a proton donor and a base is a proton acceptor in a chemical process.
brownian movement Motion of minute particles suspended in liquid.
BTU British thermal unit; measurement of heat.
buffer (1) Storage area used to temporarily hold information being transferred between two devices or between a device and memory; often a special register or a designated area of memory; (2) a solution of a weak acid and one of its salts that resists change in pH; usually used to maintain a constant pH for a reaction in solution.
buffer solution Solution that has a specific pH value and is resistant to pH change by addition of acids or bases.
bug Error in a program.
bullous Referring to a bubble or a bladder.
by-product material Radioactive material arising from controlled fission.
byte Group of binary digits usually operated upon as a unit and usually 8 bits long; in ASCII code, one character occupies one byte of memory and the maximum decimal integer that can be stored in an 8-bit byte is 255.
calyx (*pl.* **calyces**) Cuplike structure in the kidney that receives urine.
canaliculus Small canal or channel.
carbohydrate Compound consisting of carbon, hydrogen, and oxygen, such as sugars and starches.
carboxylic acids Organic molecules with the $-\overset{\overset{\displaystyle O}{\|}}{C}-OH$ functional group, which have acidic properties because of this functional group.
carcinogen Substance stimulating the formation of cancer.
carcinoma Malignant tumor; consisting of connective tissue enclosing epithelial cells.
cardiomyopathy Subacute or chronic disorder of the heart muscle.
carrier Quantity of an element mixed with radioactive isotopes of that element in order to facilitate chemical operations.
carrier free Adjective describing a nuclide that is free of its stable isotopes.
carrier proteins Macroscopic amounts of nonlabeled proteins present with trace amounts of radiolabeled proteins.
cathode Negative electrode.
cathode-ray tube (CRT) Electronic vacuum tube attached to a screen where information is displayed.
cation Positively charged ion.
cauda equina End of the spinal cord containing the nerves that supply the rectal area.
central nervous system That part of the nervous system containing the brain, spinal cord, and nerves.
central processor unit (CPU) Unit of a computing system that includes the circuits controlling the interpretation and execution of instructions—the computer proper, excluding I/O and other peripheral devices.
centrifuge (1) To rotate or spin at high speed for separation; (2) instrument for rotating or spinning samples at high speed.
cerebral radionuclide angiogram, cerebral radioangiogram (CRAG) Rapid sequential scintiphotos of the blood vessels of the brain.
cerebrospinal fluid (CSF) Fluid found in the cavities of the brain, brainstem, spinal cord, and meninges.

charged-particle accelerators Device used to electronically accelerate any charged particle. See also *cyclotron* and *electron accelerator*.
chelate Ligand that has two or more potential bonding sites.
chemical equation Symbolic statement describing a process and showing the stoichiometric relationships among the individual species involved in the process.
chemical equilibrium State of lowest energy for a chemical system undergoing a chemical reaction.
chemical reactions Processes that result in chemical change of the participant molecules.
chemistry Study of matter and the changes that matter undergoes.
chloramine-T *N*-chloro-4-methylbenzenesulfonamide sodium salt; an oxidizing agent used in radioiodination of proteins.
chlormerodrin Diuretic containing mercury.
cholecystokinin Hormone secreted by the small intestine; stimulates contraction of the gallbladder.
choroid plexus Membrane lining the ventricles of the brain, concerned with formation of cerebrospinal fluid.
chromatography Method of chemical analysis where the solution to be analyzed separates into component parts; some types are gel permeation chromatography, paper chromatography, and affinity chromatography.
cistern Fluid reservoir; enclosed space.
cloud chamber Chamber where the paths of ionizing radiation can be observed.
COBOL (commercial and business oriented language) High-level incremental compiler language primarily suited to business applications.
coefficient Constant by which a variable or other quantity is multiplied in an equation.
collagen Protein found in bone and cartilage.
collimators Shielding device used to confine radiation to a narrow beam.
colloid Molecules in a continuous medium that measure between 1 and 100 nm in diameter.
colorimetry Measurement of color.
colostomy Artificial opening in the colon.
column generator Column device using a parent radionuclide adsorbed to a support in a column; the daughter radionuclide is usually obtained by elution of the column with a solution that interacts with the daughter but not with the parent.
competitive protein binding Type of competitive binding radioassay in which the specific reactor substance is a native nonimmunologic protein.
compile To produce a binary-code program from a program written in source (symbolic) language, by selection of appropriate subroutines from a subroutine library, as directed by the instructions or other symbols of the source program; the linkage is supplied for combining the subroutines into a workable program, and the subroutines and linkage are translated into binary code.
compiler Program used to compile assembly code or source code.
compound Distinct substance formed by a union of two or more elements in definite proportions by weight.
Compton scatter One process by which a photon loses energy through collisions with electrons.
computer Programmable electronic device that can store, retrieve, and process data.
concentration Strength of substance in a solution.
congenital Existing at birth.
conjugate acid Remainder of a basic compound after it has either accepted a proton or donated an electron pair in a chemical process.
conjugate base Remainder of an acidic compound after it has either donated its acidic proton or accepted an electron pair in a chemical process.
conversion electron Orbital electron that has been excited (ionized) by internal conversion of an excited atom.
coordinate covalent bond Covalent bond formed by two atoms in which one atom donates both electrons for the bond.
core memory Main memory storage used by the central processing unit, in which binary data are represented by the switching polarity of magnetic cores.
corticosterone Compound isolated from the adrenal cortex.
cortisol Adrenocortical hormone.
Coulomb's law Basic law of electrostatics, which states that

$$F = \frac{q_1 q_2}{4\pi\epsilon r^2} \quad \text{or} \quad F = \frac{qq'}{r^2}$$

covalent bond Chemical bond formed by sharing a pair of electrons by two nuclei.
covalent compound Compound held together by covalent bonds.
CPU See *central processor unit*.
CRAG See *cerebral radionuclide angiogram*.
crash *Hardware crash* is the complete failure of a particular device, sometimes affecting the operation of an entire computer system; *software crash* is the complete failure of an operating system characterized by some failure in the system's protection mechanisms.
critical organ (1) Organ of interest; (2) organ most affected by a technique.
cross-reactivity Reaction of a molecule with an immunoglobulin directed toward another substance.
CRT See *cathode-ray tube*.
crystallography Study of the crystal structure of a molecule.
curie Standard measure of rate of radioactive decay; based on the disintegration of 1 gm of radium or 3.7×10^{10} disintegrations per second.
daughter radionuclide Decay product produced by a radionuclide. The element from which the daughter was produced is called the "parent."
debugger Program to assist in tracking down and eliminating errors that occur in the normal course of program development.
debusser Device used to erase material from a computer or recording tape.
decay Radioactive disintegration of a nucleus of an unstable nuclide.
decay factor Fraction of radionuclei that have decayed in a specified period of time, according to the following formula:

$$\tau = \frac{0.693}{T_{1/2}}$$

decay schemes Diagram showing the decay mode or modes of a radionuclide.

deiodinate Removal of iodine from a compound.

delayed neutrons Neutrons that are emitted in a radioactive process at an appreciable time after fission.

dementia Mental deterioration from disease of the brain.

denaturation Change in chemical and physical properties from the normal state, usually irreversible.

deuterons Nucleus of a deuterium atom (^2_1H) containing one proton and one neutron.

diabetes mellitus Pathologic condition with an absolute or relative insulin deficiency accompanied by elevated levels of glucose in the blood and urine.

diagnostic (1) Referring to determination of the disease; analysis of symptoms; (2) pertaining to the detection and isolation of a malfunction (hardware) or mistake (software).

dialysis Process for separating crystalloids and colloids in solution by the difference in their rates of diffusion through a semipermeable membrane.

diastole Relaxation and dilation of the heart.

diethylenetriaminepentaacetic acid (pentetic acid, DTPA) Chelating agent that can be labeled with ^{99m}Tc and used for scintigraphy.

digit Character used to express one of the positive integers.

digital computer Device that operates on discrete data, performing sequences of arithmetic and logical operations on these data.

digitalis Cardiotonic agent from the *Digitalis* plant leaf.

diphosphonate Organic phosphate compound that can be labeled with ^{99m}Tc and used for scintigraphy.

direct-memory access Access to data in any location independent of sequential prohibitions.

disintegration General process of radioactive decay, usually measured per unit time; *dps* is disintegrations per second, and *dpm* disintegrations per minute; *dps* is equal to counts per second *(cps)* divided by the efficiency of the detector; *dpm* is equal to counts per minute divided by the efficiency of the detector.

disk Form of rotating memory consisting of a platter of aluminum coated with ferrous oxide that can be magnetized or read by a read/write head in proximity to the surface; most common form of bulk memory device.

diuretic Substance that promotes the secretion of urine.

diverticulum Blind pouch; usually in the intestine.

DMA See *direct memory access.*

DMSA 2,3-Dimercaptosuccinic acid; a chelating agent that can be labeled with ^{99m}Tc for imaging.

dose Amount of ionizing radiation absorbed by a specific area or volume or by the whole body.

DTPA See *diethylenetriaminepentaacetic acid.*

dysplasia Abnormality of development.

dyspnea Difficulty in breathing.

ECAT Emission computerized axial tomography.

edema Excess fluid in the body.

edetic acid (ethylenediaminetetraacetic acid, EDTA) Chelating agent.

editor Program to permit data or instructions to be manipulated and displayed. Most commonly used in the preparation of new programs or in the revision and correction of old programs.

EDTA See *edetic acid.*

elastic scattering Scattering caused by elastic collisions between nuclei that result in a conservation of the systems kinetic energy.

electrochemical process Chemical process involving oxidation and reduction of the reaction constituents.

electrolyte Substance that forms ions when dissolved in water.

electrolytic reactions Oxidation-reduction reactions.

electrometer Electrostatic instrument for measuring difference in potential.

electron Elementary particle of an atom with a charge of negative one and a mass of 9.1×10^{-28} grams.

electron accelerators Machine used to accelerate electrons using potential differences.

electron capture Method of radioactive decay in which the nucleus captures an orbital electron, which then interacts with a proton effectively negating the proton and transmuting the nucleus to that of another element.

electron configuration Refers to the space relationships of electrons in an atom.

electronegativity Tendency of a neutral atom to acquire electrons, measured relative to that of fluorine.

electronic structure Structure of the orbital electrons in an atom that satisfies the quantum mechanical Schrödinger equation.

electron microscope Microscope where an electron beam forms an image on a fluorescent screen.

electron spin resonance (ESR) Spectroscopic technique that determines structural features of a molecule based on electron resonance in a magnetic field.

electron volt (eV) Kinetic energy gained by an electron passing through a potential difference of one volt.

electrophoresis Liquid paper chromatography carried out under the influence of an electric field.

element Pure substance consisting of atoms of the same atomic number that cannot be decomposed by ordinary chemical means.

elution Separation by solvent extraction.

embolism Matter that blocks a blood vessel.

empiric, empirical Referring to practical experience.

empirical formula Chemical formula that reflects only the simplest molar ratio of the elements in the compound, not the actual molar ratio.

emulsion (1) Mixture of two liquids, one suspended within another; colloid system; (2) suspended mixture where one of the components is gelatin-like.

endocrinology Study of hormonal secretion and of the endocrine glands.

endogonic Intake of energy.

endoscope Instrument, tubular in nature, carrying an illumination source, inserted into a body cavity to permit visual inspection.

endosteum Membrane lining of a hollow bone.

endotoxin Poison from dead bacterial cells; formed while cells are living.

energy levels Quantum levels of an atom satisfying the Schrödinger equation that are allowed levels for electron location.

enzyme Protein catalyzing specific transformation of material.

eosinophil (1) Cell stained readily by eosin; (2) white blood cell characterized by a two- or three-lobed nucleus and cytoplasm containing large granules.

epidemiology Study of disease and its rate of occurrence, manner of spread, and prevalence.

epigastrium Space in the abdomen just below the ribs.

epiphysis (1) Portion of bone between the shaft and the cartilage, (2) pineal gland.

epithelium Cells of skin and mucous membrane.

equilibrium State of equality between two opposing substances.

equilibrium constant True constant that relates the concentration of products and reactants in a reversible chemical system when no further net change is occurring in those concentrations.

equivalent Weight of a chemical species that contains either one mole of electrons and one mole of replaceable hydrogen, or combines with exactly 8 grams of oxygen.

ergometer Instrument used for measuring energy expended.

erythrocyte Red blood cell.

erythrocytosis Increase in red blood cells from a known stimulant.

erythroid Reddish in color.

erythropoiesis Formation of erythrocytes.

esters Organic compound formed by the action of an acid with an alcohol; contains the functional group

$$-\overset{\overset{\displaystyle O}{\|}}{C}-O-C\!\!\begin{array}{l}\diagup\\ -\\ \diagdown\end{array}$$

estrogenic hormone Hormone producing female characteristics.

ether Organic compound containing a C—O—C linkage.

ethylenediaminetetraacetic acid (EDTA) See *edetic acid*.

etiology Study of the causes of disease.

exergonic Release of energy.

exposure rate Rate of exposure to radioactivity usually measured in units of rads per hour.

extirpation Complete removal.

extractor Device that removes something; liquid that removes another substance with it.

extranuclear Referring to the space in an atom outside of the nucleus.

families Sets of elements that have the same valence-shell electronic configurations.

fast neutron Neutron that has a minimum energy of 100 keV.

ferrokinetics Study of iron within the body.

fibrinolysis Dissolution or splitting of fibrin.

film badge Photographic film shielded from light; worn by an individual to measure radiation exposure.

fission Splitting of a nucleus accompanied by a release of energy and neutrons.

fluid thioglycollate Medium that provides conditions for growth of aerobic and anaerobic bacteria; used in microbiologic sterility testing or radiopharmaceuticals.

fluorescence Emission of light by an activated chemical complex.

FOCAL (formula calculation) High-level, conversational, interpreter language for mathematical and string variable manipulations developed for Digital Equipment Corporation (Maynard, Mass.) computers.

folate Salt of folic acid.

follicle Sac or pouchlike depression; cavity.

follicle-stimulating hormone (FSH) Anterior pituitary hormone that stimulates follicle growth in the ovaries and spermatogenesis in the testes.

foramen magnum Large opening in the occipital bone between the cranial cavity and the vertebral canal.

FORTRAN (formula translator) High-level compiler language for mathematical and scientific applications.

free radicals Chemical complexes containing an unpaired electron.

frequency Number of cycles per unit time; normal unit is hertz, or cycles per second.

functional group Portion of a molecule responsible for its specific chemical properties.

fundus Base of an organ.

fusion Nuclear process in which two discrete nuclei collide and join together forming a larger nuclide.

gamma emission Nuclear process in which an excited nuclide deexcites by emission of a nuclear photon.

gamma globulin Globulins in plasma having the slowest mobility using electrophoresis in neutral or alkaline solutions.

gastrin Hormone stimulating secretion by the gastric glands.

gastroenteropathy Disease of the stomach and intestine.

gate Electronic device capable of performing logic operations within a digital circuit. In nuclear medicine it implies a device that can provide a timing signal to the computer. This signal is usually associated with the QRS complex of the electrocardiograph.

Geiger-Müller tube Ionization chamber measuring radiation in the region where the charge produced per ionizing event is independent of the number of primary ions produced by the initial ionizing event.

gel permeation chromatography Separation of compounds because of differences in their rates of permeation of a gel, especially useful for separation of large biomolecules such as proteins.

generator Device using a parent radionuclide to obtain its product, the daughter radionuclide, usually by addition of a solution that only interacts with the daughter.

genetic effects Dominant or recessive effects on progeny.

genitourinary tract Urinary system and the sex organs.

***g* force** Centrifugal force.

globulin Simple protein found in serum and tissue.

glomerulus Small cluster of blood vessels or nerve fibers.

glucagon Pancreatic secretion that increases concentration of the blood sugars.

glucocorticoid Hormone secreted by the adrenal cortex stimulating the conversion of proteins to carbohydrates.

glucoheptonate Chelating molecule that can bind ^{99m}Tc and be used as an imaging agent.

glycogen Form in which carbohydrates are stored in animal tissue.

glycoprotein Protein and a carbohydrate that does not contain phosphoric acid, purine, or pyrimidine.

G-M tube See *Geiger-Müller tube*.

gonad Ovary or testicle; the sex gland.

graafian follicle Ovarian follicle where the ovum matures.

gram atomic weight Weight in grams of one mole of an element.

gram molecular weight Weight in grams of one mole of a chemical compound.

granulocyte White blood cell.

granuloma Tumor or neoplasm consisting of newly formed tissue induced by the presence of a foreign body or of bacteria.

gray (Gy) A new unit of absorbed dose equal to 1 joule per kilogram in any medium.

growth hormone (GH) Hormone secreted by the anterior pituitary; stimulates growth.

half-life ($T_{1/2}$, $t_{1/2}$) A term used to describe the time elapsed until some physical quantity has decreased to half of its original value.

half-reaction Term used in an electrochemical reaction to describe either the oxidation process or the reduction process as a separate entity.

half-value layer (HVL) Thickness of absorbing material necessary to reduce the intensity of radiation by one half; synonymous with half-thickness.

halogens Family of chemical elements of similar electron structure (that is, the valence shell is completely filled except for one electron)—fluorine, chlorine, bromine, iodine, and astatine.

HAM See *human albumin microspheres*.

hapten Molecule that cannot elicit immunoglobulin response by itself but can when bound to a larger carrier molecule.

hardware Physical equipment, such as mechanical, electrical, or electronic devices.

haversian system System of canals in the bones where the blood vessels branch out.

heat-sensitive printer Type of printer that imprints characters on special sensitized paper by use of heat, without the use of an ink ribbon.

helium 3 (^{3}He) Isotope of helium with an atomic weight of three unified mass units.

hemangioma Tumor of blood vessels that is nonmalignant.

hematocrit Relative percentage of erythrocytes in whole blood.

hematology Study of the diseases of blood and blood-forming organs.

hematopoietic system The blood system.

hemocytometer Instrument used to count blood cells.

hemoglobin Pigment of the blood that carries oxygen.

hemolysis Red blood cell destruction; escape of hemoglobin within the bloodstream.

hemorrhage Bleeding.

heparin Mucopolysaccharide acid that occurs in tissues, mainly the liver; used in prevention and treatment of thrombosis, bacterial endocarditis, postoperative pulmonary embolism and in repair of vascular injury; used to prevent clotting of blood.

hepatoblastomas Tumor in the liver.

hepatoma Tumor of the liver.

heptasulfide Technetium heptasulfide: $^{99m}Tc_2S_7$; coprecipitates with colloidal sulfur particles stabilized with gelatin in ^{99m}Tc-sulfur colloid preparation.

hertz Basic unit of frequency; 1 hertz (Hz) = 1 cycle per second.

hexadecimal Pertaining to the number system with a radix of 16.

hexane Alkane with the molecular formula C_6H_{14}.

HIDA *N,N′*-(2,6-dimethylphenyl)carbamoylmethyl iminodiacetic acid; can be labeled with ^{99m}Tc and used as an imaging agent.

histochemical Referring to the deposit of chemical components in cells.

histology Study of the form and structure of tissues.

hormone Chemical having a specific effect on the activity of a specific organ.

HVL See *half-value layer*.

hydrocarbon Compound containing carbon and hydrogen exclusively.

hydrolysis Processes of decomposition by the addition of water.

hydroxide The ion OH^-.

hydroxyapatite Compound $Ca_{10}(PO_4)_6(OH)_2$; inorganic constituent of bone and teeth.

8-Hydroxyquinoline (oxine) Compound that can form a complex with indium and gallium and be used to label blood cells.

hyperemia Excess blood in an organ or part of the body.

hyperglycemia Excessive sugar (glucose) in the blood.

hyperthyroidism Overactive thyroid gland.

hypoglycemia Not enough sugar (glucose) in the blood.

hypokinesia Diminished motor function.

hypopituitarism Insufficient secretion of the pituitary.

hypothalamus Part of the forebrain below the cerebrum.

hypothyroidism Insufficient activity of the thyroid.

ICU See *instruction control unit*.

iminodiacetic acid Chelating group capable of binding technetium so that it can be attached to biologically active molecules, such as HIDA.

immunoactive Immunity produced by stimulation of antibody-producing mechanisms.

immunoglobulin Type of protein, isolated from the globulin fraction of serum having a characteristic shape and the ability to bind to molecules that are not endogenous to the species producing the immunoglobulin.

immunology Study of resistance to disease or disease agents.

immunoreaction Reaction taking place between an antigen and its antibody.

incubate To provide proper conditions for growth or a reaction to occur.

inelastic collision Interaction between two particles resulting in a net loss of kinetic energy in the system.

infarct Area deprived of its blood supply because of an obstruction.

infundibular pulmonic stenosis Obstruction in the outer passage from the right ventricle, restricting blood flow.

inhibitor Substance preventing or interfering with a chemical reaction.

innominate vein Vein receiving blood from the head and neck region.

inoculate To protect against disease by injection of pathogenic microorganisms to stimulate production of antibodies.

inorganic Branch of chemistry having to do with compounds and processes that do not involve carbon.

input Transferal of data from auxiliary or external storage into the internal storage of a computer.

insulin Hormone produced in the cells of the pancreas essential for metabolism of carbohydrates.

interface Connection between two systems, such as a scintillation camera and a computer.

internal conversion Nuclear deexcitation process in which the radionuclide deexcites by transferring energy to an orbital electron.

interpreter Computer program that translates and executes each source-language statement before translating and executing the next statement.

interrupts Signals that, when activated, cause a transfer of control to a specific location in memory, thereby breaking the normal flow of control of the routine being executed. An interrupt is normally caused by an external event such as a condition in a peripheral.

interstices Small gaps between tissues or structures.

intrinsic factor (IF) Substance produced by the gastric mucosa and found in the terminal ileum that is necessary for absorption of vitamin B_{12}.

inulin Polysaccharide that on hydrolysis yields levulose, which can be used to test kidney function.

inulin clearance test Test of renal function.

inverse-square law The radiation intensity of any source decreases inversely as the square of the distance between the source and the detector.

in vitro Outside a living organism.

in vivo Within a living organism.

I/O (input/output) device Computer device that either accepts input or prints out results.

iodination Addition of iodine to a compound.

iodohippuran Agent used for renal imaging.

ion Atom or group of atoms with a net electronic charge.

ion exchange Process involving reversible exchange of ions in a solution and in a solid.

ionic compound Compound held together by purely electrostatic forces.

ionic strength One-half the sum of the terms obtained by multiplying the molarity of each ion by the square of its valence.

irradiation Application of radiant energy for therapy or diagnosis.

ischemia Insufficient blood supply because of a spasm or constriction of the artery in an organ or part of the body.

ischemic damage Damage from a constriction of the blood vessel.

islets of Langerhans Pancreatic cells secreting insulin.

isobar Nuclides that have the same total number of neutrons and protons but are different elements.

isoelectric Having uniform electric potential; thus no current is given off.

isomers Two compounds with the same molecular formulas and different structural formulas.

isopleth Graph showing frequency of an event as a function of two variables.

isotones Nuclides having the same number of neutrons but a different number of protons.

isotonic Physiologic; compatible with body tissues.

isotopes Nuclides of the same element with the same number of protons but different number of neutrons.

IUPAC Abbreviation for the International Union of Pure and Applied Chemistry.

ketone Organic molecule with a carbon-oxygen double bond separating two alkyl portions ($R-\overset{\overset{O}{\|}}{C}-R$).

Kupffer cells Part of the reticuloendothelial system; star-shaped cells attached to the walls of the sinusoids of the liver.

lacuna Small hollow cavity.

LAL See *limulus amebocyte lysate.*

language See of representations, conventions, and rules used to convey information.

law of constant composition If two (or more) elements combine chemically to form a compound, the relative weights of the constituent elements will always be in a constant proportion to each other.

law of definite proportions If two (or more) elements chemically combine to form a compound, the relative number of moles of each constituent element will be in a proportion of simple whole numbers with each other.

law of mass action The velocity of the chemical reaction is proportional to the masses of the reactants.

law of multiple proportions If two elements form more than one compound, the number of moles of one element in the first compound is proportional to the number of moles of the same element in the second compound.

law of reciprocal proportions Two chemical elements unite with a third element in proportions that are multiples of the union of the first two elements.

Le Châtelier's principle If a system is initially at equilibrium and is forced away from equilibrium when a parameter is changed, the system will spontaneously return to a new equilibrium.

LET See *linear energy transfer.*

leukocyte White blood cell, either granular or nongranular.

leukopenia Less than the normal number of white blood cells.

leukotaxine Crystalline nitrogen substance appearing when tissue is injured.

Lewis concept An acid is an electron-pair acceptor and a base is an electron-pair donor.

ligand (1) Molecule attached to a central atom using coordinate covalent bonds; (2) in radioimmunoassay an antigen or small molecule that binds to a native carrier protein.

limulus amebocyte lysate (LAL) In vitro test for pyrogens; it reacts with gram-negative bacterial endotoxins in nanogram or greater concentrations to form an opaque gel.

linear energy transfer Amount of energy lost by ionizing radiation by way of interaction with matter per centimeter of path length through the absorbing material.

lingula Small tonguelike structure.

lipid Fat and fatlike substances.

lipoproteins Combination of a lipid and a protein.

liquid-drop model Theoretical model of the nucleus that assumes a simple continuous nuclear potential and spheroid shape.

load To store a program or data in memory; to mount a tape on a device such that the read point is at the beginning of the tape; to place a removable disk in a disk drive and start the drive.

logarithm Exponent of the power of a base that equals a given number.

logit Mathematical relationship defined as $\ln \frac{y}{1 - y}$.
Lugol's solution An iodine solution.
lymphangiography Radiography of the lymph channels.
lymphocytes White blood cell with a single rounded nucleus.
lymphoma Tumor composed of lymph node tissue.
lyophilize Rapid freezing and dehydration of a substance.
lysis (1) Separation of adhesions binding different structures; (2) destruction of a cell by a specific agent; (3) abatement of disease symptoms.
machine code See *object code*.
machine language See *language*.
macro (1) Directions for expanding abbreviated text; a borderplate that generates a known set of instructions, data, or symbols; a macro is used to eliminate the need to write a set of instructions that are used repeatedly; (2) prefix meaning 'huge,' or 'of large scale.'
macroglobulin Protein of high molecular weight.
macrophage Large white blood cell; active in bacterial destruction.
magnetic field Field induced by moving electrical charges.
magnetic quantum number Quantum number (m, m_l, or M) that defines the orientation of an orbital in space.
magnetic tape A plastic-base tape in which data is imprinted magnetically.
malabsorption Inadequate absorption of nutrients in the gastrointestinal tract.
manometer Device used to measure the pressure of liquids.
mass Basic parameter of matter referring to the quantity of matter present. It is independent of the object's weight.
maximum permissible dose (MPD) Dose limitations, in rem, placed on each individual as specified by the Nuclear Regulatory Commission.
Meckel's diverticulum Saclike pouch on the small intestine.
mediastinum Space behind the breastbone containing the heart.
medulloblastoma Tumor of the brain.
megakaryocyte A cell found in the bone marrow developing into blood platelets.
melanoma Tumor characterized by dark pigmentation.
memory (1) Erasable storage in a computer; (2) pertaining to a device in which data can be stored and from which it can be retrieved.
mesenchyme Primitive tissue of the embryo.
metabolism Process for transforming foods into compounds used by the body.
metastable state Excited state of a nucleus or atom that has a measurable lifetime; also known as an isomeric state.
metastasis Spreading of a disease process from one part of the body to another.
metathesis Chemical process in which two compounds exchange constituents.
microbiologic testing Any test for bacteria, virus, or other microorganism.
microlysis Destruction of a substance into microscopic size.
micrometer (μm) One millionth of a meter; formerly "micron."
microsphere Round mass of a small size, only visible with a microscope.
migrating solvent Chromatographic solvent; used to differentially carry the unknown solute to be separated.
mitral stenosis Deformity of the mitral valve of the heart.
mnemonic Aiding the memory; use of an acronym or other pattern to aid the memory.
mobile phase Phase in chromatography that differentially carries the unknown solutes.
molal Unit of concentration associated with molality equal to the number of moles of solute per kilogram of solvent.
molality Unit of solution concentration defined as the number of moles of solute per weight (kg) of solvent.
molar Concentration unit equal to number of moles of solute per liter of solution.
molarity Measure of solution concentration defined as the number of moles of solute per volume (liter) of solution.
mole See *gram molecular weight*.
molecular formula Chemical formula that states the actual number of atoms of each constituent per molecule of the compound.
molecular weight Weight in unified mass units of one molecule of a particular chemical compound.
molecule Basic unit of a chemical compound.
molybdate Compound containing a MoO_4^{-2} group.
monatomic One atom per molecule, usually referring to elements (such as the noble gases) in their native state.
monocyte White blood cell having one rounded nucleus that increases in number during certain types of infections.
morphology Study of the structure of tissues.
MPD See *maximum permissible dose*.
mucoid (1) Mucuslike substance; (2) an animal conjugated protein.
mucosal biopsy Removal and examination of some of the tissue of the mucous membrane.
multiple-gated acquisition Composite heart-imaging technique performed by synchronizing patient's heartbeat by means of an electrocardiograph to a scintillation camera.
myeloblast A cell in the bone marrow that develops into a white blood cell.
myelofibrosis Replacement of the bone marrow by fibrous tissue.
myeloid (1) Referring to bone marrow; (2) referring to the spinal cord; (3) cell resembling a red bone marrow cell that did not originate in the bone marrow.
myocardial infarct Heart muscle damage secondary to loss of its blood supply.
myocardial ischemia Obstruction or constriction in the coronary arteries resulting in a deficiency of blood to the heart muscle.
myocardium Heart muscle.
N See *neutron number*.
naperian logarithmic system Logarithmic system using the base e, which is a mathematical constant ($e = 2.71$).
nasopharyngeal Referring to that part of the pharynx above the soft palate.
negatron Negative electron.
neonate Newborn to 4-week-old infant.
neoplasia Condition characterized by new tumors or growths.
nephrology Study of the kidney.
nephron Part of the kidney that secretes urine.
nephrosis Degeneration of the kidney.
neurinoma Enlargement of a node or tumor on a peripheral nerve.

neurohormone Hormone stimulating the mechanism of the nerves.
neurohumeral Referring to a chemical secreted by a neuron.
neurohypophysis Main part of the posterior pituitary (hypophysis cerebri).
neuron Nerve.
neuropathology Study of nervous system diseases by examination of those tissues.
neutralization Chemical reaction in which an acid and a base react to form a salt and water.
neutrino Nuclear particle emitted during positron decay.
neutron Nuclear particle that is found in the nucleus, is electrically neutral, and has a mass of one mass unit.
neutron activation Nuclear process in which a nucleus absorbs a thermal neutron and deexcites by way of gamma-ray emission.
neutron flux Measure of neutron intensity defined as the number of neutrons passing through one square centimeter of area per second.
neutron number Number of neutrons in a nucleus (symbol for neutron number is N).
neutrophil White blood cell with three to five lobes connected by chromatin and cytoplasm containing five granules.
nidus (1) Focus of infection; (2) depression in the brain surface.
noble gas Any chemical element that has a completely filled valence-shell configuration in its neutral state—helium, neon, argon, krypton, xenon, and radon.
nomogram Process of graphically changing scales using a conversion scale.
nonpolar bond Chemical bond in which a pair of electrons is equally shared by two nuclei.
nonspecific binding (NSB) Binding of the radioligand to substances or surfaces other than the specific reactor substance.
normal Concentration unit defined as the number of equivalent weights of solute per liter of solution.
normality Method of expressing concentration defined as the number of equivalent weights of solute per volume of solution.
NRC See *Nuclear Regulatory Commission*.
nuclear charge Charge of the nucleus of an atom equal to the number of protons multiplied by the charge of a proton.
nuclear fission Nuclear process in which a nucleus splits into two pieces accompanied by neutron emission and energy release.
nuclear reactor Device that under controlled conditions is used for supporting a self-sustained nuclear reaction.
Nuclear Regulatory Commission (NRC) United States government agency regulating by-product material.
nuclear stability Condition to describe a nucleus that is stable with respect to radioactive decay.
nucleons Any particle commonly contained in the nucleus of an atom.
nucleus (1) Portion of an atom containing the neutrons and the protons; (2) spheric body that is the core of a cell; (3) mass of gray matter in the central nervous system.
NUTRAN High-level computer language.
object code Relocatable machine language code.
occipital Referring to the back of the head or occiput.
Occupational Safety and Health Administration (OSHA) United States government agency regulating health standards in the workplace.
octal Pertaining to the number system with a radix of eight.
OIH See *ortho-iodohippurate*.
oleic acid (octadecanoic acid) Straight-chained organic acid with the molecular formula $C_{18}H_{36}O_2$.
oncocytoma Granular cell adenoma of the parotid gland.
orbital Energy sublevels occupied by electrons in an atom.
organic chemistry Branch of chemistry dealing with the study of the compounds of carbon.
organic compounds Any of the class of chemical compounds that contain carbon.
organomegaly Abnormal enlargement of an organ.
op code See *operation code*.
operand That which is affected, manipulated, or operated upon.
operating systems Collection of programs, including a monitor or executive and system programs, that organizes a central processor and peripheral devices into a working unit for the development and execution of application programs.
operation code Code used to start the operation of a program.
ortho-iodohippurate (OIH) Iodinated renal imaging agent.
OSHA See *Occupational Safety and Health Administration*.
osmoreceptor Specialized sensory nerve ending that (1) gives rise to sense of smell and (2) is stimulated by changes in osmotic pressures of the surrounding medium.
osseous Composed of bone.
osteoblast Immature bone-producing cell.
osteoclast Large multinuclear cell associated with destruction of bone.
osteocyte Cell lodged in flat oval cavities of the bone.
osteogenesis Bone development.
osteomyelitis Infection of the bone.
output Information transferred from the internal storage of a computer to output devices or external storage.
ovary Female reproductive gland.
oxidation Process by which a substance loses electrons in an oxidation-reduction reaction.
oxidation-reduction Chemical reaction in which electrons are transferred from one substance to another substance.
oxidizing agent Substance in an oxidation-reduction reaction that causes another substance to lose electrons.
oxine See *8-hydroxyquinoline*.
pair production Photonic deexcitation process in which a photon disintegrates into an electron-positron pair, each of which gains an equal amount of kinetic energy.
pancreas Large gland secreting enzymes into the intestines for digestion and manufacturing and secreting insulin.
papilla of Vater Prominent tissue in the duodenum where the bile duct enters the intestine.
parathormone Hormone secreted by the parathyroid gland.
parathyroid glands Four small endocrine glands on the lateral lobe of the thyroid that control calcium and phosphorus metabolism.
parenchyma Essential elements of an organ as distinguished from its framework.
parent radionuclide Radionuclide that decays to a specific daughter nuclide either directly or as a member of a radioactive series.

parotid gland Salivary gland.
pathology Study of disease based on examination of diseased tissue.
pathophysiology Study of disordered function of organs.
Pauli exclusion principle Two electrons in the same atom cannot have the exact same set of quantum numbers.
pedicle Stemlike part of attaching structure.
pellet (1) Small pill; (2) a granule.
pentetic acid (diethylenetriaminepentaacetic acid, DTPA) Chelating agent that can be labeled with ^{99m}Tc and used for scintigraphy.
peptide Low molecular weight compound containing two or more amino acids.
peptide hormone Hormones excreted by the pituitary, parathyroid, and pancreas.
perchlorate Any chemical compound that contains the ClO_4^- group.
perfusion Passage of a fluid into an organ to thoroughly permeate it.
pericardium Tissue sheath encasing the heart.
perineal region Floor of the pelvis.
period (1) In wave motion phenomena, it is the time required to complete one cyclic motion, equalizing the reciprocal of the frequency; (2) elements in a horizontal line on the periodic chart.
periodic chart Chart of the elements depicting the interrelationships among them based on their electronic configurations.
periosteal bone Bone that develops directly from and beneath the periosteum.
periosteum Thin tissue encasing bones that possesses bone-forming potential.
peripheral (1) Near the surface, distant; distal, opposite of proximal; (2) any device distinct from the central processor that can provide input or accept output from the computer.
peripheral blood Blood that circulates in the vessels that are remote from the heart.
peripheral vessels Blood vessels that are remote from the heart.
pernicious anemia Anemia from lack of secretion by the gastric mucosa of intrinsic factor, which is important to blood formation.
pertechnetate Any chemical compound containing the TcO_4^- group.
PETT Positron emission transaxial tomography.
pH Measure of the hydrogen-ion concentration in a solution; equals the negative logarithm of the hydrogen-ion concentration.
pH meter Device used to measure the pH of a solution based on the potential difference between the solution and a standard calomel electrode.
phagocyte Cell that destroys bacteria or other foreign bodies.
phagocytize To ingest cells or microorganisms by a cell (a phagocyte).
phagocytosis Destruction of bacteria or other foreign bodies by phagocytes.
phantom (1) Model of some part of the body in which radioactive material can be placed to simulate conditions in vivo; (2) a device that yields information concerning the performance of a medical imaging system.
pharmacokinetics Study of the activity of drugs and medicines.
pharmacology Study of drugs and medicine.
pharynx Back of the nasal passages and mouth; the throat.
phenols Organic compounds with the functional group OH^- attached to an aromatic ring.
phosphor Chemical compound that upon photonic absorption will deexcite slowly by emitting light.
phosphorylation Chemical process in which a molecule acquires a PO_4^{-3} group.
photocathode Negative electrode of a photomultiplier tube.
photodisintegration Disintegration event triggered by photonic interactions.
photoelectric effect Process by which photons deexcite through absorption by electrons, resulting in ionization phenomena.
photomultiplication Multiplication of the signal given off by the interaction of a photon in a scintillation detector.
photon Discrete packet of energy.
phrenic artery Artery in the diaphragm.
phylogenetic, phylogenic Referring to the developmental history of an organism or race.
physiology Study of the function of tissues or organs.
pipet (or **pipette**) (1) Device used to deliver a precise amount of a liquid; (2) the act of using such a device.
pituitary Endocrine gland located at the base of the brain; regulates growth and secretions of other endocrine glands.
PL/1 (programming language 1) High-level compiler language.
placenta Organ attaching the embryo to the uterus; the afterbirth.
placental barrier Term used to describe the semipermeable barrier interposed between the maternal and fetal blood by the placental membrane.
planimetry Measurement of plane surfaces.
plasma Fluid of the blood not including the red and white blood cells.
platelet, blood platelet, thrombocyte Small colorless disks that aid in blood clotting found in circulating blood.
plethysmography Measurement of changes in volume using a plethysmograph.
pleura Membrane lining of the chest cavity and lungs.
pleural effusion Fluid in the space that contains the lungs and the thoracic cavity.
polar covalent bond Covalent bond formed by the unequal sharing of a pair of electrons between two atoms.
polyatomic ion Ion composed of more than one atom.
polycythemia Disease characterized by an overabundance of red blood cells.
polycythemia vera (P. vera) Inherited disease characterized by increase of red blood cells and total blood volume accompanied by splenomegaly, leukocytosis, thrombocytosis, and bone marrow hyperactivity.
polymer Compound formed of simpler molecules usually of high molecular weight.
polymerization Formation of a polymer.
polypeptide Compound containing two or more amino acids linked by a peptide bond.
polyphosphate Any molecule containing the $(PO_3)_n$ group.
pons (1) Slip of tissue connecting two parts of an organ; (2) part of the base of the brain.
popliteal fossa Depression at the back of the knee.
porcine From a pig.

porta hepatis Part of the liver receiving the major blood vessels.
positron Transitory nuclear particle with a mass equal to that of an electron and a charge equal to that of a proton.
potentiometer See *voltmeter*.
precipitate Solid compound that is produced in a chemical reaction between two soluble compounds in a solution.
precordium Upper abdominal region.
pressure Force per unit area.
principle quantum number (n or n_i) Relative distance from the nucleus at which the electron will be found and also its relative energy.
processor See *central processor unit*.
proerythroblast Primitive erythrocyte.
progesterone Hormone secreted by the ovaries.
program Complete sequence of instructions and routines necessary to solve a problem.
program development Process of writing, entering, translating, and debussing source programs.
prolactin Hormone secreted by the anterior pituitary.
promonocyte Intermediate cell between the monoblast and monocyte.
prompt neutrons Neutrons from a fission event that are emitted immediately after or during the event.
proprioception Process of receiving stimulation within the tissue.
prostaglandins Substance causing strong contractions of smooth muscle and dilation of the vascular bed.
prostatic hypertrophy Enlargement of the prostate because of an increase in the size of its cells.
protease Enzyme that digests protein.
protein High molecular weight compound of many amino acids linked by peptide bonds.
proteinuria Protein in the urine.
prothrombin Protein combining with other proteins to form thrombin, a clotting agent.
proton Nuclear particle with a mass of one unified mass unit and a charge of $+1.6 \times 10^{-9}$ coulomb.
psi Pounds per square inch; unit of pressure.
pulmonary Referring to the lungs.
pulmonic stenosis Obstruction from the right ventricle, restricting the outflow of blood.
pulse-height analyzer (PHA) Instrument that accepts input from a detector and categorizes the pulses on the basis of signal strength.
pyelonephritis Inflammation of the kidney and the pelvis of the kidney.
pylorus Part of the stomach just before the duodenum.
pyogenic Pus-forming; bacterial.
pyrogen Fever-inducing substance.
pyrophosphate Chemical compound containing a $P_2O_7^{-4}$
QF See *quality factor*.
qualitative chemical analysis Determination of the identity of each constituent in a chemical system.
quality factor (QF) Linear energy transfer–dependent factor by which absorbed doses are to be multiplied to account for the varying effectiveness of different radiations.
quantitative chemical analysis Branch of chemical analysis dealing with the determination of how much of a constituent there is in a chmeical compound.
quantum mechanics Branch of physics dealing with the mathematical description of the wave properties of atomic and nuclear particles.
quantum number Value describing the location of an electron in the electronic configuration of an atom.
rad See *radiation absorbed dose*.
radial immunodiffusion Immunochemical method used for the determination of serum concentrations of physiologically important substances.
radiation absorbed dose (rad) Quantity of radiation that deposits 100 ergs of energy per gram of absorbing material.
radiation dose Quantity of radiation absorbed by some material.
radiation exposure Exposure to ionizing radiation.
radiation safety Methods of protecting workers and the general population from the deleterious effects of radiation.
radiochemistry Study of the chemistry of radioactive elements.
radiochromatography Chromatography using a NaI crystal for detection of substances labeled with a radioisotope.
radiocolloids Colloid of a solid in a liquid where the solid phase contains a radioisotope.
radiograph Image of the internal structure of objects by exposure of film to x or gamma rays; roentgenogram.
radionuclide Unstable nucleus that transmutes by way of nuclear decay.
radionuclidic purity Amount of total radioactive species in a sample that is the desired radionuclide.
radiopharmaceutical Radioactive drug used for therapy or diagnosis.
radiopharmacology Study of radioactive drugs and their therapeutic and diagnostic uses.
radiopharmacy Laboratory producing and dispensing solutions labeled with radioisotopes for therapeutic and diagnostic purposes.
radioreceptor Sensory nerve terminal stimulated by radiant energy.
rate meter Device, used in conjunction with a detector, that measures the rate of activity of a radioisotope; usually in units of counts per minute or counts per second.
RBE See *relative biologic effectiveness*.
reaction Any process resulting in a net change to the constituents of the system.
reactor See *nuclear reactor*.
read-only input (ROI) Input only from the memory or from an internal source. (Contrast *regions of interest* [*ROI*].)
read-only memory Internal acquisition of data from the memory in computers.
reagents Any chemical used in a process.
real time In computer terminology, real time refers to the actual time elapsed during the program.
real-time system System in which the computation is performed while a related physical activity is occurring and the program results are used in guiding the physical process.
receptor Sensory nerve terminal responding to stimulation by transmission of impulses to the central nervous system.
red blood cells (RBC) Any of the red cells of the blood containing hemoglobin.
redox Abbreviation for an oxidation-reduction reaction.

reducing agent Substance that donates electrons in an oxidation-reduction reaction.

reduction In an oxidation-reduction reaction, it is the process by which one substance gains electrons.

regions of interest (ROI) Portion of the data field that is to be studied. (Contrast *read-only input* [*ROI*].)

register A device capable of storing a specified amount of data such as a word. See also *accumulator*.

relative biologic effectiveness (RBE) Ratio of the biologic response derived from a particular radiation as compared to another radiation exposure.

rem See *roentgen equivalent man*.

renal cortex Smooth outer layer of the kidney.

replacement reaction Chemical process in which an ion is replaced by another species in a compound.

reticuloendothelial cells Phagocytes.

RIA See *radioimmunoassay*.

RNA Ribonucleic acid; responsible for transmission of inherited traits.

roentgen (R) Quantity of x or gamma radiation per cubic centimeter of air that produces one electrostatic unit of charge.

roentgen equivalent man (rem) Unit of radiation dose defined as the product of rad and RBE (which see).

ROI See *read-only input* and *regions of interest*.

ROM See *read-only memory*.

Rutherford scattering See *elastic scattering*.

saccule Small sac or pouch.

sagittal (1) Plane or section parallel to the long axis of the body, (2) arrowlike shape.

saline Sodium chloride in water.

saline solution, physiologic Salt solution compatible with body tissues.

salivary gland Glands secreting saliva, connected to the mouth by ducts; the three glands are the parotids, submaxillaries, and sublinguals.

Schilling test Test for primary pernicious anemia.

scintigraphic agent Substance injected to produce images of internal organs on film; usually a radioactive solution.

scintigraphy Measurement of radiation by changing the kinetic energy of an ionizing particle into a flash of light.

scintillation Flash of light produced in a phosphor by radiation.

secretin Hormone stimulating secretion of pancreatic juice and bile secreted by the duodenal mucous membrane.

secular equilibrium Parent-daughter radioisotope pair in which the parent has a much longer half-life than does the daughter radionuclide.

semiconductor Substance whose conductivity is enhanced by the addition of another substance or through the application of heat, light, or voltage.

senescent Growing old; characteristic of old age.

septal Referring to a wall or partition.

serous Referring to serum.

serum Liquid remaining after blood has clotted.

shells Energy levels in electronic configuration.

shielding Absorbing material used to attenuate ionizing radiation.

SHPP See *N-succinimidyl-3-(4-hydroxyphenyl propionate)*.

shunt Bypass, an alternate course.

SI See *specific ionization*.

sinusoid Beginning of the venous system in the spleen, liver, bone marrow, and so on, that has an irregularly shaped, thin-walled space.

sinusoidal (1) Referring to a recess or cavity; (2) referring to an abnormal channel that permits the escape of pus.

software Collection of programs and routines associated with a computer.

sol Liquid colloid solution.

solute Material dissolved into a solution.

solution Physical system consisting of one or more substances dissolved in another substance.

solvent Substance that acts as the dissolving agent in a solution.

solvent extraction Use of a second solvent to preferentially dissolve a compound out of another solution.

specific activity Unit pertaining to the disintegrations per gram of a radioisotope.

specific ionization (SI) Linear rate of energy attenuation of ionizing radiation measured in terms of the number of ion pairs produced per unit distance traveled.

specificity Ability of a substance to recognize and bind to only one other molecule.

specific reactor substance Material capable of specifically and reversibly reacting with another molecule.

spectrometer Device measuring electromagnetic-radiation characteristics in a spectrum.

spectrophotometry Use of an instrument that measures light or color by photonic transmission.

spermatogenesis Process of forming sperm.

sphincter Muscle controlling a body opening.

splanchnic Pertaining to the interior organs in any of the four great body cavities.

splenic hilum Fissure where vessels and nerves enter the spleen.

stable electron configurations Configuration of electrons about an atom in the atom's lowest energy state.

stannous ion Ion of tin in the +2 valence state.

stationary phase Chromatographic phase that does not move with the solvent front.

steatorrhea Excess fat in the feces.

stellate Star shaped.

steroid Complex molecular structure containing four interlocking rings—three contain six carbon atoms each and the fourth contains five carbon atoms.

stoichiometry Study of numerical interrelationships between chemical elements and compounds and the mathematical laws governing such relationships.

store To enter data into a device, where it can be held and from which it can be retrieved.

subarachnoid Below the membrane between the dura mater and pia mater.

subendocardial Below the endocardium.

subphrenic Below the diaphragm.

supernatant, supernate Liquid lying above or floating on a precipitated material.

survey meter Meter that measures rate of radioactive exposure, usually in units of milliroentgens per hour.

synarthrosis Immovable joint, where bones lock within one another.

synchronous Performance of a sequence of operations controlled by an external clocking device; implies that no operation can take place until the previous operation is complete.

synchronous transfer Sequenced computer program operated by an external clock that does not permit a step to proceed until the previous step is completed.

syncope Fainting.

synovia Transparent fluid found in joint cavities.

synovitis Inflammation of joint-lining membrane.

systole Contraction and expelling of blood from the heart.

target Object to be bombarded by ionizing radiation, usually in an accelerator or cyclotron.

tentorium Fibrous tissue shelf separating the cerebrum from the cerebellum.

testosterone Hormone produced by the testes, including the male characteristics.

tetrahedron Molecular geometry in which the central atom is attached to four other atoms and the bond axes are directed along the diagonals of a cube.

tetralogy of Fallot Birth defect involving deformities of the blood vessels and walls of the heart chamber.

therapeutic Referring to the treatment of disease.

therapeutic window Range of dosage of a pharmaceutical that produces a beneficial effect.

thermal neutrons Neutrons with a maximum kinetic energy of 100 keV.

thermodynamics Study of processes based on energy changes in the system.

thermoluminescent detector (TLD) Type of crystal used to monitor radiation exposure by emitting light; used in a film badge, or ring badge.

thiols Family of organic compounds containing the functional group —SH.

thoracic cage Chest cavity.

thrombin Enzyme used as a clotting agent.

thrombocyte See *platelet*.

thrombosis Formation of a blood clot.

thyroid-binding globulin (TBG) Serum protein that is the primary agent for transport of thyroid hormone.

thyroid gland Endocrine gland that regulates metabolism.

thyrotropin (TSH) Hormone stimulating the thyroid secreted by the anterior pituitary.

thyroxine Hormone of the thyroid gland; 3,5,3′,5′-tetraiodothyronine.

time sharing Method of allocating central processor time and other computer services to multiple uses so that the computer, in effect, processes a number of programs simultaneously.

titer Aliquot of titrant (solution of known concentration).

Title 10 of the Code of Federal Regulations, Part 20 (10 CFR, Part 20) *United States Nuclear Regulatory Commission Rules and Regulations, Standards for Protection against Radiation;* Title 10 of the CFR pertains to atomic energy.

titration Method of quantitative analysis in which one substance is volumetrically added to another substance with which it quantitatively reacts.

titrimetric procedures Chemical laboratory procedure for quantitative analysis by addition of solution of a known concentration to a solution of unknown concentration.

TLD See *thermoluminescent detectors*.

torcula Hollow, expanded area.

trabeculae Fibrous tissue supporting the structure of an organ.

tracer study Examination either in vivo or in vitro using a small amount of a radionuclide-labeled substance to follow its path.

transcobalamin Derivative of the cobalt-containing complex common to all members of the vitamin B_{12} group.

transferrin Serum globulin binding and transporting iron.

transient equilibrium Equilibrium reached by a parent-daughter radioisotope pair in which the half-life of the parent is longer than the half-life of the daughter.

transmutation Nuclear process by which one element is changed into another element.

transverse tomography Tangential scanning of a cross-section of an organ, done from multiple directions, and then superimposed in a specific manner.

trauma Injury, wound.

tritium Isotope of hydrogen with a mass of three unified mass units, consisting of one proton and two neutrons.

Tyndall effect Light reflected or dispersed by particles suspended in a gas or liquid.

tyrosine Amino acid present in proteins that are susceptible to radioiodination.

ultrasonic nebulizer Device used for dispersing liquids in a fine mist through the use of sound waves.

ultrasonography Use of sound waves to image an internal structure of the body.

United States Pharmacopeia (USP) Official listing of all drugs and medications.

unsaturated iron-binding capacity (UIBC) Amount of serum transferrin that is not saturated with iron.

USP See *United States Pharmacopeia*.

vaccine Dead bacteria given to build specific immunity against disease.

valence electrons Electrons in the outermost energy level.

valence state Ionization state of an element in an ionic compound.

van der Waals bond Attraction between the charged portions of two molecules, known as dipoles.

variance Degree of change.

vascular Referring to the vessels.

vascular bed Entire blood supply of an organ or structure.

vascular lesion Lesion that affects the vessels.

vasculature (1) Supply of vessels to a region; (2) vascular system.

vasculitis Inflammation of a vessel.

vasoconstrictor Something that causes the constriction of blood vessels.

venipuncture Placement of a needle within a vein.

venography Radiography of the veins using a contrast medium; phlebography.

venous thrombi Blood clots within the veins.

ventilation Process of supplying fresh air.

ventilation-perfusion ratio ($\dot{V}/\dot{Q}$ or $\dot{V}_A/\dot{Q}_C$) Comparison of functioning ventilatory space and perfused tissue within the lung; ratio of minute flow of air through alveoli to minute flow of blood through pulmonary capillaries.

ventricular Referring to a small cavity or chamber.

ventriculography Radiography of the ventricles of the brain.

vesicoureteral reflux Backward flow of the urinary bladder and urethra.

vitamin Organic compound necessary to maintain normal growth or function; found in small amounts in plants and animals.

volume (1) Amount of space occupied in three dimensions; (2) a mass storage medium that can be treated as file-structured data storage.

volt Basic unit of electrical potential equal to one joule per coulomb.

voltmeter Device used to measure potential difference in electric circuits; potentiometer.

volume dilution Dilution of a solution by addition of pure liquid solvent.

$\dot{V}/\dot{Q}$ See *ventilation-perfusion ratio*.

wavelength Length per cycle in wave-motion mechanics.

white blood cell (WBC) Type of blood cell whose nucleus determines the type of cell: lymphocyte, monocyte, neutrophil, eosinophil, basophil.

window (1) Region of interest; (2) limits of energy radiation accepted by a pulse-height analyzer.

wipe test Testing for removable contamination.

word Unit of data that may be stored in one addressable location (most minicomputers use 16-bit words).

x ray Photonic radiation originating from electronic de-excitation.

x-ray diffraction Spectroscopic method for determining crystal structure by the interaction of x rays with the atoms involved in the crystalline structure.

zipper effect Overlap of two or more images.

Z number See *atomic number*.

INDEX

B

C

D

E

F

G

I

O

P

Q

R

U

V

W

X